BRIGHT FUTURES

Guidelines for Health Supervision of Infants, Children, and Adolescents

THIRD EDITION

Editors

Joseph F. Hagan, Jr, MD, FAAP
Judith S. Shaw, RN, MPH, EdD
Paula M. Duncan, MD, FAAP

FUNDED BY
US Department of Health and Human Services
Health Resources and Services Administration
Maternal and Child Health Bureau

PUBLISHED BY
The American Academy of Pediatrics

CITE AS

Hagan JF, Shaw JS, Duncan PM, eds. 2008. *Bright Futures: Guidelines for Health Supervision of Infants, Children, and Adolescents,* Third Edition. Elk Grove Village, IL: American Academy of Pediatrics.

Printed in the United States of America.

The American Academy of Pediatrics (AAP) and its members dedicate their efforts and resources to the health, safety, and well-being of infants, children, adolescents, and young adults. The AAP has approximately 60,000 members in the United States, Canada, and Latin America.

Library of Congress Control Number: 2007929964
ISBN-13: 978-1-58110-223-9
ISBN-10: 1-58110-223-2

BF0026

PUBLISHED BY
American Academy of Pediatrics
141 Northwest Point Blvd
Elk Grove Village, IL 60007-1098
USA
847-434-4000
AAP Web site: www.aap.org
Bright Futures Web site: www.brightfutures.aap.org

Design and production by Stephen B. Starr Design Inc.

Additional copies of this publication are available from the American Academy of Pediatrics Online Bookstore at www.aap.org/bookstore.

This publication has been produced by the American Academy of Pediatrics under its cooperative agreement (U06MC00002) with the US Department of Health and Human Services, Health Resources and Services Administration (HRSA), Maternal and Child Health Bureau (MCHB).

Dedication

The Third Edition of *Bright Futures: Guidelines for Health Supervision of Infants, Children, and Adolescents* is dedicated to Morris Green, MD, original chairperson of the Bright Futures initiative and editor of the First Edition of the Guidelines. His vision and leadership continue to inspire all of us who work for brighter futures for children and families.

The Challenge of Bright Futures

...For many children and their families, each new day is an opportunity for further self-realization, enhancement of good health, and promotion of self-esteem. For millions of others, however, the future holds little promise; their health status is poor, their health risks are many, and their prospects for successfully overcoming these problems are limited. These children, and all our nation's children, deserve the attention, the encouragement, and the intervention of health professionals from many disciplines to ensure that they develop the healthy bodies, minds, emotions, and attitudes to prepare them to be competent and contributing adults.

Health supervision policies and practices have not kept up with the pervasive changes that have occurred in the family, the community, and society. It has become evident that a "new health supervision" is urgently needed to confront the "new morbidities" that challenge today's children and families.

The goal of Bright Futures is to respond to the current and emerging preventive and health promotion needs of infants, children, and adolescents. ...[T]he guidelines are an exciting response to the needs of the times, a vision for the future, and, more importantly, a direction for child health supervision well into the 21st century.

The next step will be to promote the implementation of Bright Futures in the great variety of settings and arrangements that provide opportunities for health supervision throughout this country. It is also important to further an in-depth exploration of the science of prevention and health promotion and engage health professionals, educators, and families in this venture. It is time to walk into that bright future.

—*Morris Green, MD*
Bright Futures Guidelines, 1994

Mission Statement, Core Values, and Vision of the American Academy of Pediatrics

Mission

The mission of the American Academy of Pediatrics is to attain optimal physical, mental, and social health and well-being for all infants, children, adolescents, and young adults. To accomplish this mission, the Academy shall support the professional needs of its members.

Core Values

We believe:
- In the inherent worth of all children; they are our most enduring and vulnerable legacy.
- Children deserve optimal health and the highest quality health care.
- Pediatricians are the best qualified to provide child health care.

The American Academy of Pediatrics is the organization to advance child health and well-being.

Vision

Children have optimal health and well-being and are valued by society. Academy members practice the highest quality health care and experience professional satisfaction and personal well-being.

TABLE OF CONTENTS

Bright FUTURES

What Is Bright Futures?

Bright Futures is a set of principles, strategies, and tools that are theory based and systems oriented that can be used to improve the health and well-being of all children through culturally appropriate interventions that address the current and emerging health promotion needs at the family, clinical practice, community, health system, and policy levels.

Bright Futures Mission

The mission of Bright Futures is to promote and improve the health, education, and well-being of infants, children, adolescents, families, and communities.

Development of Bright Futures

- The Bright Futures projects was initiated in 1990 by the Health Resources and Services Administration's (HRSA) Maternal and Child Health Bureau (MCHB), with additional program support from the Medicaid Bureau of the Health Care Financing Administration (now the Centers for Medicare & Medicaid Services).
- The first edition of *Bright Futures: Guidelines for Health Supervision of Infants, Children, and Adolescents* was published in 1994. The second edition was published in 2000 and was revised in 2002. Both editions were published under the auspices of the National Center for Eduction in Maternal and Child Health (NCEMCH).
- This *Bright Futures: Guidelines for Health Supervision of Infants, Children and Adolescents, 3rd Edition,* was published in 2008.
- This edition updates and revises the guidelines, incorporating current scientific knowledge in health practice.
- This edition was developed through the collaboration of 4 multidisciplinary panels of experts in infancy, early childhood, middle childhood, and adolescent health.
- This edition was reviewed by more than 1,000 health care and public health professionals, educators, parents, and child health advocates throughout the United States.

Funding of Bright Futures

Since its inception in 1990, Bright Futures has been funded by the US Department of Health and Human Services, Health Resources and Services Administration, Maternal and Child Health Bureau.

Organizations and Agencies That Participated in the Bright Futures Project Advisory Committees

Bright Futures Steering Committee

The Bright Futures Steering Committee oversees the Bright Futures Education Center efforts. The Steering Committee provides advice on activities and consultation to chairpersons and staff of the Bright Futures Education Center and the Center's Project Advisory Committee (PAC).

Joseph F. Hagan, Jr, MD (Cochairperson), American Academy of Pediatrics
Judith S. Shaw, RN, MPH, EdD (Cochairperson), Ambulatory Pediatric Association
Betsy Anderson, Family Voices
Paula Duncan, MD, American Academy of Pediatrics
Mary Margaret Gottesman, PhD, RN, CPNP, National Association of Pediatric Nurse
    Practitioners
Mary Story, PhD, RD, American Dietetic Association
Jack Swanson, MD, American Academy of Pediatrics
Eric M. Wall, MD, MPH, American Academy of Family Physicians
Christopher A. DeGraw, MD, MPH (Federal Liaison), Health Resources and Services
    Administration, Maternal and Child Health Bureau

Bright Futures Education Center Project Advisory Committee

The Bright Futures Education Center PAC provides guidance on activities and consultation to chairpersons and staff of the Bright Futures Education Center. The PAC members serve as organizational representatives on the Center PAC, reporting on Bright Futures activities to constituents and eliciting organizational interest and support. Members promote Bright Futures content and philosophy to other national, state, and local organizations, assist in increasing collaborative efforts among organizations, and promote Center activities by offering presentations and trainings to colleagues within constituent organizations.

Joseph F. Hagan, Jr, MD
American Academy of Pediatrics
Cochairperson

Judith S. Shaw, RN, MPH, EdD
Ambulatory Pediatrics Association
Cochairperson

Betsy Anderson
Family Voices

CDR Gregory S. Blaschke, MD, MPH
Section on Uniformed Services

Ann E. Burke, MD
Association of Pediatric Program Directors

Charlotte J. Burt, MA, BSN, RN
American School Health Association

Paul S. Casamassimo, DDS
American Academy of Pediatric Dentistry

Daniel L. Coury, MD
Society for Developmental and Behavioral
    Pediatrics

James J. Crall, DDS, ScD
American Academy of Pediatric Dentistry

Paula M. Duncan, MD
American Academy of Pediatrics
    Bright Futures Pediatric Implementation
    Project PAC Cochairperson

Arthur B. Elster, MD
*American Medical Association/Guidelines on
    Adolescent Preventive Services (GAPS)*

Missy Fleming, PhD
*American Medical Association/Guidelines on
    Adolescent Preventive Services (GAPS)*

Myron Genel, MD
American College of Preventive Medicine

Mary Margaret Gottesman, PhD, RN, CPNP
*National Association of Pediatric Nurse
    Practitioners
    Bright Futures Pediatric Implementation
    Project PAC Cochairperson*

Marisa I. Herran, MD
National Hispanic Medical Association

Christopher A. Kus, MD, MPH
*Association of Maternal and Child Health
    Programs*

Carole M. Lannon, MD, MPH
*AAP Steering Committee on Quality
    Improvement and Management and eQIPP
    Planning Committee*

Danielle Laraque, MD
Bright Futures Health Promotion Workgroup

Monica Marshall, PhD
Mental Health America

Kathryn Phillips-Campbell, MPH
National Business Group on Health

Richard E. Rainey, MD
BlueCross BlueShield Association

Lisa Simpson, MB, BCh, MPH
*National Initiative for Children's Healthcare
    Quality*

Mary Story, PhD, RD
American Dietetic Association

Leonard R. Sulik, MD
*American Academy of Child and Adolescent
    Psychiatry*

Myrtis L. Sullivan, MD
National Medical Association

Jack Swanson, MD
*Committee on Practice and Ambulatory
    Medicine
    American Academy of Pediatrics*

Eric M. Wall, MD, MPH
American Academy of Family Physicians

Frances J. Wren, MD
*American Academy of Child and Adolescent
    Psychiatry*

Bright Futures Education Center Federal Liaisons

Christopher A. DeGraw, MD, MPH
Health Resources and Services Administration, Maternal and Child Health Bureau

William L. Flood, MD
Indian Health Service

J. David Greenberg, MBA
Centers for Medicare & Medicaid Services

Ruth Perou, PhD
Centers for Disease Control and Prevention

David M. Stevens, MD
Health Resources and Services Administration, Bureau of Primary Health Care

CAPT Judith K. Thierry, DO
Indian Health Service

Bright Futures Pediatric Implementation Project Advisory Committee

The Bright Futures Pediatric Implementation Project PAC oversees the activities of the Bright Futures Pediatric Implementation Project. The overall goal of the project is improved health promotion and prevention practices among child and adolescent health professionals through the effective implementation of the *Bright Futures: Guidelines for Health Supervision of Infants, Children, and Adolescents.*

Paula M. Duncan, MD
American Academy of Pediatrics
Cochairperson

Mary Margaret Gottesman, PhD, RN, CPNP
National Association of Pediatric Nurse Practitioners
Cochairperson

CDR Gregory S. Blaschke, MD, MPH
Section on Uniformed Services

James J. Crall, DDS, ScD
American Academy of Pediatric Dentistry

Arthur B. Elster, MD
American Medical Association/GAPS

Missy Fleming, PhD
American Medical Association/GAPS

Joseph F. Hagan, Jr, MD
American Academy of Pediatrics
Bright Futures Education Center PAC Cochairperson

Marisa I. Herran, MD
National Hispanic Medical Association

Christopher A. Kus, MD, MPH
Association of Maternal and Child Health Programs

Carole M. Lannon, MD, MPH
AAP Steering Committee on Quality Improvement and Management and eQIPP Planning Committee

Danielle Laraque, MD
Bright Futures Health Promotion Workgroup

Kathryn Phillips-Campbell, MPH
National Business Group on Health

Richard E. Rainey, MD
BlueCross BlueShield Association

Judith S. Shaw, RN, MPH, EdD
Ambulatory Pediatrics Association
Bright Futures Education Center PAC Cochairperson

Lisa Simpson, MB, BCh, MPH
National Initiative for Children's Healthcare Quality

Myrtis L. Sullivan, MD
National Medical Association

Jack Swanson, MD
American Academy of Pediatrics
Bright Futures Users Panel

Eric M. Wall, MD, MPH
American Academy of Family Physicians

Bright Futures Project Implementation Project Federal Liaisons

Christopher A. DeGraw, MD, MPH
Health Resources and Services Administration
Maternal and Child Health Bureau

William L. Flood, MD
Indian Health Service

J. David Greenberg, MBA
Centers for Medicare & Medicaid Services

CAPT Judith K. Thierry, DO
Indian Health Service

A Bright Future for Every Child

Foreword

—Morris Green, MD, FAAP, and Judith Palfrey, MD, FAAP
June 2007

Recognizing the Social Determinants of Children's Health

More than 15 years ago, the members of the first Bright Futures team were given the task to imagine our country's health picture if every child in America could look forward to a bright future—every child, regardless of race, religion, background, income, politics, or any other factor.

Imagine a bright future for every child in America. What would it look like? Who would be part of it? Who would sustain it? How would a truly bright future for children and youth intersect with change and brighten the present and future of all in the United States? Would a bright future for children translate into a brighter future for everyone?

With those questions in their collective conscious, the group developed the Bright Futures Children's Health Charter[1] (see box on page xvi). This charter delineates the necessities and entitlements that all children deserve and, indeed, must have to look ahead to a bright future. The charter states unequivocally, the explicit connection between a wide range of social determinants and the health of children and youth.

Making a Bright Future a Reality

First published in 1994, *Bright Futures: Guidelines for Health Supervision of Infants, Children, and Adolescents* provided a standardized, well-researched way in which everyone who cares for children in any

capacity can help realize the charter's goals—one child at a time.

The guidelines were updated in 2000, and again in this third edition, to address the ever-changing landscape in which our children are living. This latest edition, for example, includes special emphasis on 2 new significant challenges: mental health and healthy weight. Woven throughout the guidelines are new discussions about cultural competence, complementary and alternative medicine, and caring for children with special health care needs.

Like previous editions, this third edition of the Guidelines outlines activities that are vital to achieving the health goals of the Children's Health Charter, setting forth specific guidance to:

- Enhance health care professionals' knowledge, skills, and practice of developmentally appropriate health care in the context of family and community.
- Promote desired social, developmental, and health outcomes of infants, children, and adolescents.
- Foster partnerships between families, health care professionals, and communities.
- Increase family knowledge, skills, and participation in health-promoting and prevention activities.
- Address the needs of children and youth with special health care needs through enhanced identification and services.

Foreword

Bright Futures Children's Health Charter[1]

- Every child deserves to be born well, to be physically fit, and to achieve self-responsibility for good health habits.
- Every child and adolescent deserves ready access to coordinated and comprehensive preventive, health-promoting, therapeutic, and rehabilitative medical, mental health, and dental care. Such care is best provided through a continuing relationship with a primary health professional or team, and ready access to secondary and tertiary levels of care.
- Every child and adolescent deserves a nurturing family and supportive relationships with other significant persons who provide security, positive role models, warmth, love, and unconditional acceptance. A child's health begins with the health of his parents.
- Every child and adolescent deserves to grow and develop in a physically and psychologically safe home and school environment free of undue risk of injury, abuse, violence, or exposure to environmental toxins.
- Every child and adolescent deserves satisfactory housing, good nutrition, a quality education, an adequate family income, a supportive social network, and access to community resources.
- Every child deserves quality child care when her parents are working outside the home.
- Every child and adolescent deserves the opportunity to develop ways to cope with stressful life experiences.
- Every child and adolescent deserves the opportunity to be prepared for parenthood.
- Every child and adolescent deserves the opportunity to develop positive values and become a responsible citizen in his community.
- Every child and adolescent deserves to experience joy, have high self-esteem, have friends, acquire a sense of efficacy, and believe that she can succeed in life. She should help the next generation develop the motivation and habits necessary for similar achievement.

[1] Green M, ed. *Bright Futures: Guidelines for Health Supervision of Infants, Children, and Adolescents.* Arlington, VA: National Center for Education in Maternal and Child Health; 1994

Prevention Works

As demonstrated by the charter, the Bright Futures initiative is rooted in the philosophy of preventive care. Bright Futures stands on the firm foundation of years and years of experimentation and experience with preventive strategies by child health care professionals, public health officials, and other community-based workers. The third edition of the Guidelines challenges families, health care professionals, insurance companies, and government agencies to make the most of the knowledge we already have. Prevention works when practiced. The third edition of the Guidelines is about putting prevention into full-scale practice for every child.

This new edition catalogues the most effective preventive interventions in children's safety and health, as agreed upon by experts in the fields of child health care, public health, government, nutrition, mental health, social work, education and more. Before being included in the new edition, each recommendation was reviewed by a panel of experts and was subject to public review. More than 1,000 experts contributed over the course of the whole project.

Foreword

Bright Futures urges everyone who cares for children to make the most of this well-founded and experience- and evidence-based knowledge so that children across the country receive equal, accessible, high-quality care.

Families Matter

Epidemiologic, sociologic, and genetic studies have increasingly shown the correlation between parental and child health, and the critical importance of a family-centered approach to child health. Many times, the most effective health messages a child receives originate in the home. Families have been partners from the beginning of the Bright Futures initiative. This third edition begins with an elegant description of who constitutes a family and a delineation of how family strengths support children and communities.

The Guidelines also reflect the Bright Futures concept of caring for children in a "medical home." A medical home is not a building, house, or hospital; it is a family-centered partnership and approach to providing high-quality, cost-effective health care that is accessible, continuous, comprehensive, coordinated, compassionate, and culturally effective.

This edition demonstrates effective partnership models that put families in control of health information and health decisions.

Families are part of the team that includes a variety of professionals and laypeople, and the community as a whole. It is only through a successful partnership between the family and others that a child can be set on the path to a bright future.

Health Promotion Is Everybody's Business

Health is the responsibility of parents, communities, child-helping individuals and organizations (including health care professionals), government agencies, and the children and youth themselves. This third edition of the Guidelines underscores the importance of seeing health in this broadest context, as healthy communities support healthy children. Communities that may be suffering because of lack of resources, cohesion, leadership, and vision may create ill health and hopelessness among children, youth, and families. This new edition of the Guidelines provides information that communities can use to raise their health consciousness.

Imagine the great strides that could be made if more communities embraced the idea of healthfulness. Until children's health is seen as everybody's business, the goals of the Bright Futures initiative will not be reached. This third edition is the road map that shows all of us the way toward a brighter future.

References

1. Green M, ed. *Bright Futures: Guidelines for Health Supervision of Infants, Children, and Adolescents.* Arlington, VA: National Center for Education in Maternal and Child Health; 1994
2. Centers for Disease Control and Prevention. Promoting oral health: interventions for preventing dental caries, oral and pharyngeal cancers, and sports-related craniofacial injuries: a report on recommendations of the Task Force on Community Preventive Services. *MMWR.* 2001;50(No RR-21):1-13

Bright Futures: A New Approach to Health Supervision for Children

The *Bright Futures: Guidelines for Health Supervision of Infants, Children, and Adolescents* describes a system of care that is unique in its attention to health promotion activities and psychosocial factors of health and its focus on youth and family strengths. It also is unique in its recognition that effective health promotion and disease prevention require coordinated efforts among medical and nonmedical professionals and agencies, including public health, social services, mental health, educational services, home health, parents, caregivers, families, and many other members of the broader community. The Guidelines address the care needs of all children and adolescents, including children and youth with special health care needs and children from families from diverse cultural and ethnic backgrounds.

In 2001, the Maternal and Child Health Bureau (MCHB) of the US Department of Health and Human Services' Health Resources and Services Administration awarded cooperative agreements to the American Academy of Pediatrics (AAP) to lead the Bright Futures initiative. When the third edition of the *Bright Futures Guidelines* project started, many separate "guidelines" advised pediatric health care professionals on how to conduct a health supervision visit. Philosophies and approaches varied with the authoring group's goals, but many shared themes were evident. Among these guidelines, the *Bright Futures Guidelines*, the AAP *Guidelines for Health Supervision*, and the American Medical Association (AMA) *Guidelines for Adolescent Preventive Services: Recommendations and Rationale*[1] were the most widely used. Although their similarities were greater than their differences, the lack of uniformity presented difficulties for health care professionals. With the encouragement and strong support of the MCHB, the AAP and its many collaborating partners set out to write this new edition of *Bright Futures Guidelines* as a uniform set of recommendations for health care professionals.

An Evolving Understanding of Health Supervision for Children

Health supervision for children has evolved tremendously in the past half century, when it was first employed to address concerns of nutrition, child rearing, and the prevention of infectious diseases. As is true of the 2 previous editions, this third edition of the *Bright Futures Guidelines* has sought to advance the health of children and youth, with focused attention to key health components and interventions. However, few studies have evaluated health supervision care in this country, and similar systems do not exist in other regional or national health care systems for comparison.

When the Bright Futures Project Advisory Committee (PAC) convened for the third edition, the members began with key questions: What is Bright Futures? How can a new edition improve upon existing guidelines? Most importantly, how can a new edition improve the desired outcome of guidelines, which is child health? The PAC turned to the previous editions of *Bright Futures Guidelines* for insight and direction.

The first edition of the *Bright Futures Guidelines*, published in 1994, emphasized the psychosocial aspects of health. Although other guidelines at the time, notably the AAP *Guidelines for Health Supervision*, considered psychosocial factors, Bright Futures emphasized the critical importance of child and family social and emotional functioning as a core component of the health supervision encounter. In the Foreword to the first edition, Morris Green, MD, and his colleagues demonstrated this commitment by writing that Bright Futures represents "…'a new health supervision' [that] is urgently needed to confront the 'new morbidities' that challenge today's children and families."[2] The third edition continues this emphasis.

The second edition of the *Bright Futures Guidelines*, published in 2000, moved the project in new directions by emphasizing that care for children could be defined and taught to both health care professionals and families. In collaboration with Judith S. Palfrey, MD, and an expert advisory group, Dr Green retooled the initial description of Bright Futures to encompass this new dimension: "Bright Futures is a vision, a philosophy, a set of expert guidelines, and a practical developmental approach to providing health supervision to children of all ages from birth to adolescence."[3] The Green and Palfrey concept of Bright Futures was further qualified in *Bright Futures in Practice: Mental Health,* by editors Michael Jellinek, MD; Mary Froehle, PhD; Bina Patel, MD; and Trina Anglin, MD, PhD; and their contributors: "Bright Futures is a national initiative to promote the health and well-being of infants, children, adolescents, families, and communities."[4] The *Pediatrics in Practice: A Health Promotion Curriculum for Child Health Professionals,*[5] derived from the Green and Palfrey second edition, described an innovative health promotion curriculum to help health care professionals and families integrate Bright Futures

principles. The developers established the following 6 core concepts of Bright Futures:

- Partnership
- Communication
- Health promotion and illness prevention
- Time management
- Education
- Advocacy

These 6 core concepts are woven throughout the health supervision guidance of the third edition.

Developing the Third Edition
The third edition of the *Bright Futures Guidelines* represents the next steps in the journey envisioned by Dr Green when he called Bright Futures, "a vision for the future" and "a direction for child health supervision well into the 21st century." Bright Futures Expert Panels, working through the Bright Futures Education Center Steering Committee, first met in September 2003 to begin the process of drafting and developing the document.

The 4 multidisciplinary Expert Panels were divided by the ages/stages of Infancy, Early Childhood, Middle Childhood, and Adolescence. Each panel was cochaired by a pediatrician content expert and a panel member who represented family members or another health profession. The 38 members of the Expert Panels were individuals who represented a wide range of disciplines and areas of expertise. These representatives included mental health experts, nutritionists, oral health practitioners, family medicine providers, nurse practitioners, family and school representatives, and members of AAP national committees with relevant expertise (eg, Committee on Psychosocial Aspects of Child and Family Health, Committee on Practice and Ambulatory Medicine, and Committee on Adolescence).

At several stages during the draft development process, the AAP conducted reviews of the draft on a secure Web site. The drafts initially were reviewed by select AAP committees, sections, and programs, and a wide variety of individuals from various organizations and agencies. Simultaneously, a multidisciplinary group of experts in children and youth with special health care needs, including families, reviewed the guidelines and submitted additional content. After each review, the Expert Panels considered all comments and revised the draft accordingly. External reviewers who represented professional organizations or institutions, and individuals with expertise and interest in this project, gave helpful and essential final comments and endorsements.

In parallel efforts, a work group that consisted of members from the Expert Panels and Committee on Practice and Ambulatory Medicine worked on revising the AAP Recommendations for Preventive Pediatric Health Care (also known as the Periodicity Schedule) to be consistent with the Guidelines. The National Center for Cultural Competence assisted the panels in ensuring that the Bright Futures Guidelines were culturally and linguistically appropriate.

Concurrently, the Expert Panels worked with other groups on the project. A Users Panel reviewed Bright Futures materials to make recommendations for reaffirmation, revision, retirement, and development of new materials. The Pediatric Implementation Project worked to identify barriers to providing preventive services by child and adolescent health care professionals and to plan for implementation in the many care delivery settings, including private offices, public health clinics, and school-based health centers.

Building on Strengths, Moving in New Directions

As work began on this edition, Dr Green joined as a guest at the first PAC meeting and spoke of the "enduring, refreshing, and contagious vitality of Bright Futures."

He challenged the PAC to consider which Bright Futures concepts could be used and further developed to drive positive change and improve clinical practice. Keeping in mind this challenge and recognizing that the science of health care for children continues to expand, the Bright Futures Guidelines developers have created a third edition that builds on the strengths of previous editions while also moving in several new directions.

An Emphasis on the Evidence Base

Dr Green urged the continued exploration of the science of prevention and health promotion to document effectiveness, measure outcomes, and promote additional research and evidence-based practice. Recognizing that guidelines could not be legitimately promulgated without identifying, assessing, and citing the evidence base for pediatric care, the PAC urged the Expert Panels to identify evidence-based research related to preventive services.

The Expert Panels invested time and energy not only to identify such evidence but also to interpret and apply it. Next, staff and consultants from the AAP Section on Epidemiology conducted literature reviews, and the panels used and referenced summary work done by others to judge evidence whenever possible. Finally, an Evidence Panel, composed of members of the section on Epidemiology, designed and conducted systematic research on the Bright Futures recommendations. All panels drew from expert sources, such as the Cochrane Collaboration,[6] the US Preventive Services Task Force,[7] professional organizations' policy and committee work, the National Guideline Clearinghouse,[8] and Healthy People 2010.[9] In areas where research and practice are changing rapidly or are investigational, the Expert Panels referred to expert groups for the most up-to-date information. (See the Rationale and Evidence chapter for further details on this process.)

See the Recommendations for Preventive Pediatrics Health Care in Appendix C.

A Pledge to Work Collaboratively With Families and Communities

This edition of the *Bright Futures Guidelines* envisions that health supervision care will be carried out in a variety of settings and in collaboration with health care professionals from many disciplines, families, parents, and communities. New evidence, new community influences, and emerging societal changes dictate the form and content of necessary health care for children. All who care for children are challenged to construct new methodologies and systems for excellent care.[10] This edition of the *Bright Futures Guidelines* involves families and parents by recognizing the strengths that families and parents bring to the practice of health care for children and by identifying resources and educational materials specifically for families.

A Recognition That the Health Supervision Must Keep Pace With Changes in Family, Community, and Society

In any health care arrangement, successful practices create a team composed of families, health care professionals, and community experts to learn about and obtain helpful resources. In so doing, they also identify gaps in services and supports for families. The team shares responsibility with, and provides support and training to, families and other caregivers, while also identifying and collaborating with community resources that can help meet family needs. This edition of the Guidelines places special emphasis on 3 areas of vital importance to caring for children and families.

- **Care for children and youth with special health care needs.** Children and youth with special health care needs, ranging from mild to very complex, comprise a large segment of the general child population. The MCHB defines this population as children

"…who have or are at increased risk for chronic physical, developmental, behavioral, or emotional conditions, and who require health and related services of a type or amount beyond that required generally."[11] In 2000, the MCHB found that more than 9 million children in the United States have special health care needs.[12] National surveys find that between 13% and 23% of all children have a special health care need.[13-15] This means that 1 of every 5 households includes a child with a developmental delay, chronic health condition, or some form of disability.

Bright Futures uses 2 essential interventions throughout the Guidelines to promote wellness and to identify differences in development, physical health, and mental health for all children. They are (1) screening and ongoing assessment and (2) health supervision and anticipatory guidance. Both of these interventions rely on a partnership with the family.

Bright Futures also gives health care professionals (1) tools to screen for special health care needs, (2) a body of knowledge that is necessary to provide for the care of the children they have identified, including an awareness of critical community resources, and (3) encouragement to build partnerships with families. Bright Futures' strength-based approach maximizes the abilities of all children as they participate in everyday life.

Health supervision and anticipatory guidance are often overlooked in caring for children and youth with special health care needs. Careful health supervision is important to prevent secondary disability. However, the impact of *specialness* or extensive health care needs should not overshadow the *child*. The child or youth with special health care needs shares most health supervision requirements with her peers, including immunizations, nutrition and physical activity, screening for vision and hearing, school adjustment, and automobile or gun safety, among many other topics.

Family-centered care that promotes strong partnerships and honest communication among all parties (families, children, adolescents or youth, and health care professionals) is critical in caring for all children. It is especially important when caring for children and youth with special health care needs, who tend to require visits with health care professionals more frequently than other children and because most children with special health care needs now live normal life spans. The partnership between health care professionals and families increases in value over time, especially when families feel comfortable asking questions, providing insight and perspectives, and seeking advice.

- **Cultural competence.** Culture and ethnicity frame the patterns of beliefs, practices, and perceptions as to "health" and "illness"[16]; the roles of individuals within a family; the nature of the relationship between the health care professional, the child, and family members; health care-seeking behaviors; and the use of complementary and alternative care. Cultures form around language, gender, disability, sexual orientation, religion, or socioeconomic status. Even people who have been fully acculturated within mainstream society can maintain values, traditions, communication patterns, and child-rearing practices of their original culture. Immigrant families, in particular, face additional stressors, such as social isolation from family and traditional social networks, differences in cultural beliefs and values, voluntary versus involuntary immigration, cultural change

and adjustment, and the drive to achieve specific personal and family goals.

- **Complementary and alternative care.** Collaboration with families in a clinical practice is a series of communications, agreements, and negotiations to ensure the best possible health care for children. In the Bright Futures vision of family-centered care, families must be empowered as care participants. Their unique ability to choose what is best for their children must be recognized. Families do all they can to protect their children from sickness or harm.

The Bright Futures health care professional must be aware of the disciplines or philosophies that are chosen by the child's family, especially if the family chooses a therapy that is unfamiliar or a treatment belief system that the health care professional does not endorse or share. Families may seek second opinions or services in traditional pediatric medical and surgical care fields or may choose care from alternative or complementary care providers. *Alternative therapies* generally replace conventional treatments. *Complementary therapies* are used in addition to conventional treatments. Families generally seek *additional* care from other disciplines rather than *replacement* care.

Practitioners of traditional or allopathic medicine and complementary and alternative care are driven and guided by the mandate to do no harm and to do good. Just because a chosen therapy is out of the scope of standard care does not define it as harmful or without potential benefit. Therapies can be safe and effective, safe and ineffective, or unsafe. The AAP Committee on Children with Disabilities suggests that "to best serve the interests of children, it is important to maintain a scientific perspective, to provide balanced advice about therapeutic options, to guard against bias, and to establish and maintain a trusting relationship with families."[17] Providers of standard care need not be threatened by such choices.

The use of complementary and alternative care is particularly common when a child has a chronic illness or condition, such as autism. Alternative treatments are increasingly described on the Internet, with no assurance of safety or efficacy. Parents often are reluctant to tell their health care professional about such treatments, fearing disapproval. Health care professionals should ask parents directly, in a nonjudgmental manner, about the use of complementary and alternative care.[18]

Consultation with colleagues who are knowledgeable about complementary and alternative care might be necessary. Discussion with a complementary and alternative care therapist also may be useful, and conversations with the child's family will enhance the care of the child by all providers. Keeping such conversations family centered can only strengthen the therapeutic relationship with the family.

References

1. American Medical Association. *Guidelines for Adolescent Preventive Services (GAPS): Recommendations and Rationale.* Elster AB, Kuznets NJ, eds. Baltimore, MD: Williams & Wilkins; 1994

2. Green M, ed. *Bright Futures: Guidelines for Health Supervision of Infants, Children, and Adolescents.* Arlington, VA: National Center for Education in Maternal and Child Health; 1994

3. Green M, Palfrey JS, eds. *Bright Futures: Guidelines for Health Supervision of Infants, Children, and Adolescents.* 2nd ed. Arlington, VA: National Center for Education in Maternal and Child Health; 2002

4. Jellinek M, Patel BP, Froehle MC, eds. *Bright Futures in Practice: Mental Health: Practice Guide—Volume 1.* Arlington, VA: National Center for Education in Maternal and Child Health; 2002

5. Bernstein H. *Pediatrics in Practice: A Health Promotion Curriculum for Child Health Professionals.* New York, NY: Springer Publishing Company; 2005

6. The Cochrane Collaboration: The Reliable Source of Evidence in Health Care. Available at: http://www.cochrane.org/. Accessed June 7, 2007

7. US Preventive Services Task Force. *The Guide to Clinical Preventive Services: Report of the United States Preventive Services Task Force.* 3rd ed. Washington, DC: International Medical Publishing; 2002

8. US Department of Health and Human Services, National Guideline Clearinghouse. Available at: http://www.guideline.gov/. Accessed June 7, 2007

9. US Department of Health and Human Services. *Healthy People 2010: Understanding and Improving Health.* 2nd ed. Washington, DC: Government Printing Office; 2000

10. Schor EL. Rethinking well-child care. *Pediatrics.* 2004;114:210-216

11. Newacheck PW, Strickland B, Shonkoff JP, et al. An epidemiologic profile of children with special health care needs. *Pediatrics.* 1998;102:117-123

12. Centers for Disease Control and Prevention. National Survey of Children with Special Health Care Needs and Local Area Integrated Telephone Survey (SLAITS). Atlanta, GA: Centers for Disease Control and Prevention; 2001

13. US Department of Health and Human Services, Health Resources and Services Administration, Maternal and Child Health Bureau. The National Survey of Children with Special Health Care Needs *Chartbook 2001.* Rockville, MD: US Department of Health and Human Services; 2004

14. Chevarley F. Utilization and Expenditures for Children with Special Health Care Needs. Research Findings No. 24. Rockville, MD: Agency for Healthcare Research and Quality; 2006

15. Williams TV, Schone EM, Archibald ND, Thompson JW. A national assessment of children with special health care needs: prevalence of special needs and use of health care services among children in the military health system. *Pediatrics.* 2004;114:384-393

16. Anderson LM, Scrimshaw SC, Fullilove MT, Fielding JE, Normand J. Culturally competent healthcare systems. A systematic review. *Am J Prev Med.* 2003;24(3 Suppl):68-79

17. American Academy of Pediatrics, Committee on Children with Disabilities. Counseling families who choose complementary and alternative medicine for their child with chronic illness or disability. *Pediatrics.* 2001;107:598-601

18. Sibinga EM, Ottolini MC, Duggan AK, Wilson MH. Parent-pediatrician communication about complementary and alternative medicine use for children. *Clin Pediatr (Phila).* 2004;43:367-373

Acknowledgments

The third edition of *Bright Futures: Guidelines for Health Supervision of Infants, Children, and Adolescents* could not have been created without the leadership, wise counsel, and unstinting efforts of many people. We are grateful for the valuable help we received from a wide variety of multidisciplinary organizations and individuals.

Under the leadership of Peter C. van Dyck, MD, MPH, associate administrator for Maternal and Child Health (MCH), Health Resources and Services Administration, the project has benefited from the dedication and guidance of many MCH Bureau staff, especially Christopher A. DeGraw, MD, MPH, the Bright Futures project officer, and M. Ann Drum, DDS, MPH, Research, Training, and Education director.

We owe particular gratitude to Modena Wilson, MD, MPH, and Tom Tonniges, MD, for their vision, creativity, and leadership as we began our work in drafting the third edition. Their contributions were invaluable in establishing the foundation and momentum for the AAP national Bright Futures initiative. In addition, Dr Wilson's leadership of the evidence review process was essential.

Mary Margaret Gottesman, PhD, RN, CPNP, Jack Swanson, MD, Polly Arango, Frances Biagioli, MD, Marilyn Bull, MD, Barbara Deloian, PhD, RN, CPNP, Martin M. Fisher, MD, Edward Goldson, MD, Bonnie Spear, PhD, RD, and J. Lane Tanner, MD, were always available to us as our core consultants. Their continual review helped ensure that our recommendations would be relevant to practice and applicable to the community setting.

We are extremely grateful to the 4 multidisciplinary Expert Panels for their tremendous commitment and contributions in developing the third edition of the Guidelines.

We also wish to acknowledge the significant contributions of AAP staff, who work diligently to ensure the success of Bright Futures.

Throughout the process of developing and revising this edition of the Guidelines, we relied on numerous experts who reviewed sections of the document, often multiple times. Their careful review and thoughtful suggestions improved the Guidelines immeasurably. In fall 2006, the entire document was posted on the Bright Futures Web site for external review. During this time, we received more than 1,200 comments from more than 500 health care and public health professionals, educators, parents, and child health advocates throughout the United States. We are most grateful to those who took the time to ensure that the Guidelines are as complete and scientifically sound as possible.

We would like to specifically acknowledge the help that the National Center for Cultural Competence gave us by reviewing the sections of the book and assisting with incorporating information on cultural competency.

We are also grateful to Morris Green, MD, and Judy Palfrey, MD, editors of earlier editions of the Guidelines; Audrey Nora, MD, MPH, Woodie Kessel, MD, MPH, David Heppel, MD, Denise Sofka, RD, MPH, Trina Anglin, MD, PhD, and the late Vince Hutchins, MD, MPH, of the MCHB; J. David Greenberg, MBA, of the Medicaid Bureau, and the late William Hiscock; and Katrina Holt, MPH, MS, RD, Pamela Mangu, MD, Meri McCoy-Thompson, MA, and many other staff of the National Center for Education in Maternal and Child Health, for their many contributions to the Bright Futures efforts throughout the past 2 decades. Their passion and commitment has significantly advanced the field of well child care.

—*Joseph F. Hagan, Jr, MD, FAAP; Judith S. Shaw, RN, MPH, EdD; and Paula M. Duncan, MD, FAAP; Editors*

Bright Futures Expert Panels

Infancy
Marilyn J. Bull, MD (Cochairperson)
Barbara Deloian, PhD, RN, CPNP
  (Cochairperson)
Deborah Campbell, MD
George J. Cohen, MD
Kevin J. Hale, DDS
Penelope K. Knapp, MD
Beth Potter, MD
Karyl Rickard, PhD, RD
Melissa C. Vickers, MEd, IBCLC, RLC

Early Childhood
Polly Arango (Cochairperson)
J. Lane Tanner, MD (Cochairperson)
Joseph M. Carrillo, MD
Nan Gaylord, PhD, RN, CPNP
Peter A. Gorski, MD, MPA
Michael A. Ignelzi, Jr, DDS, PhD
Christopher A. Kus, MD, MPH
Donald B. Middleton, MD
Cynthia S. Minkovitz, MD
Madeleine Sigman-Grant, PhD, RD

Middle Childhood
Edward Goldson, MD (Cochairperson)
Bonnie A. Spear, PhD, RD (Cochairperson)
Scott Cashion, DDS
Jane A. Corson, MD
Beth A. MacDonald
Eve Spratt, MD
Howard L. Taras, MD
Anne Turner-Henson, DSN, RN

Adolescence
Frances Biagioli, MD (Cochairperson)
Martin M. Fisher, MD (Cochairperson)
Pamela Burke, PhD, RN, BC-FNP, PNP
Arthur B. Elster, MD
Alma L. Golden, MD (Federal Liaison)
Katrina Holt, MPH, MS, RD
M. Susan Jay, MD
Jaime Martinez, MD

Amy V. Mellencamp, EdD
Vaughn Rickert, PsyD
Scott Smith, DDS

Bright Futures Evidence Panel
Modena H. Wilson, MD, MPH (Chairperson)
Michael deCastro Cabana, MD
Elizabeth A. Edgerton, MD, MPH
Virginia A. Moyer, MD, MPH
Michael Silverstein, MD, MPH

Bright Futures Children and Youth With Special Health Care Needs Panel
Betsy Anderson (Cochairperson)
Joseph F. Hagan, Jr, MD (Cochairperson)
Richard C. Antonelli, MD
Polly Arango
Marion T. Baer, PhD
William Cooley, MD
Christopher A. DeGraw, MD, MPH
  (Federal Liaison)
Paula Duncan, MD
Mary Margaret Gottesman, PhD, RN, CPNP
Monique R. Fountain-Hanna, MD, MPH, MBA
  (Federal Liaison)
Beth A. MacDonald
Merle McPherson, MD, MPH (Federal Liaison)
Judith S. Shaw, RN, MPH, EdD
Bonnie Strickland, PhD (Federal Liaison)

Bright Futures Users Panel
Jack Swanson, MD (Chairperson)
Betsy Anderson
Bruce Bedingfield, DO
Anita Berry, MSN, CNP/APN
CDR Gregory S. Blaschke, MD, MPH
James J. Crall, DDS, ScD
Paula M. Duncan, MD
Missy Fleming, PhD
Mary Margaret Gottesman, PhD, RN, CPNP
Marisa I. Herran, MD
Philip G. Itkin, MD
Myrtis L. Sullivan, MD
Eric M. Wall, MD, MPH

American Academy of Pediatrics Staff

Vera Frances "Fan" Tait, MD
Principal Investigator

Edward P. Zimmerman, MS
Coprincipal Investigator

Darcy Steinberg-Hastings, MPH
Coprincipal Investigator and Director

Jane Bassewitz, MA
Bright Futures Program Manager

Mary Crane, PhD, LSW
Manager, Committees and Sections

Jean Davis, MPP
*Director, Division of Community-based
    Initiatives*

Marge Gates
CME Assistant

Rachael Hagan
Program and Marketing Specialist

Sandi King, MS
*Director, Division of Publishing and
    Production Services*

Laura Murray, MPH, CHES
Manager, Bright Futures Program Manager

Linda Paul, MPH
Manager, Bright Futures Program Manager

Ngozi Onyema, CHES
Coordinator, Committees and Sections

Julie Raymond
Program Assistant, Bright Futures

Maryjo Reynolds
Product Manager, Bright Futures

Sandy Szott
Program Assistant, Bright Futures

Effie Tonkovic
Program Assistant, Bright Futures

Linda Walsh, MAB
*Director, Division of Healthcare Finance and
    Quality Improvement*

Jennifer Pane
Senior Medical Copy Editor

Jill Rubino
Medical Copy Editor

University of Vermont Faculty, Staff, and Students

Rachael McLaughlin,
Project Coordinator, Bright Futures

Erica Crall
Grace Chi
Wendy Davis, MD
Heather Lesage
Kristen Norris
Douglas Shaw

Captus Communications, LLC Staff

Anne Brown Rodgers
Health Writer and Editor

Deborah S. Mullen
Donna Xander

What Is Bright Futures?

An Introduction to the third edition of *Bright Futures: Guidelines for Health Supervision of Infants, Children, and Adolescents*

Bright Futures is a set of principles, strategies, and tools that are theory based, evidence driven, and systems oriented that can be used to improve the health and well-being of all children through culturally appropriate interventions that address their current and emerging health promotion needs at the family, clinical practice, community, health system, and policy levels.

Bright Futures is…

…a set of principles, strategies, and tools…

The Bright Futures principles acknowledge the value of each child, the importance of family, the connection to community, and that children and youth with special health care needs are children first. These principles assist the health care professional in delivering, and the practice in supporting, the highest quality health care for children and their families.

Strategies drive practices and health care professionals to succeed in achieving professional excellence. Bright Futures can assist pediatric health care professionals in raising the bar of quality health care for all our children, through a thoughtfully derived process that will allow them to do their jobs well.

This book is the core of the Bright Futures tools for practice. It is not intended to be a textbook, but a compendium of guidelines, expert opinion, and recommendations for health supervision visits. Other available Bright Futures tools include the *Bright Futures in Practice* series, which provides in-depth discussions of Nutrition, Oral Health, Physical Activity, and Mental Health. A *Bright Futures Toolkit* will be designed, as a companion to this book, to assist health care professionals in planning and carrying out health supervision visits. It contains numerous charts, forms, screening instruments, and other tools that increase practice efficiency and efficacy.

…that are theory based, evidence driven…

The rationale for a clinical decision can balance evidence from research, clinical practice guidelines, professional recommendations, or decision support systems with expert opinion, experience, habit, intuition, preferences, or values. Clinical or counseling decisions and recommendations also can be based on legislation (eg, seat belts), common sense not likely to be studied experimentally (eg, sunburn prevention), or relational evidence (eg, television watching and violent behavior). Most importantly, clinical and counseling decisions are responsive to family needs and desires or patient-centered decision making. It follows that much of the content of a health supervision visit is the theoretical application of scientific principles in the service of child and family health.

Certainly, strong evidence for the effectiveness of a clinical intervention is one of the most persuasive arguments for making it a part of child health supervision. On the other hand, if careful studies have shown an intervention to be ineffective or even harmful,

Introduction

few would argue for its inclusion. Identifying and assessing evidence for effectiveness was a central element, and a key challenge, of the work involved in developing this edition's health supervision recommendations. The multifaceted approach we used is described in greater detail in the Rationale and Evidence chapter.

...and systems oriented...

In the footsteps of Green and Palfrey[1] (the developers of the earlier editions of the *Bright Futures Guidelines*), we created principles, strategies, and tools as part of a Bright Futures system of care. That system goes beyond the schema of individual health supervision visits and encompasses an approach that includes continuous improvements in the delivery system that result in better outcomes for children and families. Knowing what to do is important; knowing how to do it is essential.

A systems-oriented approach in a Bright Futures practice means moving beyond the "status quo" to become a practice where redesign and positive change are embodied every day. Methods for disseminating and applying Bright Futures knowledge in the practice environment must be accomplished with an understanding of the health care system and environment.

...that can be used to improve the health and well-being of all children...

The care described by Bright Futures contributes to positive health outcomes through health promotion and anticipatory guidance, disease prevention, and early detection of disease. Preventive services address these child health outcomes and provide guidance to parents and children, including children and youth with special health care needs.

These health outcomes, which represent physical and emotional well-being and optimal functioning at home, in school, and in the community, include:

- Attaining a healthy weight and body mass index, and normal blood pressure, vision, and hearing
- Pursuing healthy behaviors related to nutrition, physical activity, safety, sexuality, and substance use
- Accomplishing the developmental tasks of childhood and adolescence related to social connections, competence, autonomy, empathy, and coping skills
- Having a loving, responsible family that is supported by a safe community
- For children with special health care needs or chronic health problems, achieving self-management skills and the freedom from real or perceived barriers to reaching their potential

...through culturally appropriate interventions...

Culture is a system of shared values and beliefs and learned patterns of behavior that are not defined simply by ethnicity or race. A culture may form around sexual orientation, religion, language, gender, disability, or socioeconomic status. Cultural values are beliefs, behaviors, and ideas that a group of people share and expect to be observed in their dealings with others. These values inform interpersonal interactions and communication, influencing critical aspects of the provider-patient relationship, such as body language, touch, communication style and eye contact, modesty, responses to pain, and a willingness to disclose mental or emotional distress.

Cultural competence (the set of values, behaviors, attitudes, and practices within a system, organization, and program or among individuals that enables them to work effectively cross-culturally) is intricately linked to the concept and practice of "family-centered care." Family-centered care in Bright Futures honors the strengths, cultures, traditions, and expertise that everyone brings to a respectful family-professional partnership. With this approach to care, families feel they can make decisions, with providers at different levels, in the care of their own children and as advocates for systems and policies that support children and youth with special health care needs. Cultural competence requires building relationships with community cultural brokers who can provide an understanding of community norms and links to other families and organizations, such as churches or social clubs.

...that address their current and emerging health promotion needs...

Among the health issues in current child health practice, 2 issues stand out as major concerns for families, health care professionals, health planners, and the community—promoting healthy weight and promoting mental health. Healthy People 2010[2] targets these issues with a number of recommended interventions and goals, and they are highlighted as **Significant Challenges to Child and Adolescent Health** throughout this edition of the *Bright Futures Guidelines*.

Most authorities agree that lifestyle choices strongly influence weight status and that effective interventions are family based and begin in infancy. The choice to breastfeed, the appropriate introduction of solid foods, and family meal planning and participation lay the groundwork for a child's lifelong eating habits. Parents also influence lifelong habits of physical activity and physical inactivity. Through Bright Future's guidance on careful monitoring, interventions, and anticipatory guidance about nutrition, activity level, and other family lifestyle choices, health care professionals can play an important role in promoting healthy weight for all children and adolescents.

A 1999 Surgeon General's report described mental health in childhood and adolescence as the achievement of expected developmental, cognitive, social, and emotional milestones and of secure attachments, satisfying social relationships, and effective coping skills.[3] Citing the Methodology for Epidemiology of Mental Disorders in Children and Adolescents (MECA) Study, the Surgeon General's report also estimated that almost 21% of children aged 9 to 17 years had a diagnosable mental or addictive disorder that was associated with at least minimum impairment.

Bright Futures provides multiple opportunities for promoting healthy weight and family mental health in the regular and periodic health supervision visits. Child health care professionals champion a strength-based approach, helping families identify their assets that enhance their ability to care for their child and guide their child's development.

... at the family level...

The composition and context of the typical or traditional family has changed significantly over the past 2 decades. Fewer children now reside in a household with their biological mother and father and with only one parent working outside the home. Today, the term "family" is used to describe a unit that may comprise a married nuclear family; cohabiting family; single-parent family, blended family, or stepfamily; grandparent-headed household; single-gender parents; commuter or long-distance family; foster family; or larger community family with several individuals who share the caregiving and parenting responsibilities. Each of these family constellations presents unique challenges to child rearing for parents as well as children.

Families are critical partners in the care of children.[4] A successful system of care for children is family centered and embraces the medical home and the dental home concepts. In a Bright Futures partnership, health care professionals expect that families come to the partnership with strengths. They acknowledge and reinforce those strengths and help build others. They also recognize that all (health care professionals, families, and children) grow, learn, and develop over time and with experience, information, training, and support. This approach also includes

Introduction

encouraging opportunities for youth that have been demonstrated to correlate with positive health behavior choices. For some families, these assets are strongly ingrained and reinforced by cultural or faith-based beliefs. They are equally important in all socioeconomic groups. Most families can maximize these assets if they are aware of their importance.

In the *Bright Futures Pocket Guide*,[5] Green and colleagues note the importance of fostering communication and building effective partnerships among the child, the family, the health care professional, and communities. They enumerate 6 steps for building these partnerships:

1. Model and encourage open, supportive communication with the child and family.
2. Identify health issues through active listening and "fact finding."
3. Affirm strengths of child and family.
4. Identify shared goals.
5. Develop a joint plan of action based on stated goals.
6. Follow up to sustain the partnership.

Collaboration with families in a clinical practice is a series of communications, agreements, and negotiations to ensure the best possible health care for the child. In the Bright Futures vision of family-centered care, families must be empowered as care participants. Their unique ability to choose what is best for their children must be recognized.

...the clinical practice level...

To further define the diversity of practice in the care of children, it is important to consider the community of care that is available to the family. The clinical practice is central to providing health supervision. Practices may be small or large, private or hospital affiliated, or in the public sector. A rural solo practice, suburban private practice of one or several

physicians and nurse practitioners, children's service within a multidisciplinary clinic, school-based health center, dental office, community health center, and public health clinic are all examples of practices that provide preventive ser-vices to children. Each model consists of health care professionals with committed and experienced office or clinic staff to provide care for children and their families.

To adequately address the health needs, including oral health and emotional and social needs, of a child and family, child health care professionals always will serve as care coordinators. Health care professionals, working closely with the family, will develop a centralized patient care plan and seek consultations from medical, nursing, or dental colleagues, mental health care professionals, nutritionists, and others in the community, on behalf of their patients, and will facilitate appropriate referrals when necessary. Care coordination also involves a knowledge of community services and support systems that might be recommended to families. At the heart of the Bright Futures approach to practice is the notion that every child deserves a medical and dental home.

A medical home is defined as primary care that is accessible, continuous, comprehensive, family centered, coordinated, compassionate, and culturally effective.[6] In a medical home, a child health care professional works in partnership with the family and patient to ensure that all the medical and nonmedical needs of the patient are met. Through this partnership, the health care professional can help the family and patient access and coordinate specialty care, educational services, out-of-home care, family support, and other public and private community services that are important to the overall health of the child and family.

Nowhere is the medical home concept more important than in the care of children and youth with special health care needs. For families and health care professionals alike, the implications of caring for a child or youth

At the heart of the Bright Futures approach to practice is the notion that every child deserves a medical and dental home.

with special health care needs can be profound.

The dental home[7] provides risk assessment and an individualized preventive dental health program, anticipatory guidance, a plan for emergency dental trauma, comprehensive dental care, and referrals to other specialists. (For more information on this topic, see the Promoting Oral Health theme.)

... and the community, health system, and policy levels.

One of the unique and core values of Bright Futures is the commitment to advocacy and action in promoting health and preventing disease, not only within the medical home but also in partnership with other health and education professionals and others in the community. This core value rests on a clear understanding of the important role that the community plays in influencing children's health, both positively and negatively. Communities in which children, youth, and families feel safe and valued, and have access to positive activities and relationships, provide the essential base on which the health care professional can build to support healthy behaviors for families at the health supervision visits. Understanding the community in which the practice or clinic is located can help the health care professional learn the strengths of that community and how to use and build on those strengths. Data on community threats and assets provide an important tool that providers can use to prioritize action on specific health concerns.

The Bright Futures comprehensive approach to health care also encompasses continuous improvements in the overall health care delivery system that result in enhanced prevention services, improved outcomes for children and families, and the potential for cost savings.

Bright Futures embodies the concept of synergy between health care professionals, who provide health promotion and preventive services to individual children and families, and public health professionals, who develop policies and implement programs to address the health of populations of children at the community, state, and national levels. Bright Futures has the opportunity to serve as a critical link between the health of individual children and families and public policy health goals. Healthy People 2010,[2] for example, is a comprehensive set of disease prevention and health promotion objectives for the nation over the first decade of the 21st century. Its major goals are to increase the quality and number of years of healthy life and to eliminate health disparities. In its Leading Health Indicators, Healthy People 2010 enumerates the 10 most important health issues for the nation:

- Physical activity
- Overweight and obesity
- Tobacco use
- Substance abuse
- Responsible sexual behavior
- Mental health
- Injury prevention
- Environmental quality
- Immunizations
- Access to care

Many of the themes for the Bright Futures Visits were chosen from these leading health indicators to synchronize the efforts of office-based or clinic-based health supervision and public health efforts. This partnership role is explicitly mentioned in the American Academy of Pediatrics (AAP) policy statement on the pediatrician's role in community pediatrics, which recommends that pediatricians "...should work collaboratively with public health departments and colleagues in related professions to identify and decrease barriers to the health and well-being of children in the communities they serve. In many cases, vitally needed services already exist in the community. Pediatricians can play an

Introduction

extremely important role in coordinating and focusing services to realize maximum benefit for all children."[8] This is true for all health care professionals who provide clinical primary care for infants, children, and adolescents.

Who Can Use Bright Futures?

The themes and visits described in Bright Futures are designed to be readily applied to the work of child health care professionals and practice staff who directly provide primary care, and the parents and youth who participate in these visits. One of the greatest strengths of Bright Futures is that its content and approach resonate with, and are found useful by, a wide variety of professionals and families who work to promote child health. A recent evaluation of Bright Futures found that, although the guidelines themselves are written in a format to be particularly useful for health care professionals who work in clinical settings, they have been adopted and adapted by public health professionals as the basis for population-based programs and policies, by policy makers as a standard for child health care, by parent groups, and by educators who train the next generation of health care professionals in a variety of fields.[9]

The health care of well or sick children is practiced by a broad range of professionals who take responsibility for a child's health care in a clinical encounter. These health care professionals can be pediatricians, family medicine physicians, pediatric and family nurse practitioners, nurses, dentists, nutritionists, physical and occupational therapists, social workers, mental health care providers, physician assistants, and others. Bright Futures does not stop there, however. These principles and recommendations have been designed with many partners in mind because these professionals do not practice in a vacuum. They work collaboratively with other health care professionals and support personnel as part of the overall health care system.

A quick look at the key themes that provide cross-cutting perspectives on all the content of Bright Futures will reveal how collaborative work contributes to the goals. The discussions for each age group will be helpful to all health care professionals and families who support and care for children and youth.

How Is Bright Futures Organized?

The richness of this third edition of the *Bright Futures Guidelines* reflects the combined wisdom of the child and adolescent health care professionals and families on the Bright Futures Infancy, Early Childhood, Middle Childhood, and Adolescence Expert Panels. Each Panel and many expert reviewers carefully considered the health supervision needs of an age group and developmental stage. Their work is represented in several formats in the Guidelines:

- The first major section of the Guidelines is the **Health Promotion Themes.** These thematic discussions highlight issues that are important to families and health care professionals across all the developmental stages.

  These Health Promotion Themes are designed for the practitioner or student who desires an in-depth, state-of-the-art discussion of a certain child health topic with evidence regarding effectiveness. These comprehensive discussions also can help families understand the context of their child's health and support their child's and family's health. Information from the 4 Expert Panels about these themes as they relate to specific developmental stages from birth to early adulthood was blended into each Health Promotion Theme discussion.

- The second major section of the Guidelines is the **Visits.** In this section, practitioners will find the core of child health supervision activities, described as Bright Futures Visits (Box 1).

Introduction

Bright Futures Health Supervision Visits, from the Prenatal Visit to the Late Adolescent Visit, are presented in accordance with the AAP Periodicity Schedule,[10] which is the standard for preventive care for infants, children, and adolescents and is used by professional organizations, federal programs, and third-party payers.

Each visit within the 4 ages and stages of development begins with an introductory section that highlights key concepts of each age.

The visits sections are designed to be implemented as state-of-the-art practice in the care of children and youth. The visits describe the essential content of the child and family visit and interaction with the child and adolescent health care professional and the health care system in which the service is provided.

This clinical approach and content can be readily adapted for use in other situations where the health and development of children at various ages and stages is addressed. This might include home visiting programs or helping the parents of children in Head Start or other child care or early education programs understand their children's health and developmental needs. Colleagues in public health or health policy will find the community- and family-based approach embedded in the child and adolescent health supervision guidance. Educators and students of medicine, nursing, dentistry, public health, nutrition, and others will find the *Bright Futures Guidelines* and the supporting sample questions and anticipatory guidance useful in understanding the complexity and context of health supervision visits and in appreciating the warmth of the patient contact that the Bright Futures approach ensures.

Implementing Bright Futures

Carrying out Bright Futures means making full use of all the Bright Futures materials. For child health care professionals who wish to improve their skills, Bright Futures has developed a range of educational materials that complement the Guidelines. For example, the case-based *Pediatrics in Practice: A Health Promotion Curriculum for Child Health Professionals*[11] has 6 modules that address the

See Recommendations for Preventive Pediatric Health Care in Appendix C.

BOX 1

A Bright Futures Visit

A Bright Futures Visit is an age-specific health supervision visit that uses techniques described in this edition of the *Bright Futures Guidelines*, although modifications to fit the specific needs and circumstances of communities and practices are encouraged. The Bright Futures Visit is more family driven, and is designed to allow practitioners to improve their desired standard of care. This family-centered emphasis is demonstrated through several features:

- Solicitation of parental and child concerns.
- Surveillance and screening.
- Assessment of strengths.
- Discussion of certain visit priorities for improved child and adolescent health and family function over time. Sample questions and anticipatory guidance for each priority are provided as starting points for discussion. These questions and anticipatory guidance points can be modified or enhanced by each health care professional using Bright Futures.

Introduction

core components of Bright Futures: health, partnership, communication, health promotion, time management, and education and advocacy. The *Bright Futures in Practice* manuals provide detailed guidance on selected topics, including mental health, nutrition, oral health, and physical activity.

As previously mentioned, a *Bright Futures Toolkit* will be designed as a companion to this book to allow the health care professionals who wish to improve their practices or services to efficiently and comprehensively carry out new practices and practice change strategies. The tools will be compatible with suggested templates for the electronic health record (EHR); however, using the Toolkit will not require an EHR. Potential tools and resources will be identified and will contain elements designed to ensure that the valuable visit time will be sufficient to address the family's questions and agenda, the child's needs, and the prioritized anticipatory guidance recommended by the Bright Futures Expert Panels. Elements of the Toolkit may include:

- A Bright Futures Visit Questionnaire, which a parent or patient completes before the practitioner begins the visit.
- Screening tools, which allow health care professionals to screen children and youth for certain conditions at specific visits.
- A Bright Futures Visit Chart Documentation Form, which corresponds to the *Bright Futures Guidelines* tasks for that visit and the information that is gleaned from the parent questionnaire.
- The Bright Futures Preventive Services Prompt Sheet, which affords an at-a-glance compilation of work that is done over multiple visits to ensure completeness and increase efficiency.

- Parent/Child Anticipatory Guidance Materials, which reinforce and supplement the information discussed at the visit. These materials guide the health care professional in that they contain general principles and instructions for how the health care professional can communicate information with families.
- Practice Management Tools, to facilitate practice operations and administration. Information on scheduling, including recall and reminder systems, documentation of immunizations, coding options, and other practice management activities, are essential to the success of Bright Futures health supervision within the practice or clinic.
- Community Resources, providing a template to link Bright Futures practices and clinics to referral sources. As every community is unique, creating a practice Community Resources Guide allows the child health care provider to identify community assets for families, build partnerships with other community services, and facilitate referrals when needed.

Using Bright Futures to Improve the Quality of Care

This edition of the *Bright Futures Guidelines* presents an expanded implementation approach that builds on change strategies for office systems. This approach allows child health care professionals who deliver care that is consistent with Bright Futures to engage their office staff, families, public health colleagues, and even community agencies in quality improvement activities that will result in better care.[13-17]

A project that focused on implementation strategies for health supervision visits for children from birth to age 5 years examined the impact on office practices and care delivered using the Bright Futures approach and philosophy. The project addressed 6 critical and measurable characteristics (AAP, unpublished data):

- Delivery of preventive services
- Use of structured developmental screening
- Use of strength-based approaches and a mechanism to elicit and address parent and youth concerns
- Establishment of community linkages that facilitate effective referrals and access to needed community services for families and collaboration with other child advocates
- Use of a recall and reminder system
- Use of a practice mechanism to identify children with special health care needs and ensure that they receive preventive services

The program found that using the Bright Futures approach involved all the office staff in improvements that were important to patient care and demonstrable on chart audit. Many of the changes did not involve additional work but rather a more coordinated approach. Practices learned actionable changes from each other as they progressed.

In addition to the focus on systematic improvement, using Bright Futures has other potential benefits as well. Health care professionals may use the data they gather to satisfy future recertification requirements. In addition, as health insurers link reimbursement to documentation of the delivery of quality preventive services, child health care professionals will have ready access to the data that demonstrate the high caliber of their work.

Introduction

References

1. Green M, Palfrey JS, eds. *Bright Futures: Guidelines for Health Supervision of Infants, Children, and Adolescents.* 2nd ed rev. Arlington, VA: National Center for Education in Maternal and Child Health; 2002

2. US Department of Health and Human Services. *Healthy People 2010: Understanding and Improving Health.* 2nd ed. Washington, DC: Government Printing Office; 2000

3. Substance Abuse and Mental Health Services Administration. *Mental Health: A Report of the Surgeon General.* Rockville, MD: Substance Abuse and Mental Health Services Administration, US Department of Health and Human Services; 1999

4. Denboba D, McPherson MG, Kenney MK, Strickland B, Newacheck PW. Achieving family and provider partnerships for children with special health care needs. *Pediatrics.* 2006;118:1607-1615

5. Green M, Palfrey JS, eds. *Bright Futures: Guidelines for Health Supervision of Infants, Children and Adolescents. Pocket Guide.* 2nd ed Rev. Arlington, VA: National Center for Education in Maternal and Child Health; 2002

6. American Academy of Pediatrics, Medical Home Initiatives for Children With Special Health Care Needs Project Advisory Committee. The medical home. *Pediatrics.* 2002;110:184-186

7. Hale KJ, American Academy of Pediatrics Section on Pediatric Dentistry. Oral health risk assessment timing and establishment of the dental home. *Pediatrics.* 2003;111:1113-1116

8. Rushton FE, American Academy of Pediatrics, Committee on Community Health Services. The pediatrician's role in community pediatrics. *Pediatrics.* 2005;115:1092-1094

9. Zimmerman B, Gallagher J, Botsko C, Ledsky R, Gwinner V. *Assessing the Bright Futures for Infants, Children and Adolescents Initiative: Findings from a National Process Evaluation.* Washington, DC: Health Systems Research Inc; 2005. Available at: http://www.altarum.org. Accessed August 16, 2007

10. American Academy of Pediatrics, Committee on Practice and Ambulatory Medicine. Recommendations for preventive pediatric health care. *Pediatrics.* 2000;105:645-646

11. Bernstein H. *Pediatrics in Practice: A Health Promotion Curriculum for Child Health Professionals.* New York, NY: Springer Publishing Company; 2005

12. Elster AB, Kuznets NJ. *AMA Guidelines for Adolescent Preventative Services (GAPS): Recommendations and Rationale.* Batimore, MD: Williams & Wilkins; 1994

13. Margolis PA, Lannon CM, Stuart JM, Fried BJ, Keyes-Elstein L, Moore DE Jr. Practice based education to improve delivery systems for prevention in primary care: randomised trial (published online ahead of print February 6, 2004). *BMJ.* 2004;328:388 doi:10.113b/bmj.38009-706319.47

14. Bordley WC, Margolis PA, Stuart J, Lannon C, Keyes L. Improving preventive service delivery through office systems. *Pediatrics.* 2001;108:e41. Available at: http://www.pediatrics.org/cgi/content/full/108/3/e41. Accessed June 6, 2007

15. Klein JD, Allan MJ, Elster AB, et al. Improving adolescent preventive care in community health centers. *Pediatrics.* 2001;107:318-327

16. Ozer EM, Adams SH, Lustig JL, et al. Increasing the screening and counseling of adolescents for risky health behaviors: a primary care intervention. *Pediatrics.* 2005;115:960-968

17. Shaw JS, Wasserman RC, Barry S, et al. Statewide quality improvement outreach improves preventive services for young children. *Pediatrics.* 2006;118:e1039-1047. Available at: http://www.pediatrics.org/cgi/content/full/118/4/e1039. Accessed June 6, 2007

An Introduction to the Bright Futures Health Promotion Themes

As the content and structure of the age-specific sections evolved, it became increasingly clear that a number of themes were emerging repeatedly across the developmental stages. These themes are of key importance to families and health care professionals in their common mission to promote the health and well-being of children from birth through adolescence.

As a result, the *Bright Futures Guidelines* developers decided to extract these discussions from the Visits section and create a new Health Promotion Themes section. This decision accomplishes 2 objectives. Not only does it streamline the Visits sections and reduce redundancy, but it serves to highlight these key themes and provide an opportunity for focused discussion.

These Health Promotion Themes discussions are designed for the health care professional or student who desires an in-depth, state-of-the-art discussion of a certain child health topic with evidence regarding effectiveness of health promotion interventions at specific developmental stages from birth to early adulthood. These comprehensive discussions also can help families understand the context of their child's health and support their child's and family's health.

Ten issues are covered in the following section of the *Bright Futures Guidelines*, including the 2 identified as **Significant Challenges to Child and Adolescent Health:** Promoting Healthy Weight and Promoting Mental Health. The Health Promotion Themes are:

- Promoting Family Support
- Promoting Child Development
- Promoting Mental Health
- Promoting Healthy Weight
- Promoting Healthy Nutrition
- Promoting Physical Activity
- Promoting Oral Health
- Promoting Healthy Sexual Development and Sexuality
- Promoting Safety and Injury Prevention
- Promoting Community Relationships and Resources

Promoting Family Support

Theme 1

INTRODUCTION

The Family: A Description

We all come from families.

Families are big, small, extended, nuclear, multi-generational, with one parent, two parents, and grandparents.

We live under one roof or many.

A family can be as temporary as a few weeks, as permanent as forever.

We become part of a family by birth, adoption, marriage, or from a desire for mutual support.

As family members, we nurture, protect, and influence each other.

Families are dynamic and are cultures unto themselves, with different values and unique ways of realizing dreams.

Together, our families become the source of our rich cultural heritage and spiritual diversity.

Each family has strengths and qualities that flow from individual members and from the family as a unit.

Our families create neighborhoods, communities, states, and nations.

— DEVELOPED AND ADOPTED BY THE YOUNG CHILDREN'S CONTINUUM OF THE NEW MEXICO STATE LEGISLATURE
JUNE 20, 1990

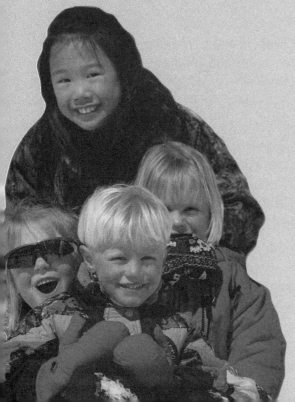

The health and well-being of infants, children, and adolescents depend on their parents and other caregivers—their families. Focusing on the family's growth and development along with the growth and development of the child is a central activity of Bright Futures for all health care professionals. It is the basis of the partnership with parents and families. Putting this approach into practice at health supervision visits involves:

- Being aware of the composition of the family
- Assessing parental well-being
- Asking about and addressing parent concerns
- Identifying and building on parents' and families' strengths
- Assessing the family's well-being

- Providing information, support, and access to community resources
- Delivering family-centered care in the medical home[1]

The Family Constellation

Just as every child is different, so is every family. Families can include one child and one parent or guardian, or several children plus parents or guardians that range in age from adolescents to senior citizens. They might be extended families, foster families, adoptive families, or blended families with stepparents and stepchildren. Parents can be married or unmarried couples, single parents, or parents who live apart and share child-rearing responsibilities. Parents may be gay or lesbian couples.[2,3] The family unit can be relatively static, or it can be quite changeable if parents divorce or remarry or if outside caregivers change.

In some families, grandparents play a central role in the daily care of young and growing children. Intergenerational parenting is a growing trend as grandparents and other family members assume the care for children whose birth parents are not present or not capable of caring for their children because of extended work-related absences, illness or death, drug use, neglect, abandonment, or incarceration.

Although it has predictable patterns, the family reshapes its daily life and support systems with the birth of each child in a way that fits with its unique mix of strengths and challenges. For families living in difficult situations, such as poverty, divorce, separation, or illness, resiliency varies tremendously and is not always predictable. Two themes that are common to all families are that parents want the best for their children and that significant change or stress that affects one family member affects all members.

Health care professionals should be aware of the type of family to which a child belongs and should be sensitive to cultural differences among families, including racial, ethnic, and language differences, as well as gender and age differences of the parents or caregivers. The health care professional and family form a partnership in the medical home that is based on respect, trust, honest communication, and cultural competence. Becoming a culturally effective professional requires changing the ways of thinking about, understanding, and interacting with the world.[4] Health care professionals can better understand their patients and facilitate communication if they integrate the family's cultural background into the general health assessment.[5] (For more information on this topic, see the Bright Futures Introduction.)

The Role of Fathers

Providers of pediatric health care most often interact with mothers, because women are typically the primary caregivers of children in our culture. As a result, the involvement of fathers in the care of their children traditionally has not received great emphasis in pediatric training. Social changes in this country have altered traditional father roles substantially, however, and parents now share more in the care of their children. Moreover, a growing number of single fathers today are raising children on their own, with 6% of children being raised in single-father households in 2003.[6] A variety of "nonnuclear" family arrangements also are on the rise, in which the primary father figure is a stepfather, fiancé, grandfather, or other extended family member.[5] At the same time, more children than ever are growing up in "father-absent," mother-only, families (26% in 2003).[6] For all these reasons, health care professionals must increase their understanding of the fathers, as well as the mothers, of their patients.[5]

Research on the impact of a father on his child's development and psychological

The health care professional and family form a partnership in the medical home that is based on respect, trust, honest communication, and cultural competence.

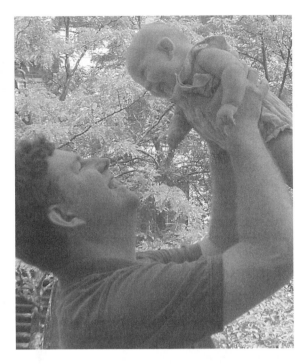

growth has shown a range of important effects on the child's well-being, cognitive development, social competence, and later school success.[7,8]

Health care professionals should consider the potential effects of their own influence on paternal involvement in the care of their children. When inviting a father to become an integral part of his new infant's health supervision visits, the health care professional is sending a clear message about his importance to the child's long-term health and development.[9] When both parents attend health supervision visits, the health care professional can observe how the parents work together with their child and where important differences exist that can affect the care and support of the child. Encouraging fathers to attend health supervision visits gives the health care professional an opportunity to gain insight through direct observation and inquiry into the following:

- The nature of the father's involvement with the child, including his views, concerns, and questions

- Some aspects of his support for the mother (and consequently support for the mother-child relationship)
- The father's general physical and mental health
- Cultural values that can contribute to the father's role and involvement with his child

Supporting Families With Special Needs
Adoption

Adoption is a broad term that can include international or domestic arrangements, adoption from foster care, placement with relatives other than parents (kinship care), open adoptions, adoption from biologic families, and adoption within and across ethnic and cultural groups. Health care professionals can play a supportive role by helping families with the many issues associated with adoption. For example, families who are pursuing an international adoption may need support in dealing with unknown developmental and cognitive status or the risk of infectious diseases for the children,[10] foreign travel, and numerous rules that often require exceptional parental patience and persistence.

Adoption presents special challenges and lifelong transitions for the adopted child, his biologic family, and his adoptive family. All adopted children need a thorough assessment of their physical, emotional, and psychological needs at the time of adoption and as they develop because of their increased risk for developing behavioral, emotional, and social problems. Children who are placed into families from foster care may exhibit behaviors that reflect their earlier abandonment or neglect. They might behave more like children younger than their own age because their childhood experiences have been atypical. Adopted children who are of a different race or ethnicity than their parents may encounter identity issues.

...families who are pursuing an international adoption may need support in dealing with unknown developmental and cognitive status or the risk of infectious diseases for the children, foreign travel, and numerous rules that often require exceptional parental patience and persistence.

As the child develops, parents commonly have ongoing questions and uncertainties related to the adoption. Thus, the continuity of care, developmental monitoring, and openness to the parent's questions that are offered by the pediatric health care professional become all-important sources of support for adoptive parents.

Health care professionals also can offer vitally important anticipatory guidance on the development of the child's perspectives on adoption. The adopted child will not be aware of the difference between biologic and adoptive families before the age of 3 years. In developmentally determined steps throughout childhood and adolescence, he will gain an understanding of what it means to be adopted. Parents who have adopted young children should be advised to introduce the words "adoption" and "adopted" as soon as the child begins to develop language, and to elaborate, for the child, the personal story of his birth and adoption in positive, developmentally appropriate terms, thus providing the child with an opportunity to integrate the concept into his thinking from an early stage. For some school-aged children, perceptions of a sense of loss and self-esteem issues can occur during middle childhood. A struggle with concepts of identity can arise during adolescence. Health care professionals also can emphasize to families the need to provide children with truthful information regarding the adoption process, a discussion that is best initiated with parents during the child's early years.[11]

Foster Care

Each year in the United States, more than 275,000 children are placed in foster care as a result of abuse or neglect,[12] with more than 500,000 children in the foster care system at any time.[13] These "out-of-home placements" for children who are unable to remain with their birth parents can be temporary or extended. Foster care ultimately may lead to family reunification; permanent severance of parental custody, thereby creating the possibility of adoption by another family; or a cycle of moving in and out of foster care until the child reaches adulthood. Children may be placed with caregivers who are relatives,[14,15] with nonrelative foster families, in a treatment or therapeutic foster care home, or in a group or congregate care home. Recent data clearly show that children in foster care have special needs.

- Most foster children are victims of abuse or neglect and did not experience a stable, nurturing environment during their early life.
- Slightly more than half of the children return to their parent or principal caregiver.[16]
- The length of time in foster care varies, but, on average, 36% of the children are in foster care for less than 1 year, 20% are in foster care between 1 and 2 years, and 27% are in foster care from 2 to 4 years.[16]
- In a study of 1,635 children in foster care in Philadelphia, PA, 41% of children had 3 or more foster care placements during the year of observation.[17]
- Thousands of children live in an informal version of foster care, in which they live with relatives other than parents. Relatives who provide this "kinship care" usually receive no training or financial support for doing so. Additionally, children in kinship care are not guaranteed the special protection or monitoring that is provided to children in official foster care programs.[14]

Children who are placed in foster care during the years of active brain development are at risk of developing special health concerns. An environment that is devoid of age-appropriate stimulation, nurturing, and

Slightly more than half of foster children return to their parent or principal caregiver.

communication affects an infant's cognitive and communication skills and alters attachment relationships. (For more information on this topic, see the Promoting Mental Health theme.) Young children who are placed in foster care because of parental neglect can experience profound and long-lasting consequences on all aspects of their development (eg, poor attachment formation, understimulation, developmental delay, poor physical development, and antisocial behavior).

Placements into foster care that occur between the ages of 6 months and about 3 years, especially if prompted by family discord and disruption, can result in subsequent emotional disturbances in the child because of the young child's limited capacity for understanding the constraints of time and place that accompany the foster care experience. The development of these disturbances depends on the nature of the attachment relationships before and after separation from the biologic parent(s) and the child's response to stress. If separation from biologic parents during the first year of life (especially during the first 6 months) is followed by good-quality care, placement in foster care may not have a deleterious effect on social or emotional functioning.[14]

Several developmental issues are important to consider for young children in foster care:

- The impact of abuse, neglect, and inadequate or multiple foster care placements on brain development
- The nature of the attachment relationships before and after separation from the biologic parent(s)
- The young child's limited capacity for understanding the constraints of time and place that accompany the foster care experience
- The child's response to stress

In addition to these mental health care concerns that can lead to later problems, including difficulty in forming adult relationships, many children in foster care have unmet physical health care needs, including missed immunizations, poor medical history, undiagnosed infections or illnesses, and undiagnosed developmental delays. (For more information on this topic, see the Promoting Child Development theme.) Foster parents often are excluded from supports and information that are provided to birth or adoptive parents about their children's health and development. They often do not have any background information on the children in their care and may have to suddenly deal with a health crisis that they did not anticipate. Health care professionals need to create partnerships and processes to support these needs. The foster child's caseworker is an important resource.

Health care professionals have a responsibility to comprehensively assess, treat, refer, and advocate for these vulnerable children and their caregivers.[13] By acknowledging the emotional rewards and challenges of foster parenting and addressing the multiple needs and concerns of foster families, health care professionals can greatly assist foster parents and the children in their care.

Families With Adolescent Parents

Adolescent parents face a variety of specific challenges. Along with their need to build a nurturing relationship with their infant, they also often want to return to school and attempt to reengage with their previous friends and activities. They often lack resources, including ready transportation to health care appointments.

In most cases, the adolescent parent lives with her own parents, and the grandparent shares some aspects of child care and child rearing. The health care professional's inquiry into the individual roles of different family caregivers, including the baby's father if the relationship is continuing, will provide an opportunity to discuss individual needs and expectations. The result can be especially

By acknowledging the emotional rewards and challenges of foster parenting and addressing the multiple needs and concerns of foster families, health care professionals can greatly assist foster parents and the children in their care.

PROMOTING FAMILY SUPPORT

powerful when the adolescent and her parent meet to discuss their roles, differences, and mutual goals.

Many adolescents adapt well to parenting when they have a supportive and encouraging environment. Focusing on their specific parenting strengths in front of other family members during visits and providing anticipatory guidance will build confidence as well as competence. These young parents also may be helped by parenting classes, peer support programs, home visitation programs, and other community support services. Schools with onsite child care and programs for adolescent parents are wonderful resources if they are available in the community.[18,19]

Children and Youth With Special Health Care Needs

The US Department of Health and Human Services' Maternal and Child Health Bureau (MCHB) defines children and youth with special health care needs as children "…who have or are at increased risk for chronic physical, developmental, behavioral, or emotional conditions, and who require health and related services of a type or amount beyond that required generally."[20] In 2000, the MCHB found that more than 9 million children in the United States have special health care needs.[21] National surveys find that between 13% and 23% of all children have a special health care need.[21-23] This means that 1 of every 5 households in the United States includes a child with a developmental delay, a chronic health condition, or some form of disability.

Health care professionals who have pediatric patients with special health care needs should seek to understand the family's composition and social circumstances and the impact that the special needs have on family functioning. Family-centered care that promotes positive relationships and honest

communication among all parties (families, children, and health care professionals) is critical. Because children and youth with special health care needs tend to require visits with health care professionals more frequently than their siblings and because most children with these special needs now live normal life spans, families find it especially important to build strong partnerships with the health care professionals who see their children, to feel comfortable asking questions and seeking advice as they face transitions and decision points along the continuum of their child's health care. Health care professionals can assist the family in helping the child reach her potential by focusing on the strengths of the child and her family.

The lives of the parents, siblings, and other caregivers are affected by the child's medical care and the need for episodic or recurrent hospitalizations, specialized procedures, and treatments; the child's interactions with multiple specialists and other service providers, including the education system; and the financial impact of the child's condition on the family. Helping families identify natural support networks and community resources

Health care professionals who have pediatric patients with special health care needs should seek to understand the family's composition and social circumstances and the impact that the special needs have on family functioning.

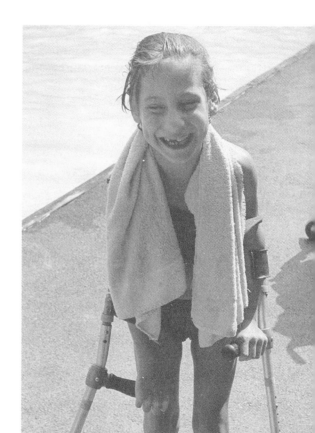

is essential. Peer and community networks can provide support not only for medical concerns but also for logistical and emotional issues. Community resources can include respite care for the child, home visitor programs, early intervention programs, family resource and support centers, libraries, faith-based organizations, Parent-to-Parent and other parenting support groups, and recreation centers.[24] (For more information on this topic, see the Promoting Community Relationships and Resources theme.) These resources may be more easily accessed if the child or youth with special health care needs is cared for in a medical home.

Recognizing the Impact of Environment on Families

Many parents may not have control over their home environment because of living arrangements or because culture or gender roles make it difficult for women to influence the behaviors of men or for younger parents to contradict teachings and practices of elders. (For more information on this topic, see the Promoting Safety and Injury Prevention theme.) The health care professional can work with parents to develop strategies for ensuring a healthy living environment for the benefit of their child's health and well-being. Neighbor-hood and community environments directly support or challenge the well-being of families and the goals that parents have for their children.

Special consideration may be needed for immigrant or refugee families, especially in relation to legal status, which can affect their children's access to health care and housing. Homeless families or families living in shelters also require assistance with medical, mental health, housing, education, and social welfare systems.

The health care professional should work with families and professional and community resources to help families create and maintain a healthy, safe environment for their children.

Inadequate housing, whether due to poor construction or disrepair, insect or rodent infestation, proximity to environmental hazards (eg, gas stations, transportation depots, waste storage sites, factories, refineries, and chemical plants), or individual lifestyle behaviors (eg, smoking), can pose a serious health risk to children living in that environment. Mold exposure,[25] indoor air pollutants from the combustion of wood, gas, oil, kerosene, propane, and other fuels and their contaminant by-products induce respiratory symptoms and exacerbate asthma. Smoke from candle and incense is another important source of particulate emissions into the air. Cultural and religious or spiritual rituals often use candles or incense, which also are popular in home décor. Exposure to lead that is deposited in soil also may occur near gas stations, bus or train terminals, factories, or refineries.[26] Family members who are exposed to lead through their occupations can carry lead into the home on their clothing. Older housing remains an important risk for lead exposure. Homes that were built before 1940 have a 68% risk of containing a lead hazard; those built between 1940 and 1959 have a 43% risk.[27] Folk or ritualistic use of elemental mercury among Latin American and Afro-Caribbean cultures can pose a risk to children because of inhalation of large amounts of vapor.[28]

Forming an Effective Partnership With Families

Family-Centered Care

The health care professional plays an important role in supporting the child's health by promoting healthy family development. She also can be helpful to a child and his family in ways that go beyond the provision of expert, sensitive health care. An effective partnership includes information, support, and links to community resources. Halfon et al[29] found that most parents of young children were

The health care professional should work with families and professional and community resources to help families create and maintain a healthy, safe environment for their children.

satisfied with their well child care. The mean global satisfaction rating is 86.9 (SE 6.1). Approximately 94% of parents of young children reported asking all their questions during the last checkup, and 88% reported adequate time with the health care professional during the last well child visit.[29]

Getting to know the family requires knowing household members and the relatives who play important roles in the child's life. Although a visit naturally focuses on the child who is present, the health care professional also must understand that, in many cases, at least one additional child may be in the home, and that the age and health condition of that sibling can affect both the child being examined and the family as a whole.

By knowing the family or asking questions, the health care professional will have a better sense of the health and well-being of the child and his family. Examples of relevant questions are as follows:

- Is your new baby in the family drawing attention away from your 3-year-old?
- Are older siblings, perhaps adolescents, adding to your family's stress?
- Does a brother or sister with special health care needs require intensive daily care?
- Is your child one of many children in the family, or is he an only child?
- Who cares for your child during the day? Do you care for other people's children in your home?
- Do you or your children participate in neighborhood or community activities (eg, parent groups or playgroups)?

Information about the person who cares for the child and how the care is provided also is important for the health care professional. Child care arrangements can fluctuate during the child's early years. Whether parents and other caregivers agree or disagree on issues related to the child's care gives the health care professional insight into sources

of stress and uncertainty for parents. How the siblings are adjusting and how the parents' relationship is faring under the pressure of the many needs of the young child are relevant to the well-being of the child and family. Knowledge about parental vulnerabilities, such as physical or mental illness, provides additional insights for the health care professional.

An American Academy of Pediatrics (AAP) Task Force on the Family policy statement summarizing the literature and professional experience shows the importance of family-centered care.[5] In family-centered care, health care professionals recognize that the family is the constant in a child's life, while health care and other professionals are involved on an as-needed basis. In partnership with the family, the health care professional can promote family, as well as child, development. A central theme of family-centered care is the strong and respectful partnership between a child's family and the health care professional. This bond promotes meaningful communication, which leads to mutual decision making and a medical home where the patient, family, and health care professional are free to discuss all issues and can expect their issues to be addressed. The elements of a successful family-professional partnership are mutual commitment, respect, trust, open and honest communication, cultural competence, and an ability to negotiate.

COMPLEMENTARY AND ALTERNATIVE CARE

Collaboration with families in a clinical practice is a series of communications, agreements, and negotiations to ensure the best possible health care for the child. In the Bright Futures vision of *family-centered* care, families must be empowered as care participants. Their unique ability to choose what is best for their children must be recognized. Families do all they can to protect their children from sickness or harm.

A central theme of family-centered care is the strong and respectful partnership between a child's family and the health care professional. This bond promotes meaningful communication, which leads to mutual decision making and a medical home where the patient, family, and health care professional are free to discuss all issues and can expect their issues to be addressed.

The Bright Futures health care professional must be aware of the disciplines or philosophies that are chosen by the child's family, especially if the family chooses a therapy that is unfamiliar or a treatment belief system that the health care professional does not endorse or share. Families may seek second opinions or services in traditional pediatric medical and surgical care fields or may choose care from alternative or complementary care providers. Families generally seek *additional* care from other disciplines rather than replacement care. *Alternative therapies* generally replace conventional treatments. *Complementary therapies* are used in addition to conventional treatments. Health care professionals should seek to determine whether complementary and alternative therapies indeed improve the standard therapies being used by a family. Families should be empowered to say whether they choose not to carry out prescribed treatments. They must be assured that the health care professional will not take offense at their choice, but will work to choose therapies that are acceptable to the family, appropriate to the problem, and safe and effective in the shared goal of the child's best health.

Practitioners of traditional or allopathic medicine and complementary and alternative care are driven and guided by the mandate to do no harm and to do good. Just because a chosen therapy is out of the standard scope of care does not define it as harmful or without potential benefit. Therapies can be safe and effective, safe and ineffective, or unsafe. The AAP Committee on Children with Disabilities suggests that "to best serve the interests of children, it is important to maintain a scientific perspective, to provide balanced advice about therapeutic options, to guard against bias, and to establish and maintain a trusting relationship with families."[30] Providers of standard care need not be threatened by such choices.

The use of complementary and alternative care in children is particularly common when a child has a chronic illness or condition, such as autism. Alternative treatments are increasingly described on the Internet, with no assurance of safety or efficacy. Parents are often reluctant to tell their health care professional about such treatments, fearing disapproval. Health care professionals should ask parents directly about the use of complementary and alternative care.[31] The health care professional's approach to this subject is equally important (ie, ask in a nonjudgmental manner to allow free discussion about the claims, hopes, and potential harm, if any, of such treatments).

The health care professional should discuss with the family its goals and reasons for the choice of alternative therapies and ask whether the family culture or religion prohibits or recommends certain health care procedures. Faith-based or religious therapeutic systems are likely to be very important to the family and its sense of health and well-being. The following issues may be considered in these discussions:

- What additional benefit is the family seeking? Are these benefits solely within the realm of complementary and alternative care, or has the traditional care plan overlooked an essential family need?
- Are treatment interactions likely? This issue is especially important if herbal, nutritional, or homeopathic remedies are planned. Just as adverse drug-drug interactions must be avoided, interactions between medically prescribed drugs and complementary and alternative remedies also must be considered.
- Are the proposed interventions generally safe? Are the therapies generally applied to children or is their use typically for adults? Are child-specific safety data available? Are they safe for the specific child's condition?

The health care professional should discuss with the family its goals and reasons for the choice of alternative therapies and ask whether the family culture or religion prohibits or recommends certain health care procedures.

- Will the intervention take away from other interventions? All therapeutic interventions have a monetary and time cost. Will therapies compete with one another? If so, how will the family address conflicting or overwhelming demands?

In developing a treatment plan for the child with the family, health care professionals can:

- Provide families with a range of treatment options.
- Educate the family on the importance of the proposed (standard) medical therapy and discuss the treatment in the context of the family's perception of the severity of their child's problem or illness, and the meaning of illness to the family.
- Avoid dismissing complementary and alternative care in ways that suggest a lack of sensitivity or concern for the family's perspective.
- Recognize the feeling of being threatened or challenged professionally and guard against becoming defensive.
- Identify and use reliable reference sources and colleagues to ensure up-to-date information regarding the efficacy and risks of complementary and alternative care in children.
- Consult with colleagues who are knowledgeable about complementary and alternative care, or with an alternative care therapist.

Ask about stress in the family (including intergenerational stress) or in the parents' relationship.

Parental Well-Being

Some aspects of parenting are specific to the developmental stage of the child, but several general issues have an impact on families with children at all ages.

- The physical and emotional health of the parents, siblings, and other family members

- The physical safety and emotional tone of the home environment and neighborhood
- The family's cultural beliefs
- Parenting beliefs, education, and strategies
- The parents' ability to deal with life's stresses

All these issues have significant implications for the successful development of the children in the family. To assess parental well-being, the health care professional can:

- Observe the parents' pleasure and pride in their child.
- Note any indications of their general level of anxiety, overload, irritability, self-doubt, or depression.
- Ask about stress in the family (including intergenerational stress) or in the parents' relationship.
- Discuss the parents' work, its satisfactions for them, and the conflicts that arise between work and home.
- Ask about parents' physical and mental health, including current substance use, and stress the importance of preventive health care for them.
- Ask about parents' sources of support, including personal, financial, and community.
- Ask about other environmental stressors, including poverty, illiteracy, community violence, housing insecurity, or lack of heat and food.

In discussing these issues, it is best if the health care professional uses open-ended questions rather than closed-ended questions. Closed-ended questions require only defined answers, such as "yes" or "no." Open-ended questions, such as, "Tell me how you manage to raise 2 children on your own," are designed to encourage discussion. They often begin with what, when, where, or why.

Family Stress and Change

Major family changes and chronic family stressors are among the most prevalent and important influences on the developmental and psychological well-being of young children. In addition to parental separation and divorce, major changes can include birth of a child with special health care needs or a diagnosis of such needs, change to single-parent status, remarriage, death of a parent or other family member, or moving to a new family home. Family issues, such as parental substance abuse, domestic violence, and parental depression, dramatically affect the child's developmental progress. These parental issues may not come up in the course of the usual pediatric history taking, but they can seriously impair parents' ability to provide a healthy environment for a growing child. For children of all ages, the goal after such an event is to return to a life that is secure and predictable, with ensured or reestablished close ties to loved ones.

Health care professionals can support parents during these challenging times through awareness of family events and focused monitoring of the child's and the family's adaptation.[5] The health care professional's most important intervention may be to help parents develop problem-solving skills. These skills will serve them well in managing important stressors or navigating periods of change or crisis. Suggesting strategies, posing questions, and providing tools are 3 ways that health care professionals can encourage these discussions of child, parent, and family well-being and safety within the family. A 2000 study of children aged 4 to 35 months showed that the majority of parents believe that questions about family, safety, and emotional well-being are appropriate questions for professionals to ask.[32]

PARENTAL DEPRESSION

The mental health of all adult caregivers is important and should be addressed by the

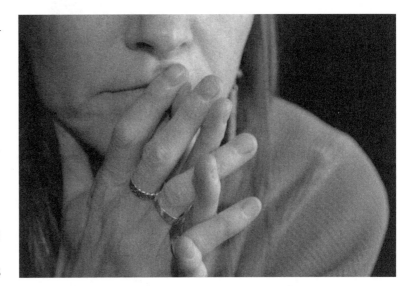

health care professional. Maternal depression has received most of the attention, but that is due to the paucity of data on paternal depression.

Depression is common. The lifetime prevalence of major depressive disorders is 16.6%.[33] Many women experience baby blues, which is an extremely common reaction following delivery of an infant. It usually appears suddenly on the third or fourth day after delivery. "An estimated 70% of all new mothers experience this emotional letdown, and it generally does not impair functioning. About 10% of new mothers experience some degree of postpartum depression. Women who have had severe premenstrual syndrome are more likely to suffer from it."[34]

Parental depression or isolation is one of the greatest risk factors for child behavioral and mental health problems. Identifying maternal depression is especially important during early childhood because of the vulnerability of young children. For the child, short-term behavioral reactions to maternal depression can include withdrawal, reduced activity, reduced self-control, clinginess, increased dependency, increased aggression, poor peer relationships, greater difficulties

For the child, short-term behavioral reactions to maternal depression can include withdrawal, reduced activity, reduced self-control, clinginess, increased dependency, increased aggression, poor peer relationships, greater difficulties adapting to school, and general unhappiness.

adapting to school, and general unhappiness. Long-term effects on the child include a significantly higher chance of developing an affective disorder.[35]

Screening for Depression
Health care professionals sometimes can observe signs of depression in the mother, such as a lack of energy, chronic fatigue, feelings of hopelessness, low self-esteem, poor concentration, or indecisiveness. A mother may say that she is feeling blue or experiencing somatic symptoms, such as insomnia, hypersomnia, poor appetite, or overeating. Culturally specific manifestations of depression also may occur, and the health care professional should seek to learn about those factors in relation to the populations served. Mothers can be willing to talk with their child's health care professional about their own state of well-being, but only in the context of a trusting relationship with a health care professional who demonstrates care and concern for her as well as for her child.[36]

Certain risk factors, such as poverty, chronic maternal health conditions, domestic violence, substance abuse, and marital discord, should alert health care professionals to the higher likelihood of maternal depression and greater risk for the child's development.[37,38] A history of illicit drug use or alcohol or tobacco use during pregnancy should be explored. Health care professionals should be aware that parents of children with special health care needs may go through periods of mourning, which has features similar to depression.

The health care professional can ask questions about possible depression, such as:

- How would you describe your mood in the past 2 weeks?
- Do you find that you no longer get pleasure out of activities that you enjoyed in the past?

Questionnaires, such as the brief Edinburgh Postnatal Depression Scale,[39] also

> Mothers can be willing to talk with their child's health care professional about their own state of well-being, but only in the context of a trusting relationship with a health care professional who demonstrates care and concern for her as well as for her child.

may be useful. For parents who are experiencing depression, the health care professional can:

- Provide understanding and support.
- Ask how the depressive symptoms interfere with everyday life, including caring for the child.
- Explore problems and stressors, including use of alcohol or tobacco, during pregnancy.
- Ask about a past history of depression and treatment.
- Assess the severity of the depression, including risk for suicidal behavior.
- Offer to speak with other family members to better understand the parent's situation and to encourage support.
- Refer to a mental health professional when appropriate.
- Refer to parent's primary care professional.

Parents with depressive symptoms should be asked directly about whether they have had suicidal thoughts. Parents who continue to have such thoughts should be asked if they have a plan to harm themselves. Positive responses to these questions require an immediate mental health evaluation.

SUBSTANCE ABUSE
Substance abuse by parents or other family members can have significant negative effects on the children in the family. Alcohol and other drug abuse also can affect the parents' ability to attend to their children's emotional needs and safety. Impaired judgment resulting from alcohol and other drug abuse leads to inconsistent parent-child interactions and poor parenting. Financial problems are often an additional result of substance abuse. Health care professionals can be alert to the signs of impairment and refer parents for help. In screening for substance abuse, the health care professional can ask, "Is there anyone in the family whose use of alcohol or other drugs worries you?"

DOMESTIC VIOLENCE

Domestic violence, also sometimes called "intimate partner violence," is prevalent across all socioeconomic groups. Estimates range from 960,000 incidents of violence against a current or former spouse, boyfriend, or girlfriend per year[40] to 3 million women who are physically abused by their husband or boyfriend per year.[41] Each year, more than 3 million children witness violence between their parents.[42] Substantial evidence has accumulated regarding the toxic effects of domestic violence on the child. Infants and toddlers who witness violence in their homes or community show excessive irritability, immature behavior, sleep disturbances, emotional distress, fear of being alone, and regression in toileting and language. In school-aged children, overall functioning, attitudes, social competence, and school performance are often affected negatively. Moreover, the presence of violence in the home creates a significant risk of participation in youth violence activities even if the child is not a victim of the family abuse.[43] Abuse of the child is far more likely to happen in families in which violence exists between the parents.[44,45]

Health care professionals must be alert to the signs of domestic violence and be prepared to ask questions in a sensitive manner about the safety of all family members. They also should discuss options that are available to parents who are being abused. Health care professionals should understand that women can be afraid to divulge that they have been abused by a partner because they fear violent reprisals or losing the children.[46]

Routine assessment should focus on early identification of all families and victims of domestic violence, regardless of whether they have symptoms. The health care professional can ask the following questions:

- Do you feel you live in a safe place?
- In the past year, have you ever felt threatened in your home?
- In the past year, has your partner or other family member pushed you, punched you, kicked you, hit you, or threatened to hurt you?

A detailed description of possible assessment questions and interventions in the primary care pediatric context are provided in *Bright Futures in Practice: Mental Health*[47] and at the Family Violence Prevention Fund Web site (http://endabuse.org/).[48]

SEPARATION AND DIVORCE

Today, more than 1 million children per year are newly involved in parental divorce. Overall, 50% of marriages end in divorce every year. The likelihood that a child will be in a family that goes through a divorce is higher than 1 in 3[5]; children also have a 1 in 3 chance of experiencing a second divorce.[49] According to Sammons and Lewis,[50] "By 2010, more than half of school-aged children will have spent substantial time living with a single parent or in a stepfamily."

The process of separation or divorce, parental dating, and stepfamilies or blended families requires many periods of adjustment for the child or adolescent, and separation and divorce are associated with many negative reactions for all members of the family. Practical concerns, such as plans for child care, support, custody, and emergency contacts, should be clarified. The health care professional should assess the child's reaction to the separation or divorce and refer a poorly adapting child for counseling.

If the family doesn't stay intact, the health care professional can seek to decrease negative effects for the parents and child by being an important resource and support for both the child and the parents. This can be done by[49]:

- Encouraging open discussion about separation and divorce with and between parents
- Emphasizing ways to deal with children's reactions

If the family doesn't stay intact, the health care professional can seek to decrease negative effects for the parents and child by being an important resource and support for both the child and the parents.

- Acting as the child's advocate
- Offering support and age-appropriate advice to the child and parents regarding reactions to divorce, especially guilt, anger, sadness, and perceived loss of love
- Referring families to mental health resources with expertise in divorce if necessary

Understanding and Building on the Strengths of Children and Youth

In addition to helping their children avoid unsafe and unhealthy behaviors, parents can foster healthy development in their children by promoting positive physical, ethical, and emotional behaviors and development. Four positive attributes are particularly related to decreased risk-taking behaviors among youth. (For more information on this topic, see the Promoting Child Development theme.) Strength-based parenting fosters opportunities and growth in the following areas[51-54]:

Adolescents who are involved in extracurricular and community activities and whose parents are authoritative, rather than authoritarian or passive, appear to progress through adolescence with relatively little turmoil.

- **Connectedness.** This concept refers to relationships with caring adults, relationships with other children and youth, and belonging. Research demonstrates the

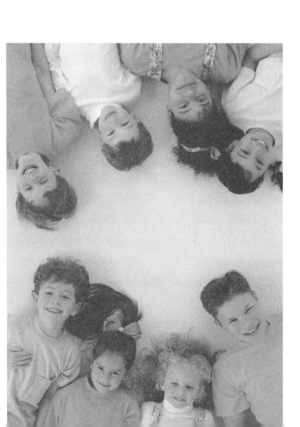

value of parental involvement and quality parent-adolescent communication on healthy adolescent development.[55-57] Adolescents who are involved in extracurricular and community activities and whose parents are authoritative, rather than authoritarian or passive, appear to progress through adolescence with relatively little turmoil.[57]

- **Competence and mastery.** Children and youth who have a chance to gain skills and knowledge grow in competence. For instance, young children learn to sit, walk, and talk. By school age, children have acquired the ability to share, take turns, and listen. For school-aged children and youth, school success becomes an important marker for mastery. Other accomplishments in areas such as the arts, athletic activities, and community service are equally important examples of this attribute. The specific areas of accomplishment may be determined by family and community cultural values. Parents, extended family, educators, and mentors can be most helpful in assisting children and youth find and participate in activities they enjoy.

- **Autonomy and independence.** Autonomy is a goal for youth as they mature to adulthood. Children who have experience with making decisions throughout childhood and who have guidance from their parents and guardians in these efforts are well-positioned to make this transition effectively. It is crucial to encourage appropriate self-care and self-advocacy for children with special health care needs. The rate at which children and youth are expected to make decisions and the areas over which families cede control may vary with the values and culture of the family.

- **Empathy.** Being able to understand the feelings of others is an important developmental task for children and youth to accomplish by adulthood. Young children can demonstrate empathy as generosity when they help at home with age-appropriate tasks or play with younger siblings and neighbors. In adolescents, this skill often manifests itself in babysitting, relationships with peers, or volunteer activities with a community or faith-based group.

Attention to these developmental tasks is equally important in children with special needs because it puts the emphasis on universal themes that are possible in almost all children as they grow. Growing in independence and having the opportunity to do things for others are 2 of the developmental tasks that often require focused effort for youth who have health issues, but these youth also benefit greatly from the chance to emphasize their progress on these developmental tasks of all children.

Family Culture and Behaviors

Understanding and building on the strengths of families requires health care professionals to combine well-honed clinical interview skills with a willingness to learn from families. Families demonstrate a wide range of beliefs and priorities in how they structure daily routines and rituals for their children and how they use health care resources. These attitudes often reflect traditional family or cultural influences, which are important for health care professionals to understand if they hope to work in effective partnership with families to maximize the health and development of their children. Consider the following:

- **Daily routines and rituals.** These include mealtimes, food choices, sleep schedules, bowel and bladder elimination habits, general cleanliness and personal hygiene, attention to dental health, tolerance for risk-taking activities, customary ways of expressing illness or distress, and parental or family use of tobacco, alcohol, or illicit drugs. For example, family meals are associated with language acquisition and literacy in young children, as well as higher dietary quality and psychological health in children and adolescents.[58] Children can thrive in families with widely varying traditions of health beliefs and practices. Emotional support, structure, and safety are the key ingredients of the environments and routines for young children at home.[59] When families hold to routines or rituals that seem to cause or exacerbate a problem, the health care professional should learn more about the history of the routine within the family and, possibly, within the family's culture.

- **Culture, beliefs, and behaviors connected with health and illness.** Families tend to use available health care resources for their young children based on their knowledge, beliefs, traditions, and past experiences with health systems. Visiting a health care professional on behalf of their child reflects a family's desire to seek help or share concerns. At the same time, the family might view typical clinical guidance or use medications in unexpected ways. One family might believe that only a prescription or a shot will help, whereas another might first consult community elders and then combine medicine from the drugstore with traditional healing methods. This makes it important for health care professionals who serve children and families from backgrounds other than their own to listen and observe carefully, to learn from the family, to build trust and respect, and not to assume that a safety checklist will be followed (not out of ignorance or disrespect, but rather out of adherence to tradition and past experience). Health

Families demonstrate a wide range of beliefs and priorities in how they structure daily routines and rituals for their children and how they use health care resources.

care professionals also should understand that families and cultures tend to approach the concept of disability and chronic conditions in different ways. If possible, the presence of a staff member who is familiar with a family's community and fluent in the family's language is helpful during these discussions.

- **Nutrition and physical activity.** Families should emphasize physical activity and healthy eating behaviors early in a child's life. Parents can be positive role models by eating healthfully themselves, participating in physical activity with their children, and performing physical activity themselves. Both regular physical activity (see the Promoting Physical Activity theme) and healthful dietary behaviors (see the Promoting Healthy Nutrition theme) are essential to prevent a sedentary lifestyle and to avoid excessive pediatric weight gain (see the Promoting Healthy Weight theme). Food insecurity and hunger (see the Promoting Healthy Nutrition theme) are problems for an increasing number of families. Health care professionals should identify any problems the family may have in obtaining nutritious food and connect families with appropriate community resources (see the Promoting Community Relationships and Resources theme) when needed.

- **Health behaviors.** Parents are powerful role models for their children. From wearing seat belts and bicycle helmets to modeling community involvement, anger management, or responsible drinking, parents play a significant role in influencing their children's and adolescents' health and risk behaviors.[60]

- **Television, computer, and media viewing.** Television viewing is an established daily routine in most families. Preschool-aged children spend most of their waking *sedentary* time watching

Parents can be positive role models by eating healthfully themselves, participating in physical activity with their children, and performing physical activity themselves.

television. One third of American children aged 2 to 7 years have televisions in their bedrooms.[61] The impact of television viewing (but not other media) on young children has been examined. Although school readiness appears to be increased among low-income children who watch informative television programs and fewer cartoons,[62] most effects are not positive. Studies have shown positive influences of age-appropriate, curriculum-based educational television on children's cognitive abilities and school readiness.[63] One study found that preschoolers who viewed educational television shows had higher grades in high school and read more books than those who did not.[64] On the other hand, television viewing patterns have raised concern because of the effects of media violence and physical inactivity on children and adolescents. Media violence is the most investigated negative factor associated with content, with research indicating that it can contribute to aggressive behavior, desensitization to violence, nightmares, and fear of being harmed.[65-69]

Preschoolers are unable to distinguish between fantasy and reality, making them vulnerable to the influence of the content of shows (eg, violence) and to advertising, particularly if show characters are used to promote products.[66]

For other forms of electronic media, only limited information exists for benefit or harm. "Few data exist regarding how learning-oriented electronic media products are used in the daily lives of young children, let alone their effect on children."[63]

Health care professionals should support the recommendation that children younger than 2 years should not watch television or videos at all, and children older than 2 years should watch no more than 1 to 2 hours of educational programming per day.[70] Sufficient information does not exist to make recommendations for other media use with young children.

- **Smoking, drinking, and substance use.** It is important to discuss with parents their attitude toward drugs or alcohol use, and ask how they plan to talk about drugs and alcohol with their children and adolescents.[71] Children and adolescents can be affected by substance abuse directly (when they use substances themselves, are exposed in utero, or are exposed through the air, such as smoke from crack cocaine) or indirectly (when they experience the consequences of substance use by family members or other adults). Parental alcoholism increases the risk of adolescent alcoholism because of genetic and environmental factors.[72]

Promoting Family Support: The Preconception and Prenatal Periods

In recent years, information on issues that are important to a woman's health before and during pregnancy has helped focus attention on the importance of these periods to the health of her children.

The Preconception Period

Health care professionals who offer preconceptional or interconceptional guidance to older adolescent girls, young adult women, and families during health supervision visits contribute to healthy pregnancies, healthy infants, and healthy outcomes for adults. Maternal health and well-being are vital to a safe pregnancy and the birth of a healthy baby. A nutritious diet and physical activity before pregnancy benefit the mother and fetus during pregnancy and delivery. Educating prospective parents (those having

unprotected intercourse as well as those who are actively planning a pregnancy) about the benefits of making health-promoting choices, particularly related to the use of tobacco, alcohol, illicit drugs, and medications, including over-the-counter medicines and herbal preparations that have potential teratogenic effects, before conception can significantly improve pregnancy outcomes for mother and infant. Adequate amounts of folic acid should be advised for women who are contemplating pregnancy.

The Prenatal Period

Prenatal care is effective in improving the health of mother and baby and is the major factor in preventing infant death and disease.[73] Women who receive early prenatal care generally have better birth outcomes than those who do not.[74]

Establishing a trusting relationship between the health care professional and the family during this time, when many families need and welcome support, can be especially productive. Pregnancy is a time of initial family adaptation, which can predict later parental coping. The health care professional can gather basic information about the family and its values, beliefs, prior experiences, goals, and concerns and can provide reassurance and key information about what to expect during the newborn period. Discussing expectations and concerns with the health care professional allows parents to share their excitement and sort out their concerns. Guidance that is provided to families also should be personalized by acknowledging their beliefs, values, experiences, and needs, and should be interwoven in discussions with parents. Engaging members of the family and community who provide natural support and guidance to new mothers (eg, grandmothers, aunts, and other older women) also is important because it can help foster compliance with health care.

Discussing expectations and concerns with the health care professional allows parents to share their excitement and sort out their concerns.

Optimally, during the last trimester of pregnancy, expectant parents should schedule a visit with the health care professional who will care for their baby after birth. Provided that parents have sufficient literacy and that materials are written in easily understandable words in their primary language, a printed questionnaire that parents can complete in the waiting room before the appointment can suggest issues that should be emphasized during the visit. For some families, illustrated or non-text materials or a brief review of the questionnaire with a staff member may be more appropriate.

An essential component of this initial visit is to introduce the role of parents as the primary decision makers for their child and to emphasize the valuable role family has in ensuring the child's health and well-being. Whenever possible, the health care professional should encourage families to participate actively in the decision-making process. In some families, the grandparents, or a family member other than the parents, may be the decision makers. Therefore, any discussions about decision making for the child should include eliciting how decisions are made within the family and with whom information should be shared.

Education is particularly powerful during the prenatal period. It is an ideal time to advise prospective parents on:

- Lifelong health issues, such as the importance of a healthy diet, physical activity, and dental health (for more information on this topic, see the Promoting Healthy Nutrition, Promoting Physical Activity, and Promoting Oral Health themes)
- The importance of using seat belts and avoiding alcohol, drugs, or tobacco or any other environmental toxicants or hazards
- The importance of the prenatal care visits; appropriate rate of weight gain during pregnancy; appropriate nutrient

Pregnancy complications are often secondary to common underlying medical and dental conditions, such as obesity, diabetes, hypertension, and periodontal disease.

intake; healthy hygiene practices, including hand washing; preparation for childbirth; and sibling preparation and the presence of the father, partner, or other family member during delivery
- Immediate postpartum care issues, including benefits of breastfeeding, rooming-in, newborn metabolic and hearing screening, risks and benefits that are associated with early hospital discharge, and planning for the care of mother and baby after birth
- Other newborn infant care topics, including safe sleep practices, infant temperament, holding and cuddling the baby, sibling precautions, and using an appropriate car safety seat for the baby
- Safety issues, such as the presence of guns in the home and exposure to lead, tobacco, and mercury (for more information on this topic, see the Promoting Safety and Injury Prevention theme)

REDUCING PREGNANCY COMPLICATIONS

Pregnancy complications are often secondary to common underlying medical and dental conditions, such as obesity, diabetes, hypertension, and periodontal disease. Prevalent adult habits can have adverse effects on a developing fetus. Preventable causes of developmental disability include prenatal exposure to teratogens, such as alcohol, and environmental toxins, such as tobacco smoke. Fetal alcohol syndrome, the most common known cause of mental retardation in the United States, is entirely preventable. Because no known amount of alcohol is safe for the developing fetus, women who may become pregnant because they are having unprotected intercourse or are actively trying to become pregnant should be counseled to avoid alcohol during the preconception period and throughout pregnancy.

Smoking during pregnancy and exposure to secondhand smoke are significant contributors to infant mortality, low birth weight, and sudden infant death syndrome. (For more information on this topic, see the Promoting Safety and Injury Prevention theme.) Health care professionals should encourage women who smoke to stop before they become pregnant and should give them information about smoking cessation programs and community resources. Extended or augmented smoking cessation counseling (5 to 15 minutes) that uses messages and self-help materials that are tailored to pregnant smokers, when compared with brief generic counseling interventions alone, substantially increases abstinence rates during pregnancy, and leads to higher birth weights. Although relapse rates are high in the postpartum period, which increases the baby's chances of being exposed to secondhand smoke, "reducing smoking during pregnancy is likely to have substantial health benefits for the baby and the expectant mother."[75]

Although health care professionals should caution families about avoiding or limiting environmental exposures that pose a risk to the developing fetus, they also should recognize that some environmental factors, such as poor housing, pollution, or poverty, can be beyond the family's control. Health care professionals' involvement with community advocacy for better living conditions can be a way to influence the health of mothers and infants. (For more information on this topic, see the Promoting Community Relationships and Resources theme.)

In the periconceptional period (before and during pregnancy), converging events can have a significant impact on the developing fetus with resulting lifelong consequences. Infants who have been exposed to outside environmental factors, maternal substance use, secondhand smoke, malnutrition, or caregiver neglect are at increased risk for morbidity or death. The *triple risk model* delineates how 3 elements—a vulnerable fetus or infant, a critical developmental period (preconception and during pregnancy),

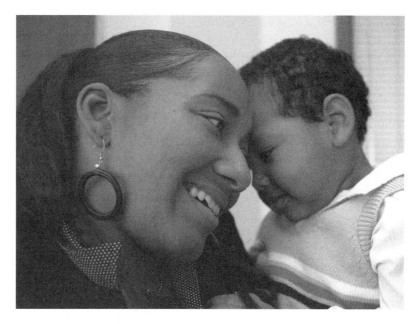

and exogenous stressors (maternal and other environmental factors)—intersect, with the potential to harm or kill the fetus or neonate. This model provides an important conceptual framework as the infant moves through other critical developmental periods after birth.[76]

Promoting Family Support: Infancy— Birth to 11 Months

Ideally, parents care for their infants with the support and assistance of others. Being cognizant of the family's culture, the health care professional should ask about caregiver roles and responsibilities of the parents and other important adults in the child's life.

The family's home setting can have a major influence on parental well-being when parents and other caregivers feel alone and have limited opportunity for social interaction. Living in rural areas with distance between neighbors, in an inner city area that seems unsafe, or in a suburban neighborhood with uninterested neighbors can cause a new parent to feel unwanted or unimportant. A mother who feels comfortable with working outside the home or being a stay-at-home

Being cognizant of the family's culture, the health care professional should ask about caregiver roles and responsibilities of the parents and other important adults in the child's life.

…the child's transition into more active and mobile activities can provide the father with new terms of engagement on familiar ground.

mom, as well as with the emotional support of her partner, can have a positive effect on an infant's emotional development.[8]

Fathers (whether biologic fathers, adoptive fathers, stepfathers, or foster fathers) also are important caregivers and teachers for their infants. A father's participation in infant care is enhanced if he is present at delivery, has early infant contact, and learns about his newborn's abilities. New fathers should learn that they have a unique role, distinct from that of the mother, in caring for and parenting the infant. For families who have recently arrived in this country, any changes in gender roles can be more difficult than for those who are more acculturated. The health care professional may need to discover the roles for fathers in the family's culture and build on them in discussions of other possible roles.

Because more than 50% of mothers in the United States currently work full-time outside the home, the responsibility for providing infant care and developmental stimulation of the infant is often shared by others.[77] High-quality child care provided by nonfamily members can be as nurturing and educational as parental care, but it requires responsive, loving, consistent caregiving by a few adults. Advising parents in their choice of child care options is an important role for health care professionals.

Emotional support between the parents powerfully affects adaptation to parenting. Parents can disagree and even feel angry with each other, and they should be offered help, either by the health care professional or a mental health specialist, to resolve difficulties in a positive way. Parents need to know that they should call for help immediately if they feel they may hurt each other or the baby.

Continuous attention to the quality of the parent-child relationship is an important element of health surveillance for the infant.[78] Because an infant is completely dependent on his parents, and because his learning and experience occur within the interpersonal

context of his relationships with his caregivers, the infant is vulnerable to his parents' mood states. Unanticipated events, such as illness, death, or other catastrophes, can affect the infant because the parent is upset, anxious, overwhelmed, or traumatized by the event and is unable to buffer the infant from those feelings or is unable to give the infant consistent comfort and nurturing.

Promoting Family Support: Early Childhood—1 to 4 Years

Families approach the early childhood years of each child in the family differently. With a first child, many parents still feel tentative about their new role. They often face each stage of their child's development (eg, standing, walking, babbling, holding a cup, playing, saying first words, exploring, throwing tantrums, adjusting to new faces, sleeping alone, making friends, and going to preschool) with shifting senses of worry and wonderment. Whether they are new or experienced at parenting, parents have many questions about their 1-year-old or 4-year-old child, such as, "Is it normal for her to cry every time I leave her?" "Why isn't he saying as many words as his cousin of the same age?" "How do I know if the car seat is the right size?" "When can she begin to eat regular table food?" "When should I start potty training?" "How can we find a good child care provider?"

During early childhood, fathers often become increasingly engaged with their children. This development can be the result of the toddler's decreased dependency on the mother, especially if the child was breastfed as an infant. The mother's return to full-time work outside the home can necessitate the father's increased involvement. In addition, the child's transition into more active and mobile activities can provide the father with new terms of engagement on familiar ground.

As their children move into toddlerhood, parents often are confronted with new pressures to balance the competing needs of their child and family with those of job and career. The new sensitivity of the toddler to separation from family members and the young child's continued high level of need for care make the decision to return to work all the more difficult. The child's increasing push for autonomy and the constant vigilance that is needed to ensure safety add to the stress of this period. These factors may explain evidence of increased depressive symptoms, as high as 42%, in mothers during the second year of their child's life.[79,80] The health care professional can provide valuable encouragement and support to mothers during this time by helping them understand their particular child's temperament and develop appropriate expectations for their child's developmental stage and level of understanding.

Promoting Family Support: Middle Childhood—5 to 10 Years

A child is quite different in the early years of middle childhood than in the later years. A child who gets along well with caregivers and siblings at age 5 may not do so at age 10. Caregivers and parents need to be reassured that these changes are a normal part of the child's growing independence from the family. The family should be encouraged to continue to give plenty of support, attention, and supervision as the child nears early adolescence.

In addition to evaluating parental well-being, health care professionals can encourage the parents of children in middle childhood to model healthy behaviors for their children. Encourage them not to smoke, to wear a seat belt, to consume alcohol responsibly, and never to drive after consuming alcohol. Also encourage them to maintain a healthy weight through proper nutrition and regular exercise. Family activities that include physical activity can be especially beneficial for children in this age group.

The health care professional should inquire about changes and stresses in the family, such as illness in a parent or child, job loss or other change in employment, loss of an older family member, starting school, or moving to a new school or location. Changes and stresses can have a significant impact on the child's moods, behaviors, and school performance. Children react to stress in myriad ways; some children are quite resilient, whereas others are very slow to adapt to change. (For more information on this topic, see the Promoting Mental Health theme.) Parents may need to offer extra support to their child during a particularly difficult time.

School is a key experience for children in middle childhood. Families can play a major supportive role by encouraging the child's educational experiences and being involved in school activities. Families who are new to this country and its educational system (especially those with low English proficiency) and families with children with special health care needs may need additional support and guidance to navigate the school system.

Promoting Family Support: Adolescence—11 to 21 Years

The changes that occur in contemporary family life are particularly significant for adolescents. The decreased amount of time that many parents, extended family members, and neighbors are able to spend with adolescents leads to decreased communication, support, and supervision from adults at a critical period in their development, when children are most likely to experiment with behaviors that can have serious health consequences.

Families are better able to support young people when they receive accurate information on the physical, cognitive, social, and emotional changes that occur during adolescence. Health care professionals must be aware of the support networks for young people and should know the adults who are involved in their lives and when they should be involved in health decisions.

School is a key experience for children in middle childhood. Families can play a major supportive role by encouraging the child's educational experiences and being involved in school activities.

Young people are more likely to become healthy, fulfilled adults if their families remain actively involved and provide loving parenting, needed limits, and respect for the process of developing maturity.

Parents should be encouraged to maintain an interest in their adolescent's daily activities and concerns. Families who are stressed because of economic issues, or families who are new to this country and do not understand the schools and social institutions, can have trouble staying involved in their children's lives but should be encouraged to do so. Although adolescence is characterized by growing independence and separation from parental authority, the adolescent still needs the family's love, support, and availability. Young people are more likely to become healthy, fulfilled adults if their families remain actively involved and provide loving parenting, needed limits, and respect for the process of developing maturity. Good parent-adolescent relationships can affect the development of other social relationships, including the practice of conflict resolution skills, prosocial behaviors, intimacy skills, self-control, social confidence, and empathy.[81] (For more information on this topic, see the Promoting Child Development theme.) The more assets young people demonstrate, the fewer at-risk behaviors they display.[82]

The health care professional also can affirm the parents as ethical and behavioral role models for their adolescent and can encourage parents to communicate their expectations clearly and respectfully. For adolescents who do not have a strong connection to family or other adults, health care professionals can play a pivotal role in providing key information on health issues, screening for emotional problems, and making referrals to community resources.

This same guidance needs to be given to parents of adolescents with special health care needs. The young person's special needs create demands that affect parents, the financial status of families, and family and social relationships, including relationships with siblings, but the developmental tasks of independence and mastery must receive equal attention for healthy outcomes. A coordinated focus on these developmental tasks is the work of an interdisciplinary team that can include educators and school nurses, occupational health professionals, medical social workers, parent experts, and pediatric subspecialists. Health care professionals can help families find balance in meeting the physical and psychological needs of the adolescent with special needs and other family members while maintaining normal family routines and rituals.[83] Informal and formal support networks are key factors to supporting families with adolescents who have a chronic illness, a disability, or other risk factors. Community resources, financial support, and emotional, spiritual, and informational support help families cope and be resilient.[83]

References

1. American Academy of Pediatrics, Medical Home Initiatives for Children with Special Needs Project Advisory Committee. The medical home. *Pediatrics*. 2002;110:184-186

2. Perrin EC, American Academy of Pediatrics, Committee on Psychosocial Aspects of Child and Family Health. Technical report: coparent or second-parent adoption by same-sex parents. *Pediatrics*. 2002;109:341-344

3. American Academy of Pediatrics, Committee on Psychosocial Aspects of Child and Family Health. Coparent or second-parent adoption by same-sex parents. *Pediatrics*. 2002;109:339-340

4. Dunn AM. Culture competence and the primary care provider. *J Pediatr Health Care*. 2002;16:105-111

5. Schor EL. Family pediatrics: report of the Task Force on the Family. *Pediatrics*. 2003;111:1541-1571

6. Fields J. *America's Families and Living Arrangements. Current Population Reports*. P20-553. Washington, DC: US Census Bureau; 2003

7. Tamis-LeMonda CS, Cabrera N. *Perspectives on Father Involvement: Research and Policy*. Social Policy Report: Society for Research in Child Development; 1999;13:1-31

8. Coleman WL, Garfield C. Fathers and pediatricians: enhancing men's roles in the care and development of their children. *Pediatrics*. 2004;113:1406-1411

9. Moore T, Kotelchuck M. Predictors of urban fathers' involvement in their child's health care. *Pediatrics*. 2004;113:574-580

10. American Academy of Pediatrics. Medical evaluation of internationally adopted children for infectious diseases. In: Pickering LK, Baker CJ, Long SS, McMillan JA, eds. *Red Book: 2006 Report of the Committee on Infectious Diseases*. 26th ed. Elk Grove Village, IL: American Academy of Pediatrics; 2006:182-188

11. Borchers D, American Academy of Pediatrics, Committee on Early Childhood, Adoption, and Dependent Care. Families and adoption: the pediatrician's role in supporting communication. *Pediatrics*. 2003;112:1437-1441

12. Bass S, Shields MK, Behrman RE. Children, families, and foster care: analysis and recommendations. *Future Child*. 2004;14:4-29

13. American Academy of Pediatrics, Committee on Early Childhood, Adoption, and Dependent Care. Health care of young children in foster care. *Pediatrics*. 2002;109:536-541

14. American Academy of Pediatrics, Committee on Early Childhood and Adoption and Dependent Care. Developmental issues for young children in foster care. *Pediatrics*. 2000;106:1145-1150

15. Beeman SK, Kim HM, Bullerdick SK. Factors affecting placement of children in kinship and nonkinship foster care. *Child Youth Serv Rev*. 2000;22:37-54

16. US Department of Health and Human Services. The AFCARS Report: Preliminary FY 2005 Estimates as of September 2006 (13). Available at: www.acf.hhs.gov/programs/cb/stats_research/afcars/tar/report13.pdf. Accessed September 13, 2007

17. Rubin DM, Alessandrini EA, Feudtner C, Mandell DS, Localio AR, Hadley T. Placement stability and mental health costs for children in foster care. *Pediatrics*. 2004;113:1336-1341

18. American Academy of Pediatrics, Committee on Adolescence and Committee on Early Childhood, Adoption, and Dependent Care. Care of adolescent parents and their children. *Pediatrics*. 2001;107:429-434

19. Meadows M, Sadler LS, Reitmeyer GD. School-based support for urban adolescent mothers. *J Pediatr Health Care*. 2000;14:221-227

20. McPherson M, Arango P, Fox H, et al. A new definition of children with special health care needs. *Pediatrics*. 1998;102:137-140

21. US Department of Health and Human Services, Health Resources and Services Adminsitration, Maternal and Child Health Bureau. *The National Survey of Children With Special Health Care Needs Chartbook 2001*. Rockville, MD: US Department of Health and Human Services; 2004

22. Chevarley FM. Utilization and Expenditures for Children with Special Health Care Needs. Research Findings No. 24. Rockville, MD: Agency for Healthcare Research and Quality; 2006. Available at: www.meps.ahrq.gov/rf24/rf24.pdf. Accessed September 13, 2007

23. Williams TV, Schone EM, Archibald ND, Thompson JW. A national assessment of children with special health care needs: prevalence of special needs and use of health care services among children in the military health system. *Pediatrics*. 2004;114:384-393

24. Singer GHS, Marquis J, Powers LK, et al. A multi-site evaluation of parent to parent programs for parents of children with disabilities. *J Early Interv*. 1999;22:217-219

25. American Academy of Pediatrics, Committee on Environmental Health. Toxic effects of indoor molds. *Pediatrics*. 1998;101:712-714

26. American Academy of Pediatrics, Committee on Environmental Health. Lead exposure in children: prevention, detection, and management. *Pediatrics*. 2005;116:1036-1046

27. Jacobs DE, Clickner RP, Zhou JY, et al. The prevalence of lead-based paint hazards in U.S. housing. *Environ Health Perspect*. 2002;110:A599-A606

28. Zayas LH, Ozuah PO. Mercury use in espiritismo: a survey of botanicas. *Am J Public Health*. 1996;86:111-112

29. Halfon N, Inkelas M, Mistry R, Olson LM. Satisfaction with health care for young children. *Pediatrics*. 2004;113(6 Suppl): 1965-1972

PROMOTING
FAMILY SUPPORT

30. American Academy of Pediatrics, Committee on Children with Disabilities. Counseling families who choose complementary and alternative medicine for their child with chronic illness or disability. *Pediatrics*. 2001;107:598-601

31. Sibinga EM, Ottolini MC, Duggan AK, Wilson MH. Parent-pediatrician communication about complementary and alternative medicine use for children. *Clin Pediatr (Phila)*. 2004;43:367-373

32. Halfon N, Olson L, Inkelas M, et al. Summary statistics from the National Survey of Early Childhood Health, 2000. National Center for Health Statistics. *Vital Health Stat*. 2002;15:1-34

33. Kessler RC, Berglund P, Demler O, Jin R, Merikangas KR, Walters EE. Lifetime prevalence and age-of-onset distributions of DSM-IV disorders in the National Comorbidity Survey Replication. *Arch Gen Psychiatry*. 2005;62:593-602

34. American Psychiatric Association. *Let's Talk Facts About Depression*. Washington, DC: American Psychiatric Association; 2005. Available at: www.HealthyMinds.org/multimedia/depression.pdf. Accessed March 1, 2006

35. Beardslee WR, Versage EM, Gladstone TR. Children of affectively ill parents: a review of the past 10 years. *J Am Acad Child Adolesc Psychiatry*. 1998;37:1134-1141

36. Heneghan AM, Mercer M, DeLeone NL. Will mothers discuss parenting stress and depressive symptoms with their child's pediatrician? *Pediatrics*. 2004;113:460-467

37. Heneghan AM, Silver EJ, Bauman LJ, Westbrook LE, Stein RE. Depressive symptoms in inner-city mothers of young children: who is at risk? *Pediatrics*. 1998;102:1394-1400

38. National Research Council and Institute of Medicine, Committee on Integrating the Science of Early Childhood Development. *From Neurons to Neighborhoods: The Science of Early Childhood Development*. Shonkoff JP, Phillips DA, eds. Washington, DC: National Academy Press; 2000

39. Cox JL, Holden JM, Sagovsky R. Detection of postnatal depression. Development of the 10-item Edinburgh Postnatal Depression Scale. *Br J Psychiatry*. 1987;150:782-786

40. Greenfeld LA. *Violence by Intimates: Analysis of Data on Crimes by Current or Former Spouses, Boyfriends, and Girlfriends*: Bureau of Justice Statistics factbook. Washington, DC: US Department of Justice, Office of Justice Programs, Bureau of Justice Statistics; 1998

41. Collins KS. *Health Concerns Across a Woman's Lifespan: The Commonwealth Fund 1998 Survey of Women's Health*. New York, NY: The Commonwealth Fund; 1999

42. Kerker BD, Horwitz SM, Leventhal JM, Plichta S, Leaf PJ. Identification of violence in the home: pediatric and parental reports. *Arch Pediatr Adolesc Med*. 2000;154:457-462

43. American Academy of Pediatrics, Task Force on Violence. The role of the pediatrician in youth violence prevention in clinical practice and at the community level. *Pediatrics*. 1999;103:173-181

44. Ross SM. Risk of physical abuse to children of spouse abusing parents. *Child Abuse Negl*. 1996;20:589-598

45. Holden GW. Children exposed to domestic violence and child abuse: terminology and taxonomy. *Clin Child Fam Psychol Rev*. 2003;6:151-160

46. American Academy of Pediatrics, Committee on Child Abuse and Neglect. The role of the pediatrician in recognizing and intervening on behalf of abused women. *Pediatrics*. 1998;101:1091-1092

47. Jellinek MS, Patel BP, Froehle MC, eds. *Bright Futures in Practice: Mental Health: Practice Guide*. Volume 1. Arlington, VA: National Center for Education in Maternal and Child Health; 2002

48. Validated Abuse Assessment Tools. In: Family Violence Prevention Fund. National Consensus Guidelines on Identifying and Responding to Domestic Violence Victimization in Health Care Settings. San Francisco, CA: Family Violence Prevention Fund; 2002. Updated 2004:39-40. Available at: www.endabuse.org/programs/healthcare/files/consensus.pdf. Accessed September 13, 2007

49. Cohen GJ, American Academy of Pediatrics, Committee on Psychosocial Aspects of Child and Family Health. Helping children and families deal with divorce and separation. *Pediatrics*. 2002;110:1019-1023

50. Sammons WAH, Lewis J. Helping children survive divorce. *Contemp Pediatr*. 2001;18:103-114

51. Fine A, Large R. A Conceptual Framework for Adolescent Health. Washington, DC: Association of Maternal and Child Health Programs and the Ntioanl Network of State Adolescent Health Coordinators; 2005. Available at: http://www.amchp.org/aboutamchp/publications/conc-framework.pdf. Accessed September 11, 2006

52. Benson PL, Leffert N, Scales PC, Blyth DA. Beyond the 'village' rhetoric: creating healthy communities for children and adolescents. *Appl Dev Sci*. 1998;2:138-159

53. Brendtro LK, Brokenleg M, Van Bockern S. *Reclaiming Youth At Risk: Our Hope for the Future*. Bloomington, IN: National Education Service; 2002

54. Murphey DA, Lamonda KH, Carney JK, Duncan P. Relationships of a brief measure of youth assets to health-promoting and risk behaviors. *J Adolesc Health*. 2004;34:184-191

55. Resnick MD. Resilience and protective factors in the lives of adolescents. *J Adolesc Health*. 2000;27:1-2

56. Resnick MD. Protective factors, resiliency and healthy youth development. *Adolesc Med*. 2000;11:157-165

57. Steinberg L. Gallagher lecture. The family at adolescence: transition and transformation. *J Adolesc Health*. 2000;27:170-178

58. Neumark-Sztainer D, Hannan PJ, Story M, Croll J, Perry C. Family meal patterns: associations with sociodemographic characteristics and improved dietary intake among adolescents. *J Am Diet Assoc*. 2003;103:317-322

59. Bradley RH, Whiteside L, Mundfrom DJ, Casey PH, Kelleher KJ, Pope SK. Early indications of resilience and their relation to experiences in the home environments of low birthweight, premature children living in poverty. *Child Dev*. 1994;65:346-360

60. Quraishi AY, Mickalide AD, Cody BF. *Follow the Leader: A National Study of Safety Role Modeling Among Parents and Children*. Washington, DC: National SAFE KIDS Campaign, April 2005

61. Roberts DF, Foehr UG, Rideout VJ, Brodie M. *Kids and Media @ the New Millennium. A Kaiser Family Foundation Report*. Menlo Park, CA: Kaiser Family Foundation; 1999

62. Wright JC, Huston AC, Murphy KC, et al. The relations of early television viewing to school readiness and vocabulary of children from low-income families: the early window project. *Child Dev*. 2001;72:1347-1366

63. Garrison MM, Christakis DA. *A Teacher in the Living Room? Educational Media for Babies, Toddlers, and Preschoolers*. Menlo Park, CA: Kaiser Family Foundation; 2005. Available at: www.kff.org/entmedia/upload/7427.pdf. Accessed March 1, 2006

64. Anderson DR, Huston AC, Schmitt KL, Linebarger DL, Wright JC. Early childhood television viewing and adolescent behavior: the recontact study. *Monographs for the Society for Research in Child Development*. 2001;66:1-147

65. Willis E, Strasburger VC. Media violence. *Pediatr Clin North Am*. 1998;45:319-331

66. American Academy of Pediatrics, Committee on Public Education. Media violence. *Pediatrics*. 2001;108:1222-1226

67. Donnerstein E. The mass media: a role in injury causation and prevention. *Adolesc Med*. 1995;6:271-284

68. Huston AC, Donnerstein E, Fairchild H, et al. *Big World, Small Screen: The Role of Television in American Society*. Lincoln, NE: University of Nebraska Press; 1992

69. Strasburger VC. *Adolescents and the Media: Medical and Psychological Impact*. Thousand Oaks, CA: Sage; 1995

70. American Academy of Pediatrics, Committee on Public Education. Children, adolescents, and television. *Pediatrics*. 2001;107:423-426

71. American Academy of Pediatrics. How to help your child or adolescent resist drugs. In: Jellinek MS, Patel BP, Froehle MC, eds. Bright Futures in Practice: *Mental Health, Volume II, Toolkit*. Arlington, VA: National Center for Education in Maternal and Child Health; 2002:148

72. Koopmans JR, Boomsma DI. Familial resemblances in alcohol use: genetic or cultural transmission? *J Stud Alcohol*. 1996;57:19-28

73. US Department of Health and Human Services, Public Health Service, Expert Panel on the Content of Prenatal Care. *Caring for our Future: The Content of Prenatal Care—A Report of the Public Health Service Expert on the Content of Prenatal Care*. Washington, DC: US Department of Health and Human Services; 1989

74. MacDorman MF, Atkinson JO. Infant mortality statistics from the 1997 period linked birth/infant death data set. *Natl Vital Stat Rep*. 1999;47:1-23

75. US Preventive Services Task Force. *Counseling to Prevent Tobacco Use and Tobacco-Caused Disease: Recommendation Statement*. Rockville, MD: Agency for Healthcare Research and Quality; 2003. Available at: www.ahrq.gov/clinic/3rduspstf/tobaccoun/tobcounts.htm. Accessed September 13, 2007

76. Filiano JJ, Kinney HC. A perspective on neuropathologic findings in victims of the sudden infant death syndrome: the triple-risk model. *Biol Neonate*. 1994;65:194-197

77. American Academy of Pediatrics. *Caring for Your Baby and Young Child: Birth to Age Five*. 4th ed. Shelov SP, Hannemann RE, eds. Elk Grove Village, IL: American Academy of Pediatrics; 2004

78. Huffman LC, Nichols M. Early detection of young children's mental health problems in primary care settings. In: DelCarmen-Wiggins R, Carter A, eds. *Handbook of Infant, Toddler, and Preschool Mental Health Assessment*. New York, NY: Oxford University Press; 2004:467-490

79. Olson AL, DiBrigida LA. Depressive symptoms and work role satisfaction in mothers of toddlers. *Pediatrics*. 1994;94:363-367

80. Lanzi RG, Pascoe JM, Keltner B, Ramey SL. Correlates of maternal depressive symptoms in a national Head Start program sample. *Arch Pediatr Adolesc Med*. 1999;153:801-807

81. Hair EC, Jager J, Garrett SB. *Helping Teens Develop Healthy Social Skills and Relationships: What the Research Shows About Navigating Adolescence*. Washington, DC: Child Trends; 2002. Available at: http://www.childtrends.org/PDF/K3_Brief.pdf. Accessed September 13, 2007

82. Scales PP, Leffert N, Lerner RM. *Developmental Assets: A Synthesis of the Scientific Research on Adolescent Development*. Minneapolis, MN: Search Institute; 1999

83. Patterson JJ, Blum RW. Risk and resilience among children and youth with disabilities. *Arch Pediatr Adolesc Med*. 1996;150:692-698

PROMOTING
FAMILY SUPPORT

Promoting Child Development

Theme 2

INTRODUCTION

Any health supervision encounter with children involves promoting healthy child development. Understanding child development and the application of its principles sets the care of children apart from that of adults. Infants must grow to be children, then adolescents, and then adults. Health promotion to ensure physical, cognitive, and social emotional health as well as to protect the child from infectious diseases and injuries (intentional and unintentional) supports the healthy development of the child. Successful health promotion efforts should take into account the developmental reality of the child now, as well as her developmental expectations for the next months and her developmental potential for growth over time.

Encouraging development of the growing child recognizes the wonder of brain development with its concurrent increases in volume, size, and synapse formation. Physical growth to support brain development is essential. Even more important are the influences of stimulation, social interactivity, family, culture, and community.

The development of the infant, child, or youth with special health care needs is addressed in separate sections within this theme. Even a child whose brain growth and function have been impaired by injury or early neglect has a developmental potential that must be discerned and supported to achieve the best possible outcome for that child.

Monitoring Child and Adolescent Development

Developmental surveillance and screening of children and adolescents are integral components of health care supervision. Surveillance of children and adolescents is a continuous and cumulative process that is used to ensure optimal health outcomes. For example, it is essential in identifying and treating children with developmental and behavioral problems. Early identification of children with developmental delay is critical for diagnosing and providing early therapeutic interventions.[1] The parents' report of current skills can accurately identify developmental delay, even though they may not

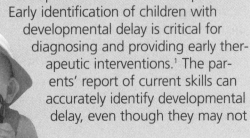

Long-term outcomes for all infants are improved when health care professionals emphasize the abilities of the infant and facilitate opportunities for the parents to have early physical contact through breastfeeding, rooming-in, holding skin-to-skin, and cuddling the infant.

recognize it as such. Standardized developmental parent-completed questionnaires make it easier for health care professionals to systematically elicit information that is reliable and valid.[1] During all encounters, health care professionals also must listen carefully to parental concerns and observations about a child's development.[2]

Comprehensive child development surveillance includes:

- Eliciting and attending to the parents' concerns
- Maintaining a developmental history
- Making accurate and informed observations of the child
- Identifying the presence of risk and protective factors
- Periodically using screening tests
- Documenting the process and findings

In monitoring development during infancy and early childhood, ongoing surveillance is supplemented and strengthened by standardized developmental screening tests that are used at certain visits (9 months, 18 months, and $2\frac{1}{2}$ years) and at other times at which concerns are identified.[1] Currently, no comprehensive developmental screening tests exist for use during the middle childhood or adolescent visits. However, several tools have been developed that are useful in screening for particular problems. For example, the Pediatric Symptom Checklist is a psychosocial screen that can be used to identify cognitive, emotional, and behavioral problems.[3] The CRAFFT is a 6-item tool that can be used to screen specifically for drug and alcohol use.[4]

Promoting Child Development: Infancy— Birth to 11 Months
The first year of life is a period of neural plasticity and rapid adjustment to stimuli that allow the infant's brain to develop to its maximum potential or not, depending on his experiences.[5]

Long-term outcomes for all infants are improved when health care professionals emphasize the abilities of the infant and facilitate opportunities for the parents to have early physical contact through breastfeeding, rooming-in, holding skin-to-skin, and cuddling the infant.[6,7]

Developmentally focused anticipatory guidance should include information on growth and development, talking and reading aloud, safety related to the child's developmental abilities and physical capabilities, sudden infant death syndrome (SIDS), coping with the stressors that make infants vulnerable to abuse (eg, infant crying and maternal postpartum depression), and parenting an infant with special or developmental health care needs. Cultural considerations influence parental perspectives about infant temperament and the parental or caregiver role in supporting the infant's self-regulation. The health care professional must try to understand the complex interrelationship of the family's beliefs, values, and behaviors, which affect how a family protects, teaches, and socializes an infant. Parents' perspectives about the needs of their children and whether they view the infant's behaviors as normal or typical for the child's age are equally important considerations. Because families vary in their responses and behaviors, the health care professional must learn about these customs and seek to understand parents' responses and behaviors, even if they differ from those expected in the community context.

Infants With Special Health Care Needs

Most infants are born healthy, but some are born early or at a low birth weight, or have special health care needs. Parents and other caregivers of an infant with special health care needs will need support and guidance in nurturing the infant and fostering family cohesion. Anticipatory guidance should be structured around the parents' goals and expectations. Specific guidance can include information on growth and development, feeding concerns, specialized health and developmental care needs for the infant, expectations for achieving developmental milestones, and any specific vulnerability that the family will need to know. The health care professional should explore with families their understanding of their infant's health condition, its impact on the family, their expectations on issues such as family supports and care coordination, and their hopes for the child. Additionally, many families may need assistance with referrals, financial assistance, and other types of supports.

The health care professional plays an important role in identifying conditions that place the infant at risk of disability and warrant immediate referral to early intervention services (Box 1). Health care professionals should note those children who require close developmental surveillance and periodic standardized developmental screening to permit the earliest identification of their need for intervention services due to other risk factors. The health care professional also plays an important and continuing role in providing informed clinical opinion in determining the child's eligibility and the scope of services that are needed by the child and family. Care coordination of screening services and follow-up in the context of the medical home are important. Professionals should, however, be aware that some families may not view early intervention as positive (eg, they may see efforts to screen and evaluate as efforts to stigmatize their child, or they may belong to a culture or religion in which differences are tolerated and accepted and are not "fixed").

Developmental surveillance, screening, and observations are important in all aspects of the child's growth and development. Formal developmental evaluation is indicated if any signs of developmental delay exist, if the parents express concern or questions about their child's development, or if the child is at risk of developmental challenges because of factors such as prematurity or prenatal exposure to alcohol, drugs, or other toxins. Many parents are aware of developmental delays or irregularities before they are told about them by a health care professional. Their concerns must be promptly responded to and appropriate evaluation must be initiated. This evaluation might begin in the primary care office or might result in an immediate referral to an early intervention program or developmental specialist.

Domains of Development

During a child's life, the most dramatic growth—physical, motor, cognitive, communicative, and social-emotional—occurs during infancy. By 1 year of age, the infant has

> **BOX 1**
>
> **Program for Infants and Toddlers with Disabilities (Part C of Individuals with Disabilities Education Act)**
>
> Children from birth to age 3 years who exhibit delays in development or are at risk are eligible under federal law for early intervention services that will foster age-appropriate development. The Program for Infants and Toddlers with Disabilities (Part C of the Individuals with Disabilities Education Act [IDEA]) assists states in operating a comprehensive, statewide program of early intervention services for infants and toddlers with disabilities, from birth through age 3 years, and their families.[8] Eligibility criteria can be found at http://www.nectac.org/topics/earlyid/partcelig.asp. A diagnosis is not necessary for enrollment in early intervention programs. Children can be on waiting lists for an evaluation while receiving services. Children from the age of 3 years to school age also are eligible for early intervention through the educational system or through developmental services.

The health care professional plays an important role in identifying conditions that place the infant at risk of disability and warrant immediate referral to early intervention services.

nearly tripled his birth weight, added almost 50% to his length, and achieved most of his brain weight. By 8 months of age, brain synapses have increased from 50 trillion to 1,000 trillion, and remain there through early childhood.[9] During the remainder of childhood and adolescence, the brain is actively engaged in developing and refining the efficiency of its neural networks, especially in the prefrontal cortex, the critical brain region responsible for decision making, judgment, and impulse control. This dynamic process of neuronal maturation continues into early adulthood.[10]

Outcomes for infants who are prenatally exposed to toxins (eg, alcohol, lead, and illicit drugs) are largely determined not by the degree of exposure but by the quality of the nurturing environment.[5] Studies on early brain development confirm the importance of positive early experiences in the formation of brain cell connections. These early experiences, especially parent-child interactions, have a significant impact on a child's emotional development and learning abilities.

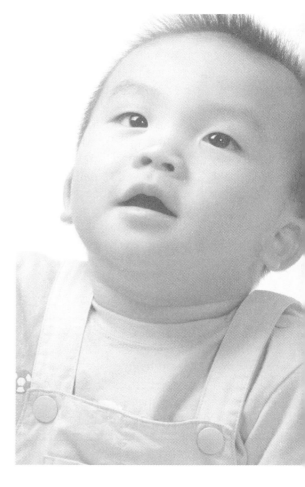

> When parents provide consistent and predictable daily routines, the infant learns to anticipate and trust his environment.

GROSS MOTOR SKILLS

From birth to the end of the first year of life, major changes occur in the infant's gross motor skills. As tone, strength, and coordination improve sequentially from head to heel, the infant attains head control, rolls, sits, crawls, pulls to stand, cruises, and may even walk by 1 year of age. Delays in gross motor milestones, asymmetry of movement, or muscle hypertonia or hypotonia should be identified and evaluated for early intervention referrals. Within the framework of back-to-sleep guidelines,[11] it is important to promote age-appropriate and safe opportunities for tummy-time play to allow young infants to master their early motor skills.

FINE MOTOR SKILLS

Hand-eye coordination and fine motor skills also change dramatically during infancy. These abilities progress from reflexive grasping to voluntary grasp and release, midline play, transferring an object from one hand to the other, shaping the hand to an object, inferior then superior pincer grasp, using the fingers to point, self-feeding, and even marking with a crayon by 1 year of age. Babies should be given opportunities to play with toys and food to advance their fine motor skills.

COGNITIVE, LINGUISTIC, AND COMMUNICATION SKILLS

Environmental factors influence the infant's developing brain significantly during the first year of life. When parents provide consistent and predictable daily routines, the infant learns to anticipate and trust his environment. An infant's brain development is affected by daily experiences with parents and other caregivers during feeding, play, consoling, and sleep routines.[12]

At birth, newborns already hear as well as adults do, but their responses can be difficult for parents to understand. Newborns should have a screening test for hearing before discharge from the hospital, or should be screened before 1 month of age if not born in a hospital. Thereafter, hearing should be screened regularly and whenever parents express concern about hearing and/or language development. Newborns can recognize their parents' voices at birth. By 3 days of age, they can distinguish their mother's voice.

Newborns also have color vision, can see in 3 dimensions, and can track visually. Close up, they show a preference for the pattern of human faces. Visual acuity progresses rapidly from newborn hyperopia to adult levels of 20/20 vision when the child is 5 to 6 years of age. Newborns copy facial expressions from birth, use the emotional expressions of others to interpret events, and understand and use gestures by 8 months of age. By 8 weeks, babies coo; by 6 to 8 months, they begin to babble with vowel-consonant combinations; and by 1 year, they usually speak a few single words. The normal range for the acquisition of these pre-linguistic skills is broad. Beyond babbling, progress depends in part on the language stimulation a child receives. Children who are talked to and read to frequently by loving parents or caregivers have nearly 300 words at age 2 years, a higher number than often acquired by those who have not had this stimulation.

Reading is important for all children, including infants. Health care professionals should educate parents about how to read to infants, the importance of language stimulation, including singing songs to infants and children, reading to them, and talking to them. They also need to understand the transition from the parent talking about pictures in a book to engaging the child in reciprocally talking and pointing to pictures in a book.

Health care professionals also should identify feeding issues related to oromotor function and coordination because these are integral to early pre-linguistic and later communication skills. Special discussions could be used with parents who are unable to communicate verbally or who have a child with special communication needs (such as a child with a hearing loss) to help the parents support normal language development in their children. Exposure to live language has been shown to have a positive impact on early child development, whereas television screen exposure increasingly shows adverse effects.[13,14]

Children who live in print-rich environments and who are read to during the first years of life are more likely to learn to read on schedule than children who are not exposed in this way.[15] Giving an age- and culturally appropriate book to the child, along with anticipatory guidance to the parent about reading aloud, at each health supervision visit from 6 months to 5 years, has been shown to improve the home environment and the child's language development, especially in children at socioeconomic risk.[16-21] Parents should make reading with their children part of the daily routine. Reading together in the evening can become an important part of the bedtime ritual beginning in infancy and continuing for years. Books and reading encourage development in multiple domains and are especially important for cognitive and linguistic development.[17-19] Book-handling skills in young children also reflect fine motor skills, and parent-child reading promotes social and emotional development as well. Reading to a young child is often a source of great warmth and good memories for parents and children alike. Parents can use books in various ways, and health care professionals can emphasize to parents with low or no literacy skills that having conversations with their young children about the pictures in books (ie, interactive

PROMOTING CHILD DEVELOPMENT

Health care professionals should educate parents about how to read to infants, the importance of language stimulation, including singing songs to infants and children, reading to them, and talking to them.

reading) also is an important way to encourage language development (Box 2).

> ## BOX 2
> ### Promoting Literacy
> To help parents promote healthy language and cognitive development in young children, *Bright Futures* recommends anticipatory guidance on reading aloud at every health supervision visit from 6 months to 5 years and encourages giving a book at these visits, whenever possible, especially for children at socioeconomic risk.
>
> Many organizations make books available at low or no cost for distribution. For example, Reach Out and Read (http://www.reachoutandread.org) is a national nonprofit organization that promotes early literacy by making books a routine part of pediatric primary care so that children grow up with books and a love of reading.[18,19] Information on trainings, technical assistance, and start-up funding for these books is available for practices or clinics that are interested in implementing a Reach Out and Read program.

SOCIAL-EMOTIONAL SKILLS

As parents learn to recognize their infant's behavior cues for engagement and disengagement or distress, and consistently respond appropriately to their infant's needs (eg, being fed when hungry or comforted when crying), babies learn to trust and love their parents.

Children with special health care needs may not exhibit the same responses as other children. This difficulty can cause parents to feel inadequate because they cannot discern their child's needs. Helping a family recognize even the small gains their child is making provides support to the family and acknowledges the progress and growth in their child with special needs.

By 3 months of age, infants may interact differently with different people. At about 8 months, an infant shows social referencing, looking to his parents in ambiguous or unfamiliar situations to figure out how to respond. At about the same age, his capacity to discriminate between familiar and unfamiliar people shows itself as stranger anxiety. By 14 months, he develops enough assurance and communication ability to contain his stranger anxiety and deal successfully with a new person. During the first year, the infant's social awareness advances from a tendency to cry when he hears crying, to attempts to offer food, initiate games, and even take turns by 1 year. As autonomy emerges, babies may begin to bite, pinch, and grab what they want. Health care professionals should tell parents to anticipate these infant behaviors and advise on consistent, appropriate (firm but gentle) responses to redirect the infant's behavior.

Different cultures may have various expectations about the age at which children will achieve socially mediated milestones. It is, therefore, important to ask not only what the child can do but also what the family expects and allows.

Separation Anxiety

Parents need to know that infants as young as 4 to 5 months of age may be anxious, when they are separated from their parents, to meet strangers or even familiar relatives. Even grandparents need to allow the infant to warm up to them before taking the infant from the mother. This anxiety peaks at about 8 months. This is not a rejection but a normal developmental phase.

Providing time for the infant to get to know a new caregiver in the presence of the mother, before separation, is critically important. There must be consistency in this relationship. Transitions will be easier if a child is encouraged to have a special stuffed animal, blanket, or similar favorite object, which she holds on to as an important companion.

As parents learn to recognize their infant's behavior cues for engagement and disengagement or distress, and consistently respond appropriately to their infant's needs (eg, being fed when hungry or comforted when crying), babies learn to trust and love their parents.

Young children use this *transitional object* to comfort them. Transition is often as difficult for the parent as it is for the child. If the parent is going back to work or school and using child care on a consistent basis, the parent often feels a combination of intense longing for the child, intense guilt, and jealousy. The mother is frequently afraid the infant will love the caregiver more than she loves the mother. Parents need to be reassured that they will remain the most important people to their infant's happiness, well-being, and health. The infant may have intense emotions, including crying and irritability, that are saved for times when she is within the safe embrace of her mother. These expressions reflect the intensity of attachment to the mother. Guidance for both the child and parent may be needed to ease transitions and promote healthy adaptations.

Child Care

In recent decades, interest in child care issues has increased as a growing number of women have entered the labor force and as child care arrangements have reflected the changing needs and interests of contemporary American families.[22] Regardless of the location or person providing care, young children benefit when they receive high-quality care. Care that fosters children's healthy development should be offered by caregivers who relate consistently to the children; who are available, physically and emotionally, to respond to each child's needs and interests; and who provide care in a clean, safe, nurturing, and stimulating environment. The fewer children cared for by each provider, the better the situation is for the child. Infant care should have no more than 3 children per provider. Parents should ask whether their child care centers adhere to national standards and are accredited by organizations such as the National Association for the Education of Young Children (www.naeyc.org).[23]

Developmental Highlights of Infancy

THE INFLUENCE OF CULTURE ON DEVELOPMENT

Health care professionals should understand that what are often considered "milestones" are less "stones" than "markers," and that these markers shift according to upbringing. The timing for acquisition of any developmental task is determined by surveying many infants to determine the range of accomplishment dates. The populations surveyed are typically the population of convenience. So "milestones" must be understood as *normed to a population*. (However, it is important to note that children are still held to the same standards once they reach kindergarten. Therefore, once a child reaches preschool age, developmental differences should be viewed in light of overall population means.) Table 1 presents examples of milestones that are reached at different ages for different ethnic groups.

TABLE 1			
Developmental Milestones by Age and Ethnicity, Months[24]			
Task	**Anglo**	**Puerto Rican**	**Filipino**
Eat solid food	8.2	10.	16.7
Use training cup	12.0	17.1	21.9
Use utensils	17.7	26.5	32.4
Eat finger foods	8.9	9.4	9.5
Wean	16.8	18.2	36.2
Sleep by self	13.8	14.6	38.8
Sleep all night	11.4	14.5	32.4
Choose clothes	31.1	44.2	33.1
Dress self	38.2	44.2	39.2
Play alone	25.0	24.8	12.3
Toilet trained (day)	31.6	29.0	20.4
Toilet trained (night)	33.2	31.8	34.2

Helping parents understand their infant's temperament and their own can help them respond effectively to their infant.

SELF-REGULATION

Infants generally are born with unstable physiologic functions. With maturation and sensitive caregiving, physiologic stability, temperature regulation, sustained suck, coordinated suck, swallow, breath sequences, and consistent sleep-wake cycles will improve. During the first year, the infant's ability to self-regulate (eg, transition from awake to sleep) and modulate his behavior in response to stress are influenced by the environment, particularly by the consistency and predictability of the caregivers. The consistency and predictability of infant feedings and encouragement for regular sleep helps establish an infant's diurnal pattern of waking and sleeping. The infant also develops ways to calm himself and expands his ability to selectively focus on a particular activity. Large individual differences exist in self-regulatory abilities. Infants who are born with special health care needs, such as those who are of low birth weight or small for gestational age, or those born to mothers with diabetes or who abused drugs or alcohol during pregnancy, are at particular risk of problems with self-regulation.

A major component of infant health supervision consists of counseling parents about their infant's temperament, colic, temper tantrums, and sleep disturbances. The "goodness of fit" between parents and infant can influence their interaction. Helping parents understand their infant's temperament and their own can help them respond effectively to their infant.

Crying is stressful for families and frustrating for parents. Health care professionals will want to help parents discover calming techniques and understand that a certain amount of crying is inevitable. Parents should consider who they can ask for help if they are having trouble coping or if they fear they might harm their baby.

SLEEP

Parents need guidance on differentiating between active and quiet sleep because they may assume their infant is getting adequate sleep when taken to the mall, taken to a party, or left in a carrier or swing all day. During these times, infants are more apt to be in active sleep. Active sleep alone is not adequate for appropriate rest and often results in a fussy baby. Health care professionals should help parents understand their infant's need for a consistent, predictable, quiet sleep location, including for nap time. Table 2 presents the key characteristics of various infant states. Table 3 lists typical infant sleep patterns.

SUDDEN INFANT DEATH SYNDROME

Sudden infant death syndrome is the sudden, unexplained death of an infant younger than 1 year. Most SIDS-related deaths occur between the ages of 2 and 4 months.[25] Numerous studies have identified the following independent risk factors for SIDS:

- Young maternal age
- Maternal smoking during pregnancy (mothers who smoke have an approximately fivefold increase in SIDS risk for their infants)
- Exposure to secondhand cigarette smoke
- Inadequate prenatal care
- Low birth weight or premature birth
- Prone sleep position for infant
- Infant sleeping on a soft surface
- Bed sharing (infant sleeping with parent or other adult)
- An overheated infant
- Male gender

Three of these risk factors are under parental control during infancy: (1) avoidance of cigarette smoke, (2) where the child sleeps and on what type of surface, and (3) in what position he sleeps.

TABLE 2
Key Characteristics of Various Infant States[26]

Infant States	Characteristics
Quiet sleep	Very difficult to awaken; regular respirations; little movements; may startle
Active sleep	May awaken and go back to sleep; body movements, eyelid movements; irregular respirations
Drowsy	Increasing body movements, eyelid opening; more easily awakened for a feeding but may return to sleep with comforting
Alert	Alert expression, open eyes, surveys surroundings, especially faces; optimum state for feedings
Active alert	Beginning to fuss and show need for a change; if needs are not met, escalates to crying
Crying	Crying that lasts for more than 20 seconds; usually infant can be comforted with holding, feeding, or diaper change; exploring the duration, intensity, and frequency of crying is needed to determine strategies for interventions

TABLE 3
Typical Infant Sleep Patterns and Sleep Location[26-28]

Activities	Birth to 3 Months	3 to 6 Months	6 to 9 Months	9 to 12 Months	12 to 18 Months	18 to 48 Months
Average sleep in 24 h	14 h	13 h	13 h	13 h	12-13 h	12-13 h
Range of sleep in 24 h	12-16 h	12-15 h	10-14 h	10-14 h	12-14 h	12-14 h
Night awakenings	Depends on feeding routine	2-3	1-3	1-2	0-1	0
Number of naps	Depends on feeding routine	2-4 naps/d (am/pm)	2 naps/d (am/pm)	1-2 naps/d (am/pm)	1-2 naps/d	1 nap/d
Length of naps	1-3 h	2-3 h each	1-3 h each	1-3 h each	1-3 h each	1-2 h each
Sleep location	Bassinette or crib in parents' room	Bassinette or crib in parents' room	Crib	Crib	Crib	2-3 y in own bed

PROMOTING CHILD DEVELOPMENT

Personal experience and beliefs significantly influence a family's acceptance of specific messages regarding infant sleep position and sleep location.

Room Sharing and Bed Sharing

Parent and infant sleeping practices are influenced by custom and family traditions,[29,30] and these sleep patterns often are among the last traditions to change in immigrant and minority families.

Room sharing, defined as an infant sleeping in the parents' room in a separate sleep space, is a common practice in many cultures worldwide. In many cultures, sharing a room is viewed as a part of the parents' overall commitment to their children's well-being. African American families, for example, view sharing a room as normal, unrelated to perceived infant sleep problems, attachment concerns, breastfeeding, or household crowding.[31] White parents who share a room with their infants, in contrast, more frequently cite infant sleep problems as the reason for this practice. Increasing evidence shows that room sharing is associated with a reduced risk of SIDS.

Sleep practices in which parents and infants share a bed also are common in many cultures. Bed sharing can take the form of mother, father, and baby together in the same bed, to mother and baby together with father sleeping elsewhere, to all family members in the same bed. Advocates of this practice cite its importance in facilitating breastfeeding, promoting parent-infant attachment, and allowing parents to quickly comfort a fussy infant. Opponents express concerns about safety and that bed sharing promotes an unhealthy attachment between the parent and child and can impede the child's progress toward independence.

A review of the dangers associated with placing children younger than 2 years in adult beds include overlying by a parent, sibling, or other adult sharing the bed; wedging or entrapment of the child between the mattress and another object; head entrapment in bed railings; and suffocation on water beds or because of clothing or bedding causing oronasal obstruction.[27,32,33] The issue of parents lying on the infant has received extensive study.[30]

Sleep Position

Despite the recommendation of supine sleep position for infants, approximately 17% of babies continue to be placed in the prone position for sleep.[34] Prone sleep position is used more often by African American families and in child care settings; it is a contributing factor to the disparate SIDS rates. Side lying, an alternative sleep position that is practiced by many families who are concerned about using the prone position, carries a twofold higher risk for SIDS because of the significant probability that the infant will roll from the side position to the prone position during sleep.

Infants who are accustomed to sleeping supine who are placed in the prone position or on their side to sleep are at higher risk for sudden infant death than infants who usually sleep in the prone or side position.[35] The risk of death due to SIDS is 7 to 8 times higher for infants who are put to sleep on their side or in the prone position if they typically are placed in a supine position for sleep.[35]

Reducing Sudden Infant Death Syndrome Risks

Personal experience and beliefs significantly influence a family's acceptance of specific messages regarding infant sleep position and sleep location.[36,37] The health care professional should learn the family's views about infant sleep, room sharing, and bed sharing to appropriately tailor SIDS prevention and risk reduction counseling. The American Academy of Pediatrics (AAP) Task Force on Infant Sleep Position and Sudden Infant Death Syndrome reviewed the evidence and compiled the following recommendations to reduce the risk of SIDS[11]:

- Supine sleep position is safest for every sleep; side sleeping is not advised.
- Use a firm sleep surface.
- Avoid placing soft objects and loose bedding in cribs, bassinets, and playpens.
- Do not smoke during pregnancy.
- Do not allow smoking in the child's environment.
- A separate but nearby sleep environment is safest for the infant.
- Avoid overheating the infant; do not over bundle the infant or set the room temperature too high.
- Use of home monitors does not prevent SIDS.

- Parents or other caregivers should not share a bed with the infant if they smoke or are using drugs or alcohol or taking medications that cause drowsiness or fatigue or induce a deep sleep.
- Parents and caregivers should not sleep with their infant on a sofa, couch, or water bed.

DISCIPLINE, BEHAVIORAL GUIDANCE, AND TEACHING

The interaction between the parents and their infant is central to the infant's physical, cognitive, social, and emotional development, as well as her self-regulation abilities. The infant brings her temperament style, physical attentiveness, health, and vigor to this interaction.

Parents need to understand the differences among discipline, teaching, and punishment so that they can introduce appropriate measures for correcting and guiding their infant's behavior.

DEVELOPMENTAL MILESTONES AT A GLANCE — INFANCY[38]				
Age	Gross Motor	Fine Motor	Cognitive, Linguistic, and Communication	Social-Emotional
2 Months	Head up 45° / Lift head	Follow past midline / Follow to midline	Laugh / Vocalize	Smile spontaneously / Smile responsively
4 Months	Roll over / Sit—head steady	Follow to 180° / Grasp rattle	Turn to rattling sound / Laugh	Regard own hand
6 Months	Sit—no support / Roll over	Look for dropped yarn / Reach	Turn to voice / Turn to rattling sound	Feed self / Work for toy (out of reach)
9 Months	Pull to stand / Stand holding on	Take 2 cubes / Pass cube (transfer)	Dada/Mama, nonspecific / Single syllables	Wave bye-bye / Feed self

KEY
Black Color: 50% to 90% of children pass this item.
Green Color: More than 90% of children pass this item.

These norms are taken from the DENVER II, and are based upon the administration and interpretation as set forth in the DENVER II Training Manual (copyright 1992).

These milestones are provided as a reference only. Reference to these milestones does not take the place of a standardized measurement of healthy child development or discourage a developmental discussion with a health care provider.

PROMOTING CHILD DEVELOPMENT

Parental concerns are highly accurate markers for developmental disability, and it is essential for the health care professional to be sensitive to these concerns.

Parents need to understand the differences among discipline, teaching, and punishment so that they can introduce appropriate measures for correcting and guiding their infant's behavior. It is important to discuss distraction as a developmentally appropriate discipline for infants. It also may be beneficial to discuss strategies to prevent the need for disciplinary measures by avoiding overtiredness through consistent daily routines for feeding and sleep and by providing a developmentally appropriate safe home environment.

Parents' ability to respond appropriately to their child's behavior is determined by their own life stresses, their past experiences with other children, their knowledge, their temperament, their own experiences of being nurtured in childhood, and other responsibilities, such as other children in the household, work, and daily household tasks. Their perceptions of the infant also can influence the interaction. These perceptions come from their own expectations, needs, and desires, as well as from the reaction of other people to the child.

The infant's emotions also can be affected by the emotional health of the caregivers. Depression is common in many mothers of infants and can seriously impair the baby's emotional and even physical well-being. Babies of depressed mothers show delays in growth and development, diminished responsiveness to facial expressions, reduced play and exploratory behaviors, and decreased motor skills.[39-41] Parental substance abuse can have similar negative effects. Health supervision for the child must include monitoring the emotional health of the parents or primary caregivers. The health care professional should recognize and provide assistance if parents demonstrate or acknowledge their difficulty in responding to their infant's needs.

Promoting Child Development: Early Childhood—1 to 4 Years

At the beginning of this developmental period, a child's understanding of the world, people, and objects is bound by what he can see, hear, feel, and manipulate physically. By the end of early childhood, the process of thinking moves beyond the "here and now" to incorporate the use of mental symbols and the development of fantasy. For the infant, mobility is a goal to be mastered. For the active young child, it is a mechanism for exploration and increasing independence. The 1-year-old child is beginning to use the art of imitation in her repetition of familiar sounds and physical gestures. The 4-year-old child has mastered most of the complex rules of the languages that are spoken in the home and can communicate thoughts and ideas effectively.

The toddler is beginning to develop a sense of himself as separate from his parents or primary caregivers. By the end of early childhood, the well-adjusted child, having internalized the security of early bonds, pursues new relationships outside of the family as an individual in his own right. Understanding and respecting this evolving independence is a common parental challenge.

Young Children With Special Health Care Needs

Health care professionals who take care of children between the ages of 1 and 4 years have a responsibility to diagnose special health care needs. Because children in this age group grow and progress rapidly, parents anticipate and analyze how their child is reaching developmental milestones such as walking, talking, and socializing. When parents express concerns about how their child is developing, the health care professional should listen and observe carefully. A "wait and see" attitude will not suffice, particularly if the child falls into an at-risk group. A proactive approach is essential.

Several tools are available for identifying a child with special health care needs. Parental concerns are highly accurate markers for developmental disability, and it is essential for the health care professional to be sensitive to these concerns. If developmental delay or disability is suspected, a referral should be made to an appropriate early intervention program or developmental specialist for evaluation. If significant developmental delay or disability is confirmed, the child should be referred to an early intervention program that is matched to the child's and family's needs. With the appropriate services in place, the primary health care professional provides a medical home for the child and, in partnership with the family, assists with ongoing care planning, monitoring, and management across agencies and professionals. The primary care practice team carries out these activities by providing care coordination services. Complicating factors, such as family finances, access to resources, parental health and well-being, and sibling issues, also should be considered. Families whose young children have special health care needs usually find that referrals to parent-to-parent support programs are helpful. (For more information on this topic, see the Promoting Community Relationships and Resources theme.)

Domains of Development

GROSS AND FINE MOTOR SKILLS
The physical abilities of children in the 1- to 4-year age range vary considerably. Some are endowed with natural grace and agility; others demonstrate less fine-tuning in their physical prowess, yet they "get the job done." As a fearless and tireless explorer and experimenter, the toddler is vulnerable to injury, but appropriate adult supervision and a physically safe environment provide the child with the freedom to take controlled risks.

Many children do not live in safe environments. Parents may try to provide a safe environment within the confines of their own dwelling, but the immediate community may be characterized by violence, substandard housing conditions, overcrowding, or residence in a shelter. Health care professionals who are aware of these circumstances can better support parents' efforts to find developmentally appropriate surroundings and experiences that allow their children to safely develop their motor skills.

COGNITIVE, LINGUISTIC, AND COMMUNICATION SKILLS
Young children learn through play. If the toddler experienced nurturing and attachment during infancy, she now has a strong base from which to explore the world. The self-centered focus of the young child is related less to a sense of selfishness than to a cognitive inability to see things from the perspective of others. The child's growth in understanding the world around her is evidenced by her linguistic development (ie, by her capacity for naming and remembering the objects that surround her and her ability to communicate her wishes and feelings to important others).

Young children live largely in a world of magic; they often have difficulty differentiating what is real from what is make-believe. Such fantasies, unless scary to the child, are to be expected and encouraged at this stage of development. Some children have imaginary friends. Many children engage in elaborate fantasy play. Learning to identify the boundaries between fantasy and reality and developing an elementary ability to think logically are 2 of the most important developmental tasks of this age.

Parents and other caregivers need to provide a safe environment for these young learners to explore. Children need access to a variety of tools (books and toys) and experiences. They need opportunities to learn through trial and error, as well as through planned effort. Their seemingly endless string

Their seemingly endless string of repetitive questions can test the limits of the most patient parents. These queries, however, must be acknowledged and responded to in a manner that not only provides answers but also validates and reinforces the child's curiosity.

of repetitive questions can test the limits of the most patient parents. These queries, however, must be acknowledged and responded to in a manner that not only provides answers but also validates and reinforces the child's curiosity.

The development of language and communication during the early childhood years is of central importance to the child's later growth in social, cognitive, and academic domains. Communication is built upon interaction and relationships. The greater the nurturing and the stronger the connection between parents and child, the greater the child's motivation to communicate will be, first with gestures and then with spoken language. Interactive play and reading are wonderful forums for language enhancement.

Language

Language development usually is described in 3 separate categories: (1) speech (ie, the ability to produce sound, a concept that encompasses rhythm, fluency, and articulation); (2) expressive language (ie, the ability to convey information, feelings, thoughts, and ideas through verbal and other means, including facial expressions, hand gestures, and writing); and (3) receptive language (ie, the ability to understand what one hears and sees). Children can have problems in one area but not in another. Exposure to books and reading aloud during the time that precedes the formal teaching and learning of reading is central to language development. Typical expressive and receptive language acquisitions in the early years include the following:

Exposure to books and reading aloud during the time that precedes the formal teaching and learning of reading is central to language development.

- **Between the ages of 12 and 18 months,** children make the leap from sound imitation and babbling to the acquisition of a few meaningful words (eg, Dada, Mama, mine, shoe). Through repeated use, these first words teach them how words are used in communication. At the same time that the child gains expressive language, he also shows increased comprehension of simple commands (eg, "say bye-bye") and the names of familiar people and objects. Toddlers expand their communicative repertoire through a variety of gestures (eg, pointing, waving, and playing "pat-a-cake") with and without vocalizations. The child's demonstration of "communicative intent" or proto-declarative pointing (ie, pointing to a desired object and watching to see whether the parent sees it) is an indication of normal social and language development. The absence of pointing and establishing joint attention is a red flag and merits screening for autistic spectrum disorder. At about 18 months of age, most toddlers have begun a word-learning explosion, acquiring an understanding, on average, of 9 new words every day. This pattern continues throughout the preschool years.
- **Between the ages of 18 months and 2 years,** children recognize many nouns and understand simple questions. By the age of 2 years, the expressive language of most children includes 2-word phrases, especially noun-verb combinations that indicate actions desired or observed (eg, "drink juice," "Mommy give").
- **Between the ages of 2 and 3 years,** children usually are speaking in sentences of at least 4 to 5 words. They are able to tell stories and use "what" and "where" questions. They have absorbed the rules for regular plural word forms and for the use of past tense. Their

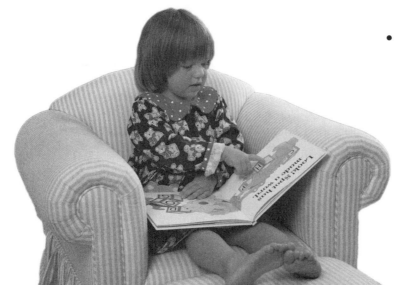

speech can still be difficult for a non-family member to understand, but it becomes increasingly clear after 3 years of age. A good rule of thumb for normal development is that 75% to 80% of a 3-year-old's speech should be intelligible to a stranger.

- **Between the ages of 3 and 4 years,** children are learning fundamental grammar rules. They have a vocabulary that exceeds 1,000 words, and their pronunciation should be generally understandable. They frequently ask "why" and "how" questions. Their exuberant use of language in play and social interaction often suggests a process of "thinking out loud."

Parents may ask health care professionals about the effects of being raised in a bilingual home. They can be reassured that this situation permits the child to learn both languages simultaneously as though each language was the mother tongue. If the child is experiencing language delays, however, a consistent language that is spoken by all caregivers may be preferred.

Many aspects of language development seem to be robust in that they develop normally despite environmental conditions. Certain aspects, notably vocabulary and language usage, however, depend heavily on the family and early school experiences if the child is to become proficient.[5] Thus, the young child who is exposed to an everyday environment that is rich in language through stories, word games, rhymes and songs, questions and conversation in the family and during play, and books will be well prepared for the language-laden world of school. (For more information on this topic, see the Literacy section of this theme.)

Often, hearing loss is first identified as a language delay. If hearing impairment or language delay is a concern, an audiological evaluation is recommended and a referral should be made to early intervention services to optimize language development.

SOCIAL-EMOTIONAL SKILLS
Temperament and Individual Differences
The temperamental differences that were manifested in the feeding, sleeping, and self-regulatory behaviors of the infant are transformed into the varied styles of coping and adaptation by the young child. Some young children appear to think before they act, whereas others are impetuous. Some children are slow to warm up to other people; others are friendly and outgoing. Some children accept limits and rules more easily than others. Some children are highly reactive to changes in their environment and to sensory experiences of all kinds, whereas others are less reactive. Some children tend to express themselves loudly and intensely; others are quieter. Thus, the range of normal behavior is broad.

Understanding the unique temperament profile of the child will better prepare the health care professional to assist parents and other caregivers in understanding the child's behavior, especially when the child's behavioral reactions are confusing or problematic. Discussing with parents how the child's behavior is interpreted within the family, and counseling them when concerns or conflicts emerge between the child's temperament and the caregivers' personal styles, may prevent significant problems later on.

Culture
The culture of the family and community provide a framework within which the socialization process unfolds. Children are heavily influenced by the culture, opinions, and attitudes of their families as they are "taught to act, believe, and feel in ways that are consistent with the values of their communities."[42] Culture influences the roles of parents and extended family members in child-rearing practices and the ways in which parents and other adults interact with children. Cultural groups approach parenting in different ways. In some cultures, the mother is expected to be primarily responsible for all aspects of an

Children are heavily influenced by the culture, opinions, and attitudes of their families as they are "taught to act, believe, and feel in ways that are consistent with the values of their communities."

PROMOTING
CHILD DEVELOPMENT

53

infant's or toddler's care. In other cultures, the care and nurturing of children is shared among mother, father, and extended family, including aunts, uncles, grandparents, and cousins. This wide circle of caregivers also may have responsibility for disciplining and making other decisions about a child's upbringing.

The increasingly self-aware young child grapples with complex issues, such as gender roles, peer or sibling competition, cooperation, and the difference between right and wrong within this cultural milieu. Aggression, acting out, excessive risk taking, and antisocial behaviors can appear at this time. Caregivers need to respond with a variety of interventions that set constructive limits and help children achieve self-discipline. Fun-filled family activities, such as playing games, reading, vacations, or holiday gatherings, serve as reminders of the joy and laughter the child brings to all. Ultimately, healthy social and emotional development depends on how children view themselves and the extent to which they feel valued by others. The quality of the parent-child relationship is the foundation for emotional well-being and the emerging sense of mastery and self-esteem.

> **Ultimately, healthy social and emotional development depends on how children view themselves and the extent to which they feel valued by others.**

Developmental Highlights of Early Childhood

SELF-REGULATION AND DAILY LIVING TASKS
During the early childhood years, the relative dominance of biologic rhythms is reduced through the development of self-control. Satisfactory self-control allows children to respond appropriately to events in their lives through delaying gratification until important facets of the situation are considered, modulating their responses, remaining calm, focusing on the task, recognizing that their responses have consequences, and behaving in the expected manner to comply with rules and expectations established by their significant caregivers.[43,44] Usually, these behaviors begin to manifest by 2 to 3 years of age.

Children with inadequate self-control can be impulsive or hyperactive, heightening concerns for safety. At the opposite extreme, children with excessive self-control tend to be anxious or have fixed behaviors. Of course, behavior varies so that a child may exhibit a great variety of behaviors at any given time in response to the same external cues.

Mastering activities in daily life shows that the child is moving toward achieving self-control. Chief among these are learning how to calm herself (which is needed to establish a regular sleep pattern), feed herself, toilet train, and take the major step of attending school. Health care professionals should actively prepare parents and their toddlers for achieving these milestones through discussing these topics and, when concerns persist after counseling, make referrals for appropriate consultation.

SLEEP
By the end of the first year of life, most children should be able to sustain or return to sleep throughout the night, and most parents should allow children to regulate their own nighttime sleep patterns. A consistent bedtime routine that promotes relaxation (eg, bath, book, or song) and the use of a transitional object are extremely helpful. Toddlers and preschoolers generally sleep 8 to 12 hours each night. Exact duration of nighttime sleep varies with the child's temperament, activity levels, health, and growth. The duration and timing of naps will affect nighttime sleeping. Most children awaken from sleep at times during the night, but can return to sleep quickly and peacefully without parental intervention. Sleep problems sometimes reflect separation fears on the part of both parents and children. Parents who feel especially anxious, depressed, or frightened can be reluctant to permit their young child to exercise self-control over sleep patterns at night. Children from 1 to 4 years of age should be allowed to sleep through the night

without a nighttime feeding. Dreams and nightmares can accompany active stages of sleep beginning at these ages. At such times, children may require reassurance that they are protected from the dangers that stir their imagination and intrude upon their calm sleep. Changes, such as acute illness, birth of siblings, and visits from friends and relatives, also can interfere temporarily with established sleep routines. Disorders, such as obstructive sleep apnea, and parasomnias, such as sleepwalking, can begin during these early years, and health care professionals should consider such a possibility in any child who has persistent sleep difficulties.

If health care professionals ask about sleep patterns at each of the visits during early childhood, they will gain rich insights into the child's and family's development. When parents have concerns about their child's sleep, the health care professional should explore, in more depth, the child's daytime behavior, temperament, and mood, as well as events, experiences, conditions, and feelings of family members. Although most issues lend themselves to open dialogue and counseling within the primary care relationship, some conflicts may require further exploration and intervention by a developmental-behavioral or mental health specialist.

TOILET TRAINING

For a child to successfully toilet train, he must have the cognitive capacity to respond to social cues and the neurologic ability to respond to bowel and bladder signals. Parents often want advice about when and how to toilet train a child. The first discussion about toilet training is best introduced at around the 18 Month Visit. Such early counseling can prevent harmful battles between the parents who might be focused on early toilet training and the child who is not yet physically or cognitively ready. In-depth discussion usually begins at the 2 Year Visit. The health care professional should explore the

parents' thoughts about this task and provide guidance to fill in the gaps.

Control of urination and bowel movements is a major step forward in developmental integrity. Successful completion of this task is a source of pride and respect for both the child and the parents.

Daytime control usually is achieved before nighttime dryness. Bed-wetting (nocturnal enuresis) is a common disorder with many possible therapies.[45] It is much more common in boys and deep sleepers. Enuresis should be investigated if a child continues to wet the bed after age 7 years, if bed-wetting results in problems within the family, or if infection or anatomical abnormalities are suspected. Fortunately, with time, the majority of all children with enuresis develop nighttime urination control.[46] Bowel control is usually completely achieved by age 3 years.

SOCIALIZATION

When provided the opportunity, toddlers and preschoolers acquire socialization skills and the ability to appropriately interact with other children and adults. Social interaction in early childhood promotes comfort and competence with relationships later in life. The social competencies are developmental assets[47,48] and, therefore, should be encouraged in children of these ages. Social competencies include planning and decision making with others, positive and appropriate interpersonal interactions, exposure to other cultures and ethnicities, behavioral resistance to inappropriate or dangerous behavior, and peaceful conflict resolution. Young toddlers will observe these behaviors in others, and preschoolers will begin to practice them. They also are inclined to internalize positive or negative attitudes toward themselves and others. Children note differences between groups of people (eg, they express understanding of racial identity as early as 3 years[49]), but they do not ascribe a value; they learn that from the adults in their environments. Opportunities for social interaction can be encouraged in the home with visitors, in play

For a child to successfully toilet train, he must have the cognitive capacity to respond to social cues and the neurologic ability to respond to bowel and bladder signals.

groups, in faith-based organizations, and in public places, such as the park, child care, or preschool.

DISCIPLINE, BEHAVIORAL GUIDANCE, AND TEACHING

Discipline is one tool parents can use to help modify and structure a child's behavior. It encompasses both positive reinforcement of admired behavior (eg, praise for picking up toys) and negative reinforcement of undesirable behavior (eg, a time-out for fighting with a sibling). The eventual incorporation of a functional sense of discipline that reinforces social norms is critical to the child's development. Although often thought of in negative terms, good discipline helps a child fit into the daily family schedule and makes childhood and child rearing pleasant and fun.

Family structure, values, beliefs, and cultural background influence approaches to behavioral guidance and teaching. Health care professionals should discuss with the parents how they were disciplined, how that discipline made them feel, and the most and least effective methods of discipline. In all families and cultures, discipline is a process whereby caregivers and other family members teach the young child, by instruction and example, how to behave and what is expected of her. What the child learns at this stage, and how the parent-child interactions surrounding discipline take form, can have long-term effects on the child's and family's development.

Exploring the roles that siblings play in development also should be addressed. The methods parents use to guide siblings in helping to raise the other family members should be reviewed. The special requirements of children and youth with special health care needs and foster care or adopted children are best discussed openly with all the family members, so that everyone is aware of parental expectations.

Although parents often look to the health care professional as a resource for developing

strategies related to behavioral guidance and teaching, many cultures also look to family, particularly elders, for such guidance and teaching. In most cases, discussions with parents regarding behavioral guidance should explore the parents' goals for the child, as well as the meaning behind the behaviors they wish to modify. Consideration of the child's developmental capacities and temperament profile should be a key component of this discussion. For instance, parents of a 2-year-old child frequently overestimate the child's capacity to integrate rules into everyday behavior, based on their observations of the child's growing understanding of language. With respect to temperament, parents can misinterpret a child's intense and reactive responses as intentionally oppositional rather than as part of her inborn behavioral style. Through explaining these developmental attributes, the health care professional plays a crucially important role in helping parents understand the meaning of their child's behavior, and in assessing the developmental readiness of the child to absorb new lessons about behavioral expectations.

Discussion of discipline is a high priority for the Bright Futures 15 Month and 18 Month Visits because it is important, for later child development, to establish a positive and successful foundation of parent-child interactions regarding behavior. Established negative behaviors can be extremely difficult to change, and, without help, many parents are not able to see the long-term effects of both

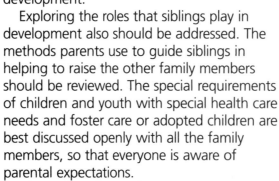

...the health care professional plays a crucially important role in helping parents understand the meaning of their child's behavior, and in assessing the developmental readiness of the child to absorb new lessons about behavioral expectations.

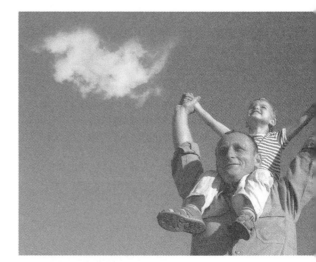

their child's behavior and their own choices in guiding them.

At times, the behavior of the child pushes all parents to their emotional limits. Health care professionals should remind parents to avoid meeting the child's anger with their own anger; this reaction teaches the wrong lesson. Many adverse behaviors, such as aggressive acts in the school-aged child have their roots in behavior established in early childhood. Maintaining a sense of humor and taking time away can help parents deal with stressful events. Discussing dilemmas and sharing frustrations with other involved adults are important in maintaining a sense of perspective and humor during difficult periods with the young child.

General features of effective behavioral guidance include several essential components, all of which are necessary for successful discipline[50]:

- A positive, supportive, loving relationship between the parents and child (children want to please their parents)
- Clear expectations communicated to the child in a developmentally appropriate manner
- Positive reinforcement strategies to increase desired behaviors (eg, having fun with the child and other family members sets the stage to reward and reinforce good behaviors with time together in enjoyable activities)
- Removal of reinforcements or use of logical consequences to reduce or eliminate undesired behaviors

Parents can increase the likelihood of achieving their behavioral goals for their child by establishing predictable daily routines and providing consistent responses to their child's behavior. Especially during early childhood, consequences should be administered within close temporal proximity to the target behavior and, if possible, related to the behavior (eg, bring the child in from playtime if she is

throwing sand when asked not to).[50] Some families (eg, first-time parents or adolescent parents) experience pressure from elders to use harsh or physical means of punishment. Culturally, it may be inappropriate to ignore what an elder has proposed. Parents may feel conflicted when they attempt to use new or different methods of discipline that are not supported within their families or communities.

Parents can use the following techniques to help foster good behavior in their child:

- Praise the child frequently for good behavior. Specific acknowledgement (rather than global praise) helps teach the child appropriate behaviors (eg, "Wow, you did a good job putting that toy away!" rather than "Great!"). Time spent together in an enjoyable activity is a valuable reward for desired behavior.
- Communicate expectations in positive terms. By noting when the child is doing something good, parents will help the child understand what they like and expect. Words such as, "I like it when you play quietly with your brother," or "I like that you climb into your car seat when I ask you to," are nonjudgmental statements and communicate to the child that these are behaviors the parents like.
- Model and role-play the desired behaviors.
- Prepare the child for change in the daily routine by discussing upcoming activities and expected behaviors.
- State behavioral expectations and limits for the child clearly and in a developmentally appropriate manner. These expectations should be few, realistic, and consistently enforced.
- Allow the child time for fun activities, especially as a reward for positive behaviors.
- Remove or avoid the places and objects that contribute to unwanted behavior.

Parents can increase the likelihood of achieving their behavioral goals for their child by establishing predictable daily routines and providing consistent responses to their child's behavior.

- Use time-out or logical consequences to deal with undesirable behavior.
- Promote consistent discipline practices across caregivers.
- Avoid responding to the child's anger with anger; this reaction teaches the wrong lesson and may escalate the child's response.
- Take time to reflect on their own physical and emotional response to the child's behavior so that they can choose the most appropriate discipline technique.

Conventional disciplinary methods do not work well with children with certain physical or developmental conditions. The following examples illustrate the point that "one size does not fit all" with respect to behavioral guidance:

- Children with poor communication skills often use behavior as a means of communication; caregivers should make every effort to help them develop more effective communication skills.
- Children who have hyperacute responses to their sensory environment require proactive interventions.

Because corporal punishment is no more effective than other approaches for managing undesired behavior in children, the AAP recommends that parents be encouraged and assisted in developing methods other than spanking in response to undesired behavior (Box 4).[50] Other forms of corporal punishment, such as shaking or striking a child with an object, should never be used. Referral to high-quality parenting programs and counseling should be considered for children with difficult behavioral problems.

LITERACY
Learning to read and write is a complex process that takes time. It requires that children have good, consistent relationships with caring adults who provide one-on-one

interactions and who support the development of oral language. Literacy begins in infancy, when parents and other caregivers talk to their baby, and, in early childhood, when toddlers learn to communicate through language, explore their world through imaginary play, and listen to stories, whether read from books or spoken in an oral tradition. Because young children are active learners, they find joy in exploring and learning the meaning of language and communicating in increasingly sophisticated ways as they move toward literacy.

Parents' and health care professionals' expectations for a young child's literacy accomplishments should be based on developmentally appropriate activities, such as the encouragement of talking, singing, and imaginative play; simple art projects; easy access to books; and frequent reading times. Reading and writing are so linked to development, relationships, and environment that children will vary greatly in when and how

Literacy begins in infancy, when parents and other caregivers talk to their baby, and, in early childhood, when toddlers learn to communicate through language, explore their world through imaginary play, and listen to stories, whether read from books or spoken in an oral tradition.

> **BOX 4**
> **Discipline: Key Messages for Parents**
> - Discipline means teaching, not punishing.
> - All children need guidance, and most children need occasional discipline.
> - Discipline is effective when it is consistent; it is ineffective when it is not consistent.
> - Parents' discipline should be geared to the child's developmental level.
> - Discipline is most effective when the parent can understand the child's point of view.
> - Discipline should help a child learn from his mistakes. The child should understand why he is being disciplined.
> - Disciplinary methods should not cause a child to feel afraid of his parents.
> - A parent should not physically discipline a child if the parent feels out of control.

they learn to read and write. This is true for other complex skills as well.

The National Research Council[51] has identified phonological awareness, shared book reading, and speech-to-print connection as key concepts underlying early literacy. Health care professionals can support literacy by encouraging parents to tell stories, create or visit environments filled with books, find a place at home for imaginary play and art projects, ask their child questions and invite him to talk about his ideas, model literacy behavior by reading newspapers or books daily, and set aside quiet times each day for reading with their child (eg, just before bed). By encouraging parents at every health supervision visit to find age-appropriate ways of incorporating books and reading aloud into children's daily routines, the health care professional can give parents a way to help their children grow up associating books with positive parental attention. These discussions also can help parents understand the role that child care and preschool programs play in helping children get ready to read and write.[52]

The health care professional's office should reflect reading as a priority, with a specific area set aside to encourage imaginative play, a place with a collection of quality books and magazines where children can look at books or be read to, and a place with information about community libraries and adult and family literacy opportunities. (For more information on this topic, see Box 2 of this theme.) The Reach Out and Read Program has increased the likelihood that parents will read to their children even among families at risk due to low-literacy among parents.[20,21,53] By giving a book at every health supervision visit from 6 months to 5 years, especially to children at socioeconomic risk, the health care professional can increase the frequency of parental reading aloud, improve the home environment, and help parents increase children's language development.[20,21]

PLAY

A hallmark of the passage through early childhood is the emergence and steady elaboration of play activities. For the young toddler, play centers on direct explorations into the surrounding world, including the manipulation of objects to create interesting outcomes (eg, the sounds that banging a pot may produce or the interesting results of pouring water into a sandbox). With the development of language, from around age 18 months, play becomes progressively more reflective of the child's remembered experiences and imagined possibilities, as enacted through symbolic play. Thus, a doll comes to represent a living, imaginary person who can be fed, bathed, or scolded—just as the young child has personally experienced in real life.

In *representational* or *symbolic play*, which usually is evident by 2 years of age, the child has a new way of "replaying" the events in her life. Unlike real life, play allows her to control the events and their outcomes. Challenging experiences can be better understood through their re-creation as play. Play can enable the child to better cope with stressful experiences by "taking charge" and developing a preferred story. Confusing or difficult experiences can be mastered through practice in experimentation and planning that play permits.

Many children at this age become attached to *transitional objects* and use them to help them fall asleep, comfort them when they are hurt or upset, and join them in their world of make-believe. The transitional object is a prime example of how the child's active imagination plays a central role in development toward independence and self-regulation.

From 3 to 5 years of age, the child's developmental gains in language and speech, cognitive ability, and fine and gross motor skills allow for increasingly complex forms of play. Play becomes an important modality for practicing and enhancing a broad range of skills,

With the development of language, from around age 18 months, play becomes progressively more reflective of the child's remembered experiences and imagined possibilities, as enacted through symbolic play.

PROMOTING CHILD DEVELOPMENT

such as the motor skills and spatial understanding that comes with building with blocks or working with puzzles.

Play is a critical part of development, and toys are a critical part of play. Health care professionals often are asked to recommend appropriate toys for their patients. Toys should be educational and should promote creativity. Parents and health care professionals should avoid toys that make loud or shrill noises, toys with small parts, loose strings, cords, rope, or sharp edges, and toys that contain potentially toxic materials. Toys that promote violence, social distinctions, gender stereotypes, or racial bias also should be avoided. Video games are not recommended for young children, but, if used, they should be screened for inappropriate content. Health care professionals should advise parents on distinguishing between safe and unsafe toys, choosing toys that help promote learning, and using books and magazines to read and play together.[54]

Play provides a window into many aspects of the child's developmental progress and into how she is attempting to understand the events, transitions, and stresses of everyday life. Parents and other caregivers should recognize the importance of play for the development of their young children. Play requires that children feel secure and that the play environment be sufficiently protected from intrusion and disruption. Parent-child play, in which the child takes the lead and the parent is attentive and responsive, elaborating but not controlling the events of play, is an excellent technique for enhancing the parent-child relationship and language development. When typical play is missing or delayed, the health care professional should consider the possibility of a developmental or emotional disorder, possible significant stresses in the child's environment, or both. The child's relationship to the family pets, if any, should be discussed and should include queries about attachment, responsibilities for pet care, and pet safety.

Play provides a window into many aspects of the child's developmental progress and into how she is attempting to understand the events, transitions, and stresses of everyday life.

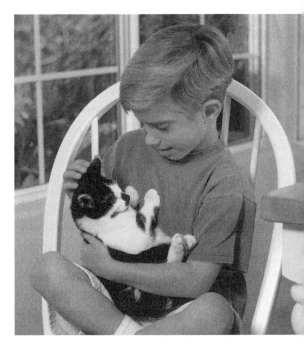

SEPARATION AND INDIVIDUATION

By the child's first birthday, he has likely secured a reasonably firm sense of trust that his primary caregivers are reliable, protective, and encouraging. In turn, the young toddler should begin to feel as though he can trust others enough to feel comfortable in communicating his feelings, needs, and interests. From this base of emotional security, the young child can dedicate his second year to begin growing increasingly independent from his caregivers—in actions, words, and thoughts. Periodically checking in with his parents for guidance and reassurance about safe and socially acceptable limits, the toddler waffles between testing bold new behaviors and demanding to be consoled and protected. During this stage of development, parents can help their child by providing safe opportunities for freedom and encouragement with support. As the young child develops increasing comfort in exploring time, space, and relationships with adults and peers, he begins to discover more about his own identity, effectiveness, and free will. The more positive experiences a preschool-aged child enjoys with other children and adults, the better prepared he becomes for his subsequent adventures at school.

CHILD CARE

According to the Child Health USA 2004 Report, 63% of mothers with preschool-aged children were in the labor force (either employed or looking for employment) in 2003, with 70% of these mothers employed full-time.[55] Working mothers use a variety of child care arrangements. For example, family members are a common source of child care. A US Census Bureau report reveals[22] that 40% of preschool-aged children are cared for by a relative, 23% by day care centers, nursery schools, preschools, federal Head Start programs, kindergarten, and grade schools, and 14% by family day care providers and nonrelatives (eg, babysitters, nannies, and housekeepers). Child care arrangements vary across states, ages, health status, and family income levels. Children from lower-income families are less likely to be cared for in centers than children from higher-income families, and are more likely to be in the care of relatives.[56]

Families with young children, especially those living at or near the poverty level and those with several children in child care, often find that child care costs strain their budget, requiring them to balance competing family needs. Although federal subsidies for child care exist, most communities have waiting lists for openings. The health care professional and support staff who are familiar with community resources and sensitive to families' financial struggles can guide families as they make child care decisions.

Because child care for children with special health care needs is the most difficult to find and is in the shortest supply in most communities, a family's search for suitable child care can be frustrating and can sometimes cause a parent to stop working. This problem is compounded for families with low incomes,

children who have more severe special health care needs, or both. In these situations, the health care professional and staff can help families by understanding their unique needs and the available community resources. The health care professional and staff also can work with the child care provider to ensure that the setting is appropriate and the staff has the training necessary to give the child a safe and healthy environment.

Preschools should never have more than 10 children per teacher. Providers for children with special health care needs may require specialized training and support. Parents should inquire whether their preschools adhere to national standards and are accredited by organizations such as the National Association for the Education of Young Children (www.naeyc.org).[23]

Quality child care gives young children valuable opportunities to learn to relate effectively with peers and adults, to explore the diverse physical and social world, and to develop confidence in their abilities to learn new skills, form trusting bonds of friendship, and process information from a variety of sources. Health care professionals should learn about the health, developmental, and behavioral issues of their patients as they are manifested in child care. Health care professionals can integrate this information in their assessment, counseling, and advocacy for children and families in their practice and their community. The more sources of insight into the child's life the health care professional has, the better prepared he will be to support the child's health and development as she takes her first steps beyond the family. Many health care professionals provide formal consultative services to child care centers in their communities.

SCHOOL READINESS

At the end of the early childhood developmental stage, the young child and his parents will begin the transition into kindergarten.

Quality child care gives young children valuable opportunities to learn to relate effectively with peers and adults, to explore the diverse physical and social world, and to develop confidence in their abilities to learn new skills, form trusting bonds of friendship, and process information from a variety of sources.

PROMOTING
CHILD DEVELOPMENT

The child will be challenged to demonstrate developmental capacities, including:

- Language and speech that is sufficient for communication and learning
- Cognitive abilities that are necessary for learning sound-letter associations, spatial relations, and number concepts
- Ability to separate from family and caregivers (especially for the child who has not already participated in preschool activities)
- Self-regulation with respect to behavior, emotions, attention, and motor movement
- Ability to make friends and get along with peers
- Ability to participate in group activities
- Ability to follow rules and directions
- Skills that others appreciate, such as singing or drawing

However, too many children today enter kindergarten significantly behind their peers in 1 or more of these abilities. Problems in self-regulation of emotions and behavior and problems in maintaining attention and focus are common at kindergarten entry and predict future educational and social problems.[57]

In an extensive survey, kindergarten teachers reported that roughly half of kindergartners have difficulty following directions because of poor academic skills or problems with working in a group.[58] Racial and ethnic disparities have been shown to exist at kindergarten entry in terms of children's readiness to learn.[59]

Social and emotional development during early childhood (which was neglected in past research on school readiness) has been shown to be strongly connected to later academic success. Qualities that are crucial to learning and are dependent on early emotional and social development include self-confidence, curiosity, self-control of strong emotions, motivation to learn, and the ability to make friends and become engaged in a

Qualities that are crucial to learning and are dependent on early emotional and social development include self-confidence, curiosity, self-control of strong emotions, motivation to learn, and the ability to make friends and become engaged in a social group.

social group.[5] Box 5 lists risk factors for school readiness.

The goal of having every child ready for school is a task that encompasses all of early childhood and depends on the efforts of everyone involved in the care of the young child during his first 5 years. Throughout these years, the health care professional plays a vital role in promoting this goal through assessing and monitoring the:

- General health of the child, including vision and hearing
- Child's developmental trajectory

BOX 5
Monitoring Risk Factors for School Readiness

Child-based risk factors. Readily apparent disabilities are found in a small proportion of those entering school (around 2%). Less-obvious special needs, due to specific learning disabilities, mild mental retardation, or emotional and social maladjustments, are found in nearly 20% of children.[60]

Family-based risk factors. Risk factors may begin very early in childhood and include low maternal education, single-parent status, poverty, low parental literacy, households with few or no books or other reading materials, and English as a second language.[61] Family habits related to television viewing also may affect school readiness. It appears that the mediators that influence readiness are the content (with children's informational shows more enhancing than general audience shows) and context (characteristics of the household) rather than television itself.

School-based risk factors. Schools may fail to recognize or accommodate the special health problems, developmental needs, and significant cultural differences of their incoming students.[62]

DEVELOPMENTAL MILESTONES AT A GLANCE — EARLY CHILDHOOD[38-63]

Age	Gross Motor	Fine Motor	Cognitive, Linguistic, and Communication	Social-Emotional
1 Year	•Stand alone •Pull to stand	•Put block in cup •Bang 2 cubes held in hands	**•Imitate vocalizations and sounds** **•Babbling*** •1 word	**•Protodeclarative pointing*** •Wave bye-bye •Imitate activities •Play pat-a-cake
15 Months	•Walk backwards •Stoop and recover •Walk well	•Scribble •Put block in cup	**•1 word*** •3 words	•Drink from cup •Wave bye-bye
18 Months	•Walk up steps •Run •Walk backwards	•Dump raisin, demonstrated •Tower of 2 cubes •Scribble	•Point to at least 1 body part •6 words •3 words	•Remove garment •Help in house
2 Years	•Throw ball overhand •Jump up •Kick ball forward •Walk up steps	•Tower of 6 cubes •Tower of 4 cubes	•Name 1 picture •Combine words •Point to 2 pictures	•Put on clothing •Remove garment
2½ Years	•Throw ball overhand •Jump up	•Imitate vertical line •Tower of 8 cubes •Tower of 6 cubes	•Know 2 actions •Speech half understandable •Point to 6 body parts •Name 1 picture	•Wash and dry hands •Put on clothing
3 Years	•Balance on each foot 1 second •Broad jump •Throw ball overhand	•Thumb wiggle •Imitate vertical line •Tower of 8 cubes •Tower of 6 cubes	•Speech all understandable •Name 1 color •Know 2 adjectives •Name 4 pictures	•Name friend •Brush teeth with help
4 Years	•Hop •Balance on each foot 2 seconds	•Draw a person with 3 parts •Tower of 8 cubes	•Define 5 words •Name 4 colors •Speech all understandable	•Copy a cross (+) •Copy a circle

KEY

Black Color: 50% to 90% of children pass this item.

Green Color: More than 90% of children pass this item.

*Absence of these milestones should trigger screening for autism.

These norms are taken from the DENVER II, and are based upon the administration and interpretation as set forth in the DENVER II Training Manual (copyright 1992).

These milestones are provided as a reference only. Reference to these milestones does not take the place of a standardized measurement of healthy child development or discourage a developmental discussion with a health care provider.

PROMOTING CHILD DEVELOPMENT

- Emotional health of the child and family, especially when based on the health care professional's long-term knowledge of child-family relationships
- Child's social development (both skills and difficulties)
- Specific child-based, family-based, school-based, and community-based risk factors

Health care professionals have a unique opportunity to recognize problems and, when possible, to intervene early with effective referral for both specific services and general evaluation so as to enhance the child's readiness for learning by the start of school. Intervention services for eligible children can begin at birth and continue through age 21 years. For details on eligibility and services, refer to the US Department of Education's Office of Special Education and Rehabilitative Services (http://www.ed.gov/about/offices/list/osers).

Promoting Child Development: Middle Childhood—5 to 10 Years

The middle childhood years are typically a stable period, without the dramatic physical, cognitive, and social changes that occur in the other developmental stages. It is an important transitional period during which children build on the skills developed in the various domains of early childhood in preparation for adolescence. Middle childhood is an important time for families to help

> **Middle childhood is an important time for families to help children consolidate and strengthen their cognitive and emotional attributes, such as communication skills, sensitivity to others, ability to form positive peer relationships, self-esteem, and independence.**

children consolidate and strengthen their cognitive and emotional attributes, such as communication skills, sensitivity to others, ability to form positive peer relationships, self-esteem, and independence. These attributes will help them cope with the stresses and potential risks of adolescence.

Families and health care professionals also can provide enormous support for children's healthy physical development. They can work with communities to ensure that children have access to safe, well-supervised play areas, recreation centers, team sports and organized activities, parks, and schools. For children to flourish, communities must provide carefully maintained facilities to help their bodies and minds develop in a healthy way. Health care professionals can support their guidance by advocating for community facilities available to all children. (For more information on this topic, see the Promoting Community Relationships and Resources and the Promoting Physical Activity themes.)

Children and Youth With Special Health Care Needs

Middle childhood is a critical time for children with special health care needs to adapt successfully to their condition. During this period, they continue to define their sense of self and improve their ability to care for their own health. Children adapt best to chronic illness when health care professionals, families, schools, and communities work together to foster their emerging independence. Inclusion in school and community life allows children with special health care needs to feel valued and to integrate their specific care needs with other aspects of their lives. It also is important to discuss family perspectives, because families may have various beliefs and values regarding the independence of children with special health care needs based on culture and history.

When families have children with special health care needs, the other children in the

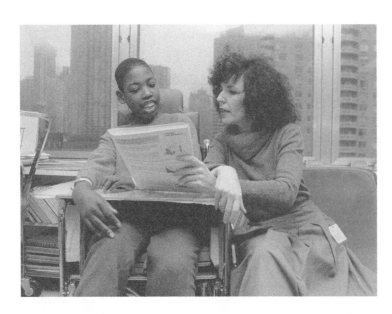

family will be introduced to the possibility that their sibling can have different challenges because of the disability and circumstances. Families may have to deal with certain difficult tasks, such as hospitalizations or painful tests, illness, and possibly death. Parents and child care providers should be sensitive to these issues and responsive to the needs of the medically fragile child and the healthy siblings. At the same time, children with special health care needs should not be given special privileges simply because of their condition. Instead, outlining rules and responsibilities is extremely important for the child's development and the family's functioning. Child care providers and teachers can play an important supportive role and be a source of information for the parents and the children.

Domains of Development

GROSS AND FINE MOTOR SKILLS

Major increases in strength and improvements in motor coordination occur during middle childhood. These changes contribute to the child's growing sense of competence in relation to his physical abilities and enhance his potential for participating in sports, dance, gymnastics, and other physical pursuits. A child's participation in sports or other physical activities can reinforce positive interaction skills that will serve the child throughout his life. Children develop at slightly different rates depending on their unique physical characteristics and experiences. Efforts to maintain good physical health and exercise patterns are important to achieving and maintaining a healthy weight. Monitoring the child's growth patterns and conducting periodic physical examinations to assess growth and development are important components of health supervision. Close monitoring for overweight and obesity should be included in these visits. (For more information on this topic, see the Promoting Healthy Weight theme.)

COGNITIVE, LINGUISTIC, AND COMMUNICATION SKILLS

Children's readiness to learn in school depends on cognitive maturation as well as their individual experiences. During middle childhood, the child moves from magical thinking to more logical thought processes. The synthesis of basic language, perception, and abstraction allows the child to read, write, and communicate thoughts of increasing complexity and creativity. Progress can appear subtle from month to month, but it is dramatic from one school year to the next. As the child's cognitive skills grow, she matures in her ability to understand the world and people around her and to function independently. Occasionally, children will be impaired in their development because of learning problems, behavior problems, or both. The health care professional can offer support by ensuring screening and evaluation for any suspected delays.

The major developmental achievement of this age is self-efficacy, or the knowledge of what to do and the confidence and ability to do it. Success at school is most likely to occur when this achievement is encouraged by parents and valued by families. Families who reward children with enthusiasm and warmth for putting forth their best effort ensure their steady educational progress and prepare them to use their intelligence and knowledge productively. Through awareness of individual learning styles, including the need for necessary accommodations, parents and teachers can adapt materials and experiences to each child. School success is an important factor in the development of a child's self-esteem. In families in which parents have had unsuccessful educational experiences or have had limited education, support from health care professionals and others in the community is critical in supporting their children through the educational process.

During middle childhood, the child moves from magical thinking to more logical thought processes.

SOCIAL-EMOTIONAL SKILLS

As children become increasingly independent and demonstrate initiative, they develop their own sense of personhood (Table 4). They begin to discern where they "fit" among their peers and in their family, school class, neighborhood, and community. When the "fit" is good and comfortable, children see themselves as effective and competent members of their family, group, team, school, and community. When the "fit" is tenuous or poor, the dissonance can be a source of distress and can predispose children to emotional disorders with long-term consequences. (For more information on this topic, see the Promoting Mental Health theme.) Ongoing support for the child provides the best opportunity for acceptance and forms the basis for a strong self-worth. Support is especially important for children with special health care needs.

Children need both the freedom of personal expression and the structure of expectations and guidelines that they can understand and accept. Families should provide opportunities for the child to interact with other children in play environments without excessive adult interference. However, not all cultures accept this perspective. The health care professional and the family should discuss these issues. Most experts believe that children benefit from the experience of independent play with peers. Unfortunately, some neighborhoods or living arrangements restrict these opportunities. In addition, some children with special health care needs may need adaptive equipment or facilities to allow for inclusive play experiences. Children also need to have positive interactions with adults, reinforcing their sense of self-esteem, self-worth, and belief in their capability of personal success.

The child's "self" evolves in a social context. Health care professionals can help families understand this dynamic and encourage specific roles for the children within the family. Parents who consciously assess their child's emotional maturity and role in the family at each birthday will appreciate the changes that have occurred subtly over time.

Children with special health care needs will have emotional maturity that is appropriately reflective of their needs, developmental level, and physical challenges (Table 4). Parents should be encouraged to appreciate the individual maturity level of their child. As a result, they can celebrate the child's evolving autonomy by granting new privileges. Parents who match each new entitlement with a new responsibility signal their respect for the child's growing capability to contribute to the family and the community.

Developmental Highlights of Middle Childhood

MORAL AND SPIRITUAL DEVELOPMENT

The child's development as an individual involves an understanding of the life cycle—birth, growth and maturation, aging, and death. He becomes increasingly aware that an individual's life fits into a larger scheme of relationships among individuals, groups of people, other living creatures, and the earth itself. School-aged children become keenly interested in these topics, especially if they experience life events such as the birth of a sibling or the death of a grandparent. Children also become aware of violent death, on the highways or on street corners. When a death occurs, parents should be encouraged to discuss the loss with their children and provide assistance to children who are having difficulty with the grieving process.

As children experience these events and learn to view their personal encounters as part of a larger whole, families and communities provide an important structure. These experiences provide children with a basic foundation of value systems and encourage them to examine their personal actions in the context of those around them.

> He becomes increasingly aware that an individual's life fits into a larger scheme of relationships among individuals, groups of people, other living creatures, and the earth itself.

TABLE 4

Social and Emotional Development in Middle Childhood

Topics	Key Areas
	(Key areas in italics are especially important for children with special health care needs.)
Self	**Self-esteem:** • Experiences of success • Reasonable risk-taking behavior • Resilience and ability to handle failure • Supportive family and peer relationships **Self-image:** • Body image, *celebrating different body images* • Prepubertal changes; initiating discussion about sexuality and reproduction; *prepubertal changes related to physical care issues*
Family	**What matters at home:** • Expectation and limit setting • Family times together • Communication • Family responsibilities • Family transitions • Sibling relationships • *Caregiver relationships*
Friends	**Friendships:** • Making friends, *friendships with peers with and without special health care needs* • Family support of friendships, *family support to have typical friendship activities, as appropriate*
School	**School:** • Expectation for school performance, *school performance/ defined in the Individualized Education Program (IEP)* • Homework • Child-teacher conflicts, *building relationships with teachers* • *Parent-teacher communication* • Ability of schools to address the needs of children from diverse backgrounds • Awareness of aggression, bullying, and victimization • Absenteeism
Community	**Community strengths:** • Community organizations • Religious groups • Cultural groups **High-risk behaviors and environments:** • Substance use • Unsafe friendships • Unsafe community environments • *Particular awareness of risk-taking behaviors and unsafe environments, because children may be easily victimized*

PROMOTING
CHILD DEVELOPMENT

The relationship between values, competence, self-esteem, and personal responsibility needs to be modeled and affirmed by the child's parents, teachers, and communities. Parents need to help their child maintain a balance of responsibilities at school and home, time spent with family and friends, extracurricular and community activities, and personal leisure. Achieving this balance is essential for healthy development. Competence and self-esteem are strengthened when a child is recognized for working hard in school, successfully completing chores and special projects, and participating in school and community activities.

Promoting Child Development: Adolescence—11 to 21 Years

Adolescence is a dynamic experience, not a homogenous period of life. Adolescents differ widely in their physical, social, and emotional maturity because they enter puberty at different ages, progress at different paces, and experience different challenges in their developmental trajectories. To complicate the adolescent experience, parents also can experience changes in health, employment, geographic relocation, marital relationships, or the health of their parents and other family members.

Viewing adolescence in stages—early adolescence (11 to 14 years of age), middle adolescence (15 to 17 years of age), and late adolescence (18 to 21 years of age)—yields a better understanding of physical and psychological development and potential problems. The nature, length, and course of typical adolescent development can be viewed differently by families because cultural expectations for independence and self-sufficiency can differ. The health care professional should discern from families how they view this stage of life and note potential conflicts between the family's cultural values and those of the developing adolescent.

Youth With Special Health Care Needs

As children with special health care needs enter adolescence and experience puberty, growth, and physical and emotional development, new levels of functionality in the face of their special need can bring important and remarkable gains in independence and autonomy. Alternatively, limitations related to their illness can further underscore their physical dependence, which can limit the development of emotional independence. The adolescent may fear that his condition precludes autonomy.

Careful assessment of medical conditions, strengths and risk-taking behaviors, followed by sensitive discussions of the youth's perceived needs and goals, can assist the adolescent with a special health care need to maximize physical development and support the attainment of full emotional development and maturity.

Stages of Adolescence

Three key transitional domains (physiological, psychological, and social) can be used to chart adolescent changes and challenges (Table 5).

Domains of Development

GROSS AND FINE MOTOR SKILLS
Pubertal growth brings completion of physical development. Adult height and muscle mass are attained. Increasing size and

As children with special health care needs enter adolescence and experience puberty, growth, and physical and emotional development, new levels of functionality in the face of their special need can bring important and remarkable gains in independence and autonomy.

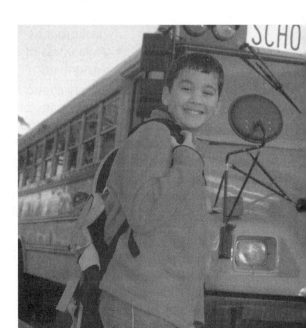

TABLE 5

Domains of Adolescent Development

	Early Adolescence (11 to 14 Years)	Middle Adolescence (15 to 17 Years)	Late Adolescence (18 to 21 Years)
Physiological	Onset of puberty, growth spurt, menarche (females)	Ovulation (females), growth spurt (males)	Growth completed
Psychological	Concrete thought, preoccupation with rapid body changes, sexual identity, questioning independence, parental controls remain strong	Competence in abstract and future thought, idealism, sense of invincibility or narcissism, sexual identity, beginning of cognitive capacity to provide legal consent	Future orientation, emotional independence, unmasking of psychiatric disorders, capacity for empathy, intimacy, and reciprocity in interpersonal relationships, self-identity, recognized as legally capable of providing consent,[64] attainment of legal age for some issues (eg, voting) but not all issues (eg, drinking alcohol)
Social	Search for same-sex peer affiliation, good parental relationships, other adults as role models; transition to middle school, involvement in extracurricular activities; sensitivity to differences between home culture and culture of others	Beginning emotional emancipation, increased power of peer group, conflicts over parental control, interest in sexual relationships, initiation of driving, risk-taking behavior, transition to high school, reduced involvement in extracurricular activities, possible cultural conflict as adolescent navigates between family's values and values of broader culture and peer culture	Individual over peer relationships; transition in parent-child relationship, transition out of home; may begin preparation for further education, career, marriage, and parenting
Potential Problems	Delayed puberty; acne; orthopedic problems; school problems; psychosomatic concerns; depression; unintended pregnancy; initiation of tobacco, alcohol, or other drug use	Experimentation with health risk behaviors (eg, sex, drinking, drug use, smoking), auto crashes, menstrual disorders, unintended pregnancy, acne, short stature (males), conflicts with parents, overweight, physical inactivity, poor eating behaviors, eating disorders (eg, purging, binge eating, and anorexia nervosa)	Eating disorders, depression, suicide, auto crashes, unintended pregnancy acne, smoking, alcohol or drug dependence

PROMOTING CHILD DEVELOPMENT

strength are accompanied by enhanced coordination of both gross and fine motor skills. The boy or girl who can barely make the high-school junior varsity basketball team as a ninth grader has the agility and strength necessary for varsity performance by 10th or 11th grade. Motor development continues into the final stage of development.

COGNITIVE, LINGUISTIC, AND COMMUNICATION SKILLS

Success in school contributes substantially to the adolescent's self-esteem and progress toward becoming a socially competent adult. The National Longitudinal Study for Adolescent Health[65] found that school performance and choice of free-time activities were the most important determinants for every risky behavior studied, regardless of socioeconomic status, race, or type of household (ie, 1 parent vs 2 parents). Students who have a high academic self-concept tend to be more motivated to achieve, more engaged in school, and more hopeful about their future. Parental involvement and expectations and participation in extracurricular activities enhance adolescent academic achievement and educational attainment. Health care professionals should encourage conversations between parents and their adolescent children on these issues.

Adolescents who feel connected to their school and who have a high academic self-concept are motivated to achieve. Peer relationships also influence adolescents' attitudes. Adolescents whose peers have or are perceived to have higher educational aspirations tend to be more engaged in school and to have higher hopes for continuing their education. Conversely, adolescents who work more than 20 hours a week tend to have a lower level of engagement in school.[66] The health care professional should encourage youth to participate in extracurricular activities. Factors such as disability and limited English proficiency can interfere with school success and need attention.

Parental involvement and expectations and participation in extracurricular activities enhance adolescent academic achievement and educational attainment.

Some adolescents make the academic and social transition from middle school to high school easily. Others find this transition overwhelming, with an impact on motivation, self-esteem, and academic performance.

The Centers for Disease Control and Prevention (CDC) National Center for Health Statistics estimates that among children 3 to 17 years of age, 8% have a learning disability.[67] Children with a fair or poor health status were 5 times as likely to have a learning disability than children with an excellent or a very good health status.[67] Students with learning disabilities can have difficulty with academics as well as social relationships. These students are more prone to depression and a lack of confidence.[68] Health care professionals should screen youth for declining grades and attendance issues, signs of learning disorders, and social adjustment concerns. Depending on the specific school district policies, heath care professionals can interact with the school nurse, psychologist, counselor, or administrator to identify and address academic, social, and emotional difficulties that can interfere with school success.

SOCIAL-EMOTIONAL SKILLS

A consistent, supportive environment for the adolescent, with graded steps toward autonomy is necessary to foster emotional and social well-being. This supportive environment requires the participation of the family, school, health care professional, and community, as well as the adolescent himself.[69] Parents will struggle for a balance for their child between restrictions that are designed to protect him and freedom that is intended to enhance growth. The adolescent will struggle for this balance, too.

The emotional well-being of adolescents is tied to their sense of self-esteem. High self-esteem is generally associated with feelings of life satisfaction and a sense of control over one's life, whereas low self-esteem is correlated with lower reports of happiness and higher reports of feeling as if one is not in control of one's life. Adolescents who demonstrate good social and problem-solving skills also usually have enhanced self-esteem because these skills increase their sense of control over their world. This asset is essential in deriving the ability to handle stress and cope with challenging situations.

Another important developmental milestone that is critical to emotional well-being is the adolescent's growing sense of self. Long hours spent talking, grooming, being alone, and rushing to be part of a group—any group—are all part of the adolescent's search for a conception of self. Intelligence, in the narrow sense of the term, also is significant to the cognitive self. During adolescence, the individual has to learn the accumulated wisdom of society. As the adolescent becomes facile in using concepts and abstractions, he begins to combine new ideas in new ways to arrive at creative solutions.

Normal fluctuations of mood now are the adolescent's responsibility. With increasing autonomy, he may become unwilling to share feelings and, to a point, unconsciously seek to avoid dependence on family for mood modulation. Like other skills he acquires, managing feelings of sadness and anxiety requires guidance, practice, and experience.

During the course of adolescence, the increasingly autonomous and socially competent youth finds his place in family and community. Social competence is defined as the degree to which significant others rate an individual as successful in solving and completing social tasks.[70] The specific behaviors that characterize social competence will vary with the situation in which the adolescent is functioning.[71] Socially competent youth are able to decode and interpret social cues and consider alternative responses, along with their consequences.

To function in an adult world, a youth must become aware of his relations to others and learn the personal impact of relationships on his daily function. Accordingly, he must appreciate the effects and impact of his actions toward others if relationships are to be mature and reciprocal. Understanding how others might interpret a situation, recognizing another's predicament, and comfortably appreciating another's feelings are new and important experiences. Empathy must be achieved for healthy adult relationships to flourish.

The adolescent's social and emotional skills also are influenced by the young adult's growing interactions with the wider community through travel, higher education, volunteer activities, or structured job experiences. These activities can help adolescents realize that they have meaningful roles and can contribute productively to society. Through these activities, youth learn the importance of general adherence to rules and authority. External mandates are internalized in an appreciation of right or wrong and consequences.

Developmental Highlights of Adolescence

ASSETS

Health advocates have begun to look at the family and community factors that promote healthy development. This "asset" model, or strength-based approach, provides a broader perspective on adolescent development than the more traditional "deficit" model, which looks at the problems experienced by adolescents and develops preventive interventions (Table 6). The asset model reinforces

TABLE 6

Comparison of Asset and Deficit Models

Asset Model	Deficit Model
Positive family environment	Abuse or neglect
Relationships with caring adults	Witness to domestic violence
Religious and spiritual anchors	Family discord and divorce
Involvement in school, faith-based organization, or community	Parents with poor health habits
	Unsafe schools
Accessible recreational opportunities	Unsafe neighborhood

health-promoting interactions or social involvement (eg, good parent-adolescent communication and participation in extracurricular activities) and assists adolescents and their parents in setting goals to achieve healthy development.

Research demonstrates the value of parental involvement and quality parent-adolescent communication on healthy adolescent development.[72-74] Adolescents whose parents are authoritative, rather than authoritarian or passive, and who are involved in extracurricular and community activities appear to progress through adolescence with relatively little turmoil.[75]

MODELS OF CARE

Onsite integrated health services in the schools—with referrals to health care professionals and community agencies (including mental health centers) for supplementary services—are evolving as one way to deliver adolescent health care in medically underserved areas. In some situations, the school-based health center is the medical home for the youth enrolled in the center. School-based health centers can be especially effective in ensuring immunizations, promoting sports safety, and providing access for students with special health care needs. All services and programs should work to improve communication between school and home so that parents stay involved in their adolescents' lives away from home and learn effective strategies to deal with some of the challenges that their children face.

Health care professionals should ask young people how they learn about healthy living. Health promotion programs in schools help adolescents establish good health habits and avoid those that can lead to morbidity and mortality. Health promotion curricula can include family life education and social skills training, as well as information on pregnancy prevention, abstinence, conflict resolution, healthy nutritional practices, and avoidance of unhealthy habits such as the use of tobacco products, alcohol, or other drugs. Referrals to appropriate, culturally respectful, and accessible community resources also help adolescents learn about and address mental health concerns, nutrition and physical health, and sexual health issues. When young people decide to seek assistance beyond their family, those resources should provide appropriate confidential counseling and support to them in making healthy choices while encouraging good communication with parents and family.

When young people decide to seek assistance beyond their family, those resources should provide appropriate confidential counseling and support to them in making healthy choices while encouraging good communication with parents and family.

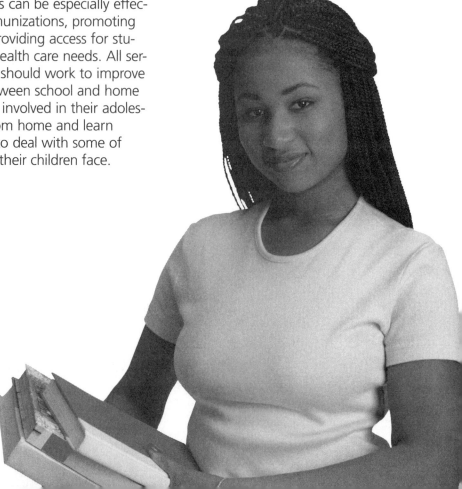

PROMOTING CHILD DEVELOPMENT

References

1. Council on Children with Disabilities; Section on Developmental Behavorial Pediatrics; Bright Futures Steering Committee; Medical Home Initiatives for Children with Special Needs Project Advisory Committee. Identifying infants and young children with developmental disorders in the medical home: an algorithm for developmental surveillance and screening. *Pediatrics.* 2006;118:405-420: Erratum in: *Pediatrics.* 2006;188:1808-1809

2. Glascoe FP, Dworkin PH. The role of parents in the detection of developmental and behavioral problems. *Pediatrics.* 1995;95:829-836

3. Jellinek MS, Patel BP, Froehle MC, eds. *Bright Futures in Practice: Mental Health. Tool Kit—Volume 2.* Arlington, VA: National Center for Education in Maternal and Child Health; 2002

4. Knight JR, Sherritt L, Shrier LA, Harris SK, Chang G. Validity of the CRAFFT substance abuse screening test among adolescent clinic patients. *Arch Pediatr Adolesc Med.* 2002;156:607-614

5. National Research Council and Institute of Medicine, Committee on Integrating the Science of Early Childhood Development. *From Neurons to Neighborhoods: The Science of Early Childhood Development.* Shonkoff JP, Phillips DA, eds. Washington, DC: National Academy Press; 2000

6. Dodd VL. Implications of kangaroo care for growth and development in preterm infants. *J Obstet Gynecol Neonatal Nurs.* 2005;34:218-232

7. Feldman R, Eidelman AI, Sirota L, Weller A. Comparison of skin-to-skin (kangaroo) and traditional care: parenting outcomes and preterm infant development. *Pediatrics.* 2002;110:16-26

8. Shackelford J. State and jurisdictional eligibility definitions for infants and toddlers with disabilities under IDEA. NECTAC Notes No. 21. Chapel Hill: The University of North Carolina, FPG Child Development Institute, National Early Childhood Technical Assistance Center; 2006. Available at: http://www.nectac.org/%7Epdfs/pubs/nnotes21.pdf. Accessed March 1, 2006

9. Shore R. What have we learned? In: *Rethinking the Brain: New Insights into Early Development.* New York, NY: Families and Work Institute; 1997:15-55

10. Weinberger DR, Elvevag B, Giedd JN. *The Adolescent Brain: A Work in Progress.* Washington, DC: The National Campaign to Prevent Teen Pregnancy; 2005

11. American Academy of Pediatrics, Task Force on Sudden Infant Death Syndrome. The changing concept of sudden infant death syndrome: diagnostic coding shifts, controversies regarding the sleeping environment, and new variables to consider in reducing risk. *Pediatrics.* 2005;116:1245-1255

12. Gorski PA. Contemporary pediatric practice: in support of infant mental health (imaging and imagining). *Infant Ment Health J.* 2001;22:188-200

13. American Academy of Pediatrics, Committee on Public Education. Children, adolescents, and television. *Pediatrics.* 2001;107:423-426

14. Wright JC, Huston AC, Murphy KC, et al. The relations of early television viewing to school readiness and vocabulary of children from low-income families: the early window project. *Child Dev.* 2001;72:1347-1366

15. Atkinson PM, Parks DK, Cooley SM, Sarkis SL. Reach Out and Read: a pediatric clinic-based approach to early literacy promotion. *J Pediatr Health Care.* 2002;16:10-15

16. High PC, LaGasse L, Becker S, Ahlgren I, Gardner A. Literacy promotion in primary care pediatrics: can we make a difference? *Pediatrics.* 2000;105:927-934

17. Sharif I, Rieber S, Ozuah PO. Exposure to Reach Out and Read and vocabulary outcomes in inner city preschoolers [published erratum appears in *J Natl Med Assoc.* 2002;94(9)]. *J Natl Med Assoc.* 2002;94:171-177

18. Weitzman CC, Roy L, Walls T, Tomlin R. More evidence for reach out and read: a home-based study. *Pediatrics.* 2004;113:1248-1253

19. Mendelsohn AL, Mogilner LN, Dreyer BP, et al. The impact of a clinic-based literacy intervention on language development in inner-city preschool children. *Pediatrics.* 2001;107:130-134

20. Needlman R, Silverstein M. Pediatric interventions to support reading aloud: how good is the evidence? *J Dev Behav Pediatr.* 2004;25:352-363

21. Needlman R, Toker KH, Dreyer BP, Klass P, Mendelsohn AL. Effectiveness of a primary care intervention to support reading aloud: a multicenter evaluation. *Ambul Pediatr.* 2005;5:209-215

22. Overturf Johnson JO. *Who's Minding the Kids? Child Care Arrangements: Winter 2002.* Washington, DC: US Census Bureau; 2005 (Current Population Reports. Household Economic Studies p70, 101)

23. American Academy of Pediatrics, Committee on Early Childhood, Adoption, and Dependent Care. Quality early education and child care from birth to kindergarten. *Pediatrics.* 2005;115:187-191

24. Carlson VJ, Harwood RL. What do we expect? Understanding and negotiating cultural differences concerning early developmental competence: the six raisin solution. *Zero to Three.* 1999;20:19-24

25. National SIDS/Infant Death Resource Center. What is SIDS? Available at: http://www.sidscenter.org/WhatIsSIDS.pdf. Accessed September 4, 2007

26. Barnard KE. *Beginning Rhythms: The Emerging Process of Sleep Wake Behaviors and Self-Regulation.* Seattle, WA: NCAST, University of Washington; 1999

PROMOTING
CHILD DEVELOPMENT

27. Carno MA, Hoffman LA, Carcillo JA, Sanders MH. Developmental stages of sleep from birth to adolescence, common childhood sleep disorders: overview and nursing implications. *J Pediatr Nurs*. 2003;18:274-283

28. Scheers NJ, Rutherford GW, Kemp JS. Where should infants sleep? A comparison of risk for suffocation of infants sleeping in cribs, adult beds, and other sleeping locations. *Pediatrics*. 2003;112:883-889

29. Bornstein MH. *Cultural Approaches to Parenting*. Hillside, NJ: Lawrence Erlbaum; 1991

30. Harkness S, Super CM, Keefer CH, van Tiijin N, van der Klugt E. *Cultural Influences on Sleep Patterns in Infancy and Early Childhood*. Atlanta, GA: American Association for the Advancement of Science; 1995

31. Brenner RA, Simons-Morton BG, Bhaskar B, Revenis M, Das A, Clemens JD. Infant-parent bed sharing in an inner-city population. *Arch Pediatr Adolesc Med*. 2003;157:33-39

32. Nakamura S, Wind M, Danello MA. Review of hazards associated with children placed in adult beds. *Arch Pediatr Adolesc Med*. 1999;153:1019-1023

33. Unger B, Kemp JS, Wilkins D, et al. Racial disparity and modifiable risk factors among infants dying suddenly and unexpectedly. *Pediatrics*. 2003;111(2):e127-e131. Available at: www.pediatrics.org/cgi/content/full/111/2/e127. Accessed May 4, 2007

34. Willinger M, Ko CW, Hoffman HJ, Kessler RC, Corwin MJ. Factors associated with caregivers' choice of infant sleep position, 1994-1998: the National Infant Sleep Position Study. *JAMA*. 2000;283:2135-2142

35. Li DK, Petitti DB, Willinger M, et al. Infant sleeping position and the risk of sudden infant death syndrome in California, 1997-2000. *Am J Epidemiol*. 2003;157:446-455

36. Sivan Y, Reisner S, Amitai Y, Wasser J, Nehama H, Tauman R. Effect of religious observance on infants' sleep position in the Jewish population. *J Paediatr Child Health*. 2004;40:534-539

37. Willinger M, Ko CW, Hoffman HJ, Kessler RC, Corwin MJ. Trends in infant bed sharing in the United States, 1993-2000: the National Infant Sleep Position study. *Arch Pediatr Adolesc Med*. 2003;157:43-49

38. Frankenburg WK, Dodds J, Archer P, et al: DENVER II Training Manual, 1992. Denver Developmental Materials. Denver, CO

39. Diego MA, Field T, Hart S, et al. Facial expressions and EEG in infants of intrusive and withdrawn mothers with depressive symptoms. *Depress Anxiety*. 2002;15:10-17

40. Diego MA, Field T, Hernandez-Reif M, Cullen C, Schanberg S, Kuhn C. Prepartum, postpartum, and chronic depression effects on newborns. *Psychiatry*. 2004;67:63-80

41. Field T. Early interventions for infants of depressed mothers. *Pediatrics*. 1998;102(5 Suppl E):1305-1310

42. Bowman BT. Educating language minority children: challenges and opportunities. *Phi Delta Kappan*. 1989;71:118-120

43. Kopp CB. Antecedents of self-regulation: a developmental perspective. *Dev Psychol*. 1982;18:199-214.

44. Raffaelli M, Crockett LJ, Shen YL. Developmental stability and change in self-regulation from childhood to adolescence. *J Genet Psychol*. 2005;166:54-75

45. Thiedke CC. Nocturnal enuresis. *Am Fam Physician*. 2003;67:1499-1506

46. Evans GD. *Bedwetting*. Gainesville, FL: Department of Family, Youth, and Community Sciences, Florida Cooperative Extension Service, Institute of Food and Agriculture Sciences, University of Florida; 2003. Available at: http://edis.fas.ufl.edu/pdffiles/HE/HE79400.pdf. Accessed September 13, 2007

47. Search Institute. Developmental Assets. Minneapolis, MN: Search Institute; 1997. Available at: http://www.search-institute.org/assets. Accessed September 5, 2007

48. Scales P, Leffert N, Lerner RM. *Developmental Assets: A Synthesis of the Scientific Research on Adolescent Development*. Minneapolis, MN: Search Institute; 1999

49. Biles B. Activities that promote racial and cultural awareness. *Family Child-Care Connections*. 1994;4:1-4. Available at: http://web.aces.uiuc.edu/vista/pdf_pubs/CHILDCARE.PDF. Accessed September 13, 2007

50. American Academy of Pediatrics, Committee on Psychosocial Aspects of Child and Family Health. Guidance for effective discipline. *Pediatrics*. 1998;101:723-728. Erratum in: *Pediatrics*. 1998;102-433

51. Burns MS, Griffin P, Snow CE. *Starting Out Right: A Guide to Promoting Children's Reading Success*. Washington, DC: National Academy Press; 1999

52. Podhajski B, Nathan J. Promoting early literacy through professional development for childcare providers. *Early Educ Dev*. 2005;16:1-5

53. Zuckerman BS, Klass P. Doctors Promoting Child Development with Books. Available at: http://www.ced.org/docs/report/report_ivk_zuckerman_2006.pdf. Accessed September 5, 2007

54. Glassy D, Romano J, American Academy of Pediatrics, Committee on Early Childhood, Adoption, and Dependent Care. Selecting appropriate toys for young children: the pediatrician's role. *Pediatrics*. 2003;111:911-913

55. US Department of Health and Human Services, Health Resources and Services Administration, Maternal and Child Health Bureau. *Child Health USA 2004*. Rockville, MD: US Department of Health and Human Services; 2004. Available at www.mchb.hrsa.gov/mchirc/chusa_04/-pdf/eo4.pdf. Accessed September 13, 2007

56. Capizzano J, Adams G, Sonenstein F. *Child Care Arrangements for Children Under Five: Variation Across States*. Washington, DC: Urban Institute; 2000

57. Raver CC. *Emotions Matter: Making the Case for the Role of Young Children's Emotional Development for Early School Readiness*. Ann Arbor, MI: Society for Research in Child Development; 2002

58. Rimm-Kaufman SE, Pianta RC, Cox MJ. Teachers' judgments of problems in the transition to kindergarten. *Early Child Res Q*. 2000;15:147-166

PROMOTING CHILD DEVELOPMENT

59. Rouse C, Brooks-Gunn J, McLanahan S. School readiness: closing racial and ethnic gaps: introducing the issue. *Future Child*. 2005;15:5-14

60. Farran DC, Shonkoff JP. Developmental disabilities and the concept of school readiness. *Early Educ Dev*. 1994;5:141-151

61. West J, Flanagan KD, Germino-Hausken E. *America's Kindergartners: Findings from the Early Childhood Longitudinal Study, Kindergarten Class of 1998-99* Fall 1998. Washington, DC: US Department of Education, National Center for Education Statistics; 1998. Publication No. NCES 2000070

62. Meisels SJ. Assessing readiness. In: Pianta RC, Cox MJ, eds. *The Transition to Kindergarten*. Baltimore, MD: Paul H Brookes; 1999:39-66

63. Coplan J. *Early Language Milestone Scale*. 2nd ed. Austin, TX: Pro-Ed Inc; 1993

64. English A, Kenney KE. *State Minor Consent Laws: A Summary*. 2nd Ed. Chapel Hill, NC: Center for Adolescent Health & The Law; 2003

65. Resnick MD, Bearman PS, Blum RW, et al. Protecting adolescents from harm. Findings from the National Longitudinal Study on Adolescent Health. *JAMA*. 1997;278:823-832

66. Redd Z, Brooks J, McGarvey AM. Educating America's Youth: What Makes a Difference. Washington, DC: Child Trends; 2002

67. Bloom B, Dey AN. Summary health statistics for U.S. children: National Health Interview Survey, 2004. *Vital Health Stat 10*. 2006;Feb(227):1-85

68. US Department of Education. *Helping Your Child Through Early Adolescence for Parents of Children from 10 through 14*. Washington, DC: US Department of Education. Available at: http://www.ed.gov/parents/academic/help/adolescence/adolescence.pdf. Accessed September 5, 2007

69. Irwin CE. The adolescent, health, and society: from the perspective of the physician. In: Millstein SG, Peterson AC, Nightingale EO, eds. *Promoting the Health of Adolescents: New Directions for the Twenty-first Century*. New York, NY: Oxford University Press; 1993:146-150

70. Dodge KA. A social information processing model of social competence in children. In: Perlmutter M, ed. *Minnesota Symposium on Child Psychology*. Vol 18. Hillsdale, NJ: Lawrence Erlbaum Associates; 1986:77-125

71. Hair EC, Jager J, Garrett SB. *Helping Teens Develop Healthy Social Skills and Relationships: What the Research Shows About Navigating Adolescence*. Washington, DC: Child Trends; 2002

72. Resnick MD. Protective factors, resiliency and healthy youth development. *Adolesc Med*. 2000;11:157-165

73. Resnick MD. Resilience and protective factors in the lives of adolescents. *J Adolesc Health*. 2000;27:1-2

74. Steinberg L. Gallagher lecture. The family at adolescence: transition and transformation. *J Adolesc Health*. 2000;27:170-178

75. Steinberg L, Lamborn SD, Dornbusch SM, Darling N. Impact of parenting practices on adolescent achievement: authoritative parenting, school involvement, and encouragement to succeed. *Child Dev*. 1992;63:1266-1281

PROMOTING
CHILD DEVELOPMENT

Promoting Mental Health

Theme 3

INTRODUCTION

Establishing mental health and emotional well-being is arguably the core task for the developing child and those who care for the child. Because cultures may differ in their conceptions of mental health, it is important for the health care professional to learn about the family members' perceptions of a mentally healthy individual and their goals for raising their children. In their shared work to raise a child, parents, family, community, and professionals commit to fostering the development of that child's sense of connectedness, self-worth and joyfulness, intellectual growth, and the many brain functions that define mental health. Shonkoff et al[1] describe that marvelous process of the child's development of mental health in their book *From Neurons to Neighborhoods*. Because of its overwhelming importance to overall health and because mental health risks and problems are all too common, promoting mental health has been identified as 1 of 2 themes with special significance.

Each Bright Futures visit addresses the physical and mental health of the child or adolescent. Although consideration of physical abnormalities or nutritional needs may come easily to the practitioner, proper and effective techniques to consider and assess a child's and family's mental health are not integral to the current standard of care.

This edition of the *Bright Futures Guidelines*, therefore, highlights opportunities for promoting mental health in every child, beginning in this section and continuing to include specific suggestions in each of the visits.

Mental health can be compromised at many critical times in development. The health care professional, therefore, is challenged to promote mental health in activities that are aimed at prevention, risk assessment, and diagnosis and to offer an array of appropriate interventions. Common risk factors for child behavioral and mental health problems include[2]:

- Genetic risk factors (eg, congenital developmental disability)
- Chronic medical illness

- Social risk factors
  - Poverty or homelessness
  - Exposure to domestic violence
- Family risk factors
  - Maternal depression and social isolation
  - Separation or divorce
  - Chronic physical or mental illness in family members
  - Substance abuse by a family member
- Skills deficiencies
  - Lack of parenting knowledge or performance deficits
  - Child social skills deficits
  - Masked school failure and learning disability

Common challenges to child, adolescent, and family mental health are further described in this theme by age of highest prevalence.

Bright Futures in Practice: Mental Health[3] expertly and extensively addresses child and family mental health. Diagnostic criteria, treatment options, diagnostic coding, and selected assessment tools are included. The mental health book also describes, in greater detail, the mental health disorders discussed in this edition of the *Bright Futures Guidelines*, along with many other disorders not mentioned here. Issues discussed here were chosen to provide facts and contextual information that are essential to the work of the health care professional in the primary care setting.

The American Academy of Pediatrics (AAP) *The Classification of Child and Adolescent Mental Diagnosis in Primary Care (DSM-PC)*[4] can aid health care professionals in diagnosing and treating common mental disorders by helping them determine the degree of severity of a behavioral or mental problem and when to refer to a mental health specialist or an early intervention program.

Half of all the lifetime cases of mental illness begin by the age of 14 years, which means that mental disorders are chronic diseases of the young.

Prevalence and Trends in Mental Health Problems Among Children and Adolescents

Half of all the lifetime cases of mental illness begin by the age of 14 years, which means that mental disorders are chronic diseases of the young.[5] An estimated 21% of US children and adolescents aged 9 to 17 years have a diagnosable mental health disorder that causes at least some impairment,[6] and the underdetection of mental health problems in pediatric practice has been well documented and recognized.[7,8] In any given year, fewer than 1 in 5 of these youth receive needed treatment.[7] For many youth, mental health problems may lead to the juvenile justice system. A high rate of psychiatric disorders (66% of boys and 75% of girls) exists among youth in juvenile justice facilities; about half were addicted to, or had abused, substances.[9]

Screening and Referral

Primary care practitioners are ideally situated to begin the process of identifying children with problem behaviors that might indicate mental disorders. They meet with children and families at regular intervals, so this frequent access to a primary care medical home is more available than access to specific mental health services. Building a solid collaboration among the health care professional and other service providers (eg, psychiatrists, psychologists, social workers, and therapists) and agencies (eg, schools, mental health agencies, state departments of health, agencies serving children and youth with special health care needs, and child protection services) improves the effectiveness of support for children and, ultimately, the possibilities of positive outcomes for the children. (For more information on this topic, see the Promoting Community Relationships and Resources theme.) This need is illustrated by the fact that although psychosocial problems identified in pediatric offices increased from 6.8% to 18.7% in the 17-year period of 1979-1996,[10] health care professionals often have limited access to professionals with appropriate training and skills to assist them with behavior screening, treatment, and referral issues.[11]

Pediatric behavioral, developmental, and mental health issues are more common than childhood cancers, cardiac problems, and renal problems combined. However, research has repeatedly shown that primary care physicians recognize less than 30% of children with substantial dysfunction.[12] This lack of recognition is due to the necessary brevity of pediatric appointments and stigma associated with mental health concerns, which results in hesitancy to bring up subject areas where no "quick fix" exists. However, in some cases, the primary care practitioner can assess the child's problem and provide appropriate and successful intervention. In other instances, when a problem is identified outside of the realm of her expertise, the practitioner must be able to refer the family to experts who can provide a complete evaluation and treatment plan. The health care professional should try to determine whether the nature of the problem falls within her areas of interest and expertise before offering interventions.

Existing screening tools can help the health care professional recognize possible mental health concerns. For example, periodic screening for maternal depression has been recommended and found to be feasible during an infant health supervision visit.[13,14] It is important to consider autism spectrum disorders (ASDs) for 15-month-old children in routine developmental surveillance; in addition, specific screening tools are available and appropriate for the 18 and 24 Month Visits.[15] One of the most efficient ways for health care professionals to improve the recognition and treatment of psychosocial problems in children and adolescents is by using a mental health screening test, such as the 35-item Pediatric Symptom Checklist (PSC)[3] or the more brief PSC-17,[16] which can be completed in the waiting room by a parent. A positive score on the PSC suggests the need for further evaluation.

Screening does not provide a diagnosis for a mental health disorder, however. Screening indicates the severity of symptoms, assesses the severity within a given time period, and provides a way to begin a conversation about mental health issues. Health care professionals must be adept at identifying mental health concerns and determining whether they are leading to impaired functioning at home, school, with peers, or in the community. Providing education to the patient and parent about mental health disorders, symptoms, causes, and treatments is an important first step to help the family take charge of its management if a disorder does exist, avoid placing blame, and allow for reasonable expectations to be set.

Health care professionals also can improve access to high-quality care for mental health disorders,[17] although, before seeing the child or adolescent or the parent, they should decide whether to provide in-office treatment or refer the patient. Training and past experience will guide this decision, but time constraints to provide ongoing management also are a consideration.[18] The presence of a trusting relationship between the child, adolescent, or parent and the health care professional often predicts a successful treatment or referral process. Child health care professionals in primary care should assess their ability to manage mild, moderate, and severe emotional problems with or without consultation. The level of health care professional competence, clinical need, and availability of mental health referral should help dictate the conditions for referral. Referral may be appropriate in the following situations:

- Emotional dysfunction is evident in more than one of the 3 critical areas of the child's or adolescent's life—home, school, and peers.
- The patient is acutely suicidal or has signs of psychosis.

The presence of a trusting relationship between the child, adolescent, or parent and the health care professional often predicts a successful treatment or referral process.

PROMOTING MENTAL HEALTH

- Diagnostic uncertainty exists.
- The patient has not responded to treatment.
- The parent requests referral.
- The adolescent's behavior creates discomfort for the health care professional, potentially precluding an objective evaluation (eg, adolescents with acting-out or seductive behaviors).
- The patient, or her family, has a social relationship with the treating health care professional.

When the possibility of referral has been brought up early in the process, acceptance of mental health treatment may be better. The health care professional should discuss with the family members their views on referral to a mental health professional and acknowledge that stigma often is associated with such referral. Understanding how the family's culture can affect the view of treatment for mental health issues, and knowing resources that will support those views, can greatly enhance the success of the referral process. The health care professional should learn how the family's culture views emotional and behavioral problems and should connect the family with culturally appropriate services.

Many syndromes that are primarily neurologic, genetic, or developmental in nature will include mental health symptoms or conditions.

Children and Youth With Special Health Care Needs

Children and adolescents with chronic health conditions require special consideration concerning their mental health needs. Many syndromes that are primarily neurologic, genetic, or developmental in nature will include mental health symptoms or conditions. Other chronic health conditions share comorbidity with mental health diagnoses. Attention to these components of the child's or adolescent's special health care need is a basic and essential part of her care.

In addition, any chronic health condition brings stressors to both child and family.

These diagnoses, while secondary to the medical problem, are essential components of the child's health. Health care professionals who care for children and youth with special health care needs must be alert to complications of anxiety, depression, or problems of adjustment. These components of care can be found in the medical home model of care.[19]

Promoting Mental Health and Emotional Well-Being: Infancy—Birth to 11 Months

Infant mental health is the flourishing of a baby's capacity for warm connection with his parents. The interaction between parent and infant is central to the infant's physical, cognitive, social, and emotional development, as well as to his self-regulation abilities. The infant brings his strengths to this interaction, in terms of temperamental style, physical attractiveness, health, and vigor. The ability of the parents to respond well is determined by their life stresses, their past experiences with children, their knowledge, and their own experiences of being nurtured in childhood. Their perceptions of the infant also can color the interaction. These perceptions derive from their own expectations, needs, and desires, as well as from the projection of other people's characteristics onto the child.

The infant's emotions may be affected by the emotional and physical health of the caregiver.[20] Depression is common in many mothers of infants and can seriously impair the baby's emotional and even physical well-being because of neglect of the infant's needs and lack of reinforcement to the infant's engagement cues. Parental substance abuse can have similar effects. Health supervision for the child must, therefore, include monitoring the emotional health of the parents or primary caregivers.

Patterns of Attachment

Attachment describes the process of interrelation between a child and her parent, and is central to healthy mental and emotional development. Attachment is influenced by parental, child-related, and environmental factors. Health care professionals can teach parents the importance of the quality of their interaction with their infant and the impact of attachment on the development of the child's sense of self-worth, comfort, and trust.

Health care professionals should observe the attachment style and pattern during clinical encounters with infants and parents. They should give anticipatory guidance to assist families in enhancing secure development.

Three patterns of attachment have been described in infants and young children—*secure attachment, insecure and avoidant attachment,* and *insecure attachment characterized by ambivalence and resistance* (Box 1).

Challenges to the Development of Mental Health

INFANT WELL-BEING

Signs of possible problems in emotional well-being in infants include the following:

- Poor eye contact
- Lack of brightening on seeing parent
- Lack of smiling with parent or other engaging adult
- Lack of vocalizations
- Not quieting with parent's voice
- Not turning to sound of parent's voice
- Extremely low activity level or tone

- Lack of mouthing to explore objects
- Excessive irritability with difficulty in calming
- Sad or somber facial expression (evident by 3 months of age)
- Wariness (evident by 4 months of age; precursor to fear, which is evident by 9 months of age)
- Dysregulation in sleep
- Physical dysregulation (eg, vomiting or diarrhea)
- Poor weight gain

BOX 1
Attachment Patterns

Secure attachment
Parent: Is sensitive, responsive, and available
Child: Feels valued and worthwhile; has a secure base; feels effective; feels able to explore and master, knowing that parent is available; and becomes autonomous

Insecure and avoidant attachment
Parent: Is insensitive to child's cues, avoids contact, and rejects
Child: Feels no one is there for him; cannot rely on adults to get needs met; feels he will be rejected if needs for attachment and closeness are shown and, therefore, asks for little to maintain some connection; and learns not to recognize his own need for closeness and connectedness

Insecure attachment characterized by ambivalence and resistance
Parent: Shows inconsistent patterns of care; is unpredictable; may be excessively close or intrusive and then push away; and seen frequently with depressed caregiver
Child: Feels he should keep adult engaged because he never knows when he will get attention back; anxious; dependent; and clingy

---

Health care professionals can teach parents the importance of the quality of their interaction with their infant and the impact of attachment on the development of the child's sense of self-worth, comfort, and trust.

PROMOTING MENTAL HEALTH

If the infant appears to have problems with emotional development, the health care professional should determine the degree to which the parents may be experiencing depression, post-traumatic stress disorder (PTSD), substance abuse, or domestic violence. A mental health professional or a child health care professional who is skilled in developmental behavior should then evaluate the parent-child interaction.

CHILD MALTREATMENT AND NEGLECT

Child maltreatment or abuse can occur in any family. Without identification and intervention, unchecked acute and chronic stressors in a household can lead to child neglect or abuse.

Many factors are associated with child maltreatment, including the following:

- A child who is perceived by parents to be demanding or difficult to satisfy
- An infant who is diagnosed with a chronic illness or disability
- A family who is socially isolated, without community support
- Mental health issues with one or both parents that have not been diagnosed and treated
- A parent with career difficulties, who may see the newborn as an impediment or burden

Infants and toddlers are at higher risk for abuse and neglect than older children. Children who are younger than 3 years account for more than one third of all maltreated children. Forty-one percent of fatally abused children are younger than 1 year.[21] A disproportionate number of these children are in families that live in poverty and experience familial disruption. Their families live in high-risk environments and frequently confront substance abuse, mental or physical illness, family violence, or inadequate living conditions. More than half of reports to child

protective services are for child neglect, yet this often can go undetected because the physical and emotional findings can be subtle.

Health care professionals should learn to recognize infants who are being abused or are at risk for abuse by the mother, father, or other member of the household. If abuse is suspected, the health care professional should ask direct questions in a respectful way to determine whether any kind of abuse might be occurring. Any unexplained bruises or other signs of abuse should be thoroughly investigated.

Abuse and neglect at this early stage have long-term effects on brain development and increase the likelihood of behavioral disorders in the child. The earlier in life the child is subjected to neglect or physical or emotional abuse, and the longer the abuse continues, the greater the risk to her emotional and behavioral development. Recognizing the risk of maltreatment or abuse to the child's healthy physical and mental development is as vital as recognizing a nutritional deficiency or toxin exposure. Physical and mental abuse during the first few years of a child's life can cause her to develop hypervigilance and fear. An infant who is under chronic stress can respond with apathy, poor feeding, withdrawal, and failure to thrive. When the infant is under acute threat, the typical "fight" response to stress can change from crying to temper tantrums, aggressive behaviors, or inattention and withdrawal. The child can become psychologically disengaged, leading to detachment and apathy. This response, in turn, has an impact on the child's ability to form healthy trusting relationships with adults and peers. Studies show that, as children get older, those who have been abused or neglected are more likely to perform poorly in school, to commit crimes, and to experience emotional problems, sexual problems, and alcohol or substance abuse.[22]

If abuse is suspected, the health care professional should ask direct questions in a respectful way to determine whether any kind of abuse might be occurring.

Bright FUTURES

PROMOTING MENTAL HEALTH

SHAKEN BABY SYNDROME

Shaken baby syndrome (SBS), also referred to as "shaken impact syndrome," is the nonaccidental traumatic injury that results from violent shaking of an infant or child. Head injury from SBS is the leading cause of death and long-term disability in children who are physically abused.[23,24] Victims typically are infants younger than 1 year, most often younger than 6 months. Infants who cry excessively, have difficult temperaments or are "colicky," or who are perceived by their caregivers to require excessive attention are at increased risk. Male infants, infants with very low birth weight, premature babies, and children with disabilities are at highest risk for SBS or physical violence.

SBS often has its roots in unrealistic expectations and parents' lack of understanding of infant development, which contribute to frustration, stress, limited tolerance, and resentment toward the infant. Parents of hospitalized or chronically ill children experience increased levels of stress, anxiety, exhaustion, depression, perceived loss of control, anger, grief, chronic sorrow, and poor adjustment. Normal behaviors for an infant, such as crying, can be frustrating, especially for parents who are sleep deprived, depressed, or experiencing other stresses. At times, most parents feel frustrated and confused if their infant exhibits any of the following:

- Cries and can be consoled only with constant holding or rocking
- Cries and is not consoled with holding, rocking, or other parent efforts
- Will not go to sleep easily, or awakens at the slightest sound and then will not return to sleep
- Stays awake for extended periods or is perceived to need constant attention
- Has feeding difficulties, such as
  - Spitting up after almost every feeding or vomiting frequently
  - Poor oromotor skills, poor sucking, or feed refusal, or takes more than 30 to 40 minutes for a feeding

- Is hungry all the time or eats a large amount and then spits up
- Takes only short naps during the day and then is fussy in the early evening

The stressed parent or caregiver may be unaware of the infant's vulnerability. Injury can occur when the parent is frustrated by the child's normal, but irritating, behavior. Health care professionals should listen to how the family is coping with their new infant, lack of sleep, their infant's crying, and other concerns. Asking how the parent reacts to these situations can reveal that the baby has been shaken or slapped or is at risk of being shaken. In this case, health care professionals should firmly educate the parents on the dangers of SBS and give them alternative strategies for helping the infant to stop crying, go to sleep, or feed as expected.

Community resources, such as home visiting programs,[25] early intervention services, and educational programs, should be offered to support the parents. It also is important to know about local and state reporting requirements regarding suspected child mistreatment. Health care professionals are mandated reporters and should err on the side of bringing concerns to authorities who will then investigate the issues. It is best practice to share concerns with the family and to explain to the family the legal obligation to report. In general, reporting without the family's knowledge is counterproductive because it can lead the family to further distrust the health care system.

CARING FOR THE FAMILY FACING INFANT ILLNESS OR DEATH

Caring for the parents and family of a sick or disabled child challenges the support and crisis intervention skills of the health care professional. Advances in medical science mean that an increased number of families are experiencing preterm birth or prenatal diagnosis of a significant health condition in the infant.

Head injury from Shaken Baby Syndrome is the leading cause of death and long-term disability in children who are physically abused.

PROMOTING MENTAL HEALTH

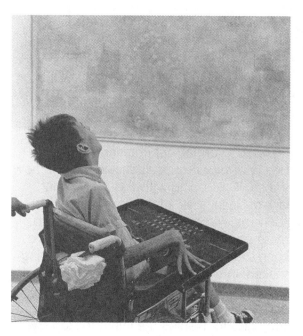

Hope, empowerment, and parent-professional partnerships are important factors in the adaptation and healing after a high-risk birth or the birth of a child with a disability.

The premature birth or an infant's illness at delivery may mean separating the infant from the mother and family, thereby impeding the attachment process. The health care professional should recognize and validate the range of responses and the strengths and needs of parents as individuals. The extended family of grandparents and relatives, as well as individual and community beliefs, values, and expectations, affect a parent's ability to adapt to having a low birth weight or sick infant.

Hope, empowerment, and parent-professional partnerships are important factors in the adaptation and healing after a high-risk birth or the birth of a child with a disability. Parents benefit from guidance and practical tools for their day-to-day living. Referrals to support groups and culturally appropriate community networks of support, combined with practical information, provide important support for families.

When parents have an infant with a disability or serious health problem, health care professionals must recognize that they will go through a process of grieving and mourning

for the anticipated and idealized child. Parents need support to understand that this is a normal and necessary process if they are to be able to form a close attachment to their infant. If their infant is critically ill, parents must learn to deal with life and death decisions and uncertainty, and understand the realities of medical decision making. Parents' responses can involve chronic or recurrent sorrow and sadness, regardless of the infant's clinical condition or level of health care need. The health care professional should be aware of specific red flags, such as symptoms of acute depression, agitation, or inability to carry out normal daily responsibilities, which should prompt referral for immediate medical or mental health care. The health care professional also should assess the parent-infant relationship for signs of inappropriate attachment, excessive perceived child vulnerability, parental guilt, and infant abuse or neglect involving the infant or other children. The health care professional also should seek to understand parents' personal strengths and the strengths they may access that are related to their cultural and religious beliefs.

Some parents tend to be permissive toward a child with a medical illness and are reluctant to set disciplinary boundaries. This reaction can happen because a parent feels sad for the child, but it also can lead to behavioral difficulties. These children sometimes are in the greatest need of a predictable structure regarding rules because other aspects of their life are not predictable.

Promoting Mental Health and Emotional Well-Being: Early Childhood—1 to 4 Years

Mental health in early childhood is tightly bound to healthy development in the child, healthy relationships within the family, and strong support for both child and family in the community. Between the ages of 1 and 4 years, the child makes remarkable advances in his abilities to rely on himself, direct his energies, and interact with others. Building from a secure base of trust in his family, his growing autonomy leads to new explorations and a beginning identity as a distinct and capable person. Within the context of a positive and supportive parent-child relationship, this new growth toward autonomy and self-determined initiative forms the basis for self-esteem, curiosity about the world, and self-confidence. Steady gains are made, as well, in the capacity for self-control and more effective regulation of strong emotions, including anger, sadness, and frustration. Maturation in emotional development, along with new communicative skills, sets the stage for dramatic growth in social understanding and behavior. Child care programs become the arenas for practice in social interaction and in learning to share with others and to express needs and feelings. From home and child care experiences, the child develops important early realizations regarding morality and fair play.

The increasingly self-aware young child grapples with complex issues, such as gender roles, peer or sibling competition, cooperation, and the difference between right and wrong. The temperamental differences that were manifested in the feeding, sleeping, and self-regulatory behaviors of the infant are transformed into the varied styles of coping and adaptation that are demonstrated by the young child. Some young children appear to think before they act; others are impetuous. Some children are slow to warm up, whereas others are friendly and outgoing. Some accept limits and rules more easily than others. The range of "normal" behavior is broad and highly dependent on the match between the child's and the caregiver's styles. Aggression, acting out, excessive risk taking, and antisocial behaviors can appear at this time. Caregivers need to respond with a variety of interventions that set constructive limits and help children achieve self-discipline. Ultimately, healthy social and emotional development depend on how children view themselves and the extent to which they feel valued by others.

Mental health and behavioral concerns can coalesce around a particular behavioral symptom in the child. The health care professional will want to consider underlying child-based factors, which are described in more detail in later sections. In addition, physical, psychological, and social issues of a parent can affect the child's emerging sense of self in relation to others, and must be considered in attempting to understand the origin of a child's behavior. Important parental issues include the parents' state of physical and mental health, their temperament, their past and present stressors, and their experiences as a child with their own parents.

Patterns of Attachment

Patterns of attachment between child and parent can be observed in early childhood and are useful in predicting healthy development as well as predicting behavioral problems and disorders in the child.[26] As independence and autonomy take center stage for the child, issues of caring, connectedness, and trust become increasingly important for a family. Health care professionals should seek to understand the family's perceptions of these issues from their personal and cultural perspectives to effectively assess strengths and concerns for the child's development.

As the child's world expands during this developmental stage, she will begin to interact regularly with other adults beyond her parents, including aunts and uncles, grandparents, day care providers, and preschool teachers. She will develop patterns of attachment with these adults as well. Secure and loving attachment in these relationships can help ensure her healthy development.

The range of "normal" behavior is broad and highly dependent on the match between the child's and the caregiver's styles.

PROMOTING MENTAL HEALTH

Challenges to the Development of Mental Health

BEHAVIORAL PATTERNS

When a child's behavioral patterns and responses seem chronically off track from those expected for his age, the health care professional should assess the following:

- Developmental capacities of the child, especially those connected with the challenges that provoke the concerning behavior
- Physical health conditions that might influence the child emotionally and behaviorally
- Temperament and sensory-processing abilities of the child
- The relationship between the child and the conditions and demands of the child's caregiving environment
- The quality of the parent-child relationship and security of the attachment
- Family understanding of the child's behavior, specifically regarding the child's underlying feelings and motivations, and the family's responses to the behavior
- Broader contextual circumstances, including family stress, family change, cultural expectations and influences, and child care or preschool experiences
- Depression in the child

The health care professional can gain a detailed understanding of the child's behavior in a particular situation in an ABC (Antecedents, Behavior, Consequences) approach,[27] which consists of asking the parents or other caregiver who saw what happened to explain in detail:

- The *antecedents*, or the conditions and circumstances in which the behavior occurs (eg, biting mainly occurs at preschool when the child is asked to stop playing)
- The *behavior* itself

- The *consequences* of the behavior for the child, and for others affected, both immediate and long-term

The parents' explanations for *why* the child is behaving in a certain way are key to understanding their reactions to the child's difficulties. Personal and cultural norms, views on how development proceeds, and theories of motivation will affect how the parent evaluates the child's behavior. This *ABC* approach avoids misleading generalizations about a particular behavior and focuses on the unique elements of the child, his relationships with family, peers, or caregivers who are important to him, and the contexts for the behavior.

When concerns about behavior are noted, the health care professional might ask the parent, "Who cares for your child during the day?" Young children may "act out," exhibit aggressive behaviors, or hurt other children because they are not supervised directly or are not disciplined in an appropriate and positive manner. They may be exhibiting negative behaviors because they spend time with someone else who acts poorly. This can occur even when the child is in a quality child care environment if the program or caregiver isn't a "good fit" for the child's temperament or personality. Asking about the child's environment or asking for the parent's permission to speak to the caregiver directly can lead to enlightening discussions that may enable the health care professional to offer effective guidance.

Table 1 shows ways that certain domains of influence can contribute, individually or in combination, to the development of behavioral problems and disorders in early childhood. By exploring these 4 domains of influence with the parent, the health care professional can better understand the behavioral problem, recognize the strengths that are inherent in the child, and assist the parent and other caregivers in making adjustments when needed. Parents have expressed

The parents' explanations for why the child is behaving in a certain way are key to understanding their reactions to the child's difficulties.

eagerness for their child's health care professionals to spend more time with them on behavioral concerns.[28] This approach to identifying strengths, anticipating developmental challenges, and solving behavioral problems will be extremely helpful in supporting and counseling families. This evaluation is best done at the primary care level. Health care professionals can then assess the efforts that parents make in response to guidance and the effect of those efforts on the child to determine the need for further mental health referral. The time and attention the primary

care provider gives to these concerns facilitate the parents' acceptance of a mental health referral when indicated.

Families from different cultures have differing developmental and behavioral expectations for their children. Begin any discussion of these issues with a dialogue about what parents expect and why. Understanding these expectations will help the health care professional provide effective and appropriate support to the parents.

TABLE 1

Domains of Influence

Examples of Behavioral Concerns	Developmental/ Health Status	Temperament and Sensory Processing[29]	Family-Child Interactions	Other Environmental Influences
Bedtime struggles: •Trouble getting the child to sleep •Difficulties with night waking	Does the child's capacity to calm herself and transition into a sleep state seem unusually delayed for that child's age? Are specific health conditions involved? Was there a recent illness?	What is the influence of the child's temperament, especially: •Biologic regularity? •Adaptability? •Reactivity to sensory input?	Has the family provided a predictable and developmentally appropriate ritual for helping the child settle into sleep? Does the family allow her to fall asleep on her own? Is the child feeling insecure because of lack of adequate time with the parent? What are the family's expectations regarding where the child sleeps? Does the child have a transitional object?	Is there a quiet room for sleeping that is free of television and sibling activities? (For families living in small spaces, this may be unattainable.) Are there any changes or tensions in the family that are likely to be felt by the child, such as the mother returning to work, a change in child care, or a new sibling?
Resistance to toilet training	Is the child developmentally ready, including showing interest? Is there any suspicion of painful defecation or constipation?	What is the influence of the child's temperament, especially: •Biologic regularity? •Reactivity to sensory input? •Distractibility?	Is the parent's approach in sync with the child's developmental status and temperament? Are there culturally based expectations that are forming the parents' expectations? Is there undue pressure or are there negative reactions from parents and others? Are there any signs of fearfulness by the child?	Is toilet training being attempted during a period of major change or high stress? What are the toileting routines at child care/ preschool? Are they compatible with home routines?

TABLE 1 *(continued)*

Examples of Behavioral Concerns	Developmental/ Health Status	Temperament and Sensory Processing[29]	Family-Child Interactions	Other Environmental Influences
Excessive temper tantrums	What other means does the child have for expressing frustration and anger? Can she do so through speech? Are there developmental delays in self-care or other skills that routinely cause frustration? Are there physical causes of chronic discomfort or pain, such as eczema or chronic rhinitis? Is the child getting sufficient sleep?	What is the influence of the child's temperament, especially: •High intensity? •Negative mood? •Reactivity to sensory input? •High persistence?	What is the child trying to communicate through the tantrum? Are there specific events or interactions in the family that trigger the tantrums? How do the parents respond? Do their responses help calm the child or escalate the tantrum? Are the parents able to give support without giving in to unacceptable demands?	Are the tantrums linked to family change or stress? Are other family members also experiencing high levels of frustration? How is anger generally expressed in the family? Are the tantrums linked to a change in the child care setting or child care provider?
Chronic aggression	Are there developmental delays that contribute to chronic frustration, including deficits in expressive language and fine-motor abilities?	What is the influence of the child's temperament, especially: •Negative mood? •Highly impulsive? •Difficulty in adapting to changes in routine? •High intensity? •Unusually sensitive to sensory input? •Has she learned to attack before she is threatened?	Is the child needy or angry because emotional needs are unmet? What is the quality of the parent-child attachment? Is the child seeking attention? Is there overt or covert encouragement of aggression in the family, such as an indication that parents are proud of child being "feisty," or showing acceptance of aggression by ignoring it? Is there a parental perception that being aggressive is a survival tactic in the neighbor-hood or community?	Has the child witnessed violence and aggression, especially within her family? Has the child witnessed, or been exposed to, violence or aggression in the community or neighborhood? Has she experienced physical abuse herself, at home or in child care? Have there been significant disruptions in the life of the family that affects daily routines? Has there been unsupervised viewing of violent or mature TV or video games?
Difficulty in forming friendships	Are there developmental delays, especially in expressive language and fine-motor skills? (Social-skill deficits are a central feature of pervasive developmental disorders and autism.)	What is the influence of the child's temperament, especially: •Shy, inhibited, or slow to warm up? •Sensory processing abnormalities with hypersensitivities or hyposensitivities?	How does the child's social behavior differ within the family compared to that of peers? Does the child have a secure emotional base with the parent?	Does the child have opportunities to meet and play with other children? Are the conditions for those interactions optimal for the child? For example, many children who are shy do better with short play dates with one other child than with extended time with large groups.

PROMOTING MENTAL HEALTH

Bright FUTURES

TABLE 1 (continued)

Examples of Behavioral Concerns	Developmental/ Health Status	Temperament and Sensory Processing[29]	Family-Child Interactions	Other Environmental Influences
Excessive anxiety; can be expressed by excessive fearfulness, clingy behaviors, frequent crying, tantrums or frequent nightmares, and other sleep problems. *Separation anxiety* is developmentally normal during the first 3 years of life; thereafter, it should steadily lessen.	Are there developmental delays or disabilities that reduce the child's capacity for expression and control? Are there chronic health conditions that affect sense of comfort and security? Are there perceived risks to health by the family ("the vulnerable child syndrome")? Are there any acute health problems requiring separation from a parent?	What is the influence of the child's temperament, especially: • Shy, inhibited, slow to warm up? • Avoidance of new situations? • Difficulty in adapting to changes in routine? • Sensory processing abnormalities, with hypersensitivities?	Is there a pattern of overprotectiveness or underprotectiveness from the parent? Does the parent accurately read the child's cues and show appropriate empathy? Or, is the parent's sensitivity to cues heightened, awkward, and tense? Does the parent demonstrate the capacity to soothe the child? Is there a family history of an anxiety disorder?	Exposure to significant traumatic events (eg, witnessing domestic violence), may result in chronic anxiety, such as PTSD. Major changes in the family or ongoing family stress situations may contribute to an anxious condition.
Excessive activity and impulsivity	Are there problems with sensory input or expressive and motor output? (Regulatory disorder of motor output and sensory input can lead to impulsive motor behaviors and craving of sensory stimulation. Behavior is disorganized, unfocused, and diffuse. It can be accompanied by weaknesses in auditory or visual-spatial processing.[30])	What is the influence of the child's temperament, especially: • High activity? • High distractibility? • Low persistence and attention span?	Is the parent clearly and comfortably in charge? Does the child receive positive feedback as well as clear expectations and appropriate limits from the parent? What is the quality of the parent-child attachment? Is there affection between the parent and child or do irritation and frustration seem to predominate?	Anxiety or depression may manifest as hyperactive, impulsive behavior in the young child. Family stress and change, past traumatic experiences, and family health and mental health conditions should be explored.

EARLY IDENTIFICATION OF AUTISTIC SPECTRUM DISORDERS

With an incidence as high as 1 in 166 children, ASDs have become a major concern for all health care professionals.[31] Autism and its milder variants are a group of neurobiologic disorders that are characterized by fundamental deficits in social interaction and communication skills. A range of other developmental delays and differences exist; approximately 70% of children with ASD also have mental retardation.[32] Common behavioral features of ASD include hand flapping, rocking, or twirling; hypersensitivity to a wide range of sensory experiences such as sound and touch; and extreme difficulties in adjusting to transitions and change. The prognosis can be greatly improved with early and intensive treatment. Therefore, early identification is critical.

Health care professionals should consider the possibility of ASD as early as the child's first year of life. Infants with ASD can show little interest in being held and may not be comforted by physical closeness with their parents. They have significant limitations in social smiling, eye contact, vocalization, and social play.[3]

PROMOTING MENTAL HEALTH

89

Bright FUTURES

During the first half of the child's second year, more specific deficits are often seen. Red flags include:

- The child fails to orient to his name.
- The child shows impairment in joint attention skills (ie, the child's capacity to follow a caregiver's gaze or follow the caregiver's pointing, or the child's own lack of showing and pointing).
- The child does not seem to notice when parents and siblings enter or leave the room.
- The child makes little or no eye contact and seems to be in his own world.
- Parents complain that the child has a "hearing problem" (ie, he does not respond to speech directed at him).
- The child's speech fails to develop as expected.

Because these signs of ASD are often difficult to elicit in the context of the pediatric well visit, health care professionals must listen carefully to the observations of parents and they must have a high index of suspicion regarding ASD. The 15 and 18 Month Visits are important times to consider ASD within routine developmental surveillance. For children who exhibit any of the red flags listed earlier, the health care professional can use one of the ASD screening tests developed for primary care providers.[15]

Promoting Mental Health and Emotional Well-Being: Middle Childhood—5 to 10 Years

A well-accepted belief of current pediatric practice is that a child's overall health is significantly influenced by psychosocial factors. Middle childhood is a time of major cognitive development and mastery of cognitive, physical, and social skills. Children in this age group continue to progress from dependence on their parents and other caregivers to increasing independence and a growing interest in the development of friendships and the world around them. Children frequently compare themselves to others. During this time, children may begin to notice the cultural differences between their family and others as they begin to develop a cultural, racial, ethnic, or religious identity. Although they are initially egocentric, they become increasingly aware of other people's feelings. Concrete thinking predominates; they are concerned primarily with the present and have limited ability for abstract or future-oriented thinking. This process evolves during the middle childhood years. As children approach adolescence, their capacity for abstract thought grows, they have the ability to think and act beyond their own immediate needs, and they are better able to see the perspectives of other people.

Middle childhood also is an important time for continued development of self-esteem and in the ongoing process of attachment. All children want to feel competent and enjoy recognition for their achievements. Success at school and home is influenced by previous experience, by their ability to get along with others, and by expectations that fit their capabilities. Success also is influenced by the quality of the schools in their community and by the expectations of educators for children of their racial, ethnic, socioeconomic background, for children who are not native English speakers, or for children with special health care needs. In addition, some children experience bullying and violence at school or

> Because these signs of autism spectrum disorder are often difficult to elicit in the context of the pediatric well visit, health care professionals must listen carefully to the observations of parents and they must have a high index of suspicion regarding autism spectrum disorder.

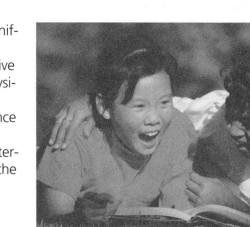

at home. These experiences can limit the child's ability to continue development of self-esteem. The health care professional should be aware of these developments and can support children and their families as they face the emerging challenges of greater independence and the awareness of others' needs, feelings, thoughts, and desires.

Children whose families are immigrants, and particularly those who live in linguistically isolated households (defined by the US Census, Bureau of the Census as a household in which no one over the age of 14 speaks English very well[33]), may be taking on responsibilities far beyond those typical for this age. For example, children may serve as interpreters for the parents in situations such as interacting with social service agencies or keeping the electric company from turning off the power. Health care professionals should assess children in these circumstances to determine whether they may be experiencing excessive stress and, if so, work with families to identify community resources to assume the roles that the school-aged children are filling.

Children with special health care needs are no different with respect to their need to belong, anxiety about self-esteem, risk-taking behavior, and coming to terms with their entrance into the expanding world outside of their family. However, their special health care needs can present limitations or challenges to a full participation in activities with their peers. Health care professionals should be aware of these issues and the risk for mental health problems and should be prepared to respond when signs of distress emerge.

Patterns of Attachment and Connection

The concept of "attachment" in infancy and early childhood is more appropriately described as "connectedness" as the child moves through middle childhood and adolescence. Defined as a strong positive connection to parents or guardians, connectedness is key to emotional well-being. The Search Institute has identified family support ("high levels of love and support") and positive family communication as important components of their 40 developmental assets. (For more information on this topic, see the Promoting Family Support theme.)

The National Longitudinal Study of Adolescent Health (AdHealth) has reported that parent-family connectedness and perceived school connectedness are protective factors against every health risk behavior, except pregnancy.[34] The physical presence of a parent at critical times, as well as time availability, is associated with reduced risk behaviors. Even more important are feelings of warmth, love, and caring from parents.

Challenges to the Development of Mental Health

Middle childhood is often the time when mental health problems first present and it is an essential time for parents to be doing all they can to promote positive social skills and reinforce desired behavior. The rate of identification of psychosocial problems and mental health disorders within a primary care setting is relatively low. Costello and Shugart[35] reported that pediatricians identify only 15% of their school-aged patients with significant behavioral or emotional disorders. Lavigne et al[36] found a lower detection rate of emotional and behavior problems in preschoolers by pediatricians as compared to problems identified by the Child Behavior Checklist and confirmed by a child psychologist.

In some situations, the health care professional can be a screener and do a thorough assessment to determine whether the child really has a problem and to refer for a more in-depth diagnostic evaluation if the screening indicates a problem. (For more information on this topic, see Bright Futures in Practice: Mental Health Toolkit.[3]) However,

Defined as a strong positive connection to parents or guardians, connectedness is key to emotional well-being.

PROMOTING MENTAL HEALTH

the reality is that only one half of families identified as needing mental health assistance will actually follow up to receive treatment. The techniques that a health care professional uses when making a referral can help break down the stigma of a mental health referral. A minimal delay between the onset of illness and treatment likely leads to the best outcome.

Attending to these issues may be especially important for those living in poverty, but most studies have not addressed the influence of culture, race, and systemic issues on outcomes. Few evidence-based treatments have taken into account the child's social context.

PROTECTIVE FACTORS

Research studies have revealed consistently strong relationships between the number of protective factors, or assets, present in young people's lives and the extent to which their mental and emotional development will be positive and successful. Children who report more assets are less likely to engage in risky health behaviors.[37] The fewer the number of assets present, the greater the possibility that children will engage in risky behaviors. Key adults in the child's life should promote a strength-based model that focuses on building these assets. Although health care professionals need to recognize deficits, they also should be helping the family develop the strengths that can contribute to a positive environment for the child.[38]

Protective factors include[39]:

- A warm and supportive relationship between parents and children
- Positive self-esteem
- Good coping skills
- Positive peer relationships
- Interest in, and success at, school
- Healthy engagement with adults outside the home
- An ability to articulate feelings

> **Children who report more assets are less likely to engage in risky health behaviors.**

- Parents who are employed and are functioning well at home, at work, and in social relationships

Increasing a child's protective factors will help him develop resiliency in the face of adversity. Resilient children understand that they are not responsible for their parents' difficulties and are able to move forward in the face of life's challenges. The resilient child is one who is socially competent, with problem-solving skills and a sense of autonomy, purpose, and future.[40]

In a child's early years of elementary school, adults need to do what they can to bolster his self-confidence because this is protective against depressive symptoms. Self-esteem is instrumental in helping children avoid behaviors that risk health and safety. In many cases, the development of self-esteem is dependent on the development of social skills. However, schools do not typically teach the development of social skills and appropriate behavior in the school setting.

Health care professionals can help parents teach their children that failure and mistakes are an inevitable but, ultimately, useful part of life. Problems with anxiety and depression commonly develop in middle childhood, but their prevalence increases remarkably in early adolescence. Early warning signs sometimes can be identified in the elementary school years so that full-blown psychiatric disorders are prevented.

LEARNING DISABILITIES AND ATTENTION-DEFICIT/HYPERACTIVITY DISORDER

The early years of elementary school are frequently the time when learning problems and learning disabilities (LDs) or attention-deficit/hyperactivity disorder (ADHD) first present. A learning disability is defined as a discrepancy between the actual academic achievement of a student and that student's intellectual potential. However, an official diagnosis of an LD usually cannot be made before the age of 7 years. Often, initial behavioral signs can mask the underlying neurodevelopmental disturbance. The health care professional should evaluate for any signs or symptoms of inattention, impulsivity, lack of focus, or poor academic performance that are not consistent with the child's potential cognitive abilities and should be prepared to counsel and to make referrals for evaluations. Early identification and intervention can have long-term positive effects for children with learning disabilities.

ADHD is one of the most commonly diagnosed mental disorders in children, affecting up to 3% to 6% of school-aged children.[3] When a child demonstrates overactivity, impulsivity, and inattention that interfere with his ability to learn, have fun, or have relationships, he should be evaluated for ADHD. Family and school skills should emphasize learning impulse control, building self-esteem, acquiring coping skills, and building social skills.

ANXIETY DISORDERS

Anxiety in childhood can be a normal feeling, but it also can lead to the appearance of symptoms that are similar to ADHD and depression. If usual coping strategies do not work or if an anxiety disorder is causing impairment in school or in relationships, these issues need to be assessed. Girls who are shy tend to be at increased risk for developing anxiety disorders,[41] and children who have experienced a recent trauma may meet criteria for PTSD.

MOOD DISORDERS

A mood disorder, such as dysthymia or depression, can lead to dysfunction in multiple areas of a child's emotional, social, and cognitive development. Mood disorders are characterized by disturbances in mood, symptoms of irritability and emptiness, and loss of interest in usual activities. They can be accompanied by reckless and destructive behavior, somatic complaints, and poor social and academic functioning.[11] A portion of prepubertal children with mood disorders have

child-onset bipolar disorder. Among prepubertal children and adolescents with bipolar disorder, a second mental health diagnosis is common, including ADHD (90% of children and 30% of adolescents), anxiety disorders (33% of children and 12% of adolescents), and conduct disorder (22% of children and 18% of adolescents). Substance use also is highly prevalent in this population.[42,43]

Frequently, a primary care provider is the main source of care for children with mild and moderate depression. All children and families need to be asked about feelings of sadness, sleep problems, and loss of interest in activities. Depression can go undetected. A simple question, such as, "When is the last time you had a really good time?", is nonthreatening but gives much information to the interviewer. Empathetic responses from the person who is conducting the interview are important. Depression screening tools and standardized instruments for behavior problems can be useful.[3]

Bipolar disorder can present in middle childhood, although it is more common in adolescence or young adulthood. Children are more likely to present in a persistently irritable mood than in a euphoric mood. Associated signs include aggressive and uncontrollable outbursts and agitated behavior that can resemble ADHD. Mood lability may be evident on the same day or over the course of days or weeks. Reckless behaviors, dangerous play, and inappropriate sexual behaviors may be present.

Further discussion of mood disorders can be found in *Bright Futures in Practice: Mental Health*[3] and in the Adolescence section of this theme.

BULLYING

Surveys indicate that as many as one half of all children are bullied at some time during their school years, and at least 10% are bullied on a regular basis.[44] Bullies come in all shapes and sizes and ages. Children usually become bullies because they are unhappy for

Attention-deficit/ hyperactivity disorder is one of the most commonly diagnosed mental disorders in children, affecting up to 3% to 6% of school-aged children.

PROMOTING MENTAL HEALTH

some reason or do not know how to get along with other children. Often, children who bully grow up to become adult bullies. Types of bullying include:

- *Verbal:* Name-calling (the most common form of bullying)
- *Physical:* Punching or pushing
- *Relational:* Purposely leaving someone out of a game or group
- *Extortion:* Stealing someone's money or toys
- *Cyber-bullying:* Using computers, the Internet, or mobile phones to bully others

Bullying hurts everyone. Victims can be physically or emotionally hurt. Witnesses also can become sad or scared by what they have seen. A child who becomes withdrawn or depressed because of bullying should receive professional help. Children who are bullied experience real suffering that can interfere with their social and emotional development, as well as their school performance. Some victims of bullying have even attempted suicide rather than continue to endure such harassment and punishment.

Most of the time, bullying does not occur in private; other children are watching 85% of the time. A health care professional who suspects that a child is the victim of bullying or that she is witnessing bullying should ask the child to talk about what is happening. Responding in a positive and accepting manner and providing opportunities to talk can foster open and honest discussion about the

Responding in a positive and accepting manner and providing opportunities to talk can foster open and honest discussion about the reasons why the bullying is occurring and about possible solutions.

reasons why the bullying is occurring and about possible solutions.

The following are suggestions for parents and health care professionals in situations of bullying[45]:

- Seek help from the child's teacher or the school guidance counselor. Most bullying occurs on playgrounds, in lunchrooms, in bathrooms, on school buses, or in unsupervised halls.
- Ask school administrators to find out about programs that other schools and communities have used to help combat bullying, such as peer mediation, conflict resolution, anger management training, and increased adult supervision.
- Ask what the child thinks should be done. What has already been tried? What worked and what did not? Health care professionals can help the child assertively practice what to say to the bully so she will be prepared the next time. The simple act of insisting that the bully leave her alone may have a surprising effect. Explain to the child that the bully's true goal is to get a response.
- Encourage a popular peer to help enforce a school's no-bullying policy.

The following are actions that adults can teach the child to do[46]:

- Always tell an adult. It is an adult's job to help keep children safe. Teachers or parents rarely see a bully being mean to someone else, but they want to know about it so they can help stop the bullying.
- Stay in a group when traveling back and forth from school, during shopping trips, on the school playground, or on other outings. Children who bully often pick on children who are by themselves because it is easier and they are more likely to get away with their bad behavior.

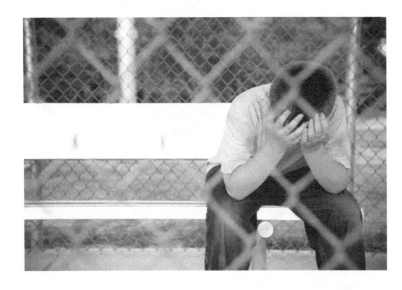

- If it feels safe, try to stand up to the bully. This does not mean the child should fight back or bully back. Instead, she can tell the bully that she does not like it and that the bully should stop. Often, children who bully like to see that they can make their target upset. Otherwise, the child should try walking away to avoid the bully and seek help from a teacher, coach, or other adult.
- A child who is being bullied online should not reply. Responding actually may make the bullying worse. Instead, she should tell a family member or another trusted adult.

EARLY SUBSTANCE USE

Almost all children eventually will find themselves in a situation in which they must decide whether they will experiment with smoking, drugs, or alcohol. Health care professionals should discuss these issues with children before they reach adolescence. Although the majority of children who experiment with substances do not develop a substance-use disorder, even occasional use can have serious consequences, such as an increased risk of health concerns, mistakes made due to impaired judgment, and motor vehicle crashes. Education about the implications of substance use must begin in middle childhood. Delaying initiation of substance use may help future substance-related problems.

Parents who smoke place their children at higher risk of smoking. Parents should think about which behaviors they would like to model for their children. Positive role modeling can be established by parents by not smoking cigarettes, banning smoking at home, limiting alcohol, and active participation and monitoring of the attitudes and behaviors of their children. Positive and honest communication between a parent and child is one of the best ways to prevent substance use. Promotion of self-esteem and avoidance of overly critical feedback can help

the child learn to resist the pressure for experimentation. If talking within the family becomes a problem, a health care professional may be able to encourage the communication.

CONDUCT DISTURBANCES

Conduct disturbances are characterized by negative or antisocial behaviors that range in severity from normal developmental variations to significant mental health disorders.[47] Symptomatic behaviors of oppositional defiant disorder can include persistent temper tantrums, arguing with adults, refusing to comply with reasonable adult requests, and annoying others.[48] Conduct disorders usually involve more serious patterns of aggression toward others, destruction of property, deceitfulness or theft, and serious violations of rules.[49]

Promoting Mental Health and Emotional Well-Being: Adolescence—11 to 21 Years

During adolescence, mental health is characterized by progression toward optimal current and future capacity and motivation to cope with stress and to be involved in personally meaningful activities and interpersonal relationships.[50] The adolescent's progression toward optimal functioning varies greatly depending on individual personality. Thus, health care professionals must identify normal ranges of development, rather than a specified outcome or end point.

The development of emotional well-being centers on the adolescent's ability to effectively cope with multiple stressors. This trait also is called psychological resilience. Effective coping includes using problem-solving strategies for emotional management, being able to match strategies to specific situations, and drawing on others as resources for social support.[50] Data supporting the strong effects of resilience on reducing risk in general, and preventing violence in particular, come from a variety of sources.[51-53] Cross-sectional data

Positive and honest communication between a parent and child is one of the best ways to prevent substance use.

PROMOTING MENTAL HEALTH

Most adolescents have at least one visit per year with their health care professional, and most behavioral, developmental, and mental health problems are first discussed in that setting.

from Vermont show a striking negative correlation between the presence of protective factors and a variety of risk behaviors.[38] National longitudinal data from the AdHealth study demonstrate a similar, powerful effect of protective factors on subsequent violence.[51] Finally, a school-based program that focused on teaching adolescents positive social development was demonstrably more effective than a more standard risk-reduction curriculum.[52] The development of resilience is a primary goal of successful adolescent development[53] and can be encouraged by a variety of counseling suggestions. Young people should be encouraged to engage in pro-social paid or volunteer community activities to develop mastery of a particular skill or activity, thus becoming more independent in responsible ways. The adolescent should experience these activities as autonomous and self-initiated. In fact, Maton[54] found that adolescents' life satisfaction and self-esteem were predicted by their level of meaningful activities independent of the social support they received from parents and peers.

Most adolescents have at least one visit per year with their health care professional, and most behavioral, developmental, and mental health problems are first discussed in that setting. Primary care can be an access point for developmental and behavioral health care, although it can be a challenge because the primary care culture focuses on acute care, whereas mental health and developmental disorders in children and adolescents tend to be chronic and relapsing. Health care professionals should know the symptoms of common mental health disorders in this population, as well as risk factors for suicide, and should ask about these symptoms during an office visit whenever appropriate.[55,56]

Compas[50] suggests a framework to assess the mental health of adolescents (Table 2). When using this framework, the health care professional should get the perspectives of the adolescent himself, as well as his parents,

teachers, and mental health professionals. Sociocultural differences are a significant factor in evaluating an adolescent's emotional well-being. Appropriate social norms within a majority culture may not be shared by youth outside that culture. Youth from culturally diverse families also may experience conflicts between values and expectations at home and those that arise from the mainstream culture and peers from other backgrounds.

Patterns of Attachment and Connection

Connectedness with parents, legal guardians, and family remains a critical component of the healthy development of adolescents. Most school-aged children and youth continue to spend time with their parents and maintain strong bonds with their parents. The risk of psychological problems and delinquency are higher in youth who are disconnected from their parents.[57] Studies document reduced risk-taking behavior among youth who report a close relationship with their parents.[51] Adolescents and their parents have to prioritize conversations and communication that balance this sense of belonging with opportunities for the youth to grow in decision-making skills and sense of autonomy. Peers and siblings also can contribute positively to the youth's sense of belonging.[57] The literature describes a positive bond with school (described as students who feel that teachers treat students fairly, are close to people at school, and feel part of their school) as a protective factor.[58]

Challenges to the Development of Mental Health

Adolescents who have major difficulties in one area of functioning often demonstrate symptoms and difficulties in other areas of daily functioning. For example, if they are having school difficulties secondary to ADHD, symptoms such as motoric activity or impulsivity will be evident at home and may interfere with other activities. Even less overt disorders, such as LDs or difficulties in peer relationships, often will manifest as a depressed mood at home, tension with siblings, or low self-esteem. Health care professionals should know the symptoms of common mental health disorders in this population, as well as risk factors for suicide, and should ask about these symptoms during an office visit whenever appropriate.[55,56]

Some prevention programs in mental health care can strengthen protective factors, such as social skills, problem-solving skills, and social support, and reduce the consequence of risk factors, psychiatric symptoms, and substance use. Unfortunately, few studies are examining the impact of prevention programs on the incidence of new mental health cases, in part because of the large number of subjects that are needed to ensure scientifically reliable findings.[59]

TABLE 2

Framework for Evaluating Adolescent Emotional Well-Being

Domain	Factors to Assess
Coping with stress and adversity	• Skills and motivation to manage acute, major life stressors and recurring daily stressors • Skills to solve problems and control emotions • Flexibility and the ability to meet the demands of varying types of stressors
Involvement in personally meaningful activities	• Skills and motivation to engage in activities • Behaviors and activities are experienced as autonomous • Self-directed involvement
Perspective of interested parties	• Perspectives of the adolescent, parents, teachers, and, if needed, the mental health care provider • Adolescent's subjective sense of well-being • Adolescent's behavioral stability, predictability, and conformity to social rules
Developmental factors	• Prior developmental milestones and issues • Variations in adolescent's cognitive, affective, social, and biologic development • Cohort differences in events and social context that affect positive mental health
Sociocultural factors	• Differences in values affect optimal development and functioning • Differences in perceived threats to positive mental health and the risk of maladjustment • Cultural protective factors, such as religion and values

Adapted from Compas BE. Promoting positive mental health during adolescence. In: Millstein SG, Peterson AC, Nightingale EO, eds. *Promoting the Health of Adolescents: New Directions for the Twenty-First Century*. New York, NY: Oxford University Press; 1993:159-179.

PROMOTING MENTAL HEALTH

Mental Health Concerns

The most common mental health problems of adolescents are mood disorders, including depression and anxiety; deficits in attention, cognition, and learning; and conduct disturbances.[47,49,60] Substance use and abuse and suicidal behavior also are significant problems during this developmental stage.

DEPRESSION AND ANXIETY

Mood disorders are characterized by repeated, intense internal or emotional distress over a period of months or years. Unreasonable fear and anxiety, lasting depression, low self-esteem, and worthlessness are associated with these conditions. The wide mood changes in adolescents challenge providers to distinguish between a mental health disorder and troubling, but essentially normal, behavior.

Depression and anxiety, with potentially different manifestations across cultural groups, are common and significant problems during this developmental period.[61] Depression is present in about 5% of adolescents at any given time. Having a parent with a history of depression doubles to quadruples a child's risk of a depressive episode. Depression also is more common among children with chronic illness and after stressful life events, such as the loss of a friend, parent, or sibling. Depression in adolescents is not always characterized by sadness, but can be seen as irritability, anger, boredom, an inability to experience pleasure, or difficulty with family relationships, school, and work.[61,62] Academic failure, substance abuse and dependency, high-risk sexual behaviors, and violence all have been linked to depression in adolescents.

When treating the depressed adolescent, the health care professional should determine past suicidal behavior or thoughts and family history of suicide. Parents should be advised to remove firearms[63] and any potentially lethal medications from the home. Access to the Internet should be monitored for suicide content in communications and Web sites. (For more information on this topic, see the Suicide section of this theme.)

Like other mental health problems, symptoms of anxiety range in intensity. For some adolescents, symptoms such as excessive worry, fear, stress, or physical symptoms can cause significant distress but not impair functioning enough to warrant the diagnosis of an anxiety disorder. The problem is classified as a disorder when symptoms significantly affect an adolescent's functioning.[3] The prevalence of any anxiety disorder among children and adolescents in the United States is about 13% in any 6-month period.[7] Studies have demonstrated a relationship between anxiety disorders and alcohol misuse in adolescents and young adults.[64] Thus, the health care professional must review the individual's risk and protective factors to better understand the adolescent's problem and make a referral.

One strategy for improving the detection of mental health problems is to screen for anxiety and depressive disorders during routine health evaluations.[65] However, screening for these disorders is controversial.

The US Preventive Services Task Force (USPSTF)[66] recommends screening adults for depression in clinical practices that have systems in place to ensure accurate diagnosis, effective treatment, and follow-up (B-level evidence). The USPSTF found limited evidence on the accuracy and reliability of screening tests in children and adolescents and limited evidence on the effectiveness of therapy in children and adolescents identified in primary care settings. Therefore, the USPSTF concluded that evidence is insufficient to recommend for or against routine screening of children or adolescents for depression, although it recommends "that clinicians maintain a high index of suspicion for mental health problems in this population."

A variety of measures can be used in the primary care setting for children and

> Depression and anxiety, with potentially different manifestations across cultural groups, are common and significant problems during this developmental period.

adolescents.[67] The health care professional should determine whether the measure was standardized on a population similar to that in his practice.

DEFICITS IN ATTENTION, COGNITION, AND LEARNING

Adolescents with deficits in attention, cognition, and learning are likely to present with an array of complaints that involve academic, psychosocial, and behavioral functioning. Placement in LD programs in the United States has tripled over the last few decades to 6% of all children who are enrolled in public schools today.[68]

Many children who have been diagnosed with ADHD continue to have difficulties throughout their adolescence and adulthood.[69] Adolescents with ADHD often have comorbid oppositional defiant disorder and conduct disorder in addition to having developmental and social problems.

CONDUCT DISTURBANCES

Conduct disturbances and disorders are manifested through the same behaviors in adolescence as they are in middle childhood. These behaviors include persistent fits of temper, arguing with adults, refusing to comply with reasonable adult requests, and annoying others,[48] aggression toward others, destruction of property, deceitfulness or theft, and serious violations of rules.[49] Substance use, interpersonal aggression, and other problem behaviors also tend to occur in adolescents with these disorders.[70]

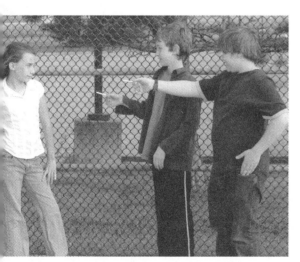

SUICIDE

Suicide is the third leading cause of death for adolescents. More than 4,000 adolescents and young adults aged 10 to 24 years committed suicide in 2001.[71] A far greater number of youth *attempt* suicide each year. Data collected in 2003 by the Centers for Disease Control and Prevention (CDC) Youth Risk Behavior Surveillance System (YRBSS) show that 16.9% of high-school students reported that they had seriously considered attempting suicide, 16.5% had made a plan, and 8.5% had made a suicide attempt.[72] Although the proportion of students who reported that they have seriously considered suicide has decreased from 29% in 1991, the proportion for reported attempted suicide has remained stable across the last decade. Suicide among adolescents has increased dramatically compared to that of the general population over the past 4 decades. Between 1960 and 2000, the suicide rate among adolescents increased 128%, compared to 2% for the general population.[71]

Health care professionals who treat suicidal adolescents should not rely solely on an adolescent's promise to not harm herself, and should involve parents and other caretakers in monitoring suicidal thoughts and gestures. Parents should be advised to remove firearms and ammunition from the home.[73] Of importance, suicide risk seems highest at the beginning of a depressive episode, so expeditious treatment or referral is crucial.[56] Although no evidence-based data indicate that psychiatric hospitalization prevents immediate or eventual suicide, the clinical consensus is that immediate hospitalization is a critical component in preventing adult and adolescent patients who are suicidal from committing suicide.[55]

SUBSTANCE USE AND ABUSE

Use or misuse of alcohol, tobacco, and other drugs is a significant health concern during adolescence.[74,75] Children of parents who abuse substances are particularly vulnerable to health or social problems.[76] Significant changes in drug awareness take place

> Health care professionals who treat suicidal adolescents should not rely solely on an adolescent's promise to not harm herself, and should involve parents and other caretakers in monitoring suicidal thoughts and gestures. Parents should be advised to remove firearms and ammunition from the home.

PROMOTING MENTAL HEALTH

between the ages of 12 and 13 years, and substance use most often begins between grades 7 and 10.[77] By late adolescence, access to substances and independence from parents contribute to the risk for substance abuse or dependence.[78] A survey by the National Center on Addiction and Substance Abuse at Columbia University[79] also has revealed a troubling connection between adolescents who smoke cigarettes and marijuana use. Adolescents who smoked

cigarettes were 14 times more likely to try marijuana and 18 times more likely to report that most of their friends smoke marijuana.

Drug misuse and dependence are major factors in adolescent deaths because they contribute to motor vehicle crashes, homicides, and suicides. Adolescents are at increased risk for unprotected sexual activity and interpersonal violence while under the influence of alcohol or other drugs. Other substances, such as smokeless tobacco or

---

BOX 2

Youth Risk Behavior Surveillance System

Since 1991, the CDC has conducted a biannual national survey of 9th- to 12th-grade high-school students. Adolescents who are in school complete the YRBSS. The actual prevalence of substance use among the general adolescent population, which includes high-school dropouts, is probably higher than that reflected in the YRBSS. Findings from the 2005 YRBSS[72] are listed below.

Alcohol
- 25.6% of students first drank alcohol (other than a few sips) before the age of 13 years.
- 74.3% of students had 1 or more drinks of alcohol in their lifetime.
- 25.5% reported episodic heavy drinking (ie, 5 or more drinks of alcohol on 1 or more occasions during the previous 30 days).
- 28.5% of these high-school students had ridden with a driver who had been drinking.

Tobacco use
- More than 50% of high-school students (54.3%) had ever tried cigarette smoking.
- 16% of students had first smoked a whole cigarette before the age of 13 years.
- 23% of students reported current cigarette use (ie, use cigarettes on 1 or more of the preceding 30 days).
- During the 30 days preceding the survey, 8% of students had used smokeless tobacco and 14% had smoked cigars.

Marijuana
- 38.4% of the high-school students reported having used marijuana, with 9.9% having tried the drug before the age of 13 years.

Cocaine
- 7.6% of students had ever used cocaine (eg, powder, "crack," or "freebase").
- 3.4% of students had used cocaine on 1 or more of the preceding 30 days.

Inhalants, heroin, methamphetamines, and nonprescription steroids
- Reported lifetime use was 12.4% for inhalants (eg, sniffing glue, breathing the contents of aerosol cans, or inhaling paints or sprays to get high, referred to as "huffing").
- 2.4% of students reported using heroin.
- 6.3% of students reported using Ecstasy.
- 6.2% of students reported using methamphetamines.
- 4.0% of students reported using steroids.

anabolic steroids, also can lead to acute or chronic health problems.

Adolescents decide to use a specific drug based on its perceived risk versus benefit and its perceived social approval versus disapproval, as well as its availability in the community. One study found that since the illicit drug epidemic originally blossomed in the 1960s, many new substances have come onto the national scene, while only a few have receded from it.[80] Because the health care professional may not be fully aware of all the illicit drugs available[81], she should talk with adolescents about the drugs of choice in their region. Data from the YRBSS also may provide valuable insights into the substance-using behaviors of adolescents (Box 2).

Screening and Intervention

Major transitions, such as puberty, moving, parental divorce, and school changes (eg, entering middle school), are associated with increased risk for adolescent substance use.[82] Adolescents, particularly those aged 12 and 13 years, should be asked whether they or their friends have ever tried, or are using, tobacco, alcohol, or other drugs. The health care professional should give anticipatory guidance as part of routine health maintenance.[83-85]

The USPSTF[66] recommends that all adolescents be screened for tobacco, alcohol, and other drug use and that "anti-tobacco messages . . . be included in health promotion counseling for children, adolescents, and young adults based on the proven efficacy of risk reduction from avoiding tobacco use." The CRAFFT is one brief screening tool that is appropriate for use in the adolescent primary care setting.[86] This screening is essential for all adolescents, including those with special health care needs. Although there may be a tendency to skip screening for children with special health care needs because of their chronic illness or developmental difference, doing so is inconsistent with the approach of the medical home.

The health care professional's screening, in combination with community prevention efforts, are important despite barriers that include limited time, low self-efficacy, and lack of reimbursement, as well as the lack of evidence that screening makes a difference.[87-92]

Success in treating a substance abuse problem is more likely if treatment is begun early. Early substance use has been correlated with an increased risk of abuse and dependence in adulthood.[93] The onset of early drinking has been associated with increased risk of alcohol-related health and social problems in adults, including dependence later in life, frequent heavy drinking, unintentional injuries while under the influence, and motor vehicle

Major transitions, such as puberty, moving, parental divorce, and school changes (eg, entering middle school), are associated with increased risk for adolescent substance use.

PROMOTING MENTAL HEALTH

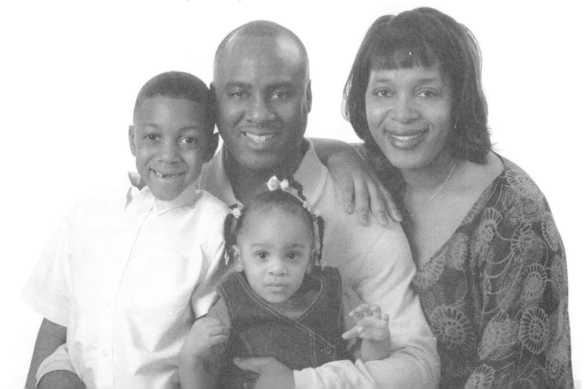

crashes.[94] Table 3 and Figure 1 illustrate 2 models for a continuum of drug use through stages.

Addiction could be viewed as a synonym for alcohol or drug dependence[95] as defined by the *Diagnostic and Statistical Manual of Mental Disorders, Fourth Edition*.[96] Alcohol or drug *dependence* is also a less stigmatizing term for adolescents.

Prevention and Protective Factors

Prevention programs have been designed for diverse target audiences in different settings. The content of prevention programs varies from didactic information about alcohol, tobacco, and other drugs to skills development for drug resistance or refusal. The prevention message needs to be consistent and from multiple sources (ie, in the home, at school, in the community, and from the medical home).[82,97] School-based smoking prevention programs with multiple compo-nents that teach resistance skills and engage youth in positive activities have been success-ful.[98] Involving families and communities and reinforcing school lessons with a clear, consistent social message that adolescent alcohol, tobacco, and other drug use is harmful, unacceptable, and illegal strengthens prevention efforts.[99]

The National Institute on Drug Abuse[82] has highlighted evidence-based examples of effective prevention that targeted risk and protective factors of drug abuse for the individual, family, and community. Based on its review of the research literature, it identified the following family protective factors:

- A strong bond between children and their families
- Parental involvement in a child's life
- Supportive parenting
- Clear limits and consistent enforcement of discipline

TABLE 3
Drug Use Severity Continuum[95]

Stage	Characteristics
Abstinence	No use.
Experimental use	Minimal use, typically associated with recreational activities, and often limited to alcohol use. Adolescents will use if the substance is available, but will not actively seek out substances.
Early abuse	More established use, often involving more than one drug, and greater frequency; adverse consequences begin to emerge. Behaviors to gain access to the substance now become evident, and persons who can supply drugs are sought out.
Abuse	Regular and frequent use over an extended period; several adverse consequences emerge.
Dependence	Continued regular use despite repeated severe consequences, signs of tolerance, and adjustment of activities to accommodate drug-seeking and drug use.
Recovery	Return to abstinence. Some youth can relapse and go through the cycle of stages again.

Adapted from Winters' hypothetical drug use problem with a severity continuum.[95]

Outside the family setting, the most salient protective factors were identified as follows:

- Age-appropriate parental monitoring (eg, curfews, adult supervision, knowing the child's friends, and enforcing household rules)
- Success in academics and involvement in extracurricular activities
- Strong bonds with prosocial institutions, such as school and religious institutions, and acceptance of conventional norms against drug abuse[82]

In 1997, Simantov et al[100] conducted a cross-sectional, school-based survey of students in grades 5 through 12. Adolescents who reported "connectedness" to their parents were least likely to engage in high-risk behaviors. Another protective factor was participation in extracurricular activities, such as exercise or after-school sports clubs. However, the positive impact of extracurricular activity was on lowering smoking, not on the risk of drinking.

FIGURE 1
Stages of Use Model[101]

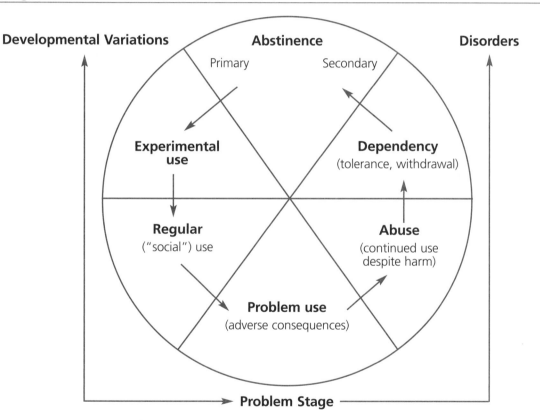

Source: Knight JR. Substance use, abuse, and dependence. In: Levine MD, Carey WB, Crocker AC, eds. *Developmental-Behavioral Pediatrics*. 3rd ed. Philadelphia, PA: WB Saunders; 1999.[101]

PROMOTING MENTAL HEALTH

References

1. Shonkoff JP, Phillips DA, eds. *From Neurons to Neighborhoods: The Science of Early Childhood Development.* Washington, DC: National Academy Press; 2000
2. Ollendick TH, Hersen M. *Handbook of Child Psychopathology.* 3rd ed. New York, NY: Plenum Press; 1998
3. Jellinek MS, Patel BP, Froehle MC, eds. *Bright Futures in Practice: Mental Health:* Volume 1 *Practice Guide* and *Toolkit,* Volume 2. Arlington, VA: National Center for Education in Maternal and Child Health; 2002
4. Wolraich M, Felice ME, Drotar D. *The Classification of Child and Adolescent Mental Diagnoses in Primary Care: Diagnostic and Statistical Manual for Primary Care (DSM-PC) Child and Adolescent Version.* Elk Grove Village, IL: American Academy of Pediatrics; 1996
5. Kessler RC, Berglund P, Demler O, Jin R, Merikangas KR, Walters EE. Lifetime prevalence and age-of-onset distributions of DSM-IV disorders in the National Comorbidity Survey Replication. *Arch Gen Psychiatry.* 2005;62:593-602
6. US Public Health Service, Office of the Surgeon General. Mental Health: *A Report of the Surgeon General.* Rockville, MD: US Department of Health and Human Services; 1999
7. National Institute of Mental Health. *Brief Notes on the Mental Health of Children and Adolescents.* Bethesda, MD: National Institute of Mental Health; 1999. Available at: www.medhelp.org/NIHlib/GF-233.html. Accessed May 15, 2007
8. Borowsky IW, Mozayeny S, Ireland M. Brief psychosocial screening at health supervision and acute care visits. *Pediatrics.* 2003;112:129-133
9. Teplin LA, Abram KM, McClelland GM, Dulcan MK, Mericle AA. Psychiatric disorders in youth in juvenile detention. *Arch Gen Psychiatry.* 2002;59:1133-1143
10. Kelleher KJ, McInerny TK, Gardner WP, Childs GE, Wasserman RC. Increasing identification of psychosocial problems: 1979-1996. *Pediatrics.* 2000;105:1313-1321
11. Perrin EC. Ethical questions about screening. *J Dev Behav Pediatr.* 1998;19:350-352
12. Glascoe FP. Increasing identification of psychosocial problems. *Pediatrics.* 2001;107:1496
13. Olson AL, Dietrich AJ, Prazar G, Hurley J. Brief maternal depression screening at well-child visits. *Pediatrics.* 2006;118:207-216
14. Spivak H, Sege R, Flanigan E, Licenziato V, eds. *Connected Kids: Safe, Strong, Secure Clinical Guide.* Elk Grove Village, IL: American Academy of Pediatrics; 2006
15. Council on Children With Disabilities, Section on Developmental Behavioral Pediatrics, Bright Futures Steering Committee, Medical Home Initiatives for Children With Special Needs Project Advisory Committee. Identifying infants and young children with developmental disorders in the medical home: an algorithm for developmental surveillance and screening. *Pediatrics.* 2006;118:405-420
16. Gardner W, Murphy M, Childs G, et al. The PSC-17: a brief pediatric symptom checklist with psychosocial problem subscales. A report from PROS and ASPN. *Ambul Child Health.* 1999;5:225-236
17. Asarnow JR, Jaycox LH, Anderson M. Depression among youth in primary care models for delivering mental health services. *Child Adolesc Psychiatr Clin N Am.* 2002;11:477-497, viii
18. Hagan JF Jr. The new morbidity: where the rubber hits the road or the practitioner's guide to the new morbidity. *Pediatrics.* 2001;108:1206-1210
19. American Academy of Pediatrics, Medical Home Initiatives for Children With Special Needs Project Advisory Committee. The medical home. *Pediatrics.* 2002;110:184-186
20. Kahn RS, Wise PH, Finkelstein JA, Bernstein HH, Lowe JA, Homer CJ. The scope of unmet maternal health needs in pediatric settings. *Pediatrics.* 1999;103:576-581
21. National Clearinghouse on Child Abuse and Neglect Information. *Child Abuse and Neglect Fatalities: Statistics and Interventions.* Washington, DC: National Clearinghouse on Child Abuse and Neglect Information; 2004
22. American Academy of Pediatrics. Some Things You Should Know About the Effects of Violence on Children. Available at: http://www.aap.org/advocacy/childhealthmonth/effects.htm. Accessed January 21, 2007
23. American Academy of Pediatrics, Committee on Child Abuse and Neglect. Shaken baby syndrome: rotational cranial injuries-technical report. *Pediatrics.* 2001;108:206-210
24. Graham DI. Paediatric head injury. *Brain.* 2001;124:1261-1262
25. American Academy of Pediatrics, Council on Child and Adolescent Health. The role of home-visitation programs in improving health outcomes for children and families. *Pediatrics.* 1998;101:486-489
26. Cassidy J. The nature of the child's ties. In: Cassidy J, Shaver PR, eds. *Handbook of Attachment: Theory, Research, and Clinical Applications.* New York, NY: Guilford Press; 1999:3-20
27. Albrecht SJ, Dore DJ, Naugle AE. Common behavioral dilemmas of the school-aged child. *Pediatr Clin North Am.* 2003;50:841-857
28. Bethell C, et al. *Partnering with Parents to Promote the Healthy Development of Young Children Enrolled in Medicaid.* New York, NY: The Commonwealth Fund; 2002
29. Carey WB, McDevitt SC. *Coping with Children's Temperament: A Guide for Professionals.* New York, NY: Basic Books; 1995
30. Zero to Three: Diagnostic Classification, 0-3: *Diagnostic Classification of Mental Health and Developmental Disorders of Infancy and Early Childhood.* Arlington, VA: Zero to Three: National Center for Clinical Infant Programs; 1994

31. American Academy of Pediatrics. Autism A.L.A.R.M. Elk Grove Village, IL: American Academy of Pediatrics; 2004. Available at: www.medicalhomeinfo.org/health/Autism%20downloads/AutismAlarm.pdf. Accessed September 13, 2007

32. National Mental Health Association. Fact Sheet: The Autistic Child. Available at: http://www.nmha.org/infoctr/factsheets/73.cfm. Accessed May 12, 2006

33. US Census Bureau. *Language Use and English-Speaking Ability: 2000*. Washington, DC: US Department of Commerce, Economics and Statistics Administration, US Census Bureau; 2003

34. Resnick MD, Bearman PS, Blum RW, et al. Protecting adolescents from harm. Findings from the National Longitudinal Study on Adolescent Health. *JAMA*. 1997;278:823-832

35. Costello EJ, Shugart MA. Above and below the threshold: severity of psychiatric symptoms and functional impairment in a pediatric sample. *Pediatrics*. 1992;90:359-368

36. Lavigne JV, Binns HJ, Christoffel KK, et al. Behavioral and emotional problems among preschool children in pediatric primary care: Prevalence and pediatricians' recognition. Pediatric Practice Research Group. *Pediatrics*. 1993;91:649-655

37. Scales P, Leffert N, Lerner RM. *Developmental Assets: A Synthesis of the Scientific Research on Adolescent Development*. Minneapolis, MN: Search Institute; 1999

38. Murphey DA, Lamonda KH, Carney JK, Duncan P. Relationships of a brief measure of youth assets to health-promoting and risk behaviors. *J Adolesc Health*. 2004;34:184-191

39. National Mental Health Association. *When a Parent Has a Mental Illness: From Risk to Resiliency—Protective Factors for Children*. Alexandria, VA: National Mental Health Association; 2007. Available at: http://www.nmha.org/index.cfm?objectid=E3397A71-1372-4D20-C807F1AOE93C2812. Accessed May 15, 2007

40. American Psychological Association, Taskforce on Resilience in Response to Terrorism. *Fostering Resilience in Response to Terrorism: For Psychologists* Working With Children. Washington, DC: American Psychological Association; 2004. Available at: www.apa.org/psychologists/pdfs/children.pdf. Accessed September 13, 2007

41. Bernstein GA, Borchardt CM, Perwien AR. Anxiety disorders in children and adolescents: a review of the past 10 years. *J Am Acad Child Adolesc Psychiatry*. 1996;35:1110-1119

42. Geller B, Luby J. Child and adolescent bipolar disorder: a review of the past 10 years. *J Am Acad Child Adolesc Psychiatry*. 1997;36:1168-1176

43. Wilens TE. *Straight Talk About Psychiatric Medications for Kids*. New York, NY: Guilford Press; 1999

44. Nansel TR, Overpeck M, Pilla RS, Ruan WJ, Simons-Morton B, Scheidt P. Bullying behaviors among US youth: prevalence and association with psychosocial adjustment. *JAMA*. 2001;285:2094-2100

45. American Academy of Child and Adolescent Psychiatry. Bullying. Facts for Families. Washington, DC: American Academy of Child and Adolescent Psychiatry; 2001. Available at: http://www/aacap.org/cs/root/facts_for_families/bullying. Accessed June 27, 2006

46. Stop Bullying Now! Are you being bullied? Washington, DC: Health Resources and Services Administration. Available at: http://stopbullyingnow.hrsa.gov/index.asp?area=areyou. Accessed June 27, 2006

47. Mezzacappa E, Earls F. The adolescent with conduct disorder. *Adolesc Med*. 1998;9:363-371

48. Forness SR, Walker HM, Kavale KA. Psychiatric disorders and treatments: a primer for teachers. *TEACHING Exceptional Children*. 2003;36:42-49

49. Dodge KA, Pettit GS. A biopsychosocial model of the development of chronic conduct problems in adolescence. *Dev Psychol*. 2003;39:349-371

50. Compas BE. Promoting positive mental health during adolescence. In: Millstein SG, Petersen AC, Nightingale EO, eds. *Promoting the Health of Adolescents: New Directions for the Twenty-first Century*. New York, NY: Oxford University Press; 1993:159-179

51. Resnick MD, Ireland M, Borowsky I. Youth violence perpetration: what protects? What predicts? Findings from the National Longitudinal Study of Adolescent Health. *J Adolesc Health*. 2004;35:424:e1-e10

52. Flay BR, Graumlich S, Segawa E, Burns JL, Holliday MY. Effects of 2 prevention programs on high-risk behaviors among African American youth: a randomized trial. *Arch Pediatr Adolesc Med*. 2004;158:377-384

53. Bell CC. Cultivating resiliency in youth. *J Adolesc Health*. 2001;29:375-381

54. Maton KI. Meaningful involvement in instrumental activity and well-being: studies of older adolescents and at risk urban teen-agers. *Am J Community Psychol*. 1990;18:297-320

55. American Academy of Pediatrics, Committee on Adolescence. Suicide and suicide attempts in adolescents. *Pediatrics*. 2000;105:871-874

56. Zametkin AJ, Alter MR, Yemini T. Suicide in teenagers: assessment, management, and prevention. *JAMA*. 2001;286:3120-3125

57. Moore KA, Halle TG. *Preventing Problems Versus Promoting the Positive: What Do We Want for Our Children?* Washington, DC: Child Trends; 1999

58. National Association of Secondary School Principals. *Breaking Ranks II: Strategies for Leading High School Reform*. Reston, VA: National Association of Secondary School Principals; 2004

59. Cuijpers P. Examining the effects of prevention programs on the incidence of new cases of mental disorders: the lack of statistical power. *Am J Psychiatry*. 2003;160:1385-1391

PROMOTING MENTAL HEALTH

60. Loeber R, Burke JD, Lahey BB, Winters A, Zera M. Oppositional defiant and conduct disorder: a review of the past 10 years. Part I. *J Am Acad Child Adolesc Psychiatry*. 2000;39:1468-1484

61. National Institute of Mental Health. *Depression in Children and Adolescents: A Fact Sheet for Physicians*. Bethesda, MD: National Institutes of Health; 2000

62. Brent DA, Birmaher B. Clinical practice. Adolescent depression. *N Engl J Med*. 2002;347:667-671

63. Brent DA, Perper JA, Allman CJ, Moritz GM, Wartella ME, Zelenak JP. The presence and accessibility of firearms in the homes of adolescent suicides. A case-control study. *JAMA*. 1991;266:2989-2995

64. Zimmerman P, Wittchen HU, Hofler M, Pfister H, Kessler RC, Lieb R. Primary anxiety disorders and the development of subsequent alcohol use disorders: a 4-year community study of adolescents and young adults. *Psychol Med*. 2003;33:1211-1222

65. Valenstein M, Vijan S, Zeber JE, Boehm K, Buttar A. The cost-utility of screening for depression in primary care. *Ann Intern Med*. 2001;134:345-360

66. US Preventive Services Task Force. *The Guide to Clinical Preventive Services: Report of the United States Preventive Services Task Force*. 3rd ed. Alexandria, VA: International Medical Publishing; 2002

67. Sharp LK, Lipsky MS. Screening for depression across the lifespan: a review of measures for use in primary care settings. *Am Fam Physician*. 2002;66:1001-1008

68. Margai F, Henry N. A community-based assessment of learning disabilities using environmental and contextual risk factors. *Soc Sci Med*. 2003;56:1073-1085

69. Barkley RA. Major life activity and health outcomes associated with attention-deficit/hyperactivity disorder. *J Clin Psychiatry*. 2002;63(Suppl 12):10-15

70. Griffin KW, Botvin GJ, Scheier LM, Doyle MM, Williams C. Common predictors of cigarette smoking, alcohol use, aggression, and delinquency among inner-city minority youth. *Addict Behav*. 2003;28:1141-1148

71. National Adolescent Health Information Center. 2006 *Fact Sheet on Suicide: Adolescents & Young Adults*. San Francisco, CA: University of California San Francisco; 2006

72. Grunbaum JA, Kann L, Kinchen S, Ross J, et al. Youth Risk Behavior Surveillance—United States, 2005. MMWR Surveill Summ. 2004;53:1-96. Available at: http://www.cdc.gov/mmwr/preview/mmwrhtml/ss5302a1.htm. Accessed May 15, 2007

73. American Academy of Pediatrics, Committee on Injury and Poison Prevention. Firearm-related injuries affecting the pediatric population. *Pediatrics*. 2000;105:888-895

74. Horgan CM. *Substance Abuse: The Nation's Number One Health Problem*. Princeton, NJ: Robert Wood Johnson Foundation; 2001

75. MacKay AP, Fingerhut LA, Duran C. *Adolescent Health Chartbook: Health, United States, 2000*. Hyattsville, MD: National Center for Health Statistics; 2000

76. Werner MJ, Joffe A, Graham AV. Screening, early identification, and office-based intervention with children and youth living in substance-abusing families. *Pediatrics*. 1999;103:1099-1112

77. National Adolescent Health Information Center. *Fact Sheet on Substance Use: Adolescents and Young Adults*. San Francisco, CA: University of California San Francisco; 2002. Available at: http://nahic.ucsf.edu//downloads/sub_use.pdf

78. Monti PM, Colby SM, O'Leary TA, eds. *Adolescents, Alcohol, and Substance Abuse: Reaching Teens Through Brief Interventions*. New York, NY: Guilford Press; 2001

79. *Report on Teen Cigarette Smoking and Marijuana Use*. New York: National Center on Addiction and Substance Abuse at Columbia University; September 2003

80. Johnston L, O'Malley PM, Bachman JG. *Monitoring the Future: National Results on Adolescent Drug Use: Overview of Key Findings, 2002*. Secondary school students. Bethesda, MD: National Institute on Drug Abuse; 2003. NIH Publication No. 03-5374

81. Office of National Drug Control Policy. Drug Facts. Available at: http://www.whitehousedrugpolicy.gov/drugfact/index.html. Accessed September 13, 2007

82. Robertson EB, David SL, Rao SA. *Preventing Drug Abuse Among Children and Adolescents*. 2nd ed. Bethesda, MD: National Institute on Drug Abuse, National Institutes of Health; 2003

83. Comerci GD, Schwebel R. Substance abuse: an overview. *Adolesc Med*. 2000;11:79-101

84. Elster AB. Comparison of recommendations for adolescent clinical preventive services developed by national organizations. *Arch Pediatr Adolesc Med*. 1998;152:193-198

85. National Adolescent Health Information Center. *Investing in Clinical Preventive Health Services for Adolescents*. Washington, DC: US Department of Health and Human Services; 2001

86. Knight JR, Sherritt L, Shrier LA, Harris SK, Chang G. Validity of the CRAFFT Substance Abuse Screening Test Among Adolescent Clinic Patients. *Arch Pediatr Adolesc Med*. 2002;156:607-614

87. Boekeloo BO, Bobbin MP, Lee WI, Worrell KD, Hamburger EK, Russek-Cohen E. Effect of patient priming and primary care provider prompting on adolescent-provider communication about alcohol. *Arch Pediatr Adolesc Med*. 2003;157:433-439

88. Cabana MD, Rand CS, Powe NR, et al. Why don't physicians follow clinical practice guidelines? A framework for improvement. *JAMA*. 1999;282:1458-1465

89. Klein JD, Allan MJ, Elster AB, et al. Improving adolescent preventive care in community health centers. *Pediatrics*. 2001;107:318-327

90. Stange KC, Woolf SH, Gjeltema K. One minute for prevention: the power of leveraging to fulfill the promise of health behavior counseling. *Am J Prev Med*. 2002;22:320-323

91. Stevens MM, Olson AL, Gaffney CA, Tosteson TD, Mott LA, Starr P. A pediatric, practice-based, randomized trial of drinking and smoking prevention and bicycle helmet, gun, and seatbelt safety promotion. *Pediatrics*. 2002;109:490-497

92. Yarnall KS, Pollak KI, Ostbye T, Krause KM, Michener JL. Primary care: is there enough time for prevention? *Am J Public Health*. 2003;93:635-641

93. Weinberg NZ, Rahdert E, Colliver JD, Glantz MD. Adolescent substance abuse: a review of the past 10 years. *J Am Acad Child Adolesc Psychiatry*. 1998;37:252-261

94. Hingson R, Heeren T, Zakocs R. Age of drinking onset and involvement in physical fights after drinking. *Pediatrics*. 2001;108:872-877

95. Winters KC. Assessing adolescent substance use problems and other areas of functioning: state of the art. In: Monti PM, Colby SM, O'Leary TA, eds. *Adolescents, Alcohol, and Substance Abuse: Reaching Teens Through Brief Interventions*. New York, NY: Guilford Press; 2001:80-106

96. Wolraich MFM. *The Classification of Child and Adolescent Mental Diagnoses in Primary Care: Diagnostic and Statistical Manual for Primary Care (DSM-PC) Child and Adolescent version*. Elk Grove Village, IL: American Academy of Pediatrics; 1996

97. Hawkins JD, Catalano RF. *Communities that Care: Action for Drug Abuse Prevention*. San Francisco, CA: Jossey-Bass Publishers; 1992

98. Child Trends. *American Teens: A Special Look at "What Works" in Adolescent Development*. Washington, DC: Child Trends; 2003

99. Drug Strategies. *Making the Grade: A Guide to School Drug Prevention Programs*. Washington, DC: Drug Strategies; 1999

100. Simantov E, Schoen C, Klein JD. Health-compromising behaviors: why do adolescents smoke or drink? Identifying underlying risk and protective factors. *Arch Pediatr Adolesc Med*. 2000;154:1025-1033

101. Knight, JR. Substance use, abuse, and dependence. In: Levine MD, Carey WB, Crocker AC, eds. *Developmental-Behavioral Pediatrics*. 3rd ed. Philadelphia, PA: Saunders; 1999:477-492

PROMOTING MENTAL HEALTH

Promoting Healthy Weight

Theme 4

INTRODUCTION

Healthy weight, because of its importance to childhood and future adult health, its interrelationships with lifestyle, behavior, the environment, and family life, and the growing prevalence of overweight and obesity, has been identified as 1 of 2 themes with special significance. Recommendations for screening, assessing, and managing healthy weight and the prevention of overweight and obesity are highlighted throughout this book.

A child's weight status is the result of a number of factors (genes, metabolism, height, behavior, and environment) working together. Two of the most important determinants are nutrition and physical activity. A balanced and nutritious diet and regular physical activity are key factors to promoting a healthy weight during childhood and throughout life. This is also true for children and youth with special health care needs who may have additional nutrition

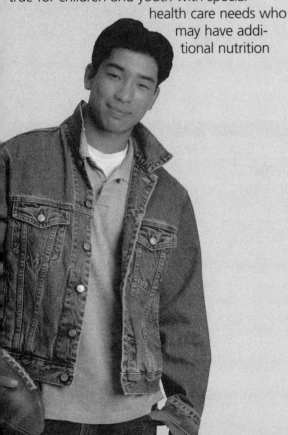

and physical activity demands specific to their condition. Therefore, readers are encouraged to review this theme, which focuses on assessing, managing, and preventing overweight and obesity, in concert with the Promoting Healthy Nutrition and Promoting Physical Activity themes.

Defining Pediatric Overweight and Obesity

An overweight child or adolescent has accrued weight beyond the healthy level for his or her age and height. Obesity represents an even greater increase of overweight. The overweight child is at risk for obesity in adolescence. Obesity places children and adolescents at risk for adverse health effects.[1]

Overweight and obesity in children and adolescents are defined by body mass index (BMI), which equals weight in kilograms divided by height in meters squared. (In the English system, BMI equals weight in pounds divided by height in inches squared, multiplied by 703.) Because children's body fatness changes as they grow, and boys and girls differ in body fatness as they mature, BMI for children, also referred to as BMI-for-age, is determined by comparing weight and height against age- and gender-specific growth charts. BMI for children and youth with special health care needs is calculated in the same manner. Table 1 provides percentiles for interpreting BMI for normal weight, overweight, and obesity in children.[2,3]

TABLE 1

Percentiles for Assessing Overweight and Obesity

Percentile	Status
<85th	Normal, or healthy, weight
≥85th but <95th	Overweight
≥95th	Obese

Prevalence and Trends of Overweight and Obesity in Children

Childhood obesity is the most prevalent pediatric nutritional problem in the United States. It occurs in all parts of the country and affects all income, racial, and ethnic groups. The nutrition and physical activity choices that lead to obesity are influenced by many factors, including lack of access to nutritious foods, individual lifestyle choices, food advertising, and a prevailing culture that promotes overeating and sedentary lifestyles. It affects as many as 15% to 30% of grade-school children and adolescents. The percentage of overweight children aged 6 to 11 years has almost quadrupled from 4% in 1970 to 19% in 2004.[4] The prevalence of overweight varies among different ethnic groups. African American, Hispanic/Latino, and American Indian children and adolescents have particularly high overweight rates.[5,6] Children also are becoming overweight at increasingly young ages. This is of concern because obesity that occurs early in life and persists throughout childhood is more difficult to treat than obesity that develops later in life. Moreover, a child who continues to be obese into adolescence is at increased risk of developing related health problems. A school-aged child who is at risk of being overweight has an increased probability of becoming an obese adolescent and adult. Obese adolescents are unlikely to attain normal adult weight.

National Health and Nutrition Examination Survey (NHANES) data show a continuing rise in overweight status among children and youth. The increase in overweight from NHANES (1988-1994) to NHANES (1999-2000) has been significant (Table 2). African American and Mexican American children are disproportionately affected by this problem. For example, among 6- to 11-year-olds, 22% of African American children and 22.5% of Mexican American children are classified as overweight compared to 17.7% non-Hispanic white children.

> The nutrition and physical activity choices that lead to obesity are influenced by many factors, including lack of access to nutritious foods, individual lifestyle choices, food advertising, and a prevailing culture that promotes overeating and sedentary lifestyles.

TABLE 2

Obesity Statistics for Children (Body Mass Index ≥95th Percentile)

Age (years)	NHANES 1988-1994 (%)	NHANES 1999-2000 (%)	NHANES 2003-2004 (%)
2-5	7.2	10.4	13.9
6-11	11.3	15.3	18.8

NHANES, National Health and Nutrition Examination Survey.
Data from Ogden CL, Flegal KM, Carroll MD, Johnson CL. Prevalence and trends in overweight among US children and adolescents, 1999-2000. *JAMA*. 2002;288:1728-1732[5]; Hedley AA, Ogden, CL, Johnson, CL, Carroll, MD, Curtin, LR, Flegal, KM. Overweight and obesity among US children, adolescents, and adults, 1999-2002. *JAMA*. 2004;291:2847-2850.[7] Ogden CC, Carroll MD, Curtin LR, McDowell MA, Tabak CJ, Flegal KM. Prevalence of overweight and obesity in the United States, 1999-2004. *JAMA*. 2006;295:1549-1555.[8]

Children and youth with special health care needs share similar risk for overweight conditions. The risk of obesity in US Special Olympics athletes, both in children and adults, is similar to that of the general population. United States Special Olympians are 3.1 times more likely to be obese than non-US participants in the Special Olympics.[9]

Obesity is associated with significant health problems in children and adolescents and is an important early risk factor for much adult morbidity and mortality. Medical problems that are common in obese children and adolescents can affect cardiovascular health (eg, hypercholesterolemia, dyslipidemia, and hypertension), the pulmonary system (eg, asthma and obstructive sleep apnea), the endocrine system (eg, hyperinsulinism, insulin resistance, impaired glucose tolerance, type 2 diabetes mellitus, and menstrual irregularity), the musculoskeletal system (eg, osteoarthritis), and mental health (eg, depression and low self-esteem).

Screening for, and Assessing, Overweight and Obesity

Infants, children, and adolescents should be considered at high risk of overweight or obesity if any of the following conditions apply:

- One or both parents are obese.
- One or more siblings are obese.
- They are from families with low incomes.
- They have a chronic disease or disability that limits mobility.

The first step in screening for weight problems is determining and interpreting a child's BMI-for-age. If he is overweight or obese, a comprehensive physical assessment is then critical to determine the appropriate interventions. Assessment also should determine whether the child's weight status is accompanied by any other disorder and whether the child has any physical limitations that will require modifications to an exercise program to make it suited to the child.[2]

A critical component of this review is the health care professional's sensitivity to cultural differences that exist in perceptions about healthy weight and body image. Scientific findings about healthy weights may not coincide with family and community beliefs about health and beauty. Discussion about family cultural perspectives is a key piece of assessing obesity in children. In addition, the motivation to make the changes needed to achieve and maintain a healthy weight may come from a variety of sources other than scientific evidence. Partnering with respected community leaders, such as elders or clergy, can encourage behavior change. Techniques for assessing and treating obesity are the same across all cultures. What differs is the way in which these actions can be approached and carried out. Culturally relevant messages can be potent for families.

If a child is overweight or obese, health care professionals also must be sensitive to the possibility that the family may be experiencing food insecurity. Food insecurity for a family means limited or uncertain availability of nutritionally adequate and safe foods, or uncertain ability to acquire appropriate foods in socially acceptable ways. Twelve percent of American households were food insecure for at least part of 2004.[10] The prevalence of food insecurity has increased steadily since 1998.[11] Food insecurity forces people to buy and consume less-expensive foods, which are often less nutrient dense but more calorically dense and higher in fat than more expensive foods. Overconsumption of nonnutritious foods is recognized as a factor in the etiology of obesity in disadvantaged populations.[12] (For more information on this topic, see the Promoting Healthy Nutrition theme.)

Children older than 2 years who are between the 85th and 95th percentile of BMI need a second-level assessment and screening for the following 5 items:

> Obesity is associated with significant health problems in children and adolescents and is an important early risk factor for much adult morbidity and mortality.

- **Family history.** Does the history include early cardiovascular disease, parental hypercholesterolemia, parental obesity, or a first- or second-generation relative with type 2 diabetes, or is the family history of these conditions unknown?
- **Blood pressure.** What is the child's or adolescent's blood pressure, based on age, gender, and height? Sustained blood pressures above the 90th percentile for age, gender, and height are considered prehypertensive, and blood pressure above the 95th percentile for age, gender, and height is considered high.
- **Fasting Lipid Profile.** Is fasting blood cholesterol level 200 mg/dL or higher? Is HDL cholesterol reduced? Are triglycerides elevated?

TABLE 3

Criteria for Metabolic Syndrome in Children and Adolescents

Measures	Criteria
BMI	>97th percentile
Triglycerides	>110 mg/dL
High-density lipoprotein cholesterol	<40 mg/dL
Systolic/diastolic blood pressure	>90th percentile for age, gender, and height
Impaired glucose tolerance	>110 mg/dL FBG >140 mg/dL OGTT

Waist circumference
  Boys
  Girls
	
	>90th percentile
	≥90th percentile

FBG, Fasting blood glucose; OGTT, oral glucose tolerance test.

- **Large change in BMI.** Has there been an increase of more than 2 to 3 points in BMI-for-age in 1 year?
- **Concern about weight.** Has the child or family expressed concerns over the child's or adolescent's weight?

If any one of these factors is present, the child should receive, or be referred for, an in-depth medical assessment and intervention to reduce weight and improve overall health.

Body Mass Index Rebound

After about 1 year of age, BMI-for-age begins to decline and continues falling during the preschool years. After it reaches a minimum at approximately 4 to 6 years of age, BMI-for-age begins a gradual increase through adolescence.

The increase in BMI that occurs after it reaches its lowest point is referred to as BMI rebound. This change is a normal pattern of growth in all children. The age when the BMI rebound occurs may be a critical period in childhood for the development of obesity as an adult. An early BMI rebound, occurring before 4 to 6 years of age, is associated with obesity in adulthood. Additional research is needed to further understand the impact of early BMI rebound on adult obesity.

Metabolic Syndrome

Metabolic syndrome is not a disease itself, but is characterized as a cluster of related diseases that has been well described in adults and is associated with increased health risks, including cardiovascular disease. Currently, no acceptable definition of the metabolic syndrome exists for children and adolescents. A 2004 study[13] in children and adolescents proposed that children having 3 or more of the criteria shown in Table 3 be defined as having metabolic syndrome. Being overweight leads to insulin resistance and hypertension, dyslipidemia, type 2 diabetes, and other metabolic abnormalities. The prevalence of metabolic syndrome increases as BMI climbs above the 95th percentile.

Results of this study suggest that metabolic syndrome is more common among children and adolescents than previously reported and that its prevalence increases directly with the degree of obesity.[13] Increasingly, data demonstrate that childhood obesity is "significantly associated with insulin resistance, dyslipidemia, and elevated blood pressure in young adulthood."[14] Thus, risk factors and pre-disease conditions (eg, insulin resistance and shortness of breath) must be identified and treated as early and as effectively as possible.

NHANES (1988-1994) data showed a 6.8% prevalence of the characteristics that define metabolic syndrome among overweight adolescents in the 85th to 94th percentiles for weight and 28.7% among obese adolescents who are in the 95th or greater percentiles for weight.[15] These rates may underestimate the current extent of the problem, because the magnitude and prevalence of childhood obesity have increased in the past decade.

Treating Overweight and Obesity

The development and persistence of overweight and obesity is based on a wide variety of factors, including age, gender, family history, developmental stage, ethnicity, and social environment. Each factor influences the treatment goal, the selection of the type of treatment, and the course of therapy. Obesity is a complex condition and, even with strict adherence to treatment recommendations, progress with weight loss can be slow. Because treatment requires a time commitment, recommended interventions must recognize family lifestyle patterns and the child's social environment.

The primary goals of treatment should relate to changing eating and physical activity habits and resolving any comorbid conditions. Interventions should be focused on encouraging dietary changes, increasing physical activity, and modifying behaviors, rather than weight loss alone. Box 1 presents the goals for intervention.

Preventing Overweight and Obesity

Because intervention programs are few, and program costs are high, the most successful intervention for promoting a healthy weight is prevention. Strategies that encourage healthy eating behaviors, regular physical activity, and reduced sedentary behaviors (eg, watching television, videotapes, or DVDs, or using the computer) are essential to helping children and adolescents achieve and maintain a healthy weight. The need for well-designed studies that examine a range of interventions remains a priority.[2] Features of

---

BOX 1
Intervention Goals

Children 2 to 18 years of age

- BMI 85th to 94th percentile: GOAL = Weight maintenance, resulting in decreasing BMI as age increases
- BMI ≥95th percentile with no comorbidity: GOAL = Weight maintenance, resulting in decreasing BMI as age increases
- BMI ≥95th percentile with comorbid conditions or severely obese: GOAL = Gradual weight loss that should not exceed 1 pound per month in children 2 to 11 years of age or 2 pounds per week in older obese children and adolescents

Source: The Expert Committee Recommendations on the assessment, prevention, and treatment of child and adolescent overweight and obesity. Supplement to *Pediatrics*. In press.[1]

---

prevention programs with successful outcomes include:

- Targeting both parents and children for behavior change
- Emphasizing the role of parents as a way to influence young children's behaviors
- Using behavior modification and education, rather than focusing on education alone
- Increasing physical activity, which is essential to long-term maintenance of weight control in children
- Reducing sedentary activities, which achieves better long-term physical activity levels than increasing structured physical activity
- Maintaining the treatment program over a long period of time

Successful outcomes also depend on action and guidance by everyone involved with a child or adolescent, from parents to health care professionals to the school and the community. Some helpful actions are listed in Box 2.

Strategies that encourage healthy eating behaviors, regular physical activity, and reduced sedentary behaviors (eg, watching television, videotapes, or DVDs, or using the computer) are essential to helping children and adolescents achieve and maintain a healthy weight.

BOX 2

Actions to Reduce Overweight and Obesity in Children and Adolescents

For the health care professional

- Plot BMI routinely for early recognition of overweight and obesity.
- Address increasing BMI percentile before it reaches 95% or higher.
- Identify "at risk" children.
    - Children whose parents are obese
    - Children with a sibling who is obese
    - Children from families with low income
    - Children with a chronic disease or disability that limits mobility
- Provide anticipatory guidance for nutrition and physical activity.

For the parents

- Act as a role model for nutrition and physical activity.
- "Special times" do not have to involve food or sedentary activities.
- Use things other than food or TV time as rewards.
- Promote physically active family time (eg, hikes, bike rides, and playing outside).
- Eat together as a family.
- Limit screen time (ie, TV, computer, and video games) to 1 to 2 hours per day.[16]
- Do not allow a TV in the child's bedroom.[17]
- Turn the TV off during mealtimes.
- Limit dining out.
- Promote water and low-fat milk consumption over juice and soda.

For schools

- Integrate nutrition and physical activity education into the school curriculum.
- Promote physical activity.
- Encourage children to walk or bike to school where it is safe to do so.
- Provide nutritious meals.
- Have recess before lunch.
- Control vending machines and encourage the sale of healthy foods in vending machines.

For the community

- Provide safe playgrounds and safe neighborhoods for bike riding, walking, and other physical activity.
- Promote physical activity outside of school.
- Identify and deliver culturally relevant messages about healthy eating and weight.

For reimbursement and legislation (insurance and policy)

- Acknowledge obesity as a medical condition so that health care professionals can be reimbursed for services.
- Provide reimbursement to health care professionals for anticipatory guidance about nutrition and physical activity.

Sources

American Academy of Pediatrics, Committee on Nutrition. Prevention of pediatric overweight and obesity. *Pediatrics.* 2003;112:424-430.[2]

American Academy of Pediatrics, Council on Sports Medicine and Fitness and Council on School Health. Active healthy living: prevention of childhood obesity through increased physical activity. *Pediatrics.* 2006;117:1834-1842.[18]

Screen Time

Although few data have been compiled on media use and its relationship to weight gain in the early childhood years, some literature describes the relationship of screen watching and weight gain for children in the middle childhood and adolescent years.[19] Children who watch 5 or more hours of TV per day were 4.6 times more likely to be overweight or obese compared with those watching 0 to 2 hours per day.[20] All media viewing, including time spent in front of a computer screen in later childhood and adolescence, correlates with weight gain.[16,21,22] This physical inactivity should be taken into consideration in determining the total media time allowed.

Concerns about screen time and obesity generally focus on 2 issues. The first is that television watching and other screen time is a sedentary activity. Obesity prevention efforts increasingly recommend that children and adolescents reduce time spent in sedentary activities as well as increase time spent in physical activity. The second concern is the effect on eating behaviors, both because children may eat while watching television or using the computer and because food advertisements and cross-promotions on television may encourage children to buy (or influence their parents to buy) and eat foods that are high in calories, fat, and sugar, and low in nutrients. One study has shown an association between increased television viewing among children and adolescents and behaviors such as increased consumption of high-fat foods.[23] A recent analysis of advertising and obesity provides an additional perspective by suggesting that, although advertising may prompt a new behavior, its main power is to maintain and reinforce existing behaviors. By supporting unhealthful nutrition behaviors (eg, snacking on high-fat, high-calorie foods), advertising reduces individuals' ability to recognize the behaviors as detrimental to their health or their desire to change the behavior.[24]

Promoting a Healthy Weight: Infancy— Birth to 11 Months

Multiple and additive risk factors are associated with childhood overweight and obesity. Intrauterine exposure, genetic makeup, and biologic, psychological, sociocultural, and environmental factors combine to influence a child's weight. Parental obesity and maternal gestational diabetes consistently predict childhood overweight.

BMI cannot be calculated from birth to 23 months of age because length is measured instead of height. Weight-for-length is an important alternative recording of infant growth.

Exclusive breastfeeding, and avoidance of overfeeding if parents bottle feed their infants, is recommended to ensure adequate growth that is not excessive. Solid foods are not introduced until 4 to 6 months of age and should be presented as both complementary foods and calorie replacement. The young infant should have multiple opportunities for supervised back and tummy time while awake, and exploration of her environment is encouraged as an age-appropriate physical activity.

Exclusive breastfeeding, and avoidance of overfeeding if parents bottle feed their infants, is recommended to ensure adequate growth that is not excessive.

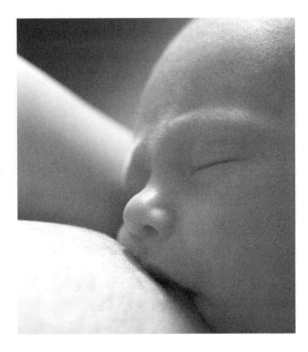

Promoting a Healthy Weight: Early Childhood—1 to 4 Years

Given the large number of significant health problems that are associated with obesity in children as age increases, the American Academy of Pediatrics (AAP) Committee on Nutrition recommends early recognition by monitoring the BMI of every child older than 2 years.[25]

Addressing rapid weight gain involves helping families initiate lifestyle changes (Box 3). The probability of an overweight 4-year-old child becoming an obese adult is about 20%. Some parents do not recognize (or accept) that their child may be gaining weight too rapidly, is overweight, or is unlikely to outgrow the overweight.

In some cultures, a large child is considered a healthy child. If families do not believe that a child is overweight, they probably will not consider changing current behaviors. Moreover, if mothers are dieting or restricting their food intake and limiting their children's access to food, the outcome is a diminished ability for the child to self-regulate food intake as well as an increased desire for the restricted foods. Interestingly, both situations can result in excessive weight gain. Many health care professionals counsel mothers to restrict food access to children, particularly young girls, in an attempt to slow weight gain. Such advice must be given judiciously so as not to hamper the child's ability to self-regulate.[25]

Early childhood is the time when a family begins to imprint its habits on a child. This is a period of opportunity for families to establish healthful eating habits and activity patterns for both children and parents. Providing and role modeling a healthy and nutritious diet, regular physical activity, and limited sedentary time is recommended. The AAP recommends no television viewing for children younger than 2 years, and no more than 1 to 2 hours per day for older children.[16] Most pediatric health care professionals

> Addressing rapid weight gain involves helping families initiate lifestyle changes.

BOX 3
A Health-Centered Approach
In its *Guidelines for Childhood Obesity Prevention Programs*, the Society for Nutrition Education notes that it is best to apply "a health-centered, rather than weight-centered, approach that focuses on the whole child, physically, mentally, and socially."

The *Guidelines* explains further by saying, "The emphasis is on living actively, eating in normal and healthy ways, and creating a nurturing environment that helps children recognize their own worth and respect cultural foodways and family traditions. It is recognized that overweight, eating disorders, hazardous weight loss, nutrient deficiencies, size discrimination, and body hatred are all interrelated and need to be addressed in comprehensive ways that do no harm."

Source: Society for Nutrition Education, Weight Realities Division. *Guidelines for Childhood Obesity Prevention Programs: Promoting Healthy Weight in Children. J Nutr Educ Behav.* 2003;35:1-4.[26]

---

include videos, computers, and TV when calculating viewing time. This "screen time" is inevitably a time of physical inactivity. Because a majority of young children spend part or all of their day in out-of-home child care programs,
parents and health care professionals should factor in their nutrition intake and physical activities in these settings.

Promoting a Healthy Weight: Middle Childhood—5 to 10 Years

Family habits that have been established for younger children can be continued and modified in the middle childhood years. Parents remain powerful role models in providing a healthy lifestyle for the family regarding food and activity. Television and other media must now be actively limited by parents and other caregivers.[27]

Out-of-home influences are becoming more important as school routine, and the behavior of peers may challenge or enrich the child's and family's habits. Media have a strong influence on food choice, and community decisions regarding school meals, food and drink vending machine policies, and physical education activities affect the child's eating and playing environment. Likewise, community resources for safe play spaces have a direct impact on obesity risk. (See Box 2.)

Promoting a Healthy Weight: Adolescence—11 to 21 Years

As with the earlier age groups, obesity during adolescence affects blood pressure, blood lipids, lipoprotein, and insulin levels. Perhaps the most widespread consequence of overweight and obesity is psychological, resulting from discrimination.[28]

The percentage of adolescents who are overweight or obese has increased considerably over the past 25 years, according to NHANES.[4] During the 1976 to 1980 survey period, 5% of adolescents aged 12 to 19 years were obese, a figure that increased to 11% during the 1988 to 1994 survey period, and to 17% during the 2003 to 2004 period.

Thus, more than 3 times as many adolescents are obese today than in 1980.[4]

Most obese adolescents have at least one additional risk factor for cardiovascular disease, such as elevated blood pressure, hyperlipidemia, or hyperinsulinemia. Adolescents who are overweight or obese are more likely to be so as adults,[29,30] and adolescent obesity has been linked to higher mortality from all causes in adulthood.[31] Racial and ethnic disparities also can be noted from obesity data.

People from various cultures may view body weight in different ways. Keeping an adolescent from being underweight may be very important to people from cultures in which poverty or insufficient food supplies are common. Families may view excess weight as healthy and may be offended if a health care professional refers to their adolescent as overweight or obese.

To reduce the risk of obesity, all foods and beverages sold or served to students in schools should meet an accepted nutritional content standard (eg, *Dietary Guidelines for Americans*[32]). However, many popular foods (foods and beverages that are not part of the federal school meal programs) that are served or sold in school cafeterias, vending machines, and school stores, and at school fundraisers are high in calories and low in nutritional value.

In addition, schools should ensure that all adolescents participate in 60 minutes of moderate to vigorous physical activity during the school day. Opportunities for physical activity through the school should be expanded, including intramural and interscholastic sports programs and other physical activity clubs, programs, and lessons.[33]

...many popular foods... that are served or sold in school cafeterias, vending machines, and school stores, and at school fundraisers are high in calories and low in nutritional value.

References

1. The Expert Committee Recommendations on the assessment, prevention, and treatment of child and adolescent overweight and obesity. Supplement to *Pediatrics*. In press

2. American Academy of Pediatrics, Committee on Nutrition. Prevention of pediatric overweight and obesity. *Pediatrics*. 2003;112:424-430

3. Himes JH, Dietz WH. Guidelines for overweight in adolescent preventive services: recommendations from an expert committee. The Expert Committee on Clinical Guidelines for Overweight in Adolescent Preventive Services. *Am J Clin Nutr*. 1994;59:307-316

4. US Centers for Disease Control and Prevention, National Center for Health Statistics. Prevalence of Overweight among Children and Adolescents: United States, 2003-2004. Available at: www.cdc.gov/nchs/products/pubs/pubd/hestats/overweight/overwght_child_03.htm. Accessed August 29, 2007

5. Ogden CL, Flegal KM, Carroll MD, Johnson CL. Prevalence and trends in overweight among US children and adolescents, 1999-2000. *JAMA*. 2002;288:1728-1732

6. Troiano RP, Flegal KM. Overweight children and adolescents: description, epidemiology, and demographics. *Pediatrics*. 1998;101:497-504

7. Hedley AA, Ogden CL, Johnson CL, Carroll MD, Curtin LR, Flegal KM. Prevalence of overweight and obesity among US children, adolescents, and adults, 1999-2002. *JAMA*. 2004;291:2847-2850

8. Ogden CL, Carroll MD, Curtin LR, McDowell MA, Tabak CJ, Flegal KM. Prevalence of overweight and obesity in the United States, 1999-2004. *JAMA*. 2006;295:1549-1555

9. Harris N, Rosenberg A, Jangda S, O'Brien K, Gallagher ML. Prevalence of obesity in International Special Olympic athletes as determined by body mass index. *J Am Diet Assoc*. 2003;103:235-237

10. United States Department of Agriculture, Economic Research Service, Briefing Rooms. Food Security in the United States. Available at: http://www.ers.usda.gov/briefing/FoodSecurity/. Accessed August 29, 2007

11. Sullivan AF, Choi E. *Hunger and Food Insecurity in the Fifty States: 1998-2000*. Waltham, MA: Center on Hunger and Poverty; 2002

12. Center on Hunger and Poverty. *The Paradox of Hunger and Obesity in America*. Waltham, MA: Center on Hunger and Poverty; 2003

13. Weiss R, Dziura J, Burgert TS, et al. Obesity and the metabolic syndrome in children and adolescents. *N Eng J Med*. 2004;350:2362-2374

14. Steinberger J, Daniels SR, American Heart Association. Atherosclerosis, Hypertension, and Obesity in the Young Committee (Council on Cardiovascular Disease in the Young) American Heart Association Diabetes Committee (Council on Nutrition, Physical Activity, and Metabolism). Obesity, insulin resistance, diabetes, and cardiovascular risk in children. *Circulation*. 2003;107:1448-1453

15. Cook S, Weitzman M, Auinger P, Nguyen M, Dietz WH. Prevalence of a metabolic syndrome phenotype in adolescents: findings from the third National Health and Nutrition Examination Survey, 1988-1994. *Arch Pediatr Adolesc Med*. 2003;157:821-827

16. American Academy of Pediatrics, Committee on Public Education. Children, adolescents, and television. *Pediatrics*. 2001;107:423-426

17. Center on Media and Child Health, Children's Hospital Boston. Issue Brief: *The Effects of Electronic Media on Children Ages Zero to Six: A History of Research*. Menlo Park, CA: The Henry J. Kaiser Family Foundation; 2005

18. American Academy of Pediatrics, Council on Sports Medicine and Fitness and Council on School Health. Active healthy living: prevention of childhood obesity through increased physical activity. *Pediatrics*. 2006;117:1834-1842.

19. Robinson TN. Television viewing and childhood obesity. *Pediatr Clin North Am*. 2001;48:1017-1025

20. Gortmaker SL, Must A, Sobol AM, Peterson K, Colditz GA, Dietz WH. Television viewing as a cause of increasing obesity among children in the United States, 1986-1990. *Arch Pediatr Adolesc Med*. 1996;150:356-362

21. Certain LK, Kahn RS. Prevalence, correlates, and trajectory of television viewing among infants and toddlers. *Pediatrics*. 2002;109:634-642

22. Anderson DR, Huston AC, Schmitt KL, Linebarger DL, Wright JC. Early childhood television viewing and adolescent behavior: the recontact study. *Monogr Soc Res Child Dev*. 2001;66:I-VIII, 1-147

23. Wong ND, Hei TK, Qaqundah PY, Davidson DM, Bassin SL, Gold KV. Television viewing and pediatric hypercholesterolemia. *Pediatrics*. 1992;90:75-79

24. Hoek J, Gendall P. Advertising and obesity: a behavioral perspective. *J Health Commun*. 2006;11:409-423

25. Kleinman RE, ed. *Pediatric Nutrition Handbook*. 5th ed. Elk Grove Village, IL: American Academy of Pediatrics, Committee on Nutrition; 2004

26. Society for Nutrition Education, Weight Realities Division. *Guidelines for Childhood Obesity Prevention Programs: Promoting Healthy Weight in Children*. J Nutr Educ Behav. 2003;35:1-4

27. Hassink SG, ed. *A Parent's Guide to Childhood Obesity: A Road Map to Health*. Elk Grove Village, IL: American Academy of Pediatrics; 2006

28. Daniels SR, Arnett DK, Eckel RH, et al. Overweight in children and adolescents: pathophysiology, consequences, prevention, and treatment. *Circulation*. 2005;111:1999-2012

29. Guo SS, Wu W, Chumlea WC, Roche AF. Predicting overweight and obesity in adulthood from body mass index values in childhood and adolescence. *Am J Clin Nutr*. 2002;76:653-658

30. Serdula MK, Ivery D, Coates RJ, Freedman DS, Williamson DF, Byers T. Do obese children become obese adults? A review of the literature. *Prev Med*. 1993;22:167-177

31. Must A, Jacques PF, Dallal GE, Bajema CJ, Dietz WH. Long-term morbidity and mortality of overweight adolescents. A follow-up of the Harvard Growth Study of 1922 to 1935. *N Engl J Med*. 1992;327:1350-1355

32. US Department of Health and Human Services and US Department of Agriculture. *Dietary Guidelines for Americans 2005*. 6th ed. Washington, DC: US Government Printing Office; 2005

33. Institute of Medicine, Committee on Prevention of Obesity. *Progress in Preventing Childhood Obesity: Focus on Schools—Brief Summary*. Washington, DC: National Academies Press; 2006

Promoting Healthy Nutrition

Theme 5

INTRODUCTION

Infancy, childhood, and adolescence are marked by rapid physical growth and development, and every child's and adolescent's health and development depends on good nutrition. Any disruption in appropriate nutrient intake may have lasting effects on growth potential and developmental achievement. Physical growth, developmental requirements, nutrition needs, and feeding patterns vary significantly in each stage of growth and development.

The dramatic increase in pediatric overweight and obesity in recent years has increased health care professionals' and parents' attention to nutrition. Along with regular physical activity, a balanced and nutritious diet is essential to prevent pediatric overweight conditions. Therefore, health care professionals are encouraged to review this Bright Futures theme in concert with the Promoting Physical Activity and Promoting Healthy Weight themes.

Key Food and Nutrition Considerations

Food and nutrition behaviors are influenced by myriad environmental and cultural forces. Health care professionals should keep these forces in mind as they work with patients and families. Three issues of particular importance are discussed here.

Culture and Food

All people belong to some kind of cultural group. Culture influences the way people look at the world, how they interact with others, and how they expect others to behave. To meet the challenge of providing nutrition supervision to diverse populations, health care professionals must learn to respect and appreciate the variety of cultural traditions related to food and the wide variation in food practices within and among cultural groups. They also need to understand how their own cultures influence their attitudes and behaviors, and the resulting implications for nutrition counseling. Sharing food experiences, asking questions, observing the food choices people make, and working with the community are important ways for health care professionals to learn about and appreciate the food and nutrition traditions of other cultures.[1]

Culture influences how people prepare food, how they use seasonings, and how often they eat certain foods. These behaviors can differ from region to region and family to family, though some traditions exist across cultures. For example, staple, or core, foods form the foundation of the diet in all cultures. Staple foods, such as rice or beans, are typically bland, relatively inexpensive, easy to prepare, an important source of calories, and an indispensable part of the diet.

Acculturation, which is the adoption of the beliefs, values, attitudes, and behaviors of a dominant, or mainstream, culture, can be a significant influence on a person's food choices. Acculturation may involve altering traditional eating behaviors to make them similar to those of the dominant culture. These changes can be grouped into 3 categories: (1) the addition of new foods, (2) the substitution of foods, and (3) the rejection of foods. People add new foods to their diets for several reasons, including increased economic status and food availability (especially if the food is not readily available in the person's homeland). Substitution may occur because new foods are more convenient to prepare, more affordable, or better liked than traditional ones. Children and adolescents, in particular, may reject traditional foods because eating them makes them feel different from the mainstream.

Culture also influences nonnutritive aspects of food practices, and any nutritional information and guidance should take these preferences and practices into account. Some ethnic practices related to diet and nutrition may focus more on the food's texture, appearance, flavor, or aroma, or on beliefs related to the complementary nature of the food items, rather than on specific nutritional value. For many people, certain foods are closely linked to strong feelings of being cared for and nurtured by their families or are a reflection of religious practices. People from virtually all cultures use food during celebrations.

In many cultures, people believe that food promotes health, cures disease, or has other medicinal qualities. In addition, many people believe that foods can help maintain a

balance in the body that is important to health. For example, many Chinese believe that health and disease are related to the balance between "yin" and "yang" forces in the body. Diseases caused by yin forces are treated with yang foods to restore balance, and vice versa. In Puerto Rico, foods are classified as hot or cold (which may not reflect the actual temperature or spiciness of foods), and people believe that maintaining a balance between these 2 types of foods is important to health.

Health care professionals can provide effective nutrition guidance by being sensitive to cultural beliefs that categorize foods in ways other than the Western scientific model, by exploring such beliefs, and by incorporating them into their guidance. When discussing their food choices, patients and their parents may respond by saying what they think the health care professional wants to hear. Health care professionals can encourage people to be more candid about their food choices by asking open-ended, nonjudgmental questions that reflect their knowledge of, and sensitivity to, these issues.

Two issues illustrate the challenges of providing nutrition supervision to people from diverse cultural backgrounds. The first, lactose intolerance, highlights the medical aspects involved. The second, attitudes toward body weight, highlights the deep-seated emotional and attitudinal aspects that are often involved.

LACTOSE INTOLERANCE
Lactose intolerance is common in people of non-European ancestry. People who are lactose intolerant may experience cramps and diarrhea when they eat moderate to large amounts of foods that contain lactose, such as milk and other dairy products. Children and adolescents may be able to avoid symptoms by consuming small servings of milk throughout the day, by consuming lactose-reduced milk, or by taking lactase tablets or

Health care professionals can provide effective nutrition guidance by being sensitive to cultural beliefs that categorize foods in ways other than the Western scientific model, by exploring such beliefs, and by incorporating them into their guidance.

drops with milk. Cheese and yogurt are often better tolerated than milk because they contain less lactose. For people who cannot tolerate any milk or dairy products in their diet, health care professionals can suggest other sources of calcium, such as dark green, leafy vegetables or canned salmon, and calcium-fortified foods, such as orange juice, tofu, or bread.

ATTITUDES ABOUT BODY WEIGHT

People from different cultures can view body weight differently. Keeping a child from being underweight can be very important to people from cultures in which poverty or insufficient food supplies are common. Families may not recognize that their child is overweight according to body mass index (BMI) tables or may view excess weight as healthy. In these cases, the families may be offended if a health care professional refers to their child as overweight or obese. (For more information on this topic, see the Promoting Healthy Weight theme.)

Food Insecurity and Hunger

Hunger describes the personal sensation that results from a lack of food and is typically felt as unpleasant or painful. Involuntary hunger results from not being able to obtain enough food and excludes hunger related to voluntary dieting, religious fasting, or the personal choice to skip a meal.

Food insecurity for a family means limited or uncertain availability of nutritionally adequate and safe foods, or the uncertain ability to acquire appropriate foods in socially acceptable ways. In contrast, food-secure households have access to sufficient food for a healthy lifestyle at all times. Twelve percent of American households were food insecure for at least part of 2004.[2] (The remaining families were food secure throughout the entire year of 2004.) The prevalence of food insecurity has increased steadily since 1998.[3]

Food insecurity may occur with or without hunger. In its most severe presentation, this problem is associated with hunger and is an indication of a serious nutritional problem and family predicament. Food insecurity without hunger is associated with increased nutritional risk.

An important deleterious effect of food insecurity is that it forces people to buy and consume less-expensive foods, which are often less nutrient dense, but more calorically dense and higher in fat than more expensive foods. As a result, the nutritional quality of the diet declines. (For more information on this topic, see the Promoting Healthy Weight theme.)

The problems of food insecurity and hunger may be difficult to detect in the primary pediatric health care setting. If disorders of growth, both underweight and overweight, are noted, health care professionals should ask about food security. Options for referral and community support are available for each developmental stage. For example, local lactation specialists or other knowledgeable health care professionals, such as *doulas* or *promotoras,* can provide follow-up care after a new mother is discharged from the hospital, and they can consult by phone or schedule visits to a hospital-based lactation clinic. Health maintenance organizations and community hospitals also are a source of infant nutrition education. The US Department of Agriculture (USDA) Special Supplemental Nutrition Program for Women, Infants, and Children (WIC) offers a food package for women who are pregnant or postpartum, women who are breastfeeding their baby, and for infants and children up to 5 years of age. Health departments offer educational services through WIC and other programs in which public health nurses or nutritionists visit families at home.

Families also may qualify for programs such as the USDA Food Stamp Program. A community food shelf or pantry can provide

Twelve percent of American households were food insecure for at least part of 2004... The prevalence of food insecurity has increased steadily since 1998.

additional food for needy families. For school-aged children and adolescents, community services expand to include free school breakfast and lunch programs and, ideally, nutritious and appealing school food services. For adolescent parents, school programs can focus on the importance of prenatal nutrition to ensure the quality of nutrition.

Partnerships With the Community

Partnerships among health care professionals, families, and communities are essential to ensure that infants and children have good nutrition and that parents receive guidance on infant and child nutrition and feeding. (For more information on this topic, see the Promoting Community Relationships and Resources theme.) Health care professionals can have a tremendous impact on decisions about feeding the family because they provide an opportunity for parents to discuss, reflect on, and decide on options that best suit their circumstances. As part of their guidance, health care professionals also can identify and contact community resources that help parents at each stage of their children's development. As a result of considerable media attention to the problem of overweight and obesity, the public has become increasingly aware of the importance of healthful eating and adequate physical activity. Communities have responded by creating educational programs that provide nutritious school lunches, access to affordable nutritious foods, and safe neighborhood opportunities for play and exercise. Health care professionals can help families learn about and participate in these opportunities. These resources are particularly important for families with limited or no literacy skills and for those with limited English proficiency.

> Partnerships among health care professionals, families, and communities are essential to ensure that infants and children have good nutrition and that parents receive guidance on infant and child nutrition and feeding.

Essential Components of Nutrition

The following essential components of nutrition are useful constructs for discussing nutrition from birth to young adulthood:

- **Nutrition for appropriate growth**— Provide adequate energy and essential nutrients to ensure appropriate growth and prevent overweight or obesity.
- **Nutrition and development of feeding and eating skills**—Choose feedings that provide all the essential nutrients and support the development of appropriate feeding and eating skills.
- **Healthy feeding and eating habits**— Establish a positive, nurturing environment and healthy patterns of feeding and eating to promote healthy eating habits that are built on variety, balance, and moderation.
- **Healthy eating relationships**— Promote healthy adult-child feeding relationships and social and emotional development.
- **Nutrition for children and youth with special health care needs**— Recognize special nutrient demands or supplemental needs for vitamins or minerals related to a child's specific and special health condition and provide these nutrition components in an effective and family-centered manner.

Promoting Nutritional Health: Preconception and the Prenatal Period

In deciding to become parents, a couple may examine many issues of lifestyle and health because they recognize that their nutrition and physical activity beliefs, habits, and practices affect not only their own health but also the health of their family and children. Obesity, smoking, alcohol, and substance use affect the family as well. Pregnant women and women who may become pregnant should be encouraged to follow a nutritious diet. Adequate intakes of certain nutrients, such as folic acid, are important even before conception.

Folic Acid

Neural tube defects are among the most common birth defects contributing to infant mortality and serious disability. Women of childbearing age can substantially reduce their risk of having babies with certain congenital malformations, including spina bifida, by taking appropriate amounts of folic acid before and during early pregnancy. Current guidelines suggest that all women of childbearing age take a daily multivitamin or multivitamin-mineral supplement containing 400 μg of folic acid.[4-7] Women who have given birth previously to a child with a neural tube defect, or those who have a history of insulin-dependent diabetes or a seizure disorder and are taking antimetabolites or antiepileptic drugs (eg, carbamazepine or valproic acid), require higher dosages of folate. The appropriate folic acid dosages continue to evolve. The most current recommendations are available from the Centers for Disease Control and Prevention (CDC).[4]

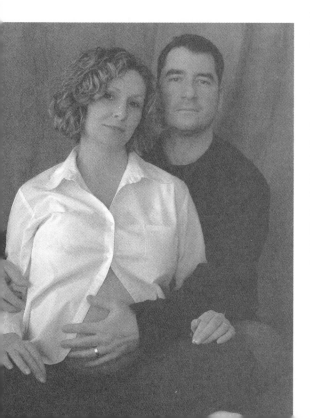

Promoting Nutritional Health: Infancy— Birth to 11 Months

Physical growth, developmental achievements, nutrition needs, and feeding patterns vary significantly in each stage of infancy. During the first 2 to 6 weeks of life, the infant primarily feeds, sleeps, and grows. The most rapid growth occurs in early infancy, between birth and 6 months of age. In middle infancy, from 6 to 9 months of age, and late infancy, from 9 to 12 months of age, rapid growth continues, but at a slower pace. By late infancy, mastery of purposeful activity complements physical maturity, and loss of newborn reflexes allows him to progress from a diet of breast milk or formula to feeding with an increasingly wide variety of flavors, textures, and foods.

Feeding practices and routines serve as the foundation for much of child and family development, as parents build many important skills. These skills include identifying, assessing, and responding to infant cues, promoting reciprocity, and building the infant's feeding and pre-speech skills. When feeding their infant, parents clarify and strengthen their sense of what it means to be a parent. They gain a sense of responsibility by caring for an infant, experience frustration when they cannot easily interpret their infant's cues, and further develop their ability to negotiate and solve problems through their interactions with the infant.

Nutrition for Growth

The infant's diet must provide adequate energy and essential nutrients for appropriate growth. Conversely, growth is an important indicator of nutritional adequacy. Although newborns may lose up to 10% of their body weight in the first week of life, they usually regain their birth weight by 7 days after birth. By the time they are 4 to 6 months old, infants typically have doubled their birth weight, gaining about 4 to 7 ounces per

> Feeding practices and routines serve as the foundation for much of child and family development, as parents build many important skills.

week. Infants typically triple their birth weight by 1 year of age, gaining about 3 to 5 ounces per week from 6 to 12 months of age.

Infants grow approximately 1 inch per month from birth to age 6 months, but the rate of growth slows from 6 to 12 months of age when infants gain about one half inch per month. Infants usually increase their length by 50% in the first year.

Infants who are fed on demand usually consume the amount they need to grow well. Growth of exclusively breastfed infants during the first 6 months exceeds that of other infants, but formula-fed infants gain more rapidly during the remainder of the first year.[8-10] The significance of this difference to future growth or risk of overweight is uncertain. Infants' growth depends on nutrition, perinatal history, and genetic factors (such as parental height, genetic syndromes, or disorders), and other physical factors.

The growth of head circumference up to 2 years of age is so closely related to growth in body length that head circumference measurements do not yield more information about a child's nutritional status than body length measures. After 2 years of age, head circumference grows so slowly that it is a poor indicator of actual malnutrition. However, in an older child, head circumference may be a good indicator of malnutrition that occurred during the first 2 years of life. Head circumference is not a good indicator of nutritional status, but it remains important in screening for microcephaly and macrocephaly because these abnormalities are not nutritional in origin.

CALORIC NEEDS

To meet growth demands, all infants require a high intake of calories and adequate intakes of fat, protein, vitamins, and minerals. Breast milk and formula provide 40% to 50% of energy from fat to meet the infant's growth and development demands. Fats

should not be restricted in the first 2 years of life. Vitamin and mineral needs, with the exception of vitamin D, usually are supplied if the infant is breastfed or if the infant receives an adequate volume of correctly prepared formula. After 6 months of age, complementary foods (solids) aid the development of appropriate feeding and eating skills for all infants and provide additional nutrients to meet the dietary reference intakes (DRIs) for breastfed infants.

VITAMIN AND MINERAL SUPPLEMENTS

A major concern in infancy is the adverse effect of early iron deficiency on psychomotor development. Iron deficiency can result in cognitive and motor deficits,[11] some of which may be reversible with iron therapy.[12] However, a recent Cochrane Review on the subject concluded that there is no clear evidence that treating young children with anemia secondary to iron deficiency will improve psychomotor development.[13] Thus, *prevention* is extraordinarily important. During the first year of life, the infants at highest risk of iron deficiency are those born prematurely, those fed formula that is not iron fortified, and those who are exclusively breastfed without iron supplements. Infants who receive only breast milk are at risk for iron deficiency by 6 months of age, and risk subsequent iron-deficiency anemia.[14-15] It is judicious to begin iron supplements of 1 mg/kg/d after 4 months of age if infants are not receiving iron-fortified complementary foods.[16] Red meat is a better source of iron than iron-fortified cereals for older infants. Infants who receive at least 500 mL (17 oz) of iron-fortified formula do not need additional iron supplementation.

The American Academy of Pediatrics (AAP) currently recommends vitamin D supplementation (400 IU per day) for breastfed infants beginning in the first few days of life.[17] Breastfed infants whose mothers are vegans or vitamin B_{12} deficient need supplements of vitamin B_{12}.

A major concern in infancy is the adverse effect of early iron deficiency on psychomotor development. Iron deficiency can result in cognitive and motor deficits, some of which may be reversible with iron therapy.

Fluoride supplementation is not indicated until after the eruption of teeth, which usually occurs at approximately 6 months of age. At that time, the pediatric health care professional or dentist will evaluate the need for fluoride supplementation based on the child's risk for of dental caries and total fluoride exposure. Adequate calcium intake is not an issue in infants who receive enough breast milk or formula. (For more information on this topic, see the Promoting Oral Health theme.)

Developing Healthy Feeding and Eating Skills

Feedings should be planned to provide all the essential nutrients and support the development of appropriate feeding and eating skills.

BREASTFEEDING

Breastfeeding is recommended for infants during at least the first year of life because of its benefits to infant nutrition, gastrointestinal function, host defense, neurodevelopment, and psychological well-being (Box 1). Breastfeeding, with a restricted maternal diet during pregnancy and lactation, may reduce the incidence of atopic illness, such as allergy or eczema, in infants who have strong family histories of these illnesses. Immediately after delivery, early and frequent physical contact, rooming-in, and exclusion of commercial formula samples enhance the duration of breastfeeding. The AAP Section on Breastfeeding recommends exclusive breastfeeding for about 6 months to maximize its benefits.[18] However, after a review of all available evidence, the AAP Committee on Nutrition recommends exclusive breastfeeding for 4 to 6 months.[12]

Because the decision to breastfeed is often made before, or early in, pregnancy, the prenatal visit offers an important opportunity to promote breastfeeding. Parents often are aware of the benefits of breastfeeding, but lack confidence in their ability to successfully breastfeed their infant. They may have questions about breastfeeding and its nutritional adequacy, their ability to know if the infant is drinking enough milk, the mother's ability to produce enough milk to satisfy the infant's hunger, or whether the mother should breastfeed if she smokes or has an underlying health condition. Mothers also express concerns about their need to return to work or school within 6 to 8 weeks after the baby's birth, or the competing needs of other children and family members. Prenatal and postpartum counseling can address these issues and also prolong the duration of breastfeeding.[19]

Parents also may raise concerns about maternal medication usage, or maternal or infant illness, and the advisability of breastfeeding. Decisions regarding the appropriateness of breastfeeding in these situations are best made on an individual basis with a health care professional. Under most circumstances, mothers can continue to breastfeed their infants or supply breast milk if the infant is unable to breastfeed directly, but a few contraindications to breastfeeding do exist. Medications taken by the mother should be individually evaluated to determine whether they can be used safely when breastfeeding. Few prescription and nonprescription medications are contraindicated for the mother who breastfeeds her baby.[20]

Cultural factors may influence breastfeeding initiation and success. Parents need practical support for breastfeeding, as well as culturally based information and guidance. A solid knowledge of the parents' culture and community will help health care professionals give parents the support, appropriate education, and guidance they need to be successful in breastfeeding their infant. (For more information on this topic, see the Promoting Community Relationships and Resources theme.)

FORMULA FEEDING

For infants who are not breastfed, iron-fortified infant formula is the recommended

Breastfeeding is recommended for infants during at least the first year of life because of its benefits to infant nutrition, gastrointestinal function, host defense, neurodevelopment, and psychological well-being.

BOX 1
Benefits of Breastfeeding

Breast milk is uniquely suited to the needs of the newborn and growing infant and provides many benefits for general health, growth, and development.

Benefits to the infant

- Breastfeeding provides ideal nutrition and promotes the best possible growth and development.
- Breastfeeding significantly decreases the incidence of diarrhea, lower respiratory tract infection, otitis media, bacteremia, bacterial meningitis, botulism, and urinary tract infection.
- Breastfeeding may be protective against Crohn's disease, lymphoma, and certain genotypes of type 1 diabetes mellitus, and delay the onset of certain allergies.[12]
- Breastfeeding lowers the risk of obesity in some populations.
- Breastfeeding promotes healthy neurologic development.
- Breastfeeding can reduce the incidence of atopic illness, such as allergy or eczema.[21]
- Breastfeeding promotes close mother-infant connection.

Benefits to the mother

- Breastfeeding increases levels of oxytocin, which results in less postpartum bleeding and more rapid uterine involution.
- Lactating women have an earlier return to pre-pregnancy weight, delayed resumption of ovulation with increased child spacing, improved postpartum bone remineralization, and reduced risk of ovarian cancer and premenopausal breast cancer.
- Lactational amenorrhea causes less menstrual blood loss over the months after delivery.

Benefits to the family

- Breastfeeding has no associated costs and requires no equipment or preparation.
- It is easy to travel with a breastfed baby because no special equipment or supplies are necessary.

Benefits to the community

- Breastfeeding reduces health care costs and employee absenteeism because of reduced childhood illness.
- Breastfeeding reduces parent absence from work and lost income.

Sources

American Academy of Pediatrics, Work Group on Breastfeeding. Breastfeeding and the use of human milk. *Pediatrics*. 2005;115:496-506.[18]

Kleinman RE, ed. *Pediatric Nutrition Handbook*. 5th ed. Elk Grove Village, IL: American Academy of Pediatrics, Committee on Nutrition; 2004.[12]

Kramer M, Kakuma R. Optimal duration of exclusive breastfeeding (Cochrane Review). In: *The Cochrane Library*. Issue 2. Oxford (UK): Software Update; 2002.[22]

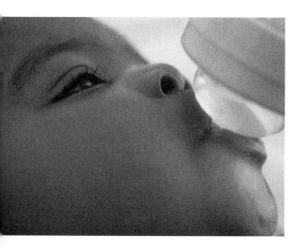

manifested by loose stools, spitting up, or vomiting, may prompt a change to soy formula, but there is little evidence to support this practice. Soy formulas may be recommended for a vegetarian lifestyle, transient lactase deficiency, and galactosemia. Soy formula should not be used for premature infants, cow's milk protein-induced enterocolitis, or the prevention of colic or allergy.[12]

FREQUENCY AND AMOUNT OF FEEDINGS

In the first months of life, breastfed infants usually feed 8 to 12 times in 24 hours (ie, approximately every 2 to 3 hours). Parents should be taught to recognize and respond to early feeding cues. As infants grow older, they typically are satisfied by larger feedings less frequently.

No recommendations exist for maximum volumes of formula at any one feeding, only for meeting total energy and fluid needs. Parents should offer 2 ounces of infant formula every 2 to 3 hours in the first week of life. If the infant still seems hungry, parents can provide more until the infant indicates that he is full. As the infant grows, a larger amount of formula should be given, and the infant should feed until he indicates that he is full. Satiety cues include turning away from the nipple, falling asleep, and spitting up milk. A newborn at the 50th percentile will consume an average of 20 oz of formula per day; the amount of formula ranges from 16 to 24 oz per day.

When he begins to sleep for longer periods at night (4 to 5 hours at about 2 months of age), the formula-fed infant will still need to feed 6 to 8 times in 24 hours. A 4-month-old infant will consume an average of 31 ounces of formula per day without complementary foods with a range of 26 to 36 oz per day. However, his intake fluctuates from day to day and week to week. During growth spurts, intake volume increases but will fall back to lesser volumes.

substitute during the first year of life.[12] Cow's milk, goat's milk, soy beverages (not soy formula), and low-iron formulas should not be used during the first year. Reduced-fat (2%), low-fat (1%), fat-free (skim), and soy milk are not recommended for infants during the first 2 years.

Health care professionals should counsel parents to avoid propping the bottle or letting their infant feed alone. This precaution will minimize the risk of choking, ear infections, early childhood caries, insufficient intake, and the missed opportunity for enhancing the parent-child relationship. To prevent early childhood caries, parents should be instructed not to put the infant to bed with a bottle or sippy cup that contains milk, juices, soda, or other sweetened liquids. (For more information on this topic, see the Promoting Oral Health theme.) Fruit juices are not needed in the infant diet during the first 6 months, but, if they are given, they should be fed by cup, not a bottle. Cereal or other foods should not be added to infant formula unless instructed by a health care professional.

A variety of specialized infant formulas have been developed for infants who cannot tolerate milk protein or lactose (eg, soy formulas, protein hydrolysates, and amino acid formulas). Health care professionals should supervise infants with milk intolerance. Intolerance to cow's milk-based formulas,

In the first months of life, breastfed infants usually feed 8 to 12 times in 24 hours (ie, approximately every 2 to 3 hours). Parents should be taught to recognize and respond to early feeding cues.

129

Infants 6 months and older generally consume 24 to 32 ounces per day, but larger infants may take as much as 42 ounces of formula per day in addition to complementary foods. Over time, the increasing volume of complementary foods is accompanied by a decreasing volume of milk.

For the newborn, hunger cues include rooting, sucking, and hand movements. In young infants, hunger cues may include hand-to-mouth movements and lip smacking. Smiling, cooing, or gazing at the parent during feeding can indicate that the infant wants more food. For older infants, hunger cues can include crying, excited arm and leg movements, opening mouth and moving forward as the spoon approaches, and swiping food toward the mouth. Crying is considered a late feeding cue and usually interferes with feeding as the infant becomes distressed and is less likely to eat well.

Infants can signal that they are full by becoming fussy during feeding, slowing the pace of eating, turning away, stopping sucking, or spitting out or refusing the nipple. Other satiety cues include refusing the spoon, batting the spoon away, and closing the mouth as the spoon approaches. As with all feeding interactions, parents should observe the infant's verbal and nonverbal cues and respond appropriately. If a food is rejected, parents should move on and try it again later rather than forcing the infant to eat or finish foods.

INTRODUCING COMPLEMENTARY FOODS

Complementary foods, commonly referred to as solids, include any foods or beverages besides human milk or formula. The AAP Committee on Nutrition states that complementary foods can be introduced in infants' diets between 4 and 6 months of age and when the infant is developmentally ready.[12] The AAP recommends exclusive breastfeeding for a minimum of 4 months, but preferably for 6 months. During the second 6 months of life, complementary foods are an addition to, not a replacement for, breast milk or infant formula.

Parents need practical guidance when they begin to introduce complementary foods. The health care professional should work with each family to determine the best time to start this exciting new phase. Infants differ in their readiness to accept complementary foods. Counseling parents on the normal progression of the development of feeding and eating skills, and the infant's related ability to safely eat, will help them succeed in and enjoy the new experience.

Waiting until the infant is developmentally ready to begin eating complementary foods makes that process, and the later transition to table foods, easier. Signs that an infant is ready to begin semisolids (pureed foods) include fading of the extrusion reflex (the tongue-thrust reflex that pushes food out of the mouth) and elevating the tongue to move pureed food forward and backward in mouth (which usually occurs between 4 and 6 months of age). An increased demand for breastfeeding that continues for a few days, is not affected by increased breastfeeding, and is unrelated to illness, teething, or changes in routine also may be a sign of readiness for complementary foods. At this stage, the infant sits with arm support and has good head and neck control. The infant can indicate his desire for food by opening his mouth and leaning forward and can indicate disinterest or satiety by leaning back and turning away.

When the infant is able to sit independently and tries to grasp foods with his palms, he is ready to progress to thicker pureed foods and soft, mashed foods without lumps. He also can begin to sip from a small cup. When the infant crawls and pulls to stand, he also begins to use his jaw and tongue to mash food, plays with a spoon at mealtime (but does not use it for self-feeding yet), and tries to hold a cup independently. At this stage, he

The American Academy of Pediatrics recommends exclusive breastfeeding for a minimum of 4 months, but preferably for 6 months.

is able to progress to ground or soft, mashed foods with small, soft, noticeable lumps (eg, finely chopped meat or poultry). At about 7 to 9 months of age, the infant learns to put objects in his mouth and will try to feed himself. At this age, the infant has developed a pincer grasp (the ability to pick up objects between thumb and forefinger). Any food the infant can pick up can be considered a finger food. Foods that dissolve easily, such as crackers or dry cereal, are good choices, but foods that can cause choking, such as popcorn, grapes, raw carrots, nuts, hard candies, and hot dogs, should be avoided.

Evidence for introducing complementary foods in a specific sequence or at any specific rate is not available. The general recommendation is that the first solid foods should be single-ingredient foods and should be introduced one at a time at 2- to 7-day intervals. The order in which solid foods are introduced is not critical as long as essential nutrients that complement breast milk or formula are provided. Pureed meats and iron-fortified cereals provide many of these nutrients for both breastfed and formula-fed infants. After the infant has accepted these new foods, parents can gradually introduce other pureed foods or soft fruits and vegetables 2 to 3 times per day and allow him to control how much he eats. Parents also can offer store-bought or home-prepared baby food and soft table foods, such as mashed potatoes or bananas. Breastfed infants are exposed to a variety of flavors through their mother's breast milk; thus, dietary variety is important not just for infants, but for their mothers as well. Mixing cereal with breast milk enhances acceptance of cereal by the breastfed infant.[23] Repeated exposures to foods enhances acceptance by both breastfed and formula-fed infants.[24]

A nutritious and balanced diet for the older infant includes appropriate amounts of breast milk or formula and complementary foods to ensure intake of all essential nutrients and to foster appropriate growth. By the end of the first year, the infant should be introduced to healthful foods, such as fruits, vegetables, whole grains, and lean meats. Foods that are high in calories, fat, and sugar, and low in essential nutrients, such as sweetened drinks, sodas, chips, and french fries, should be avoided.

Because of their high sugar and calorie content and lack of nutrients, parents should avoid giving their infants and young children carbonated soda and fruit drinks. In addition, parents should allow no more than 4 to 6 ounces of 100% fruit juice daily. Because 100% fruit juice is considered nutritious, parents may not recognize the need to limit consumption. However, fruit juice is high in calories and sugar. Consuming large quantities can contribute to pediatric overweight and obesity, diarrhea, and early childhood caries.[25]

To establish habits of eating food in moderation, infants should be allowed to stop eating at the earliest sign of unwillingness and not urged to consume more. Parents should allow the infant to control the amount of milk, formula, or complementary foods consumed based on his hunger and satiety cues. Breastfeeding can aid in establishing habits of eating in moderation because the breastfed infant has more control over the amount consumed at a feeding. Parents who feed their infant formula should be warned against encouraging the infant to finish the bottle when satiety cues are demonstrated.

Eating nutritious foods and avoiding foods that provide calories without nutrients help establish habits of eating in moderation. Furthermore, establishing regular mealtimes and snack times and avoiding continuous feeding, or "grazing," will help prevent both overweight and underweight.

…fruit juice is high in calories and sugar. Consuming large quantities can contribute to pediatric overweight and obesity, diarrhea, and early childhood caries.

HANDLING FEEDING AND EATING PROBLEMS

Parents frequently have concerns and questions about infant feeding and eating issues, and an important aspect of health supervision during this developmental stage is helping parents distinguish normal infant feeding behaviors from feeding or eating problems.

Food Sensitivities and Allergies

Food allergy or hypersensitivity is a form of food intolerance characterized by reproducible symptoms with each exposure to the offending food and an abnormal immunologic reaction to the food. Symptoms and disorders, such as irritability, hyperactivity, gastrointestinal discomfort, and asthma, have been attributed to food allergies, but true food allergies are rare. Food hypersensitivity reactions occur in 2% to 8% of infants and children younger than 3 years. Food allergy can result in symptoms affecting the gastrointestinal tract (eg, vomiting, cramps, or diarrhea), skin (eg, eczema or hives), and respiratory tract (eg, asthma), or it can result in generalized, life-threatening allergic reactions (ie, anaphylaxis). Hyperactivity is not considered a manifestation of food allergy.

Approximately 2.5% of infants will experience an allergic reaction to cow's milk in the first 3 years of life, 1.5% will have a reaction to eggs, and 0.6% will have a reaction to peanuts.[12] The most common foods associated with allergic reactions in young children are cow's milk, eggs, peanuts, soy, and wheat. Tree nuts, fish, and shellfish become more common causes of food allergy in adolescents and adults.[26] Infants who are exclusively breastfed may react to these or other food proteins that reach breast milk from the mother's diet.

Infants with a strong family history of food allergy (ie, those whose parents or siblings have or had significant allergies) may benefit from breastfeeding, particularly with regard to the development of cow's milk allergy.[27] However, another recent review concluded

that 4 months of exclusive breastfeeding did not protect against food allergy at 1 year of age.[22] Firm conclusions about the role of breastfeeding in either preventing or delaying the onset of specific food allergies are not possible at this time. In addition, though solid foods should not be introduced before 4 to 6 months of age, there is no convincing evidence that delaying their introduction beyond this period has a significant protective effect on the development of atopic disease, whether infants are fed cow's milk protein formulas or human milk.[21] Single-ingredient new foods should be introduced one at a time, and the infant should be watched for adverse reactions over several days to a week. For infants who are not at risk of food allergies, no evidence indicates that restriction or avoidance of any food is necessary.

Regurgitation, Spitting Up, and Gastroesophageal Reflux Disease

Regurgitation and spitting up are common concerns for parents. During the first year of life, particularly in the first few months, infants typically have episodes of emesis (vomiting or "wet burps") within the first 1 to 2 hours after feeding. Emesis is related to transient physiologic episodes of lowered esophageal sphincter tone with efflux of gastric contents into the esophagus. Spitting up often occurs because milk has been ingested too rapidly or as a reaction to overfeeding,

> **Infants with a strong family history of food allergy (ie, those whose parents or siblings have or had significant allergies) may benefit from breastfeeding, particularly with regard to the development of cow's milk allergy**

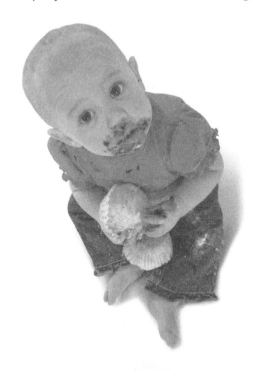

inadequate burping, or improper feeding techniques (eg, bottle propped, bottle not adequately tipped up, or shaking formula too vigorously before feeding). Approximately half of infants younger than 3 months spit up or regurgitate one or 2 times a day, with the incidence peaking between the ages of 2 to 4 months. The frequency may increase again when the baby starts solid foods. Spitting up resolves itself in most children by 12 to 24 months of age.

Frequent spitting up or significant vomiting is classified as gastroesophageal reflux (GER) and usually is harmless in infants. The clinical manifestations of gastroesophageal reflux disease (GERD) include vomiting and associated poor weight gain, apparent discomfort with eating, esophagitis, and respiratory disorders.[28] The health care professional will need to differentiate these symptoms from pyloric stenosis in some very young babies.

Providing a Nurturing and Healthy Feeding Environment

Infants need a nurturing environment and positive patterns of feeding and eating to promote healthy eating habits and build variety, balance, and moderation. In early infancy, feeding is crucial for developing a parent's responsiveness to an infant's cues of hunger and satiation. The close physical contact during feeding facilitates healthy social and emotional development.

During the first year, feeding the hungry infant helps him develop a sense of trust that his needs will be met. For optimum development, newborns should be fed as soon as possible when they express hunger. Children with special health care needs often have subtle cues that can be difficult for parents to interpret. Parents must be careful observers of the infant's behaviors, so that they can respond to their infant's needs. As infants become more secure in their trust, they can wait longer for feeding. Infants should

develop their feeding skills at their own rate. However, if significant delays occur in the development of these skills, or delays are anticipated (eg, as in the case of some children with special health care needs), a health care professional should assess the infant.

The suck-and-pause sequence in breast-feeding or infant formula feeding and behaviors such as eye contact, open mouth, turning to the parent, and even turning away provide the foundation for the first communication between the infant and parents. Difficulties in early feeding create strong emotions for the parent and can undermine parenting confidence and sense of competency. Thus, feeding difficulties must be addressed in a timely manner.

Over time, parents become more skilled at interpreting their infant's cues and increase their repertoire of successful responses to those cues. As they feed their infant, parents learn how their actions comfort and satisfy. Physical contact during breastfeeding or formula feeding strengthens the psychological bond between the mother and infant and enhances communication because it provides the infant with essential sensory stimulation, including skin and eye contact. A sense of caring and trust evolves, which lays the groundwork for communication patterns throughout life.

A healthy feeding relationship involves a division of responsibility between the parent and the infant. The parent sets an appropriate, safe, and nurturing feeding environment and provides appropriate, healthy foods. The infant decides when and how much to eat. In a healthy infant-parent feeding relationship, responsive parenting involves:

- Responding early and appropriately to hunger and satiety cues
- Recognizing the infant's developmental abilities and feeding skills
- Balancing the infant's need for assistance with encouragement of self-feeding

A healthy feeding relationship involves a division of responsibility between the parent and the infant. The parent sets an appropriate, safe, and nurturing feeding environment and provides appropriate, healthy foods. The infant decides when and how much to eat.

PROMOTING
HEALTHY NUTRITION

- Allowing the infant to initiate and guide feeding interactions

Nutrition for Infants With Special Health Care Needs

Medical problems or other special health care needs can place the infant at nutritional risk. Because this is a time of high caloric need, health care professionals should consider referring the family for specialized medical and nutrition consultation.

Not all infants are able to develop the skills for feeding and eating easily. Approximately 25% of all children have some feeding problems, and 80% of children with a developmental disability have some form of feeding problem.[29] Feeding difficulties can lead to problems in the parent-child relationship, as well as growth problems, inadequate nutrition, and significant feeding problems later in childhood. Health care professionals should address the following common concerns expressed by parents:

- Refusing food (infant cereal and purees)
- Difficulty transitioning to textures
- Gagging, choking, or vomiting with feeding
- Poor or inadequate food volume
- Poor or inadequate variety of foods, picky eating, or food jags
- Prolonged feeding time (more than 30 minutes)
- Respiratory symptoms after feeding

Infants with special health care needs are at increased risk of feeding complications, including failure to thrive, aspiration of food, and GERD. Parents of infants with special health care needs also may need extra emotional support and instruction about special techniques for positioning or special equipment. These accommodations can help overcome feeding problems and prevent suboptimal nutrition, poor weight gain, and growth deficiency.

Infants with special health care needs are at increased risk of feeding complications, including failure to thrive, aspiration of food, and gastroesophageal reflux disease. Parents of infants with special health care needs also may need extra emotional support and instruction about special techniques for positioning or special equipment.

Parents often blame themselves for their infant's feeding problem, yet the difficulty is typically related to the infant's oromotor developmental problem. Children with oromotor delay may retain primitive reflexes like the extrusion reflex and the tonic bite reflex. These behaviors can be mistakenly interpreted as food refusals. Thus, health care professionals should try to identify feeding challenges early and provide resources for evaluation, education, and support. Assessing and treating physical or behavioral feeding difficulties is best accomplished by an interdisciplinary team that may include a neurobehavioral pediatrician, dietitian, occupational therapist, speech pathologist, nurse or nurse practitioner, social worker, and psychologist. Parents should learn the different philosophies, intervention strategies, and approaches of the different programs available, as well as their costs and outcomes, before they make a decision on the best approach for their child and family.

Low birth weight infants need additional iron after the first month of life (2 mg/kg/d) until they reach 1 year of age.[12] They also may need special food (eg, preterm discharge formulas with enhanced nutrients). Infants with sequelae of prematurity, chronic lung or reactive airway disease, short bowel syndrome, cholestasis, GERD, rickets, or chronic heart, kidney, or liver disease have medical and developmental factors that will affect their growth. They may require specialized feedings with nutritional supplements, including fortifiers, vitamins, and minerals. Medication usage also may alter nutritional requirements.

Infants with special health care needs often need increased calories, but may be limited by feeding issues. Because their immune systems may be compromised, most of these infants benefit from breastfeeding (or being fed expressed breast milk). Parents may need to modify breast milk or formula or adapt their feeding techniques to ensure that infants with the following conditions achieve adequate caloric intakes:

- Prematurity and low birth weight
- Chronic respiratory or congenital heart disease
- Gastrointestinal tract disease
- Renal disease
- Neurologic disorders
- Syndromes and genetic disorders affecting growth potential, such as cystic fibrosis

Promoting Nutritional Health: Early Childhood—1 to 4 Years

Ensuring adequate nutrition during early childhood focuses on promoting normal growth by selecting appropriate amounts and kinds of foods and providing a supportive environment that allows the child to self-regulate food intake. As in all other areas of development, self-regulation of eating and its accompanying independence are major achievements during the early childhood years. Children continue their exposure to new tastes, textures, and eating experiences depending on their own developmental ability, cultural and family practices, and individual nutrient needs.

Nutrition for Growth

Most infants triple their birth weight within the first year of life and experience a significantly slower rate of weight gain after the first year, which results in a dramatic decrease in appetite and diminished food intake. This diminished intake is compensated for by eating foods with increased caloric density (ie, foods with less water content). Health care professionals can alert parents to this change when the child's height and weight are measured and plotted on the gender- and age-appropriate CDC growth and BMI-for-age charts (for children older than 2 years).

Monitoring growth measures by age allows the health care professional to determine how the child compares to others of

the same age and gender. These measures can be used to signal abnormal growth patterns. Linear growth is used to detect long-term undernutrition. Using weight-for-length until age 2 years, and BMI growth charts after that, allows the health care professional to determine underweight and overweight or obesity and whether the child is maintaining her own growth trajectory. If the child has moved up or down 2 percentile lines on the growth chart since the previous visit, the health care professional should question parents in detail about portion sizes, types of food served, and feeding frequency. Skinfold measurements for this age group are not used unless medically indicated and performed by an adequately trained technician.

As additional table foods are offered, toddlers consume foods similar to those of the entire family. Even in early childhood, dietary preferences and patterns begin to be established, and, all too often, the reported amount of milk consumed decreases significantly, while the intake of juices, fruit drinks, and carbonated sodas increases.[30] The Infant and Toddler Study suggests that, in general, young children are getting sufficient intakes of calcium.[31] However, the shift from milk to juice and soda lowers calcium intake and makes it more difficult for young children to attain the recommended calcium intake (Box 2). Fruit drinks and carbonated sodas are

Monitoring growth measures by age allows the health care professional to determine how the child compares to others of the same age and gender. These measures can be used to signal abnormal growth patterns.

BOX 2
Child Calcium Dietary Reference Intake

Children aged 1 to 3 years: 500 mg/d
Children aged 4 to 8 years: 800 mg/d

Source: Institute of Medicine. Dietary reference intakes for calcium, phosphorous, magnesium, vitamin D, and fluoride. (1997). Washington, DC: National Academies Press. 1997. Available at: http://www.iom.edu/file.asp?id =21372. Accessed August 17, 2006.[32,33]

discouraged, and 100% fruit juice is recommended at no more than 4 to 6 ounces daily.[25] Overuse may lead to excess energy intake, diarrhea, and dental caries. (For more information on this topic, see the Promoting Healthy Weight and Promoting Oral Health themes.)

A primary safety concern for preschoolers during feeding is choking or inhalation of food. The following foods should be avoided at this stage:

- Peanuts
- Chewing gum
- Popcorn
- Chips
- Round slices of hot dogs or sausages
- Carrot sticks
- Whole grapes
- Hard candy
- Large pieces of raw vegetables or fruit
- Tough meat

A basic premise is that nutrient needs should be met primarily by consuming a variety of foods that have beneficial effects on health.

To limit the risk of choking, the toddler should sit up while eating. Parents should avoid feeding a young child while in a car because, if the child should begin to choke, pulling over to the side of the road in traffic to dislodge the food is difficult.[12] Furthermore, feeding children while driving contradicts the recommendation to feed children in appropriate locations.

Because few data were available on nutrient adequacy for toddlers and preschoolers, the Institute of Medicine (IOM)[34] extrapolated values from studies of infants and adults to establish dietary reference intakes. Translating these nutrient intakes into specific food choices and portions for toddlers has not been clearly defined. However, guidelines suggest offering appropriate nutritious foods spaced into 3 meals, along with 2 or 3 snacks per day.[12] For children older than 2 years, the *Dietary Guidelines for Americans* are the primary sources of dietary guidance.[35]

Other national health organizations also have developed nutrition policy statements to

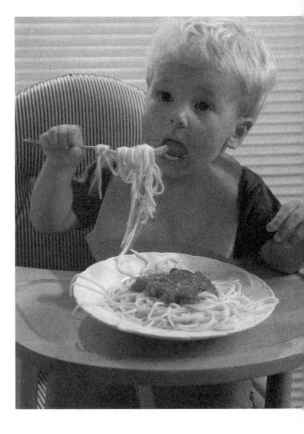

promote optimal health and reduce risk for chronic disease, and these statements can be used as well to guide food choices in children older than 2 years.[36-39] These science-based nutrition guidelines recommend a diet that includes a variety of nutrient-dense foods and beverages from the basic food groups and that limits the intake of saturated and trans fats, cholesterol, added sugars, and salt. A basic premise is that nutrient needs should be met primarily by consuming a variety of foods that have beneficial effects on health. Supplementation with vitamins and minerals is not considered necessary when children are consuming the recommended amounts of healthful foods.[40] However, health care professionals should not assume that all toddlers are getting the nutrients they need.[41] A significant number of children in the United States live in households with insufficient food.

Developing Healthy Feeding and Eating Skills

Young children often will eat sporadically over one day or several days. Over a period of a week or so, their nutrient and energy intakes balance out. Food jags (ie, favoring only one or 2 foods) and picky eating (eg, refusing to eat certain foods or not wanting foods to touch) are normal behaviors in young children. For most children, these behaviors disappear before school age if parents patiently continue to expose them to a variety of new and familiar foods. As their manipulative skills mature, preschoolers also can successfully help in food preparation, which may help them accept new foods.

Unfortunately, some parents and caregivers become discouraged and frustrated when their toddler seems to concentrate more on exploring food than eating it. This behavior reflects the emerging curiosity and independence associated with early childhood and is normal. Parents and caregivers can foster this newly found, and often assertively expressed, independence while still ensuring adequate nutrition by offering a well-balanced selection of foods and allowing children to choose the types and amounts of foods they want to eat. Parents and caregivers need to understand that recognizing the child's signals of hunger and fullness supports the child's innate ability to self-regulate energy intake and portion size. They also need to understand that a child does not have an innate ability to select only appropriate foods. Food choice remains the responsibility of the caregiver.

Mealtime provides an opportunity for wonderful parent-child interactions. These opportunities exist for the young toddler, who may be fed before the family meal, as well as for the older toddler and preschooler, who may participate in the family routine and sit at the table for a short time. Finger foods should be encouraged because they foster competence, mastery, and self-esteem. Even when the parent or caregiver is doing the feeding, the child also should be given a spoon. The 12- to 15-month-old toddler should be encouraged to use a spoon. When the child is finished eating, she should be allowed to leave the table and be placed where she can be supervised until the adults have finished their meal.

Nutrition for Children With Special Health Care Needs

Children with special health care needs generally follow similar developmental pathways as children without these challenges when they begin the process of self-feeding. However, the pace of development and the ultimate mastery of tasks will vary depending on the physical, emotional, or cognitive challenges facing the child. Health care professionals should follow children with special health care needs closely, paying particular attention to nutritional intake and physical activity.

The types of nutritional issues most common for children with special health care needs include feeding problems (eg, chewing and swallowing), slow growth, metabolic or gastrointestinal issues, and overweight or obesity. Sometimes children with special health care needs require special feeding techniques, longer periods of time to feed, or special foods (both type and texture), formulas, and feeding approaches (eg, restriction of certain foods). The health care professional can identify these issues and refer the family, as needed, to a registered dietitian or interdisciplinary team for further assessment, intervention, and monitoring.

Food jags (ie, favoring only one or 2 foods) and picky eating (eg, refusing to eat certain foods or not wanting foods to touch) are normal behaviors in young children.

137

Promoting Nutritional Health: Middle Childhood—5 to 10 Years

To achieve optimal growth and development, children need a variety of nutritious foods that provide sufficient calories, protein, carbohydrates, fat, vitamins, and minerals. By middle childhood, a child needs 3 meals and 2 to 3 healthy snacks per day. As the child's ability to feed himself improves, he can help with meal planning and food preparation, and he can perform tasks related to mealtime. Performing these tasks enables the child to contribute to the family and can boost his self-esteem. The USDA MyPyramid for Kids, which is based on the *Dietary Guidelines for Americans*, provides an easy reference on food intake and physical activity recommendations for children aged 6 to 11 years.[42]

Nutrition for Growth

> Parents need to make sure that nutritious foods are available and decide when to serve them; however, children should decide how much to eat.

Middle childhood is characterized by a slow, steady rate of physical growth. Plotting the child's BMI from 2 years of age into middle childhood allows the health care professional to note any increasing percentile changes and provide early intervention as needed to prevent childhood obesity.

CALCIUM

Calcium intake continues to be a concern during middle childhood. Nutritional intake studies indicate that few school-aged children receive adequate calcium intake. Calcium is a critical nutrient for bone health, and a higher incidence of fractures is reported in children who do not get adequate amounts of calcium. Consumption of large amounts of juice, soft drinks, or sport drinks suggests inadequate intake of milk. Children need 3 to 4 servings of calcium-rich foods per day (Box 3). One 8-ounce glass of milk provides approximately 300 mg of calcium. Health care professionals should, therefore, encourage parents to provide water, low-fat milk, and no more than 4 to 6 ounces of 100% fruit juice daily for their children to drink.

BOX 3

Child Calcium Dietary Reference Intake

Children aged 4 to 8 years: 800 mg/d

Children aged 9 to 18 years: 1,300 mg/d

Source: Institute of Medicine. Dietary reference intakes for calcium, phosphorous, magnesium, vitamin D, and fluoride. (1997). Washington, DC: National Academies Press. 1997. Available at: http://www.iom.edu/file.asp?id =21372. Accessed August 17, 2006.[32]

Developing Healthy Eating Habits

Parents and other family members continue to have the most influence on children's eating behaviors and attitudes toward foods. Parents need to make sure that nutritious foods are available and decide when to serve them; however, children should decide how much to eat. During this period, when children may be missing several teeth, it can be difficult for them to chew certain foods (eg, meat). Offering foods that are easy to eat can alleviate this problem.

Health care professionals should try to determine whether families have access to, and can afford, nutritious foods. They also should discuss families' perceptions of which foods are nutritious and their cultural beliefs about foods. Families should eat together in a pleasant environment (without the TV), allowing time for social interaction. Participation in regular family meals is positively associated with appropriate intakes of energy, protein, calcium, and many micronutrients, and can reinforce the development of healthy eating patterns.[43]

During middle childhood, mealtimes take on social significance, and children become increasingly influenced by outside sources (eg, their peers and the media) regarding eating behaviors and attitudes toward foods. In addition, they eat a growing number of meals away from home and may have expanding options for nonnutritious foods. Their eagerness to eat certain foods and to participate in nutrition programs (eg, National School Lunch programs) may be based on what their friends are doing. However, some children can have difficulty in adapting to school lunch programs. This difficulty can be because the foods are different from those at home, the foods may not conform to cultural and religious practices, they have less time to eat than they are accustomed to, or they may have difficulty serving their own plates.

Nutrition for Children With Special Health Care Needs

Dietary needs of children with special health care concerns that can affect their ability to maintain a healthy weight should be addressed with the family. Health care professionals should be aware of medications that can affect appetite, leading to weight loss or weight gain. The children may be making food choices at school, and parents may need help guiding them to make healthy choices, depending on their particular needs. Children with special health care needs can have significant nutritional challenges, leading to underweight or overweight. These challenges can be the result of behavioral disturbances or because children may need assistance with feeding. When weight gain is desired, nutritious high-calorie foods are preferred over calorie-dense "junk food." Some children may require gastrostomy tubes and fundoplications. Overweight and obesity are risks when physical activity is limited by a special health care need. Health care professionals should be aware of these challenges and be prepared to seek assistance in monitoring and facilitating appropriate nutrition.

Promoting Nutritional Health: Adolescence—11 to 21 Years

Adolescence is one of the most dynamic periods of human development. The increased rate of growth that occurs during these years is second only to that occurring in the first year of life. Nutrition and physical activity can affect adolescents' energy levels and influence growth and body composition, and the changes associated with puberty can influence adolescents' satisfaction with their appearance. Health supervision visits provide an opportunity for health care professionals to discuss healthy eating and physical activity behaviors with adolescents and their parents. (For more information on this topic, see the Promoting Physical Activity theme.)

Nutrition for Growth

As for the earlier stages of childhood, the adolescent's diet should follow the *Dietary Guidelines for Americans* and the complementary recommendations of other national health organizations.[35,39] All of these recommendations emphasize a variety of nutrient-dense foods and beverages from the basic food groups and moderation in saturated and trans fats, cholesterol, added sugars, and salt. They also emphasize meeting recommended intakes within energy needs and maintaining a healthy body weight by balancing calories from foods and beverages with calories expended through physical activity.[35]

These recommendations direct that nutrient needs should be met primarily by consuming a variety of healthful foods. In certain cases, fortified foods and dietary supplements may be useful sources of one or more nutrients that otherwise might not be consumed in the recommended amounts. However, although they are recommended in some cases, dietary supplements cannot replace a healthy diet.

For many adolescents, intake of certain vitamins (ie, folate, vitamin B_6, and vitamin A)

Adolescence is one of the most dynamic periods of human development. The increased rate of growth that occurs during these years is second only to that occurring in the first year of life.

BOX 4
Current Recommendations for Selected Nutrients

Folate

The Institute of Medicine recommends that, to reduce the risk of giving birth to an infant with neural tube defects, female adolescents who are capable of becoming pregnant should take 400 µg of folate per day from fortified foods, a supplement, or both, in addition to consuming folate-containing foods from a varied diet.[34]

Iron

The body's need for iron increases dramatically during adolescence, primarily because of rapid growth. Adolescent boys require increased amounts of iron to manufacture myoglobin for expanding muscle mass, and hemoglobin for expansion of blood volume. Although adolescent girls generally have less muscular development than adolescent boys, they have a greater risk for iron-deficiency anemia because of blood lost through menstruation. Iron-deficiency anemia in adolescents may be caused by inadequate dietary intake of iron, which results from low-calorie and extremely restrictive diets, periods of accelerated iron demand, and increased iron losses. The current Dietary Reference Intakes for iron are[12]:

- Females and males aged 9 to 13 years: 8 mg/d
- Females aged 14 to 18 years: 15 mg/d
- Males aged 14 to 18 years: 11 mg/d

Calcium

Adequate calcium intake is essential for peak bone mass development during adolescence, a period when 45% of the total permanent adult skeleton is formed. Calcium requirements increase with the growth of lean body mass and the skeleton. Therefore, requirements are greater during puberty and adolescence than in childhood or adulthood. The current calcium DRIs for children and adolescents are[32]:

- Children and adolescents aged 9 to 18 years: 1,300 mg/d
- Adolescents aged 19 years and older: 1,000 mg of calcium per day

Sources: Kleinman RE, ed. *Pediatric Nutrition Handbook*. 5th ed. Elk Grove Village, IL: American Academy of Pediatrics, Committee on Nutrition; 2004[12]; Institute of Medicine. Dietary reference intakes for calcium, phosphorous, magnesium, vitamin D, and fluoride. Washington, DC: National Academies Press; 1997[32]; Institute of Medicine. Dietary reference intakes for thiamin, riboflavin, vitamin B6, folate, vitamin B12, pantothenic acid, biotin, and choline. Washington, DC: National Academies Press. 1998;8:196-305.[34] A summary table of the DRIs is available at: http://www.iom.edu/file.asp?id=21372. Accessed August 17, 2006.[32]

and minerals (ie, iron, calcium, and zinc) is inadequate, particularly among adolescents from families with low incomes and among adolescent girls. Box 4 provides current recommendations for several nutrients of particular concern for adolescents, including folate, iron, and calcium.

Dietary excess of total fat, saturated fat, cholesterol, sodium, and sugar is common in both genders and in all income and racial and ethnic groups. Other nutrition-related concerns for adolescents include low intakes of fruits, vegetables, and calcium-rich foods, and high soft-drink consumption. Diets that are low in fruits and vegetables and high in saturated fats constitute a significant risk factor for obesity and other health problems.[44] Only 21% of adolescents report eating 5 or more servings of fruits and vegetables per day,[45] and only 62% report eating a lower-fat diet with no more than 2 daily servings of food that are typically high in fat content. Adolescent girls (71%) are significantly more likely than adolescent boys (55%) to report eating this lower-fat diet.[46] Adolescents also may engage in unsafe weight-loss methods, and some experience iron-deficiency anemia (for girls), eating disorders, hyperlipidemia, or obesity. Hunger and insufficient food resources are sometimes a concern among adolescents from families with low incomes. In addition, nutritional problems can result from pregnancy, disabilities, emotional trauma, chronic health conditions, or substance abuse.

ASSESSING THE ADOLESCENT DIET

Evaluating the dietary intake of an adolescent is a fundamental component of ongoing health supervision. It is, therefore, useful for the health care professional to gather quantitative and qualitative data about foods and beverages consumed (both common and unusual), eating patterns, attitudes about foods and eating, and other issues, such as cultural patterns and taboos associated with food.

Although good eating behaviors are an important component of a healthy lifestyle, the US Preventive Services Task Force has concluded that insufficient scientific evidence exists to recommend for or against behavioral counseling in primary care settings to promote a healthy diet.[47] Most intervention studies of adolescents have focused on nonclinical settings (eg, schools) or have used physiologic outcomes, such as cholesterol level or weight, rather than more comprehensive measures of a healthy diet.[47] However, because nutrition has such an important impact on well-being and longevity, nutritional counseling is included in preventive health care.

Developing Healthy Eating Habits

Developing an identity and becoming an independent young adult are central to adolescence. Adolescents may use foods to establish individuality and express identity. They usually are interested in new foods, including those from different cultures and ethnic groups, and may adopt certain eating behaviors (eg, vegetarianism) to explore various lifestyles or to show concern for the environment. Parents can have a major influence on adolescents' eating behaviors by providing a variety of nutritious foods at home and by making family mealtimes a priority.[48] Parents

Developing an identity and becoming an independent young adult are central to adolescence. Adolescents may use foods to establish individuality and express identity.

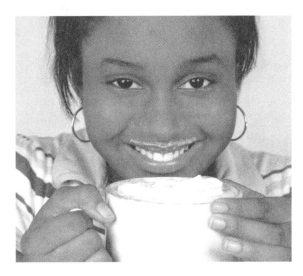

also can be positive role models by practicing healthy eating behaviors themselves.

As adolescents strive for independence, they begin to spend large amounts of time outside the home. Parents can encourage adolescents to choose nutritious foods when eating away from home.[1] Many adolescents walk or drive to neighborhood stores and fast-food restaurants and purchase foods with their own money. This situation can be especially problematic for adolescents from families with low incomes or adolescents who live in neighborhoods with many fast-food restaurants and with no grocery stores or with stores that do not sell affordable nutritious foods.

Although eating together as a family is a challenge for many adolescents and their families coping with school demands, after-school activities, and work schedules, the frequency of family meals has many positive associations. Having meals together is positively associated with intake of fruits, vegetables, grains, and calcium-rich foods, and negatively associated with soft-drink consumption. Frequency of family meals also is positively associated with more appropriate intake of energy, protein, iron, folate, fiber, and vitamins A, C, E, and B$_6$.[43] Family meals also can promote the development of healthy eating patterns that may continue into adulthood and can protect against the inadequate dietary intake reported by many adolescents.[43,49]

BODY IMAGE AND EATING DISORDERS

The physical changes that are associated with puberty can affect adolescents' satisfaction with their appearance. For some adolescent boys, the increased height, weight, and muscular development that come with physical maturation can lead to a positive body image. However, for many adolescent girls, puberty-related changes (in particular, the normal increase in body fat) may result in weight concerns. The social pressure to be thin and the stigma of being overweight can lead to unhealthy eating behaviors and a poor body image.[1] Adolescents may attempt to lose weight or avoid gaining weight by eating smaller amounts of food, foods with fewer calories, or foods low in fat. They also may forego eating for many hours; engage in excessive physical activity; take diet pills, powders, or liquids without a physician's advice; and vomit or take laxatives. Fad diets that recommend unusual and, sometimes, inadequate or unbalanced dietary patterns promise the loss of several pounds a week over a short period of time. Virtually no evidence is available about their efficacy and safety in adolescents, making such regimens a poor choice for adolescents who want to lose weight and who may underestimate the health risks associated with them.[12]

Unhealthy eating behaviors and preoccupation with body size can lead to life-threatening eating disorders (eg, anorexia nervosa or bulimia nervosa). Although eating disorders are more prevalent among adolescent girls (prevalence is 1% to 2%) than among adolescent boys, they occur in both genders across socioeconomic and racial and ethnic groups and are now seen in children (aged 10 to 12 years) as well. Major medical complications of eating disorders include cardiac arrhythmia, dehydration and electrolyte imbalances, delayed growth and development, endocrine disturbances (eg, menstrual dysfunction or hypothermia), gastrointestinal problems, oral health problems (eg, enamel demineralization or salivary dysfunction), osteopenia, osteoporosis, and protein and calorie malnutrition and its consequences. Estimates of mortality that result from anorexia nervosa vary considerably from the average estimate of 5% to 8% to as high as 20%.[50] Death may be due to cardiac arrhythmia (irregular heartbeat), acute cardiovascular failure, gastric hemorrhaging, or suicide. Bulimia nervosa can damage teeth and cause enlargement of the parotid gland.

Family meals also can promote the development of healthy eating patterns that may continue into adulthood and can protect against the inadequate dietary intake reported by many adolescents.

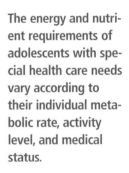

ATHLETICS AND PERFORMANCE-ENHANCING SUBSTANCES

Adolescents who engage in competitive sports can be vulnerable to nutrition misinformation and unsafe practices that promise to enhance performance. Inadequate nutritional intake and unsafe weight control methods can adversely affect performance and endurance, jeopardize health, and undermine the benefits of training. Health supervision includes the promotion of healthy eating and weight management strategies to enhance performance and endurance while ensuring optimal growth and development.[51,52]

Nutrition for Youth With Special Health Care Needs

As with earlier age groups, youth with special health care needs are at increased risk for nutrition-related health problems for the following reasons[1]:

- Physical disorders or disabilities can affect their capacity to consume, digest, or absorb nutrients.
- Biochemical imbalances can be caused by long-term medications or internal metabolic disturbances.
- Psychological stress that results from a chronic condition or physical disorder can affect appetite and food intake.
- Environmental factors are often controlled by parents, who may influence access to, and acceptance of, food.

The energy and nutrient requirements of adolescents with special health care needs vary according to their individual metabolic rate, activity level, and medical status. Once a desired energy level has been achieved, the adolescent should be routinely monitored to ensure adequate nutrition for growth and development and to make adjustments for periods of stress and illness.

The energy and nutrient requirements of adolescents with special health care needs vary according to their individual metabolic rate, activity level, and medical status.

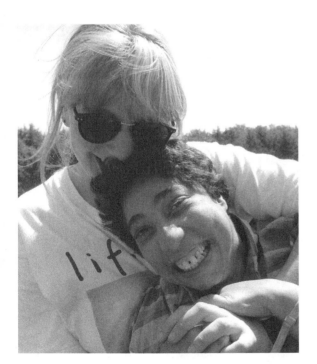

References

1. Story M, Holt K, Sofka D, eds. *Bright Futures in Practice: Nutrition*. 2nd ed. Arlington, VA: National Center for Education in Maternal and Child Health; 2002

2. United States Department of Agriculture, Economic Research Service, Briefing Rooms: Food Security in the United States. http://www.ers.usda.gov/Briefing/FoodSecurity/. Accessed March 1, 2006

3. Sullivan AF, Choi E. *Hunger and Food Insecurity in the Fifty States: 1998-2000*. Waltham, MA: Center on Hunger and Poverty; 2002

4. Centers for Disease Control: Recommendations for the use of folic acid to reduce the number of cases of spina bifida and other neural tube defects. *MMWR Recomm Rep*. 1992;41:1-7

5. Bailey LB, Rampersaud GC, Kauwell GP. Folic acid supplements and fortification affect the risk for neural tube defects, vascular disease and cancer: evolving science. *J Nutr*. 2003;133:1961S-1968S

6. Lumley J, Watson L, Watson M, Bower C. Periconceptional supplementation with folate and/or multivitamins for preventing neural tube defects. *Cochrane Database Syst Rev*. 2001(3)

7. Berry RJ, Li Z, Erickson JD, et al. Prevention of neural-tube defects with folic acid in China. China-U.S. Collaborative Project for Neural Tube Defect Prevention. *N Engl J Med*. 1999;341:1485-1490

8. Butte NF, Wong WW, Hopkinson JM, Smith EO, Ellis KJ. Infant feeding mode affects early growth and body composition. *Pediatrics*. 2000;106:1355-1366

9. Dewey KG, Peerson JM, Brown KH, et al. Growth of breast-fed infants deviates from current reference data: a pooled analysis of US, Canadian, and European data sets. World Health Organization Working Group on Infant Growth. *Pediatrics*. 1995;96:495-503

10. deOnis M, Garza C, Onyango AW, Borghi E. Comparison of the WHO Child Growth Standards and the CDC 2000 Growth Charts. *J Nutr*. 2007:137:144-148

11. Lozoff B, Jimenez E, Hagen J, Mollen E, Wolf AW. Poorer behavioral and developmental outcome more than 10 years after treatment for iron deficiency in infancy. *Pediatrics*. 2000;105:E51

12. Kleinman RE, ed, American Academy of Pediatrics, Committee on Nutrition. *Pediatric Nutrition Handbook*. 5th ed. Elk Grove Village, IL: American Academy of Pediatrics; 2004

13. Logan S, Martins S, Gilbert R. Iron therapy for improving psychomotor development and cognitive function in children under the age of three with iron deficiency anaemia. *Cochrane Database Syst Rev*. 2001;CD001444

14. Meinzen-Derr JK, Guerrero ML, Altaye M, Ortega-Gallegos H, Ruiz-Palacios GM, Morrow AL. Risk of infant anemia is associated with exclusive breast-feeding and maternal anemia in a Mexican cohort. *J Nutr*. 2006;136:452-458

15. Friel JK, Aziz K, Andrews WL, Harding SV, Courage ML, Adams RJ. A double-masked, randomized control trial of iron supplementation in early infancy in healthy term breast-fed infants. *J Pediatr*. 2003;143:582-586

16. Pizarro F, Yip R, Dallman PR, Olivares M, Hertrampf E, Walter T. Iron status with different infant feeding regimens: relevance to screening and prevention of iron deficiency. *J Pediatr*. 1991;118:687-692

17. Wagner CL, Greer FR, Section on Breastfeeding, committee on Nutrition. Prevention of rickets and vitamin D deficiency in infants, children, and adolescents. *Pediatrics*. In Press 2008 (possibly 2007)

18. American Academy of Pediatrics, Section on Breastfeeding: Breastfeeding and the use of human milk. *Pediatrics*. 2005;115:496-506

19. International Lactation Consultant Association. Clinical Guidelines for the Establishment of Exclusive Breastfeeding. Raleigh, NC: International Lactation Consultant Association, 2005. Available at: http://www.ilca.org/pubs/ClinicalGuidelines2005.pdf. Accessed March 29, 2007

20. Hale TW. *Medications and Mothers' Milk*. 12th ed. Amarillo, TX: Hale Publishing; 2006

21. Greer FR, Sicher SH, Burks AW, Committee on Nutrition, Section on Allergy and Immunology. The effects of early nutritional interventions on the development of atopic disease in infants and children: the role of maternal dietary restrictions, breastfeeding, timing of introduction of complementary foods and hydrolyzed formulas. *Pediatrics*. In Press 2008 (possibly late 2007)

22. Kramer MS, Kakuma R. Optimal duration of exclusive breastfeeding. *Cochrane Database Syst Rev*. 2002:CD003517

23. Mennella JA, Beauchamp GK. Mothers' milk enhances the acceptance of cereal during weaning. *Pediatr Res*. 1997;41: 188-192

24. Sullivan SA, Birch LL. Infant dietary experience and acceptance of solid foods. *Pediatrics*. 1994;93:271-277

25. American Academy of Pediatrics, Committee on Nutrition: The Use and Misuse of Fruit Juice in Pediatrics. *Pediatrics*. 2001;107:1210-1213

26. Sampson HA. Update on food allergy. *J Allergy Clin Immunol*. 2004;113(5):805-819; quiz 820

27. Muraro A, Dreborg S, Halken S, et al. Dietary prevention of allergic diseases in infants and small children: Part III: critical review of published peer-reviewed observational and interventional studies and final recommendations. *Pediatr Allergy Immunol*. 2004;15:291-307

28. Rerksuppaphol S, Barnes G. Guidelines for evaluation and treatment of gastroesophageal reflux in infants and children: recommendations of the North American Society for Pediatric Gastroenterology and Nutrition. *J Pediatr Gastroenterol Nutr.* 2002;35:583

29. Manikam R, Perman JA. Pediatric feeding disorders. *J Clin Gastroenterol.* 2000;30:34-46

30. Fox MK, Devaney B, Reidy K, Razafindrakoto C, Ziegler P. Relationship between portion size and energy intake among infants and toddlers: evidence of self-regulation. *J Am Diet Assoc.* 2006;106:S77-83

31. Devaney B, Ziegler P, Pac S, Karwe V, Barr SI. Nutrient intakes of infants and toddlers. *J Am Diet Assoc.* 2004;104:s14-21

32. Steering Committee on the Scientific Evaluation of Dietrary Reference Intakes, Food and Nutrition Board, Institute of Medicine. Dietary Reference Intakes for Calcium, Phosphorous, Magnesium, Vitamin D, and Fluoride. Washington, DC: National Academy Press; 1997. Available at: http://www.iom.edu/file.asp?id=21372. Accessed March 1, 2006

33. Greer FR, Krebs NF, American Academy of Pediatrics, Committee on Nutrition. Optimizing bone health and calcium intakes of infants, children, and adolescents. *Pediatrics.* 2006;117:578-585

34. Standing Committee on the Scientific Evaluation of Dietary Reference Intakes and its Panel on Folate, other B Vitamins, and Choline and Subcommittee on Upper Reference Levels of Nutrients, Food and Nutrition Board, Institute of Medicine. Dietary Reference Intakes for Thiamin, Riboflavin, Niacin, Vitamin B6, Folate, Vitamin B12, Pantothenic Acid, Biotin, and Choline. Washington, DC: National Academy Press; 1998

35. US Department of Health and Human Services, US Department of Agriculture. *Dietary Guidelines for Americans.* 6th ed. Washington, DC: US Department of Health and Human Services; US Department of Agriculture; 2005

36. Gidding SS, Dennison BA, et al. Dietary recommendations for children and adolescents: a guide for practitioners: Consensus Statement from the American Heart Association. *Circulation.* 2005;112:2061-2075

37. Daniels SR, Arnett DK, Eckel RH, et al. Overweight in children and adolescents: pathophysiology, consequences, prevention, and treatment. *Circulation.* 2005;111:1999-2012

38. American Academy of Pediatrics, Committee on Nutrition. Prevention of pediatric overweight and obesity. *Pediatrics.* 2003;112:424-430

39. Hampl JS, Anderson JV, Mullis R. Position of the American Dietetic Association: the role of dietetics professionals in health promotion and disease prevention. *J Am Diet Assoc.* 2002;102:1680-1687

40. Fox MK, Reidy K, Novak T, Ziegler P. Sources of energy and nutrients in the diets of infants and toddlers. *J Am Diet Assoc.* 2006;106:S28-42

41. Fox MK, Pac S, Devaney B, Jankowski L. Feeding infants and toddlers study: What foods are infants and toddlers eating? *J Am Diet Assoc.* 2004;104:s22-30

42. MyPyramid for Kids. Available at: www.mypyramid.gov/kids/index.html. Accessed July 4, 2006

43. Neumark-Sztainer D, Hannan PJ, Story M, Croll J, Perry C. Family meal patterns: associations with sociodemographic characteristics and improved dietary intake among adolescents. *J Am Diet Assoc.* 2003;103:317-322

44. Frazão E. The high costs of poor eating patterns in the United States. In: Frazão E, ed. *America's Eating Habits: Changes and Consequences.* Washington, DC: US Department of Agriculture, Economic Research Services; 1999:6-32

45. Grunbaum JA, Kann L, Kinchen SA, et al. Youth risk behavior surveillance—United States, 2001. *MMWR Surveill Summ.* 2002;51:1-62

46. Kann L, Kinchen SA, Williams BI, et al. Youth Risk Behavior Surveillance-United States, 1997. *MMWR CDC Surveill Summ.* 1998;47(SS-3):1-89

47. US Preventive Services Task Force. Behavioral Counseling in Primary Care to Promote a Healthy Diet: Recommendations and Rationale. Rockville, MD: Agency for Healthcare Research and Quality; 2003. Available at: www.ahrq.gov/clinic/3rduspstf/diet/dietrr.pdf. Accessed September 13, 2007

48. Neumark-Sztainer D, Story M, Perry C, Casey MA. Factors influencing food choices of adolescents: findings from focus-group discussions with adolescents. *J Am Diet Assoc.* 1999;99:929-937

49. Munoz KA, Krebs-Smith SM, Ballard-Barbash R, Cleveland LE. Food intakes of US children and adolescents compared with recommendations. *Pediatrics.* 1997;100:323-329

50. Neumarker KS. Mortality and sudden death in anorexia nervosa. *Int J Eat Disord.* 1997;21:205-212

51. Yesalis CE, Barsukiewicz CK, Kopstein AN, Bahrke MS. Trends in anabolic-androgenic steroid use among adolescents. *Arch Pediatr Adolesc Med.* 1997;151:1197-1206

52. Gomez J, American Academy of Pediatrics, Committee on Sports Medicine and Fitness. Use of performance-enhancing substances. *Pediatrics.* 2005;115:1103-1106

Promoting Physical Activity

Theme 6

INTRODUCTION

Physical activity is an essential component of a healthy lifestyle and must begin in infancy and extend throughout adulthood. Regular physical activity increases lean body mass, muscle, and bone strength and promotes good physical health. It fosters psychological well-being, can increase self-esteem and capacity for learning, and can help children and adolescents handle stress. Vigorous-intensity physical activity (eg, jogging or other aerobic exercise) generally provides more benefits than moderate-intensity physical activity.[1] Families should emphasize physical activity early in a child's life, because, as children mature, modern culture provides many temptations to adopt a sedentary lifestyle.

In recent years, a number of governmental agencies and national organizations have focused on the need for Americans to increase their physical activity levels. The US Surgeon General, the Centers for Disease Control and Prevention, and the President's Council on Physical Fitness have recognized and championed the importance of physical activity to overall health.[2-4]

Healthy People 2010 lists physical activity as a leading health indicator and includes goals to improve levels of physical activity and reduce sedentary behavior among adolescents.[5] In addition, the US Department of Health and Human Services and US Department of Agriculture's *Dietary Guidelines for Americans* recommend that children and adolescents engage in at least 60 minutes of moderate to vigorous physical activity on most days of the week, preferably daily.[1]

The dramatic rise in pediatric obesity in recent years has increased health care professionals' and parents' attention to the importance of physical activity. Along with a balanced and nutritious diet, regular physical activity is essential to preventing pediatric overweight conditions.[1,3] Therefore, health care professionals are encouraged to review this Bright Futures theme in concert with the Promoting Healthy Nutrition and Promoting Healthy Weight themes.

Physical Inactivity: A Growing Problem for Children and Adolescents

Children and adolescents live in an environment today in which opportunities for physical **inactivity** are increasingly common. Children ride to school rather than walk or bike, many schools are reducing or eliminating physical education classes and time for recess, many parents are afraid to let their children play outside, and labor-saving devices abound. Screens (television, videos, computers, and video games) are all around us, and "screen time" is an important component of daily life.

The primary sedentary behavior for preschoolers is watching television. Children 6 years and younger spend an average of 2 hours per day in front of the TV, which is about the same amount of time they spend playing outside.[6] For adolescents, time spent watching television represents the single greatest source of physical inactivity, second only to sleep.[7] Therefore, reducing the amount of time children and adolescents spend in front of a screen can provide opportunities for them to be physically active.[8] Parental awareness and assessment of screen time should encourage a balance that includes adequate time for physical activity. The American Academy of Pediatrics recommends that children younger than 2 years should not watch television, and children 2 years and older should limit media time to no more than 1 to 2 hours of quality programming daily.[9] (For more information on this topic, see the Promoting Healthy Weight Theme.)

In an environment that supports inactivity, being physically active must be a lifelong, conscious decision. Health care professionals can support children, adolescents, and families in this daily commitment by explaining why physical activity is important to overall health, providing information about community physical activity resources, and being physically active themselves.

Children and Youth With Special Health Care Needs

Children and youth with special health care needs should be encouraged to participate in physical activity, based on their ability and

> For adolescents, time spent watching television represents the single greatest source of physical inactivity, second only to sleep.

health status, as appropriate. Participating in physical activity can make their tasks of daily living easier, improve their health status, and, ultimately, reduce morbidity from secondary conditions during adulthood. Health care professionals can help parents and children select appropriate activities and duration by considering the child's needs and concerns, cognitive abilities, and social skills, as well as adaptations that will enable the child to have a positive experience.

Opportunities for physical activity should be included in the child's Individualized Education Program (IEP) at school, as well as the care plan for home services. Many organizations (eg, American Physical Therapy Association, Disabled Sports USA, and National Sports Center for the Disabled) provide information on appropriate physical activities and potential adaptations for specific conditions and disabilities. Programs such as the Special Olympics also can encourage children with special heath care needs to become involved with physical activity.[10]

Promoting Physical Activity: Infancy— Birth to 11 Months

The first year of life is marked by dramatic changes in the amount and type of physical

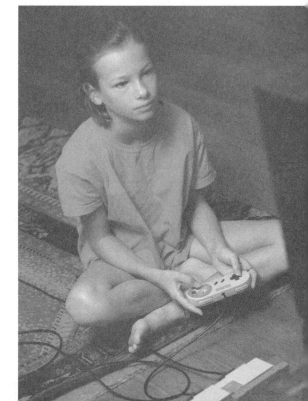

activity the infant displays. Motor skill development begins with involuntary reflexes that ensure the infant's survival. These reflexes become integrated as the infant gains voluntary control over his body. All infants usually acquire motor skills in the same order, but the rate at which these skills are acquired varies from child to child.

At each visit, the health care professional should provide parents with appropriate guidance about the child's next developmental steps to help them plan safe, educational, and appropriate physical activities (Box 1). Infants need parents and other caregivers to provide consistent, lively, and developmentally appropriate physical activity. Without adequate physical stimulation, infants adopt more sedentary behaviors and tend to roll over, crawl, and walk later than babies who enjoy physical activity with a parent or caregiver.

Part of the infant's day should be spent with a caregiver or parent who provides both systematic and spontaneous opportunities for active play and physical activity. Parents or caregivers can help the child be active through floor play, supervised "tummy time," and all daily routines, such as diapering, dressing and bathing, pulling to sit, rolling over, lifting arms over head, pulling to stand, and helping to lift a foot for a sock. Games such as pat-a-cake, peek-a-boo, and "how big is the baby?" all encourage active movement of the infant.

Giving infants freedom of movement encourages them to explore their environment and learn about their surroundings. Playpens, swings, and infant seats may be appropriate at certain times, but parents should be encouraged to let the infant move around freely with close supervision. Infant walkers and jumpers and car safety seats should not be used as positioning devices in the home. Consideration should be given to families who live in environments where they do not feel it is safe for their child to explore, such as in shelters or substandard housing. Discussions with parents who live in these environments can help them identify appropriate activities so that their child can meet the daily physical activity recommendations.

Health care professionals should caution parents not to use the television or other media to "entertain" or "educate" fussy or bored infants during the first years of life. At this stage of a child's development, television, videos, and computers are not effective tools for these purposes. Quiet play, such as reading, talking, and singing, is preferable because it helps the child appreciate the social component of physical activity and interactivity.

Infants with special health care needs may have delays in motor movement due to genetic or metabolic conditions, premature birth, developmental delays, or other causes. The health care professional should provide parents with information on Early Intervention Services for their child. These services provide support on ways to promote the infant's development within the family's daily routines.

BOX 1

Physical Activity Guidelines for Infants

- Infants should be placed in safe settings that facilitate physical activity and do not restrict movement for prolonged periods.
- Infants should be placed in settings and environments that meet or exceed recommended safety standards for performing large-muscle activities.

Adapted from National Association for Sport and Physical Education. Active start: a statement of physical activity guidelines for children birth to five years. 2002. Available at: http://www.aahperd.org/naspe/template.cfm?template=toddlers.html. Accessed March 1, 2006.[11]

Without adequate physical stimulation, infants adopt more sedentary behaviors and tend to roll over, crawl, and walk later than babies who enjoy physical activity with a parent or caregiver.

Young children with special health care needs can and should enjoy physical activity as much as any other child. Depending on the child's diagnosis and health status, such activities may need to be modified by parents, preschool teachers, child care workers, or therapists.

Promoting Physical Activity: Early Childhood—1 to 4 Years

A primary reason for promoting physical activity during early childhood is to assist young children in mastering basic motor skills.[12] As a child progresses through infancy into the toddler years, her strength and flexibility increase and she is better able to control her head and neck. Most (but not all) children develop gross motor skills in a typical sequence—walking, marching, galloping, hopping, running, traveling around obstacles, and skipping.[12] Most children also master fine motor skills (manipulation) and spatial relationships during the toddler and preschool years. Eye-hand and eye-foot coordination, balance, and depth perception develop during the preschool years as well. Physical activity can promote the mastery of these skills, all of which are important milestones in the child's development. In addition, physical activity can improve physical and mental health and is fun for the child.

Component activities that build upon each other include gross motor activity (large movement skills), stability activity, manipulative activity (small movement or fine motor skills), and rhythm activity.[12] Some activities, such as dancing, combine several of these components. Movement concepts include learning about where and how the body moves, the effort it takes to move the body (eg, time and force), and the relationship of the body to what is around it. Structured play contributes to stability, flexibility, and stamina.

Engaging young children in all forms of physical activity (active play and interactive guided play) promotes the joy of movement, the sense of control, and the ability to navigate the body through space. The most prevalent form of physical activity in early childhood is active play. Simply playing outside (eg, walking, running, climbing, and exploring the outdoor environment) is an important opportunity for physical activity. Interactive guided play, which includes

developmentally appropriate structured forms of physical activity, such as dancing or simple games, allows a caregiver to help the child master specific motor skills in a safe and supervised manner.

Physical activity in young childhood also has other benefits. An Iowa study of young children showed that physical activity contributes to optimal bone development.[13] Other research has shown that adolescents who had the highest levels of activity in their preschool years also had lower accretion of body fat.[14] Active play and interactive guided play in the young can prevent pediatric overweight and obesity,[15] and also appear to increase self-esteem and reduce symptoms of depression and anxiety during early childhood.[10]

Young children with special health care needs can and should enjoy physical activity as much as any other child. Depending on the child's diagnosis and health status, such activities may need to be modified by parents, preschool teachers, child care workers, or therapists. Young children who have significant physical or cognitive impairments usually are enrolled in Early Intervention programs where physical activity takes place as part of the routine day. Alternatively, they are in preschool or child care settings where physical movement activities are adapted to their particular disability, if necessary. Health care professionals can encourage families to ask teachers and therapists for help in integrating those activities into daily routines at home. In addition, many young children with special health care needs (depending on the type of disability) can be included in physical activities that are enjoyed by all children in the community, from playground swings and slides to preschool gymnastic and dance classes.

Promoting Physical Activity: Middle Childhood—5 to 10 Years

As children grow and develop, their motor skills increase, giving them an opportunity to participate in a variety of physical activities. Children may try different physical activities and establish one or more interests that serve as the foundation for lifelong participation in physical activity. When children have multiple options for physical activity available in the community, they can be encouraged to express their preferences, develop competencies, and find activities that fit their skills and interests.

During the middle childhood years, parents are a major influence on a child's level of physical activity. Parents should encourage their children to be physically active. Parents who also participate in physical activity with their children (eg, walking, dancing, biking, hiking, playing outside, or participating in sports such as basketball or baseball) demonstrate the importance of regular physical activity and show their children that physical activity can be fun. Children also can be influenced to participate in physical activity by other family members, peers, teachers, and people depicted in the media.

Children are motivated to participate in physical activity by having fun, by feeling competent, and through variety. Age-appropriate activities, coaching styles, and

BOX 2
Age-Appropriate Physical Activities

Age	Motor Skills Being Developed	Appropriate Physical Activities
5-6 years	Fundamental (eg, running, galloping, jumping, hopping, skipping, throwing, catching, striking, or kicking)	• Activities that focus on having fun and developing motor skills rather than on competition • Simple activities that require little instruction • Repetitive activities that do not require complex motor and cognitive skills (eg, running, swimming, tumbling, or throwing and catching a ball)
7-9 years	Fundamental Transitional (eg, throwing for distance or throwing for accuracy)	• Activities that focus on having fun and developing motor skills rather than on competition • Activities with flexible rules • Activities that require little instruction • Activities that do not require complex motor and cognitive skills (eg, entry-level baseball or soccer)
10-11 years	Transitional Complex (eg, playing basketball)	• Activities that continue to focus on having fun and developing motor skills rather than on competition • Activities that require entry-level complex motor and cognitive skills • Activities that continue to emphasize motor skill development but that begin to incorporate instruction on strategy and teamwork

techniques are important (Box 2).[10] Feelings of failure, embarrassment, competition, and boredom, and rigid structure, discourage participation.

Parents should be cautioned about relying exclusively on schools to provide physical activity for their child, particularly if the child is not involved in organized sports. Given the emphasis on academics, outdoor recess and physical education have been curtailed in many school systems.

Adequate fluid intake during physical activity is important to prevent dehydration (Box 3). The risk of dehydration becomes greater with increased heat, humidity, intensity, or duration of physical activity, body surface area, and sweating.

Promoting Physical Activity: Adolescence—11 to 21 Years

Participating in regular physical activity helps adolescents develop skills and pastimes they can enjoy throughout their lives. Like the younger child, the adolescent who participates in physical activity increases his muscle and bone strength and lean muscle mass. In addition, physical activity may help him reduce body fat and maintain a healthy body weight. Physical activity also can reduce symptoms of depression and anxiety and improve overall mood.[16] Weight-bearing physical activity contributes to building greater bone density in adolescence and helps maintain peak bone density in adulthood.[16]

Some adolescents are aware of diseases that affect their family or community (eg, obesity, diabetes, or cardiovascu-

lar disease). This awareness may make them receptive to actions that may reduce risks of these diseases. Health care professionals can consider linking exercise and physical activities with reduced risk of diseases that negatively affect their families and perhaps many people within their communities.

Adolescents have numerous options for regular physical activity, and the longer an adolescent participates in vigorous physical activity, the greater the health benefits.[16] Competitive sports appeal to some; others enjoy noncompetitive activities that provide variety and opportunities for socialization. Even those adolescents who are heavily scheduled with school, extracurricular activities, and part-time jobs can be physically active through short periods (eg, 10-minute duration) of moderate-intensity activity.

> **Physical activity also can reduce symptoms of depression and anxiety and improve overall mood.**

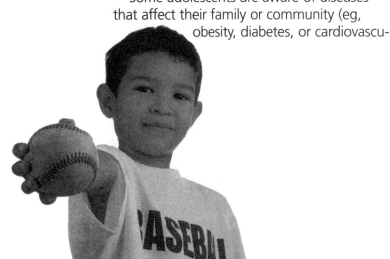

> ### BOX 3
> #### Fluid Intake During Physical Activity
> Sports drinks usually contain 6% to 8% sugar as well as replenishing electrolytes. They are generally beneficial for physical activities that last longer than 60 minutes. For brief periods of physical activity, the caloric burden of these drinks outweighs the benefits of fluid and electrolyte replacement.
>
> During extremely hot weather, outdoor physical activity should be scheduled during the coolest times of the day (ie, before 10:00 am and after 6:00 pm).[10]
>
> To avoid dehydration, children and adolescents should:
>
> - Drink before feeling thirsty, because mild dehydration occurs before thirst sets in.
> - Drink cool water (40ºF to 50ºF) before, during, and after physical activity.
>   - Drink 4 to 8 ounces of water 1 to 2 hours before physical activity.
>   - Drink 4 to 8 ounces of water every 15 to 20 minutes during physical activity that lasts longer than 1 hour.

Current recommendations note that physical activity can be accumulated through 3 to 6 ten-minute activities over the course of a day. The accumulated total of 60 minutes daily is the important variable for overall health and calorie burning. The longer an adolescent participates in vigorous physical activity, the greater the health benefits.[16]

Social and peer influences can positively or negatively affect participation in physical activities. The best physical activities are those that adolescents enjoy. In some communities, the lack of safe places for recreation requires creative alternatives for physical activity, such as using the steps at school or in apartment complexes.

During early adolescence, girls and boys can participate in competitive sports together. However, with the onset of puberty, weight and strength differences rapidly become great enough to pose a safety concern. Coed activities should be limited to non-collision sports. To promote participation and enjoyment for all adolescents, including adolescents with special health care needs, physical education teachers and coaches should establish teams based on each person's skill level, size, and strength, rather than on gender.

In the pursuit of enhanced performance, adolescents who engage in competitive sports and physical activity can be vulnerable to misinformation and unsafe practices. Pressure to achieve a "competitive edge" can encourage adolescents to experiment with ergogenic aids or performance-enhancing substances (eg, anabolic steroids, creatine, and stimulants). Many performance-enhancing substances offer no benefit, and some can adversely affect performance and endurance, jeopardize health, and undermine the benefits of training. Use of anabolic steroids is dangerous. Although they can help build muscle mass, anabolic steroids cause early closure of the epiphyseal plates, resulting in stunted growth. Adolescents who use steroids also risk sterility.

Healthy People 2010 lists physical activity as a leading health indicator and includes goals to improve levels of physical activity and reduce sedentary behavior among adolescents.[5] By encouraging increased physical activity, health care professionals, program administrators, and policy makers can help their communities achieve these goals and use community resources efficiently.[17]

Preventing injury to adolescents during physical activity is a responsibility shared by parents, physical education teachers, coaches, recreation program staff, and adolescents themselves. (For more information on this topic, see the Promoting Safety and Injury Prevention Theme.) The practices listed in Box 4 have been demonstrated to prevent sports and exercise injury.

The longer an adolescent participates in vigorous physical activity, the greater the health benefits.

PROMOTING
PHYSICAL ACTIVITY

BOX 4
Preventing Sports and Exercise Injury

- Stretch before participating in sports.
- Use appropriate safety equipment, such as batting helmets in baseball and softball, athletic supporter and cup for boys in contact sports, bicycle helmets in biking, shin guards in soccer and field hockey, wrist guards and elbow and knee pads in in-line skating, and goggles in handball and racquetball.
- Limit duration of specific, repetitive physical activities that require the use of the same muscles (eg, pitching or running).
- Set an appropriate pace when beginning an activity and be aware of early symptoms of injury (eg, increase in muscle soreness, bone or joint pain, excessive fatigue, or decrease in performance). Adolescents who experience any of these symptoms should decrease participation in physical activity until symptoms diminish, or, if the injury is severe, should cease participation temporarily.

References

1. US Department of Agriculture. *Dietary Guidelines for Americans, 2005*. 6th ed. Washington, DC: US Department of Agriculture, US Department of Health and Human Services; 2005

2. President's Council on Physical Fitness and Sports Web site. Available at: http://www.fitness.gov/. Accessed July 4, 2006

3. Centers for Disease Control and Prevention, Division of Nutrition and Physical Activity, National Center for Chronic Disease Prevention and Health Promotion. Physical Activity for Everyone: Are There Special Recommendations for Young People? Available at: http://www.cdc.gov/nccdphp/dnpa/physical/recommendations/young.htm. Accessed March 1, 2006

4. Office of the Surgeon General. *The Surgeon General's Call to Action to Prevent and Decrease Overweight and Obesity*. Rockville, MD: Office of the Surgeon General, US Public Health Service, US Department of Health and Human Services; 2001

5. US Department of Health and Human Services. Physical activity and fitness. In: *Healthy People 2010: Objectives for Improving Health*. Vol 2. 2nd ed. Washington, DC: US Government Printing Office; 2000:22-3-22-39

6. Rideout VJ, Vandewater EA, Wartella EA. *Zero to Six: Electronic Media in the Lives of Infants, Toddlers and Preschoolers*. Menlo Park, CA: Kaiser Family Foundation; 2003. Publication No. 3378. Available at: http://www.kff.org/entmedia/3378-CFM. Accessed April 10, 2007

7. Dietz WH, Strasburger VC. Children, adolescents, and television. *Curr Probl Pediatr*. 1991;21:8-32

8. Dietz WH. The obesity epidemic in young children. Reduce television viewing and promote playing. *BMJ*. 2001;322:313-314

9. American Academy of Pediatrics, Committee on Public Education. Children, adolescents, and television. *Pediatrics*. 2001;107:423-426

10. Patrick K, Spear B, Holt K, Sofka D, eds. *Bright Futures in Practice: Physical Activity*. Arlington, VA: National Center for Education in Maternal and Child Health; 2001

11. National Association for Sport and Physical Education. *Active Start: A Statement of Physical Activity Guidelines for Children Birth to Five Years*. Reston, VA: National Association for Sport and Physical Education; 2002

12. Sanders SW. *Active for Life: Developmentally Appropriate Movement Programs for Young Children*. Washington, DC: National Association for the Education of Young Children; 2002

13. Janz KF, Burns TL, Torner JC, et al. Physical activity and bone measures in young children: the Iowa bone development study. *Pediatrics*. 2001;107:1387-1393

14. Moore LL, Gao D, Bradlee ML, et al. Does early physical activity predict body fat change throughout childhood? *Prev Med*. 2003;37:10-17

15. Krebs NF, Jacobson MS. Prevention of pediatric overweight and obesity. *Pediatrics*. 2003;112:424-430

16. US Department of Health and Human Services. *Physical Activity and Health. A Report of the Surgeon General*. Atlanta, GA: The President's Council on Physical Fitness and Sports, US Department of Health and Human Services; 1996

17. Centers for Disease Control and Prevention. Increasing physical activity: a report on recommendations of the Task Force on Community Preventive Services. *MMWR Recomm Rep*. 2001;50(RR-18):1-14

Promoting Oral Health

Theme 7

INTRODUCTION

Oral health is critically important to the overall health and well-being of children and adolescents. It covers a range of health promotion and disease prevention concerns, including dental caries (tooth decay); periodontal health; proper development and alignment of facial bones, jaws, and teeth; oral diseases and conditions; and trauma or injury to the mouth and teeth. Oral health is an important and continuing health supervision issue for the health care professional.

Childhood caries (tooth decay) is a preventable and transmissible infectious disease, caused by bacteria (eg, *Streptococcus mutans or Streptococcus sobrinus*) that form plaque on the surface of teeth. The bacteria interact with sugar in foods and beverages, turning it into acids that dissolve tooth enamel, causing caries.

Caries is the most common chronic disease in children—5 times more common than asthma.[1] Left untreated, pain and infection caused by tooth decay can lead to problems in eating, speaking, and learning.[1] Forty percent of children have caries by the time they reach kindergarten,[2] and many school hours are lost each year due to dental problems related to caries.[1-3]

Several population groups are particularly vulnerable to caries. For example, children and youth with special health care needs are at increased risk. National surveys also have demonstrated that children in low-income and moderate-income households are more likely to have caries and more decayed or filled teeth than children who are from more affluent households. Even within income levels, children of color are more likely to have caries than white children.[4] Thus, sociodemographic status should be viewed as an initial indicator of risk that can be offset by the absence of other risk indicators.

Health care professionals can teach children, adolescents, and their families about oral hygiene, healthy diet and feeding practices, optimal exposure to fluoride, and timely referral to a dentist. Health care professionals also often make the initial response for oral trauma. They should keep in mind that the differential diagnosis for oral trauma includes intentional injury.[5]

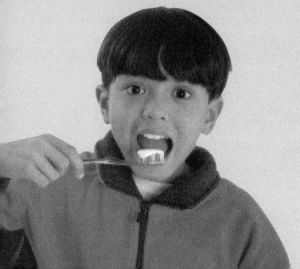

Bright Futures in Practice: Oral Health Pocket Guide (2004) provides a structured and comprehensive approach to this anticipatory guidance for the health care professional.[6] The Health Resources and Services Administration's (HRSA's) National Maternal and Child Oral Health Resource Center (www.mchoralhealth.org) also provides many valuable tools and resources for health care professionals.[7] Additional information is available at the American Academy of Pediatrics (AAP) Web site (www.aap.org).

The Importance of a Dental Home

The dental home is the "ongoing relationship between the dentist and the patient, inclusive of all aspects of oral health delivered in a comprehensive, continuously accessible coordinated and family-centered way."[8]

Box 1 describes the services that should be provided within a dental home.

The dental community (the American Dental Association, the Academy of General Dentistry, and the American Academy of Pediatric Dentistry [AAPD]) is united in encouraging families to establish a dental home by the time their child is 1 year old.[9] Having a dental home is the ideal deterrence to the development of caries, from infancy through adolescence. Early preventive dental

The dental community (the American Dental Association, the Academy of General Dentistry, and the American Academy of Pediatric Dentistry) is united in encouraging families to establish a dental home by the time their child is 1 year old.

PROMOTING ORAL HEALTH

BOX 1
Dental Home

According to the American Academy of Pediatric Dentistry (AAPD), the dental home should provide the following:

- Comprehensive oral health care, including acute care and preventive services, in accordance with AAPD periodicity schedules.
- Comprehensive assessment for oral diseases and conditions.
- An individualized preventive dental health program based on a caries risk assessment and a periodontal disease risk assessment.
- Anticipatory guidance about growth and development issues (ie, teething, thumb or finger or pacifier habits).
- A plan for acute dental trauma.
- Information about proper care of the child's teeth and gingivae. This would include prevention, diagnosis, and treatment of disease of the supporting and surrounding tissues and the maintenance of health, function, and esthetics of those structures and tissues.
- Dietary counseling.
- Referrals to specialists when care cannot directly be provided within the dental home.
- Education regarding future referral to a dentist knowledgeable and comfortable with adult oral health issues for continuing oral health care; referral at an age determined by patient, parent, and pediatric dentist.

Adopted from: American Academy of Pediatric Dentistry. *Policy on the Dental Home*. American Academy of Pediatric Dentistry; revised 2004.[9]

visits have been shown to reduce dental disease and reduce costs. For example, Savage et al[10] showed that dental costs for Medicaid-eligible children who began dental visits between the ages of 1 and 2 years were approximately 60% of the cost for children who began dental visits between the ages of 4 and 5 years.

As children and adolescents mature into adulthood, a dental home also can ensure that they receive oral health education/counseling, preventive and early intervention measures, and treatment, including treatment for periodontal care, orthodontic services, trauma, and other conditions.

Efforts to establish a dental home offer an opportunity for partnerships and foster a connection with the community. A partnership among health care professionals in primary care, dental health, public health, child care, and school settings can help ensure access to a dental home for each child during the early childhood, middle childhood, and adolescent years. (For more information on this topic, see the Promoting Community Relationships and Resources theme.)

Supplemental Fluoride

Fluoride plays a key role in preventing and controlling caries. Fluoride helps reduce loss of minerals from tooth enamel (demineralization) and promotes replacement of minerals (remineralization) in dental enamel that has been damaged by acids produced by bacteria in plaque. Regular and frequent exposure to small amounts of fluoride is the best way to protect the teeth against caries. This exposure can be readily accomplished through drinking water that has been optimally fluoridated and brushing with fluoride toothpaste twice daily.[11]

Fluoride supplementation typically is not needed in the first 6 months of life. Beginning at the age of 6 months, children should drink fluoridated community drinking water or take prescribed supplements (ie, drops or chewable tablets).[11-13] As an alternative to fluoride supplements, parents can purchase bottled water that contains fluoride.

Additional types of fluoride may be used as a primary preventive measure and, generally, are recommended for infants, children, and adolescents who are deemed to be at high risk of caries. Research has shown that the primary caries prevention effects of fluoride result from its topical contact with enamel and through its antibacterial actions. Therefore, topical agents (eg, concentrated fluoride gels, foams, and varnishes) may be used as a strategy for children who are deemed to be at elevated risk of tooth decay.[11,14]

Even if indicated, additional fluoride should be used judiciously in children 6 years and younger to minimize the risk of fluorosis (ie, overexposure to fluoride).[11] Fluorosis can come from using too much toothpaste that contains fluoride, drinking water with higher than recommended fluoride levels, and taking fluoride supplements when other sources of fluoride are available.[15] To prevent fluorosis, the primary water source(s) must be tested before parents are advised to supplement with fluoride.[16]

For adolescents, optimal fluoride levels in drinking water, combined with fluoride-containing preparations, such as toothpastes, gels, varnishes, and rinses, have significantly reduced dental decay, but caries risk remains high during this age period.[17,18] Adolescents at high risk of caries should be evaluated for topical fluoride beyond that provided by water supply and a fluoridated toothpaste.

Children and Youth With Special Health Care Needs

Children with special health care needs (eg, infants at risk of enamel demineralization and hypoplasia because of poor mineralization or osteopenia, nutritional deficiencies, or medication usage) present a unique set of concerns for oral health because they are

Fluoride helps reduce loss of minerals from tooth enamel (demineralization) and promotes replacement of minerals (remineralization) in dental enamel that has been damaged by acids produced by bacteria in plaque.

PROMOTING ORAL HEALTH

particularly prone to the development of caries. Because dental care for these children is often difficult and sometimes risky, the health care professional should refer the child to a dentist as early as possible for vigilant preventive dental care, which may alleviate the need for future surgical intervention.

Oral diseases also may have a direct and devastating impact on the general health of children with certain systemic or developmental problems or conditions. Children with compromised immunity or certain cardiac, kidney, or liver conditions may be especially vulnerable to the effects of oral diseases. Children with cognitive disabilities or developmental or neuromuscular conditions who do not have the ability to understand and assume responsibility for, or cooperate with, preventive oral health practices may be at higher risk for complications or systemic infections from oral diseases.[19]

Children and youth with special health care needs may require more help with their oral self-care routines (ie, brushing and flossing) than other children. Health care professionals should advise parents or caregivers to supervise and intervene as needed to help their children with brushing and flossing if their special needs prevent them from doing a thorough job. The child with special needs should begin dental care in the first year and visit the dentist every 6 months or more frequently as needed.

Adolescents with special health care needs may face difficulties because of their physical condition, malformations, medicines, or nutrition. They should receive regular dental care and be encouraged to take as much responsibility as possible for their own oral hygiene.

Promoting Oral Health: Infancy— Birth to 11 Months

Even though a child's teeth do not begin to appear until the middle of this developmental period, oral health is still a concern because of the potential that caries can develop during the first year of life.

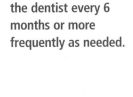

The child with special needs should begin dental care in the first year and visit the dentist every 6 months or more frequently as needed.

Oral Hygiene and Feeding Practices That Promote Oral Health

Even before the baby's birth, parents and other caregivers should make sure their own mouths are as healthy as possible to reduce transmission of caries-causing harmful bacteria from their saliva to the newborn baby's mouth. Health care professionals should educate family members or caregivers in the following ways to prevent transmission of these bacteria from themselves to the infant:

- Practice good oral hygiene and seek dental care.
- Do not share utensils, cups, spoons, or toothbrushes with the infant.
- Do not clean a pacifier in their own mouths before giving it to the infant.
- Consult with an oral health professional about the use of xylitol gum (if the adult's oral health is a concern). This gum can have a positive impact on oral health by decreasing the bacterial load in an adult's mouth.[20]

The primary teeth begin to erupt at different ages during the first year of life. An infant is susceptible to tooth decay as soon as her first teeth erupt if she has a sufficient bacterial load already present in her mouth and prolonged exposure to carbohydrates. Chalky white areas on the teeth are the first sign of dental decay. Both inadequate oral hygiene and inappropriate feeding practices that expose teeth to natural or refined sugars for prolonged periods contribute to the development of early childhood caries. Health care professionals should educate parents in the

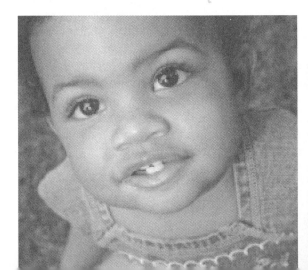

following ways to keep teeth clean and remove plaque:

- Minimize exposure to natural or refined sugars in the infant's mouth.
  - Avoid frequent exposure to foods that can lead to early childhood caries.
  - Hold the infant while feeding. Never prop a bottle (ie, use pillows or any other object to hold a bottle in the infant's mouth).
  - Do not allow the infant to fall asleep with a bottle that contains milk, formula, juice, or other sweetened liquid.
  - Avoid dipping pacifiers in any sweetened liquid, sugars, or syrups.[16]
- Use a toothbrush twice daily as soon as teeth erupt. In children younger than 2 years, the teeth should be brushed with plain water twice a day (after breakfast and before bed),[6] unless advised by a dentist to use fluoridated toothpaste based on a child's elevated dental caries risk.

To help prevent early childhood caries, parents also should take advantage of this developmental stage to establish lifelong nutritious eating patterns for the family that emphasize consumption of fruits, vegetables, whole grains, lean meats, and dairy products, and that minimize consumptions of foods and liquids high in sugars. (For more information on this topic, see the Promoting Healthy Nutrition theme.)

Oral Health Risk Assessment

In 2003, the AAP developed a policy statement, Oral Health Risk Assessment Timing and Establishment of the Dental Home, that recommended that primary care child health care professionals conduct an oral health risk assessment when a child is 6 months of age (Box 2).[21] This assessment consists of asking parents about their, and the child's, oral hygiene and looking at the child's mouth to assess the risk of caries.

The AAP recognizes that, even today, some children live in communities that lack pediatric dentists or general dentists who are able to see infants and young children. Therefore, primary care child health care professionals who care for these children may have to continue to perform periodic oral health risk assessments even after the first 6 to 12 months of age. These assessments allow health care professionals to identify children at the highest risk of oral health problems so that they can be referred to whatever limited resources are available. Some child health care professionals also may provide enhanced oral health counseling or apply fluoride varnish to help with caries prevention in

BOX 2
Pediatric Oral Health Risk Assessment
Adopted from the AAP policy statement that states that all children should undergo an oral health risk assessment beginning at 6 months of age by a qualified pediatric health care professional:

"If an infant is assessed to be in one of the following risk groups, the care requirements could be significant and surgically invasive. Therefore, these infants should be referred to a dentist as early as 6 months of age and no later than 6 months after the first tooth erupts or 12 months of age (whichever comes first) for establishment of a dental home:

- Children with special health care needs
- Children of mothers with a high caries rates
- Children with demonstrable caries, plaque, demineralization, and/or staining
- Children who sleep with a bottle or breastfeed throughout the night
- Children in families of low socioeconomic status"

In 2003, the American Academy of Pediatrics… recommended that primary care child health care professionals conduct an oral health risk assessment when a child is 6 months of age.

high-risk children.[22,23] In addition, public health professionals often assist health care professionals and families to link to a dental home.

Promoting Oral Health: Early Childhood—1 to 4 Years

The key oral health priorities of this developmental stage are the same as those of infancy, namely preventing caries and developing healthy oral hygiene habits. Early childhood also is a good time for parents, caregivers, and health care professionals to build positive dietary habits as they introduce new foods and the child establishes taste preferences. Parents may have questions during this period about pacifiers and thumb-sucking and finger-sucking behaviors that are related to teeth and jaw alignment.

Early childhood is a time in which children are exposed to new tastes, textures, and eating experiences. It is an important opportunity for parents and caregivers to firmly establish healthful eating patterns for the child and her family.

Oral Hygiene, Fluoride, and Feeding Practices That Promote Oral Health

Parents and caregivers can do much to prevent the development of caries and promote overall oral health during this period. As noted earlier, caries is an infectious disease, and parents should make sure their oral hygiene and diet meet the standards outlined here. Health care professionals should educate the family and caregivers in the following ways to reduce transmission of bacteria from themselves to the child:

- Practice good oral hygiene and seek dental care.
- Do not share utensils, cups, spoons, or toothbrushes with the child.
- Do not put the child's pacifiers in their own mouths. Clean pacifiers with mild soap and water.
- Consult with their oral health care professional about the use of gum containing xylitol (if the adult's oral health is a concern).

Health care professionals also should educate parents about ways to keep their child's teeth clean and ensure sufficient fluoride intake.

- Brush the child's teeth twice daily as soon as teeth erupt. Because young children do not have the manual dexterity to properly clean their own teeth, an adult usually must brush the teeth of preschool-aged children. When parents feel their child is doing a thorough job, they should allow the child more independence and freedom.
  - For children younger than 2 years, brush the teeth with plain water twice a day (after breakfast and before bed) unless advised by a dentist to use fluoridated toothpaste based on a child's elevated dental caries risk.
  - For children 2 years and older, brush the teeth with no more than a pea-sized amount (small smear) of fluoride toothpaste twice a day (after breakfast and before bed). The child should spit out the toothpaste after brushing, but not rinse his mouth with water. The small amount of toothpaste that remains in his mouth helps prevent tooth decay.[6] Children can be taught to floss if recommended by the dental professional.
- Make sure the child drinks fluoridated water or takes prescribed fluoride supplements.

Early childhood is a time in which children are exposed to new tastes, textures, and eating experiences. It is an important opportunity for parents and caregivers to firmly establish healthful eating patterns for the child and her family. These patterns should emphasize consumption of fruits, vegetables, whole grains, lean meats, and dairy products, and minimize consumptions of foods and liquids high in sugars. (For more information on this topic, see the Promoting Healthy Nutrition theme.)

PROMOTING ORAL HEALTH

Oral Health Risk Assessment

The AAPD recommends that, after 12 months of age, a child should be seen by a dentist every 6 months or according to a schedule recommended by the dentist, based on the child's individual needs and susceptibility to disease.[24] The AAP notes that, in the absence of a dental home program that is able to see the 1- to 4-year-old child, the primary care child health care professional should continue to perform oral health risk assessments in the 1- to 4-year-old child.

The AAPD also recommends that health care professionals use the Caries-Risk Assessment Tool (CAT) beginning at age 1 year (Table 1) as part of the oral risk assessment.[25]

Other Oral Health Issues

The health care professional should be prepared to discuss the use of pacifiers and finger sucking or thumb sucking. Finger sucking often fills an emotional need, but it can lead to malocclusion, including anterior open bite (top teeth do not overlap the bottom teeth) and excess overjet (top teeth protrude relative to the bottom teeth). The intensity, duration, and nature of the sucking habit can be used to predict the amount of harm that can occur. Positive reinforcement, including a reward system or reminder system, is the most effective way to discourage finger sucking.

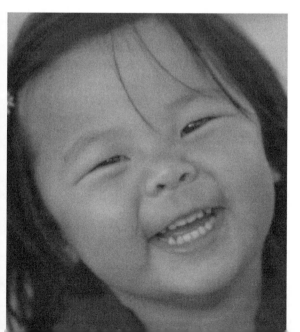

Promoting Oral Health: Middle Childhood—5 to 10 Years

During the early part of middle childhood, a child loses his first tooth and the first permanent teeth (maxillary and mandibular incisors and first molars) start to erupt. By the end of middle childhood, most of the permanent teeth have erupted. For the child, these are exciting signs of getting older. Middle childhood also is a good time for parents and caregivers to reinforce oral hygiene, optimal fluoride exposure, and positive diet habits they pursued in early childhood.

The history and physical examination performed by the health care professional should include oral health. The child also should see the dentist every 6 months or according to a schedule recommended by the dentist, based on the child's individual needs and susceptibility to disease. When the permanent molars erupt, the child's dentist should evaluate his teeth to determine the need for sealants that protect the teeth from caries.

The key oral health issues for this developmental stage are preventing caries and gingivitis, and ensuring proper development of the mouth and jaw. Reducing the risk of injury or trauma to the mouth and teeth and avoiding risk behaviors that negatively affect oral health also are important.

Oral Hygiene, Fluoride, and Nutrition Practices That Promote Oral Health

Health care professionals should educate parents in the following ways to help their child keep his teeth clean and remove plaque:

- Helping with, and supervising, the brushing of their child's teeth at least twice a day and flossing if recommended by the dental professional.
- Using only a pea-sized amount of fluoridated toothpaste to clean the child's teeth. The child should spit out the toothpaste after brushing, but not rinse his mouth with water. The small amount

The American Academy of Pediatric Dentistry recommends that, after 12 months of age, a child should be seen by a dentist every 6 months or according to a schedule recommended by the dentist, based on the child's individual needs and susceptibility to disease.

PROMOTING ORAL HEALTH

TABLE 1

American Academy of Pediatric Dentistry Caries-Risk Assessment Tool (CAT)

Risk Factors to Consider	Risk Indicators		
(For each item below, circle the most accurate response found to the right under "Risk Indicators")	High	Moderate	Low
Part 1 – History (determined by interviewing the parent/primary caregiver)			
Child has special health care needs, especially any that impact motor coordination or cooperation[A]	Yes		No
Child has condition that impairs saliva (dry mouth)[B]	Yes		No
Child's use of dental home (frequency of routine dental visits)	None	Irregular	Regular
Child has decay	Yes		No
Time lapsed since child's last cavity	<12 months	12 to 24 months	>24 months
Child wears braces or orthodontic/oral appliances[C]	Yes		No
Child's parent and/or sibling(s) have decay	Yes		No
Socioeconomic status of child's parents[D]	Low	Mid-level	High
Daily between-meal exposures to sugars/cavity producing foods (includes on demand use of bottle/sippy cup containing liquid other than water; consumption of juice, carbonated beverages, or sports drinks; use of sweetened medications)[E]	>3	1 to 2	Mealtime only
Child's exposure to fluoride[F,G]	Does not use fluoridated toothpaste; drinking water is not fluoridated and is not taking fluoride supplements	Uses fluoridated toothpaste; usually does not drink fluoridated water and does not take fluoride supplements	Uses fluoridated toothpaste; drinks fluoridated water or takes fluoride supplements
Times per day that child's teeth/gums are brushed	<1	1	2-3
Part 2 – Clinical evaluation (determined by examining the child's mouth)			
Visible plaque (white, sticky buildup)	Present		Absent
Gingivitis (red, puffy gums)[H]	Present		Absent
Areas of enamel demineralization (chalky white-spots on teeth)	More than 1	1	None
Enamel defects, deep pits/fissures[I]	Present		Absent
Part 3 – Supplemental professional assessment (Optional)[J]			
Radiographic enamel caries	Present		Absent
Levels of mutans streptococci or lactobacilli	High	Moderate	Low

Each child's overall assessed risk for developing decay is based on the highest level of risk indicator circled above (ie, single risk indicator in any area of the "high risk" category classifies a child as being "high risk").

A   Children with special health care needs are those who have a physical, developmental, mental, sensory, behavioral, cognitive, or emotional impairment or limiting condition that requires medical management, health care intervention, and/or use of specialized services. The condition may be developmental or acquired and may cause limitations in performing daily self-maintenance activities or substantial limitations in a major life activity. Health care for special needs patients is beyond that considered routine and requires specialized knowledge, increased awareness and attention, and accommodation.

B   Alteration in salivary flow can be the result of congenital or acquired conditions, surgery, radiation, medication, or age-related changes in salivary function. Any condition, treatment, or process known or reported to alter saliva flow should be considered an indication of risk unless proven otherwise.

C   Orthodontic appliances include both fixed and removable appliances, space maintainers, and other devices that remain in the mouth continuously or for prolonged time intervals and which may trap food and plaque, prevent oral hygiene, compromise access of tooth surfaces to fluoride, or otherwise create an environment supporting caries initiation.

D   National surveys have demonstrated that children in low-income and moderate-income households are more likely to have caries and more decayed or filled primary teeth than children from more affluent households. Also, within income levels, minority children are more likely to have caries. Thus, socioeconomic status should be viewed as an initial indicator of risk that may be offset by the absence of other risk indicators.

E   Examples of sources of simple sugars include carbonated beverages, cookies, cake, candy, cereal, potato chips, French fries, corn chips, pretzels, breads, juices, and fruits. Clinicians using caries-risk assessment should investigate individual exposures to sugars known to be involved in caries initiation.

F   Optimal systemic and topical fluoride exposure is based on use of a fluoride dentifrice and American Dental Association/American Academy of Pediatrics guidelines for exposure from fluoride drinking water and/or supplementation.

G   Unsupervised use of toothpaste and at-home topical fluoride products are not recommended for children unable to expectorate predictably.

H   Although microbial organisms responsible for gingivitis may be different than those primarily implicated in caries, the presence of gingivitis is an indicator of poor or infrequent oral hygiene practices and has been associated with caries progression.

I   Tooth anatomy and hypoplastic defects (eg, poorly formed enamel, developmental pits) may predispose a child to develop caries.

J   Advanced technologies such as radiographic assessment and microbiologic testing are not essential for using this tool.

---

of toothpaste that remains in his mouth helps prevent tooth decay.[6]
- Make sure the child drinks fluoridated water or takes prescribed fluoride supplements.

As children begin school and expand their horizons beyond the immediate circle of home and family, they are increasingly exposed to eating habits and foods that put them at increased risk of caries. Media, especially television, likely play a role in this increasing risk. Studies of the content of television programming show that advertisements directed at children are heavily weighted toward foods that are high in sugar, such as sweetened breakfast cereals, soft drinks, snacks, and candy.[26-28]

Parents continue to have the most influence on their children's eating behaviors and attitudes toward food. To the extent possible, parents should make sure that nutritious foods are available to their children, and they should continue to emphasize the healthful eating patterns and limitations of snacks that were established in infancy and early childhood. (For more information on this topic, see the Promoting Healthy Nutrition theme.)

Other Oral Health Issues

Finger or other sucking habits sometimes continue into middle childhood. These habits should be stopped when the permanent teeth begin to erupt. As the child begins to grow, the mouth grows, and the child should be evaluated by a dentist if malocclusion is seen.

Some children begin using tobacco during middle childhood. Therefore, the child should be encouraged not to smoke or use smokeless tobacco because it increases the risk of periodontal disease and oral cancer and poses substantial risks to overall health.

As children mature and begin to play with increased strength and vigor, both in free play

> As children begin school and expand their horizons beyond the immediate circle of home and family, they are increasingly exposed to eating habits and foods that put them at increased risk of caries.

PROMOTING ORAL HEALTH

and organized sports, the risk of injury to the mouth increases. The child and parent or caregiver should know what to do in the event of an emergency, especially if a tooth is visibly broken (chipped or fractured), displaced (luxated), or knocked completely out of the socket (avulsed). In these cases, the patient should be referred to a dentist immediately. An avulsed permanent tooth needs to be reimplanted as quickly as possible, but an avulsed primary tooth should not be reimplanted, because it likely would cause damage to developing permanent teeth.

Mouth guards worn during sports and other athletics greatly reduce the severity of accidental trauma to individual teeth by distributing the forces of impact to all of the teeth and jaws. Custom adaptations range from softening a generic plastic mouth guard in boiling water and biting into it to register a custom bite, to fabricating a guard on a custom mold. Both types work well to prevent oral trauma and differ only in cost and comfort. The protection afforded by any type of guard mandates use in both organized and leisure-time sports activity.

Promoting Oral Health: Adolescence— 11 to 21 Years

Adolescence is characterized by the loss of the remaining primary teeth and complete eruption of all the permanent teeth, including the third molars or wisdom teeth in late adolescence. Growth spurts of the facial bones occur early and then taper off as adolescence progresses. The end result is a fully established bite.

Several oral health issues from earlier developmental stages continue to be important in adolescence. For example, vigilant oral hygiene and positive dietary habits can strengthen a sound foundation for adult oral health by preventing destructive periodontal disease and dental decay. Avoiding traumatic injury to the mouth is another continuing priority. Other issues are new. For example,

adolescence brings increased susceptibility to irreversible periodontal or gum disease that may be related to hormonal and immunologic changes. A comprehensive oral hygiene regimen of brushing and flossing, combined with regular professional care, can manage this response.

Oral Hygiene, Fluoride, and Nutrition Practices That Promote Oral Health

The adolescent should be responsible for her own preventive oral health care and should have an established dental home. She should see the dentist every 6 months or according to a schedule recommended by the dentist, based on individual needs and susceptibility to disease. The dental professional also may consider diet analysis, topical fluoride applications, antimicrobial regimens, and dental sealants for high-risk patients or those with significant dental disease.

Although preventive therapy has resulted in increased numbers of adolescents with healthy teeth, caries is still common in teens and growing evidence suggests that a small percentage of adolescents account for the most severe caries.[4,17,18]

Adolescents' risk of caries may be increased by the following:

- Susceptible tooth surfaces as a result of immature enamel in newly erupted permanent teeth.
- Indifference to oral hygiene, which allows plaque to accumulate and mature.
- Frequent and unregulated exposure to high quantities of natural and refined sugars, a feature of many adolescent diets, which provides the perfect medium for caries to develop.[29,30]
- Eating disorders, such as bulimia, which can result in a characteristic erosion of the dental enamel by repeated exposure of the teeth to gastric acids.

Mouth guards worn during sports and other athletics greatly reduce the severity of accidental trauma to individual teeth by distributing the forces of impact to all of the teeth and jaws.

- Use of certain drugs, specifically methamphetamine, which has a detrimental effect on oral health. Methamphetamine abuse is associated with rampant decay that is attributed to some combination of the acidic nature of the drug, decreased saliva, tooth grinding and clenching, poor oral hygiene, and cravings for high-calorie beverages.[31]
- Frequent consumption of acidic drinks, which can directly erode the enamel.[32]

Health care professionals should educate adolescents to keep their teeth clean and remove plaque by following a comprehensive, daily home care regimen, including a minimum of twice-daily brushing with fluoride toothpaste and once-daily flossing. It is recommended that the adolescent spit out the toothpaste but not rinse with water. This regimen should be customized to each patient based on risk factors. Adolescents also should follow nutritious eating patterns that include only modest consumption of high-sugar foods (for more information on this topic, see the Promoting Healthy Nutrition theme) and should drink fluoridated water. If necessary, prescribed fluoride supplements until the age of 16 years are appropriate.[33]

Other Oral Health Issues

Adolescence is a period of experimentation and making choices. Added freedom and extension of boundaries are characteristic of appropriate supervision, but certain behaviors can lead to oral health problems. Substance use, including tobacco and drugs, can affect soft and hard tissues of the oral cavity and is linked to oral cancer.[34] Oral piercing can cause local and systemic infection, tooth fracture, and hemorrhage. Sexual behaviors can lead to infectious and traumatic consequences to the mouth. The health care professional should continue to counsel the adolescent about these nondietary behavioral factors that affect oral health.

Substance use, including tobacco and drugs, can affect soft and hard tissues of the oral cavity and is linked to oral cancer.

PROMOTING ORAL HEALTH

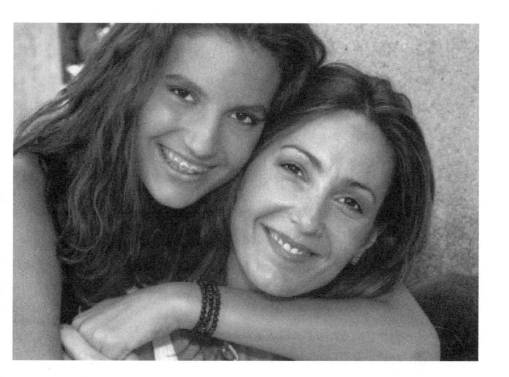

PERIODONTAL CONDITIONS

Evidence suggests that irreversible tissue damage from periodontal disease begins in late adolescence and early adulthood. Early diagnosis, prevention, and minor treatment can, in most cases, prevent irreversible damage to the periodontal structures in adulthood.[33,35] Preventing this damage obviates the need for dental restorations, which require lifelong care and monitoring.

TRAUMATIC INJURY TO THE MOUTH

Adolescents' risk of traumatic injury to the mouth may be increased by the following:

- High-risk behaviors that may involve trauma to the head and neck
- Driving crashes
- Injuries that occur as a result of participating in organized and leisure-time sports
- Unrecognized psychiatric and behavioral problems, such as bulimia or substance use
- Family or peer violence

Health care professionals should make sure that parents and adolescents know what to do and who to call if an injury occurs and a tooth is fractured or avulsed.

ORTHODONTIA

Genetically related abnormal development, premature primary tooth loss or extraction, or thumb sucking or finger sucking all can result in significant crowding and malalignment of the teeth, which can adversely affect oral health, function, and esthetics. Most orthodontic problems are not debilitating and can be resolved with appropriate treatment.[36] Preventing premature tooth loss early in life has a significant impact on minimizing space loss and the resultant crowding in adolescence.

PROMOTING ORAL HEALTH

References

1. National Institute of Dental and Craniofacial Research. *Oral Health in America: A Report of the Surgeon General*. Rockville, MD: US Department of Health and Human Services; 2000. NIH publication 00-4713

2. Pierce KM, Rozier RG, Vann WF, Jr. Accuracy of pediatric primary care providers' screening and referral for early childhood caries. *Pediatrics*. 2002;109:e82. Available at: www.pediatrics.org/cgi/content/full/109/5/e82. Accessed April 17, 2007

3. Gift HC, Reisine ST, Larach DC. The social impact of dental problems and visits. *Am J Public Health*. 1992;82:1163-1668

4. Vargas CM, Crall JJ, Schneider DA. Sociodemographic distribution of pediatric dental caries: NHANES III, 1988-1994. *J Am Dent Assoc*. 1998;129:1229-1238

5. American Academy of Pediatrics, Committee on Child Abuse and Neglect. Oral and dental aspects of child abuse and neglect. *Pediatrics*. 1999;104:348-350

6. Casamassimo PS, Holt KA, eds. *Bright Futures in Practice: Oral Health Pocket Guide*. Washington, DC: National Maternal and Child Oral Health Resource Center; 2004

7. National Maternal and Child Oral Health Resource Center Web site. http://www.mchoralhealth.org/. Accessed June 29, 2006

8. American Academy of Pediatric Dentistry. Definition of Dental Home. Chicago, IL: American Academy of Pediatric Dentistry; 2006 Available at: http://www.aapd.org/media/Policies_Guidelines/D_DentalHome.pdf. Accessed April 17, 2007

9. American Academy of Pediatric Dentistry. Policy on the Dental Home. Chicago, IL: American Academy of Pediatric Dentistry; 2004. Available at: http://www.aapd.org/media/Policies_Guidelines/P_DentalHome.pdf. Accessed April 17, 2007

10. Savage MF, Lee JY, Kotch JB, Vann WF, Jr. Early preventive dental visits: effects on subsequent utilization and costs. *Pediatrics*. 2004;114(4):e418-e423. Available at: www.pediatrics.org/cgi/content/full/114/4/e418. Accessed April 17, 2007

11. Centers for Disease Control and Prevention. Recommendations for using fluoride to prevent and control dental caries in the United States. *MMWR Recomm Rep*. 2001; 50(RR-14):1-42

12. American Academy of Pediatric Dentistry. Policy on the Use of Fluoride. Available at: http://www.aapd.org/media/Policies_Guidelines/P_FluorideUse.pdf. Accessed April 17, 2007

13. US Preventive Services Task Force Prevention of Dental Caries in Preschool Children. In: *Guide to Clinical Preventive Services, 2006: Recommendations of the US Preventive Services Task Force*. Rockville, MD: Agency for Healthcare Research and Quality; 2006. AHRQ publication 06-0588

14. American Dental Association, Council on Scientific Affairs. Professionally applied topical fluoride: evidence-based clinical recommendations. *J Am Dent Assoc*. 2006;137:1151-1159

15. Centers for Disease Control and Prevention. Surveillance for dental caries, dental sealants, tooth retention, edentulism, and enamel fluorosis—United States, 1988-1994 and 1999-2002. *MMWR Surveill Summ*. 2005;54:1-43

16. American Academy of Pediatrics, Committee on Nutrition. Nutrition and oral health. In: Kleinman RE, ed. *Pediatric Nutrition Handbook*. 5th ed. Elk Grove Village, IL: American Academy of Pediatrics; 2004:789-800

17. Kaste LM, Selwitz RH, Oldakowski RJ, Brunelle JA, Winn DM, Brown LJ. Coronal caries in the primary and permanent dentition of children and adolescents 1-17 years of age: United States, 1988-1991. *J Dent Res*. 1996;75 (spec No):631-641

18. Allukian M Jr. The neglected epidemic and the surgeon general's report: a call to action for better oral health. *Am J Public Health*. 2000;90:843-845

19. American Academy of Pediatric Dentistry. Guideline on Management of Persons with Special Health Care Needs. Chicago, IL: American Academy of Pediatric Dentistry; 2004. Available at: http://www.aapd.org/media/Policies_Guidelines/G_SHCN.pdf. Accessed April 17, 2007

20. American Academy of Pediatric Dentistry. Clinical Guideline on Infant Oral Health Care. Chicago, IL: American Academy of Pediatric Dentistry; 2004

21. Hale KS, American Academy of Pediatrics. Section on Pediatric Dentistry. Oral health risk assessment timing and establishment of the dental home. *Pediatrics*. 2003;111(5):1113-1116

22. Rozier RG. Primary care physicians enlisted to provide preventative dental services. *AAP News*. 2006;27:18

23. Rozier RG, Slade GD, Zeldin LP, Wang H. Parents' satisfaction with preventive dental care for young children provided by nondental primary care providers. *Pediatr Dent*. 2005;27:313-322

24. American Academy of Pediatric Dentistry. *Guideline on Periodicity of Examination, Preventive Dental Services, Anticipatory Guidance Counseling, and Oral Treatment for Infants, Children and Adolescents*. Chicago, IL: American Academy of Pediatric Dentistry; 2007

25. American Academy of Pediatric Dentistry. Policy on Use of a Caries-risk Assessment Tool (CAT) for Infants, Children, and Adolescents. Chicago, IL: American Academy of Pediatric Dentistry; 2006. Available at: http://www.aapd.org/media/Policies_Guidelines/P_CariesRiskAssess.pdf. Accessed April 17, 2007

26. Byrd-Bredbenner C. Saturday morning children's television advertising: a longitudinal content analysis. *Fam Consum Sci Res J*. 2002;30:382-403

27. Harrison K, Marske AL. Nutritional content of foods advertised during the television programs children watch most. *Am J Public Health*. 2005;95:1568-1574

28. Kotz K, Story M. Food advertisements during children's Saturday morning television programming: are they consistent with dietary recommendations? *J Am Diet Assoc*. 1994;94:1296-1300

29. Majewski RF. Dental caries in adolescents associated with caffeinated carbonated beverages. *Pediatr Dent*. 2001;23:198-203

30. Freeman R, Sheiham A. Understanding decision-making processes for sugar consumption in adolescence. *Community Dent Oral Epidemiol*. 1997;25:228-232

PROMOTING ORAL HEALTH

31. American Dental Association. For the dental patient ... methamphetamine use and oral health. *J Am Dent Assoc.* 2005;136:1491

32. American Academy of Pediatric Dentistry. Policy on Dietary Recommendations for Infants, Children, and Adolescents. Chicago, IL: American Academy of Pediatric Dentistry; 2006. Available at: http://www.aapd.org/media/Policies_Guidelines/P_DietaryRec.pdf. Accessed April 17, 2007

33. American Academy of Pediatric Dentistry. *Guideline on Adolescent Oral Health Care.* Chicago, IL: American Academy of Pediatric Dentistry; 2005

34. American Cancer Society. *Detailed Guide: Oral Cavity and Oropharyngeal Cancer.* Atlanta, GA: American Cancer Society; 2004

35. American Academy of Periodontology, Research, Science and Therapy Committee. Periodontal diseases of children and adolescents. *J Periodontal.* 2003;74:1696-1704

36. Proffit WR, Fields HW, Moray LJ. Prevalence of malocclusion and orthodontic treatment need in the United States: estimates from the NHANES III survey. *Int J Adult Orthodon Orthognath Surg.* 1998;13:97-106

Promoting Healthy Sexual Development and Sexuality

Theme 8

INTRODUCTION

Families have different perspectives on how sexuality should be discussed with children and adolescents (ie, who should be involved in those discussions and how much young people need to know and at what age). With respect for different individual and cultural values, health care professionals can address this important component of healthy development by integrating sexuality education into health supervision from early childhood through adolescence.[1] In the supportive environment of the medical home, health care professionals can provide personalized information, confidential screening of risk status, health promotion, and counseling for the child and adolescent. Age-appropriate, accurate resources that are related to sex education and healthy sexuality provide parents with factual information and encouragement as they educate and guide their growing child.

Health care professionals also should acknowledge and discuss the healthy sexual feelings that all children and youth have, including those with special health care needs.

Families of children with special health care needs may require additional counseling around sexual development issues to ensure a healthy understanding of their child's pubertal and sexual development.

Promoting Healthy Sexual Development and Sexuality: Infancy—Birth to 11 Months

Nurturing the development of the biological and physical foundations of healthy intimacy is an important goal that begins in infancy. These foundations require the ability to be comfortable and safe in a close physical relationship with another person. Intimacy begins in the parent's arms with good parent-child reciprocity, response to cues, management of states of arousal (eg, pain and hunger), and establishment of regular cycles of excitement and relaxation (eg, waking up and falling asleep). The infant needs to have the sense that she is valued, loved, and important for who she is.

Bright FUTURES

Establishing a sense of self early in life under-lies a child's sense of being either a girl or a boy. Parents must accept their child's gender, even if they might have hoped for a child of the other gender. Parents must communicate to their children that they are intact, beauti-ful, and well-formed. The gender of most infants is known prenatally or immediately at birth. There are endocrinologic and genetic conditions that may result in ambiguity of the external genitalia, making gender assignment difficult initially. Gender *identity*, however, is a gradual process that is based on an internal conviction of belonging to either the male or female gender. Gender identity is distinct from gender *role*, which refers to a set of behaviors through which individuals convey to the larger society that they are male or female. Children usually develop a fixed gen-der identity by $2\frac{1}{2}$ to 3 years of age, after which they emphatically perceive themselves as being either a girl or a boy.[2]

Parents often ask how to handle their infant's behavior (eg, genital touching) as the infant becomes aware of her own genitalia. This issue can be addressed as normal behav-ior with parents during the 6 and 9 Month Visits, perhaps when discussing bathing or diapering. Parents can be encouraged to practice proper naming of their infant's geni-talia (eg, penis and vagina) during diapering and bathing. It may facilitate future discus-sion between parents and their children about sexuality.

Promoting Healthy Sexual Development and Sexuality: Early Childhood—1 to 4 Years

Sexual exploration is a normal, universal, and healthy part of early childhood development. At this age, children show interest in their own, as well as others', "private" areas, and they become aware of gender differences. Their curiosity can be shown in behaviors such as playing doctor with their peers, undressing during play activities, trying to watch people when they are nude, and phys-ically touching their parents' body parts (eg, their mother's breasts). In early childhood, children also are exposed to social norms and learn boundaries regarding sexual behaviors. Personal boundaries are the presumed inter-personal distances, both physical and emo-tional, that are maintained by most people. Young children first learn personal boundaries in their families. Issues related to the timing, settings (eg, public vs private), and spectrum of sexual behaviors can best be discussed in the context of trusting relationships and open communication between the parent and the child.

The most common sexuality issues for this age group are related to bathing and showering, toileting, modesty, privacy, mas-turbation, and sexual play. Masturbation is frequently a concern for parents. A variety of behaviors can be seen, such as posturing, tightening of thighs, sexual arousal, and handling of genitals. Parent experiences, as well as cultural, religious, and family norms, influence parents' responses to their children's sexual behavior.

Sexual play between same-age peers usu-ally is lighthearted and voluntary in nature. This behavior diminishes when children are requested to stop. Sexual behavior in children can create uncertainty for the health care professional because of the potential relation-ship between child sexual abuse and sexual behavior. Consequently, it is important to understand normative sexual childhood behaviors. The less-frequent and more-concerning sexual behaviors are intrusive, such as inserting objects into the vagina or anus, or aggressive sexual behaviors. It is important that health care professionals be able to distinguish healthy and natural from concerning and distressing sexual behaviors. They should provide reassurance about nor-mal activities, provide developmentally appro-priate parameters for identifying problem behaviors, and encourage family discussions regarding sex education.

Parents must commu-nicate to their chil-dren that they are intact, beautiful, and well-formed.

PROMOTING HEALTHY SEXUAL DEVELOPMENT AND SEXUALITY

Bright FUTURES

Promoting Healthy Sexual Development and Sexuality: Middle Childhood—5 to 10 Years

Middle childhood is the time to provide accurate information to children and give them opportunities to explore, question, and assess their own and their family's attitudes toward sexuality and human relationships. At this age, the changes of puberty also can be addressed.

Health care professionals should perform a sexual maturity rating as early as ages 7 to 10 years. Health care professionals should address upcoming stages of sexual development as part of their anticipatory guidance because children and their parents can be reluctant to ask questions about normal physical development or the differences noted in their child's development compared to that of the child's peers. Normal pubertal development varies widely in the US population, and race/ethnic differences are now observed (eg, African American girls have been shown to have a higher rate of early-onset puberty than white girls).[3]

In middle childhood, children should appreciate wide variations in body shapes, sizes, and colors and acquire pride in their own body and gender. Children this age can, and should, understand that their bodies will change as they grow older. They should learn the differences between male and female genitalia, as well as the correct name and specific function of each body part. They also can learn that some body parts can feel good when touched, that it's normal to be curious about one's body, and that not all exploratory behaviors are appropriate in every place and time. Teaching about human immunodeficiency virus (HIV) infection and other sexually transmitted infections (STIs) can include discussion of their causes (eg, viruses and bacteria) and general modes of transmission.

Concepts of family, friendship, and other human relationships are core components of healthy sexuality at this stage. Children should learn to express love and intimacy in appropriate ways and to avoid manipulative or exploitative relationships. Empathy and respect for another's feelings also is an essential component of a healthy relationship, facilitated through effective communication skills. Kissing, hugging, touching, and other intimate behaviors are understood within the norms of the child and family's culture. Children need to understand their rights and responsibilities for their own bodies (eg, privacy and hygiene) and the importance of communicating fears and concerns with trusted adults. Children should know that no parent or adult has the right to tell them to keep secrets from either parent, especially when someone is touching their body inappropriately. Parents should give their child permission to tell them about any uncomfortable or threatening experiences, reassuring the child that he will be believed and will not be in trouble for telling.

Children's exposure to elements of sexuality from their peers, families of their peers, and the media (eg, news stories, advertisements, television programs, and pornography on the Internet) can influence them to make choices that may not be healthy, safe, or consistent with family values. Health care professionals can encourage parents to talk with their children about these issues and suggest tools, such as books or videos, to help open these discussions and conduct them comfortably.

Promoting Healthy Sexual Development and Sexuality: Adolescence—11 to 21 Years

Experiences with romantic relationships, exploration of sexual roles, and self-awareness of sexual orientation commonly occur during adolescence. Decisions that are associated with sexual development in the adolescent years often have important implications for health and education, as well as current and future relationships.

Health care professionals should address upcoming stages of sexual development as part of their anticipatory guidance because children and their parents can be reluctant to ask questions about normal physical development or the differences noted in their child's development compared to that of the child's peers.

Key Data and Statistics

PARENTS AND ADOLESCENT SEXUAL DECISION MAKING

A National Campaign to Prevent Teen Pregnancy survey conducted in 2004 demonstrated that:

- Adolescents aged 12 to 19 years report that parents are the greatest influence regarding sexual decision making and values (37% compared to 33% for friends, 6% for siblings, and 5% for the media).[4]
- Ninety-four percent of adolescents and 91% of parents believe that adolescents should be advised that they should not have sex before completing high school.[4]
- Nearly 87% of adolescents agree that "it would be easier for adolescents to postpone sexual activity and avoid adolescent pregnancy if they were able to have more open, honest conversation about these topics with their parents."[4]

Data from the National Longitudinal Study of Adolescent Health, sponsored by the National Institutes of Health, demonstrate that a strong parental relationship is related to an adolescent's decision to delay sexual initiation.[5] A report released by the National Campaign to Prevent Teen Pregnancy found that a strong parent-child relationship and parental supervision are associated with reduced risk of teen pregnancy. Adolescents who have a close relationship with their parents are more likely to be abstinent than those who do not, and, of those who are sexually active, are more likely to have fewer partners and to use contraception.[6] Other protective factors that are related to delayed sexual initiation include strong community support, youth who are connected to their schools and faith communities, and youth who report strong personal values or religious beliefs. Adolescents report that their own morals and values are as influential as health information in their decision to delay sex.[4]

PERCENTAGE OF YOUTH WHO REPORT HAVING HAD SEXUAL INTERCOURSE

The 2002 National Survey of Family Growth (NSFG) released by the Centers for Disease Control and Prevention in 2004, contains the following data about adolescent sexual activity[7]:

- Forty-six percent of never-married male and female adolescents aged 15 to 19 years reported that they have had sexual intercourse. This represents a significant decline in sexual involvement for male individuals from 55% reported in 1995.
- Approximately 30% of female and male adolescents aged 15 to 17 years reported having intercourse in 2002, compared to 38% for female and 43% for male adolescents in 1995.
- African American males aged 15 to 17 years reported the most remarkable decline in sexual intercourse. Their rate of sexual initiation changed from nearly 76% in 1995 to 53% in 2002.
- Older female adolescents (aged 18 to 19 years) reported stable rates of sexual intercourse at approximately 69% in 1995 and 2002, while male adolescents declined significantly from 75% (1995) to 64% (2002).

> Adolescents aged 12 to 19 years report that parents are the greatest influence regarding sexual decision making and values...

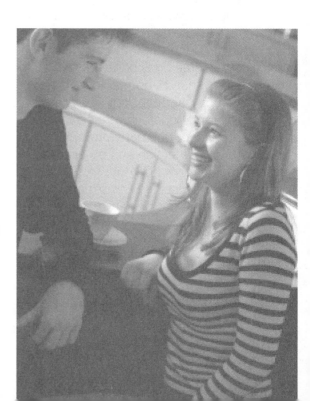

- Young adolescents (younger than 15 years) also are delaying sexual intercourse. Between 1995 and 2002, the percentage of young adolescents who reported sexual intercourse dropped from 21% to 15% among males and from 19% to 13% among females.

ONSET OF INTERCOURSE
- In 2005, according to the Youth Risk Behavior Surveillance System, the percentage of students who had sexual intercourse for the first time before the age of 13 years was 6.2% (8.8% for boys and 3.7% for girls)[8] compared to 1995, in which it was 9.0% (12.7% for boys and 4.9% for girls).[9]
- Early age of onset of sexual intercourse is associated with an increased number of partners during adolescence.[10] Young women who first had sex before age 14 years were about twice as likely to have had multiple partners than those who first had intercourse at age 16 years or later.[11]

Two thirds (66%) of the sexually experienced adolescents (aged 12 to 19 years) who participated in the 2004 National Campaign to Prevent Teen Pregnancy survey said they wished they had waited longer before having sexual intercourse.[4]

CONTRACEPTION
Data from the NSFG[7] show that education about contraceptive use may be reaching the adolescent population. Its studies report the following:

- Along with an overall decline in the percentage of sexually active adolescents, contraceptive use at first intercourse for women is much higher for those who had first intercourse between 1999 and 2002 (79%) compared to those who initiated sexual activity before 1980 (43%).
- Although the birth control pill and condoms are the most frequently used methods of contraception, use of injectable contraception and other methods is increasing.
- Between 1995 and 2002, reported condom use increased for 15- to 19-year-old sexually active, never-married males (from 64% to 71%) and females (from 38% to 54%).

PREGNANCY RATES
- The adolescent pregnancy rate in 2000 was the lowest since 1976; it declined by 27% among female adolescents aged 15 to 19 years since 1990. In 2000, the rate of pregnancy among female adolescents aged 15 to 17 years was 54 per 1,000, compared to 67 per 1,000 in 1996.[12]
- Santelli et al[13] analyzed the decline in adolescent pregnancy. Approximately 53% of the decline can be attributed to decreased sexual experience, and 47% can be attributed to greater contraceptive use.

SEXUALLY TRANSMITTED INFECTIONS
- An estimated 9 million young people (aged 15 to 24 years) develop infections that are spread primarily by sexual contact.[14] Common STIs for people in this age group are human papillomavirus (HPV), trichomoniasis, Chlamydia, herpes simplex virus, and gonorrhea.[14,15] Each type of infection has the potential for both short- and long-term consequences.
- Female adolescents are more likely than older women to become infected when exposed to STIs because their vaginal and cervical tissues are not completely mature.[16]
- An estimated 1,991 15- to 24-year-olds were newly diagnosed with acquired immunodeficiency syndrome (AIDS) in 2003, bringing the cumulative number of 15- to 24-year-olds with AIDS to 37,599 in the United States that year.[17]

The adolescent pregnancy rate in 2000 was the lowest since 1976; it declined by 27% among female adolescents aged 15 to 19 years since 1990.

Role of the Health Care Professional

Clinical care for adolescents and young adults is commonly related to concerns about sexual development, contraception, STIs, and pregnancy. Clinical encounters for acute care, health maintenance visits, or sports physicals all provide opportunities to teach adolescents and their families about healthy sexuality. Health care professionals can discuss sexual maturation, family or cultural values, communication, monitoring and guidance patterns for the family, personal goals, informed sexual decision making, and safety.

The American Academy of Pediatrics (AAP) policy statement, Sexuality Education for Children and Adolescents,[1] advises health care professionals to integrate sexuality education into the longitudinal relationship they develop through their care experiences with the preadolescent child, the adolescent, and the family. Confidential, culturally sensitive, and nonjudgmental counseling and care are important to all youth, including youth with special health care needs and nonheterosexual youth. The American College of Obstetricians and Gynecologists has a similar statement that supports the same approach.[18]

To address this issue in ways that respect values and meet the adolescent's needs, health care professionals must learn about the family's values and attitudes. Parents and health care professionals should be partners with youth in supporting healthy adolescent development and decision making. The rewards are long-term. Health care professionals, however, cannot assume that the family's values are the adolescents' values. In addition, although parents of most adolescents are concerned and available, health care professionals also must offer the best care possible to adolescents whose parents are absent or disengaged.

Counseling adolescents should include stating the advantages of delaying sexual involvement, suggesting skills for refusing sexual advances, providing information about drug and alcohol risks, and expressing encouragement for healthy decisions. Adolescents with and without sexual experience may welcome support for avoiding sex until later in their lives. Health care professionals also should support adolescents in how to have healthy relationships. In addition, health care professionals should screen for, as well as counsel against, coercive and abusive relationships for adolescents who are involved with intimate partners.[19]

Information about contraception, including emergency contraception and STIs, should be offered to all sexually active adolescents and those who plan to become sexually active. Each contraceptive method has instructions for correct use, effectiveness for preventing pregnancy, potential side effects, and long-term consequences (eg, potential bone density concerns with depot medroxyprogesterone acetate). Hormonal contraception does not protect against STIs. Emergency contraception is available to prevent pregnancy after intercourse.[20] The latex condom is the only method available to prevent the spread of HIV and can reduce the risks of some other STIs, including Chlamydia, gonorrhea, and trichomoniasis.[21] Condoms also can reduce the risk of genital herpes, syphilis, and HPV infection when the infected areas are covered or protected by the condom.

Health care professionals who care for adolescents may encounter some adolescents who are gay, lesbian, bisexual, transgendered, unsure, or uncomfortable with their sexual orientation or gender identity. Many of these youth remain unidentified and secretive because they are not comfortable enough to identify themselves and their sexual concerns. They may fear rejection or stigmatization from disclosure of their sexual orientation or gender identity issues to health care professionals. The goals for these youth are the same as for all adolescents—to promote healthy development, social and emotional well-being, and optimal physical health.[22,23]

Parents and health care professionals should be partners with youth in supporting healthy adolescent development and decision making.

Supportive, quality health care for adolescents means that adolescents must feel welcomed as individuals, regardless of social status, gender, disability, religion, sexual orientation, ethnic background, or country of origin. The health care professional must create a clinical environment in which the adolescent believes that sensitive personal issues, including sexual orientation and expression, can be discussed.[1] According to an AAP clinical report on sexual orientation and adolescents, "Sexual orientation refers to an individual's pattern of physical and emotional arousal toward other persons."[22] The health care professional must help the adolescent understand that same-sex interest and behaviors can occur at this age and that they do not define sexual orientation.[22] Clinic and practice materials, as well as personnel, can convey a nonjudgmental and safe environment for care and confidentiality for adolescents who may be experiencing same-sex attractions.[1,22,23] Nonheterosexual adolescents are sensitive to jokes, attitudes, and comments regarding their sexual orientation, and they may not feel comfortable discussing significant health history or concerns. If the health care professional cannot ensure a safe environment for these adolescents because of personal feelings or other barriers, the

adolescent should be referred to another practice or clinic with appropriate services.

As with all other patients, the adolescent should be assured that confidentiality will be protected and also should be told of the conditions under which it can be broken. In those situations of serious concern, the health care professional should help the adolescent discuss the issue with her parents or family and, if necessary, obtain additional services with mental health professionals or other health care professionals. The health care professional also should offer advice to guide these adolescents in avoiding sexual and other health risk behaviors.

Adolescents with special health care needs and their families can benefit from knowledgeable, personalized anticipatory guidance.[24] Education about normal puberty and sexuality can be augmented with information that is germane to adolescents with physical differences, especially those that directly affect sexual functioning, as well as youth with cognitive delays. The risk of sexual exploitation and the protection of youth are always critical. A focus on youth access to accurate and complete information and support for healthy decision making is key for all youth who are transitioning to adulthood.

Supportive, quality health care for adolescents means that adolescents must feel welcomed as individuals, regardless of social status, gender, disability, religion, sexual orientation, ethnic background, or country of origin.

References

1. American Academy of Pediatrics: Committee on Psychosocial Aspects of Child and Family Health and Committee on Adolescence. Sexuality education for children and adolescents. *Pediatrics*. 2001;108:498-502
2. Carver PR, Yunger JL, Perry DG. Gender identity and adjustment in middle childhood. *Sex Roles*. 2003;49:95-109
3. Herman-Giddens ME, Slora EJ, Wasserman RC, et al. Secondary sexual characteristics and menses in young girls seen in office practice: a study from the Pediatric Research in Office Settings network. *Pediatrics*. 1997;99:505-512
4. Albert B. *With One Voice 2004: America's Adults and Teens Sound Off About Teen Pregnancy*. Washington, DC: National Campaign to Prevent Teen Pregnancy; 2004. Available at: http://www.teenpregnancy.org/resources/data/pdf/WOV2004.pdf. Accessed September 5, 2007
5. Resnick MD, Bearman PS, Blum RW, et al. Protecting adolescents from harm. Findings from the National Longitudinal Study on Adolescent Health. *JAMA*. 1997;278:823-832
6. Miller BC. *Families Matter: A Research Synthesis of Family Influences on Adolescent Pregnancy*. Washington, DC: National Campaign to Prevent Teen Pregnancy; 1998
7. Abma JC, Martinez GM, Mosher WD, Dawson BS. Teenagers in the United States: sexual activity, contraceptive use and childbearing, 2002. *Vital Health Stat*. 2004;1-48
8. Eaton DK, Kann L, Kinchen S. Youth Risk Behavior Surveillance - United States, 2005. *MMWR Surveill Summ*. 2006;55: 1-108
9. Kann L, Warren CW, Harris WA, et al. Youth Risk Behavior Surveillance—United States, 1995. *MMWR Surveill Summ*. 1996;45:1-84
10. Coker AL, Richter DL, Valois RF, McKeown RE, Garrison CZ, Vincent ML. Correlates and consequences of early initiation of sexual intercourse. *J Sch Health*. 1994;64:372-377
11. Santelli LS, Brener ND, Lowry R, Bhatt A, Zabin LS. Multiple sex partners among US adolescents and young adults. *Fam Plann Perspect*. 1998;30:271-275
12. U.S. Department of Health and Human Services. Family Planning. In: *Healthy People 2010: Understanding and Improving Health*. Vol 1. 2nd ed. Washington, DC: U.S. Government Printing Office; 2000:9-3–9-34
13. Santelli JS, Abma J, Ventura S, et al. Can changes in sexual behaviors among high school students explain the decline in teen pregnancy rates in the 1990s? *J Adolesc Health*. 2004;35:80-90
14. I Am Sexually Active. Life Care Pregnancy Center Web site. Available at: http://www.pregnancylifecare.org/sexuallyactive.html. Accessed March 1, 2006
15. Centers for Disease Control and Prevention. CDC Fact Sheet. *Trichomoniasis* Web site. Available at: http://www.cdc.gov/std/trichomonas/trich.pdf. Accessed September 5, 2007
16. Shrier LA. Bacterial sexually transmitted infections: gonorrhea, chlamydia, pelvic inflammatory disease, and syphilis. In: Emans SJ, Laufer MR, Goldstein DP, eds. *Pediatric & Adolescent Gynecology*, 5th ed. Philadelphia, PA: Lippincott Williams & Wilkins; 2005:565-614
17. Centers for Disease Control and Prevention. *HIV/AIDS Surveillance Report, 2003*. Vol 15. Atlanta: Center for Disease Control and Prevention; 2003. Available at: http//www.cdc.gov/HIV/topics/surveillance/resources/reports/2003report/pdf/2003SurveillanceReport.pdf. Accessed August 18, 2007
18. American College of Obstetricians and Gynecologists. Appendix A. In: *Health Care for Adolescents*. Washington, DC: American College of Obstetricians and Gynecologists; 2003:107-108
19. National Council on Crime and Delinquency and the National Center for Victims of Crime. *Our Vulnerable Teenagers: Their Victimization, Its Consequences, and Directions for Prevention and Intervention*: Oakland, CA, and Washington, DC: National Council on Crime and Delinquency and the National Center for Victims of Crime; 2002
20. Klein JD, American Academy of Pediatrics, Committee on Adolescence. Adolescent pregnancy: current trends and issues. *Pediatrics*. 2005;116:281-286
21. Centers for Disease Control and Prevention Web site. CDC Fact Sheet. *Male Latex Condoms and Sexually Transmitted Diseases*. Atlanta, GA: Centers for Disease Control and Prevention; 2003. Available at: http://www.cdc.gov/condomeffectiveness/condoms.pdf. Accessed August 16, 2007
22. Frankowski BL, American Academy of Pediatrics, Committee on Adolescence. Sexual orientation and adolescents. *Pediatrics*. 2004;113:1827-1832
23. American College of Obstetricians and Gynecologists. Primary Care of Lesbians and Bisexual Women in Obstetric and Gynecologic Practice. In: *Special Issues in Women's Health*. Washington, DC: American College of Obstetricians and Gynecologists; 2005:61-73
24. American College of Obstetricians and Gynecologists. Access to Reproductive Health Care for Women With Disabilities. In: *Special Issues in Women's Health*. Washington, DC: American College of Obstetricians and Gynecologists; 2005:39-59

Promoting Safety and Injury Prevention

INTRODUCTION

Ensuring that a child remains safe from harm or injury during the long journey from infancy through adolescence is a constant task that requires the participation of parents and the many other adults who care for and help to raise children, and, of course, of the children themselves. Health care professionals have long recognized the importance of safety and injury prevention counseling as a tool to help educate and motivate parents in keeping their children safe. Many professional societies have bolstered these efforts by recommending guidance to prevent injuries.[1-5]

Safety and injury prevention is a topic area that covers a wide array of issues for infants, children, and adolescents. These issues can be grouped into 2 general categories:

- **Unintentional injury** continues to be the leading cause of death and morbidity among children older than 1 year, adolescents, and young adults. Although motor vehicle crashes cause the highest number of injuries, childhood injuries result from a myriad of causes, including falls, burns, firearms, recreational activities, and sports. Unintentional injuries take an enormous financial, emotional, and social toll on children and adolescents, their families, and society as a whole. Although the word *accident* is familiar, the word *injury* is preferred because it connotes the medical consequences of events that are both predictable and preventable.[6] The causes of unintentional injury-related illness and death vary according to a child's age, gender, race, geographic region, and socioeconomic status and are dependent upon developmental abilities, exposure to potential hazards, and parental perceptions of a child's abilities and the injury risk. Younger children, males, minorities, adolescents, and children who live in poverty are affected at disproportionately higher rates.[7]

- **Intentional injury,** which results from behaviors that are designed to hurt oneself or others, is a multifaceted social problem and a major health hazard for children and youth. Homicide and suicide are particularly important for the health care professional to consider because their frequency increases as children grow older. Among 1- to

21-year-olds, homicide is the second-leading cause of death, and suicide is the third-leading cause of death.[7] Intentional injuries cover a wide array of mechanisms, and the impact on children is great, no matter whether the violence is directly experienced, as in a youth attempting suicide, or is witnessed, as at home, in the community, or in the media. The association of early childhood exposure to violence and subsequent violent behaviors has been established.[8] The prevention of violence in all its forms, therefore, follows a developmental trajectory, beginning with infancy. To provide appropriate guidance and counseling, health care professionals need to be alert to the possible presence of violence in a family or to the effect of a violent environment on a child.

Safety and injury prevention are discussed in greater detail in the remainder of this themed section. Guidance on interventions and strategies to ensure safety and prevent injuries targets 3 domains: (1) the development and age of the child, (2) the environment in which the safety concern or injury takes place, and (3) the circumstances surrounding the event. The health supervision visit provides a venue to assess the parents' and the child's current safety strategies, encourage and praise their positive behaviors, provide guidance about potential risks, and recommend participation in community interventions to promote safety.

The health supervision visit also is a good venue in which to review emergency and disaster preparedness measures.[9] Information on handling emergencies, how to access local emergency care systems, and cardiopulmonary resuscitation (CPR) and first aid can be made available to all parents.

> The health supervision visit provides a venue to assess the parents' and the child's current safety strategies, encourage and praise their positive behaviors, provide guidance about potential risks, and recommend participation in community interventions to promote safety.

Health care professionals can suggest that parents do the following:

- Complete an American Heart Association or American Red Cross First Aid and CPR program.
- Have a first aid kit and know the local emergency telephone numbers. The national number for the National Poison Control Center is 800-222-1222.
- Know when to call a health care professional. (Counsel parents to call whenever they are not sure what to do.)
- Know when to go to the emergency department. (Counsel parents on when to call 911.)

Child Development and Safety

Ensuring safety and preventing injuries must be an ongoing priority for parents as their children progress from infancy through adolescence. However, the nature of their efforts evolves over time. Safety issues in infancy relate primarily to the infant's environment and interactions with parents. Parents must modify the environment to prevent suffocation, motor vehicle-related injuries, falls, burns, and other hazards. A young child's emerging independence and rapidly increasing mobility presents new safety and injury prevention challenges and necessitates further environmental modifications, or "childproofing." Parents of young children often underestimate the level of the child's motor skill development (eg, age of ability to climb) and overestimate their cognitive and sensory skills (eg, assessing the speed of an oncoming car). Integrating injury prevention counseling with developmental and behavioral discussions when talking with the family can be an effective method of delivering this important information.

The middle childhood years are a period during which safety challenges at home begin to be augmented by those outside the home (eg, at school, in sports, and with friends). During middle childhood, increasing independence allows the child to broaden his world beyond that of the immediate family. This requires good decision-making skills to stay safe and reduce the risk of injury. During adolescence, decision making about safety shifts to choices the adolescent makes about his activities, behavior, and environment.

Parents have an important role to play in keeping their children and adolescents safe through maintaining open lines of communication, balancing strong support with clear limits, and close monitoring. Strong support and close monitoring by parents have been linked with positive outcomes in children regardless of race, ethnicity, family structure, education, income, or gender.[10] Health care professionals can help parents foster openness, encourage communication with their child, and address concerns when they arise. When a risky behavior is identified, counseling can be directed toward helping the parent and child with strategies to reduce or avoid the risk, such as using appropriate protective gear (eg, seat belts, helmets, hearing protection, and sports equipment), not riding in a car or boat with someone who has been drinking, and ensuring that guns are inaccessible to children. Parents should be alert to unusual changes in behavior, such as sleep disturbances, withdrawal, aggression, sudden isolation from peer groups, or the need for unusual or extreme privacy, which can indicate that a child or adolescent is involved in high-risk situations. Risk reduction counseling is most likely to be effective when it is used in a repetitive, multi-setting approach, rather than being isolated in the medical office.[11] Partnering with the parent and sharing strategies for how to promote positive youth development, address strengths, and reduce risk-taking behaviors is an important collaborative approach as parents gradually decrease their supervisory responsibilities

and help their child transition to young adulthood.

Families and Culture in Safety and Injury Prevention

Parents often feel challenged as they try to set priorities among the many health and safety messages that are given to them by the medical community. For some families, these messages may conflict with their cultural or personal beliefs and may result in parents disregarding the health and safety recommendations. Examples include bed sharing or the use of a car safety seat. In addition, certain culturally derived medical or alternative health practices may place children at risk of injury. Cultural or gender roles, in which women are not able to tell men in the household what to do, may limit their ability to enact a safety measure. In some communities, cultural beliefs dictate that the mother or parents are not the primary decision makers or caregivers for their young children. Acknowledging the influential roles that older women (eg, grandmothers or mothers-in-law) and other elders and spiritual leaders play in guiding child care practices is key to the effective delivery of safety, injury prevention, and health promotion messages. Health care professionals should be sensitive to these cultural perspectives and alert to any potential health and safety issues that may influence the child and family. Helping parents devise alternative safety approaches may be a useful discussion topic during anticipatory guidance.

The health care professional has the dual role of helping families set priorities among the health and safety messages in the context of the child's health, developmental age, and family circumstances, as well as assisting families in implementing these recommendations within their own cultural framework. The health care professional also should recognize when health and safety information is ineffective because of cultural differences in beliefs about the care of the child. A

Risk reduction counseling is most likely to be effective when it is used in a repetitive, multi-setting approach, rather than being isolated in the medical office.

familiarity with local community public health services and state and local resources is critical to tailoring information and care recommendations to best suit the needs of the child and family. Rather than giving a parent or child an absolute requirement, the health care professional might consider where an appropriate adaptation or modification can be made to accommodate cultural and family circumstances.

Economic circumstances often affect parents' ability to alter their home to create a safer environment for their child. Children who live in poverty often live in substandard, crowded homes, in unsafe neighborhoods, and may be exposed to environmental pollution. Their parents often experience poor health, economic stresses, and discrimination. These families are least able to make the changes they want and need in their homes and communities. (For more information on this topic, see the Promoting Family Support theme.) Health care professionals should be aware of housing codes that govern safety issues (eg, hot water, window guards, and lead paint). Access to legal services for families who live in poverty has brought improvements to child health and safety. In addition, low-income families, who are least likely to be able to afford injury prevention devices, may require assistance to overcome cost barriers. Community-based injury prevention interventions are effective and are models of community partnership. (For more

information on this topic, see the Promoting Community Relationships and Resources theme.) These programs can address cultural beliefs, income barriers, and community norms to assist families to implement safety interventions, especially those that have been shown to reduce injuries (eg, car safety seats, bike helmets, smoke detectors, and window guards). Community-based interventions are more likely to be successful at reducing injuries if they are integrated into, and tailored to, the community and involve community stakeholders.[12] Trials of community programs that involve home visits to distribute free smoke alarms have reported large increases in smoke detector ownership and decreases in fire-related injuries.[13]

Children and Youth With Special Health Care Needs

Children with special health care needs may present with unique needs for safety and injury prevention. Parental supervision must be focused on the developmental level and physical capabilities of the child. Parents of children with special health care needs may have to seek alternative safety equipment, such as special car safety seats, to ensure a safe environment. Inquiring about the need for this equipment and providing information or resources may improve the quality of life for families, as in the case, for example, of a family that may not be able to travel together without such equipment.[14] Increasing parents' awareness of the potential added complexity of creating a safe environment for their child with special health care needs and guiding parents toward local and national resources are ways that the health care professional can help parents provide a safe environment.

Many children with special health care needs encounter new safety challenges as they enter school and begin to deal with the community at large. They often are vulnerable and at risk of being bullied or victimized. They also may have an increased risk

Many children with special health care needs encounter new safety challenges as they enter school and begin to deal with the community at large. They often are vulnerable and at risk of being bullied or victimized.

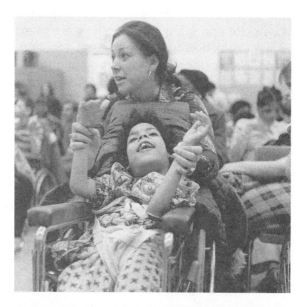

of maltreatment, including child neglect and physical or sexual abuse. Because they may rely heavily on caregivers for their physical needs and hygiene, their mental or physical limitation may impair their ability to defend themselves. Health care professionals can highlight differences between caregiving and sexual abuse, discuss the potential of bullying, and encourage parents to establish monitoring systems at home, in the community, and at school to protect their child. Planning for children with special health care needs requires understanding and anticipating the child's limitations and needs, with designated roles for family members and referral to additional community resources to ensure safety.

Safety and Injury Prevention Counseling in the Bright Futures Visit

Anticipatory guidance for safety is an integral part of the medical care of all children. Counseling needs to be directed to the parent as the role model for the child's behavior and as the person who is most capable of modifying the child's environment.[1] Counseling about some of the more effective safety and injury prevention interventions, such as using car safety seats and seat belts, spans infancy through adolescence, while other issues, such as bicycle safety, are developmentally and age specific.

Evidence from several systematic reviews confirms that injury prevention guidance is effective and beneficial. Bass et al[15] found that parents view pediatricians as respected advisors, especially on health-related issues. In 18 of the 20 studies reviewed, positive effects from injury prevention counseling included improved knowledge, improved safety behaviors, and a decrease in the number of injuries involving motor vehicles and non-motor vehicles.[15]

DiGuiseppi and Roberts[16] systematically reviewed 22 randomized controlled trials to examine the impact on child safety practices and unintentional injuries of interventions delivered in the clinical setting. The results indicate that some, but not all, safety practices are increased after counseling or other interventions in this setting. Specifically, guidance about motor vehicle car safety seat restraints for young children, smoke detectors, and maintenance of a safe hot water temperature was more likely to be followed after interventions in the clinical setting than guidance on other issues. Clinical interventions were most effective when they combined an array of health education materials and behavior change strategies, such as counseling, demonstrations, the provision of subsidized safety devices, and reinforcement.

Four safety topics that deal with ways to reduce or prevent violence have particularly strong research evidence and lend themselves to pediatric anticipatory counseling: (1) using constructive disciplining techniques and alternatives to corporal punishment[17-25] (see the Promoting Family Support theme), (2) promoting factors associated with psychological resilience among adolescents[26-29] (see the Promoting Mental Health theme), (3) preventing bullying[30-32] (see the Promoting Mental Health theme), and (4) preventing gun injury[25,33-43] (see the Safety Priority in selected Visits).

Since its peak in the mid-1990s, the epidemic of fatal youth violence has steadily declined. Many segments of society, in addition to the health care system, have contributed to this reduction.[44] Programs with proven effectiveness are described by the University of Colorado Center for the Study and Prevention of Violence (www.colorado.edu/cspv/blueprints/index.html). Information about a wide variety of violence prevention programs, ranging from public service announcements to school curricula, is available through the National Youth Violence Prevention Resource Center (www.safeyouth.org).

Recent surveys and focus groups have demonstrated that parents want to discuss community violence with their child's health

Clinical interventions were most effective when they combined an array of health education materials and behavior change strategies, such as counseling, demonstrations, the provision of subsidized safety devices, and reinforcement.

care professional.[23,45] Pediatricians also have expressed enduring interest in violence prevention counseling, although many feel inadequately trained to do so.[46] Few published studies directly address the effectiveness of health care professional counseling in violence prevention. However, the strong supporting research evidence provides a rationale for incorporating violence prevention into routine clinical practice.[47]

The effectiveness of counseling can be improved if a health care professional knows the risks specific to the local population. For example, if the major cause of morbidity in the local population is handgun-related violence, counseling about guns is appropriate. In a farming community, counseling about the risk of agricultural injury can be more pertinent. Local injury data can be obtained from state or local departments of health, and statewide fatality data are available online (www.cdc.gov/ncipc/wisqars). The astute Bright Futures health care professional will adapt these Guidelines to the child, family, and community based on a sound knowledge of the local causes, risks of injury in the child's environment, and the assessed and expressed needs of the child and family.

TIPP®—The Injury Prevention Program,[5] developed by the American Academy of Pediatrics (AAP), is a developmentally based, multifaceted counseling program that allows the health care professional to use safety surveys at strategic visits and counsel parents on unintentional injury prevention topics delineated as areas of specific risk. Parents can complete these surveys, which are distributed by office staff, in a few minutes. Based on information from the surveys, health care professionals can use different parts of TIPP to individualize and supplement their anticipatory guidance with counseling and handouts that are appropriate for the child's age and community. In an effort to better tailor anticipatory guidance, primary care practices have used kiosk systems to help delineate

specific injury risks that families might have in the home.[48] The health care professional may choose to concentrate counseling on topics with the potential for catastrophic consequences.

Connected Kids: Safe, Strong, Secure, also developed by the AAP, takes an asset-based approach to violence prevention anticipatory guidance.[49] Recommended counseling topics for each health supervision visit discuss the child's development, the parent's feelings and reactions to the child's development and behavior, and specific practical suggestions on how to encourage healthy social, emotional, and physical growth in an environment of support and open communication. Counseling can be supplemented by the use of Connected Kids brochures for parents and youth. (For more information on this topic, see the *Bright Futures Toolkit*.)

Each Bright Futures visit has established safety priorities for discussion, and sample questions are provided in the anticipatory guidance sections. The priorities and sample questions in each visit that are relevant to safety are specifically linked to the counseling guidelines in TIPP (for Infancy, Early Childhood, and Middle Childhood visits) and Connected Kids (for all visits), making it easy for the practitioner to incorporate these tools in a Bright Futures practice. In addition, the *Bright Futures Toolkit* includes many other resources that may assist the health care professional.

The Health Care Professional as a Community Advocate for Safety

The clinical setting may not be suitable for carrying out the entire range of information, modeling, resources, and reinforcement that are required to change safety practices. For some families, the effectiveness of clinical interventions can be boosted if they are delivered in concert with community efforts that involve representatives from the community to overcome language and cultural differences.

> The astute Bright Futures health care professional will adapt these Guidelines to the child, family, and community based on a sound knowledge of the local causes, risks of injury in the child's environment, and the assessed and expressed needs of the child and family.

For example, community-based educational interventions that have included clinical counseling as one component of a broader effort have shown positive effects on childhood bicycle helmet ownership and use.[50] Nationwide, bicycle helmet education campaigns and legislation, as well as improvements in helmet design, have contributed to a reduction of fatalities.[7]

Health care professionals can consider participating in fun, community-based safety activities and can support community partners to increase public awareness about safety issues and provide prevention education. In most communities, it is possible to partner with agencies such as the local fire departments, Safe Kids USA (http://www.safekids.org/members/unitedStates.html), and public health programs that work directly with families of young children. In addition, health care professionals often provide leadership for effective safety and injury prevention programs and legislation through advocacy activities and testimony at public hearings. (For more information on this topic, see the Promoting Community Relationships and Resources theme.)

Promoting Safety and Injury Prevention: The Prenatal Period

Safety and injury prevention begins in the prenatal period. Preparing for the arrival of an infant should include the purchase of an approved car safety seat and a crib that meets approved safety standards. Prospective parents also may want to consider other safety measures, such as taking an infant CPR and first aid class, getting a first aid kit, checking or installing smoke detectors, and placing the National Poison Control Center telephone number on all their telephones.

Promoting Safety and Injury Prevention: Infancy—Birth to 11 Months

Promoting safety and preventing injuries is a continuing task for parents during the first year of their child's life. Injury prevention for the infant requires careful integration of awareness of developmental skills as they are rapidly acquired and the necessary supervision and interventions to ensure the infant's safety. Parents commonly underestimate their infant's motor skills while overestimating their infant's cognitive skills and judgment. Counseling in the primary care setting is important to help parents understand the correct timing of the development of these skills so that they can focus their safety interventions most appropriately.

Although suffocation and motor vehicle crashes are the most common causes of unintentional injury and death during this age, the infant also is at risk of other injuries, including falls, fires and burns, poisoning, choking, and drowning. Each of these tragedies is preventable, and appropriate counseling can provide parents with the knowledge and strategies for reducing the likelihood that these injuries will occur. Vulnerable infants who are exposed to maternal substance use, secondhand smoke, malnutrition, lack of caregiver supervision, or caregiver neglect also are at increased risk of morbidity or death. The importance of

Injury prevention for the infant requires careful integration of awareness of developmental skills as they are rapidly acquired and the necessary supervision and interventions to ensure the infant's safety.

establishing good habits begins in infancy, and parents can be counseled about the positive value of their own behavior as a role model for their child.

Sudden Infant Death Syndrome

Sudden Infant Death Syndrome (SIDS) is the leading cause of death in infancy beyond the neonatal period. Current guidelines[51] cite evidence that the risk of SIDS is reduced when infants sleep on their backs and in their parents' room, but not in their parents' bed. (For more information on this topic, see the Promoting Child Development theme.) Pacifiers have been linked with a lower risk of SIDS. It is recommended that infants be put to sleep with a pacifier, beginning at 1 month of age. It should not be forced if the infant refuses or be reinserted once the infant is asleep.

Promoting Safety and Injury Prevention: Early Childhood—1 to 4 Years

Young children are especially vulnerable to preventable injuries because their physical abilities exceed their capacities to understand the consequences of their actions. They are extraordinary mimics, but their understanding of cause and effect is not as developed as their motor skills. Gradually, between the ages of 1 and 4 years, children develop a sense of themselves as a person who can make things happen. However, at this age, young children are likely to see only their part in the action. A 2-year-old child whose ball rolls into the road will think only about retrieving the ball, not about the danger of being hit by a motor vehicle. Caretakers of young children must provide constant supervision. They should establish and consistently enforce safety rules, recognizing that this is done more to establish a foundation for following rules because young children do not have the cognitive capacity to understand the rule, take action, and avoid the hazard.

> **Young children are especially vulnerable to preventable injuries because their physical abilities exceed their capacities to understand the consequences of their actions.**

Parents and other caregivers should be aware of potential hazards in their home, and they should create a safe environment that will allow the young child to have the freedom she needs to explore.

Parents can teach their child about personal safety at an early age. Parents should train their child how to approach authority figures (eg, teachers, police, and salesclerks) and ask them for assistance in the event she becomes lost or temporarily separated from her parents.

A 1- to 4-year-old child also does not fully understand that her actions can have harmful consequences for herself or for others, and parental guidance is, therefore, necessary to shape aggressive behaviors. Longitudinal observations have suggested that childhood aggression peaks around age 17 months and that, with adult guidance, most children learn to regulate these tendencies before school age.[52]

Promoting Safety and Injury Prevention: Middle Childhood—5 to 10 Years

Middle childhood is a time of intellectual and physical growth and development, when children become more independent. The controls and monitoring that parents provided during the early childhood years change as children get older. As children go to school, participate in activities away from home, engage in more complex and potentially dangerous physical and social activities, and encounter children and adults who are not members of their immediate families, they need to develop good judgment and other skills to function safely in their expanding environment. Safety promotion and injury prevention are central aspects of the child's education.

Preventing or lessening the effects of violence also is an ongoing concern for many children during the middle childhood years, especially those living in families or communities where violence is prevalent. Television violence also may have serious effects during this period, as children spend increasing amounts of time away from home or out of the continued supervision of a parent and have increased opportunities to watch TV.[53]

School and Community Safety

During this time, children transition from complete dependence on their parents to developing their own strategies and decision-making skills for ensuring their own safety. Nowhere is it more apparent than when children are out of the home and functioning independently in their community. The process of going to school, on errands, to a friend's house, or to a music lesson, scout meeting, or team practice can present challenges to the young child who is negotiating his environment. Walking or taking the bus, going with groups of other children, and meeting new adults all have the potential for increasing social skills and respect for others, as well as the potential to place the child in danger. This developmental stage is the time when children acquire essential interpersonal skills, including conflict resolution. School-based conflict resolution and skill-building programs have been shown to be effective.[54-56]

The health care professional should encourage parents to know the child's activities, daily whereabouts, and friends. Good communication between parent and child is essential to the child's safety. Lessons that were introduced in early childhood, such as pedestrian safety (eg, retrieving a ball from the street), dealing with authority figures, and appropriate touching by others, should continue as needed. This information does not need to be communicated specifically as a safeguard against abduction or abuse, but can be taught as developmental achievements to be praised for their own value in the growing child.[57] The message to parents is that they should safeguard their children but not generate unnecessary fear or overly restrict freedom and independence.

Ensuring a safe environment and appropriate supervision is essential for children who are home alone for any period of time. Parents should make sure the child has information about his home, including address, telephone number, and keys to the home, and a "backup" contact person if the parents are not available. Parents should insist that the child "check in" with his family. Health care professionals also can partner with child care centers, schools, after-school programs, and municipalities to enhance public awareness and modify physical environments. Speed bumps, crosswalks, the passage and enforcement of school zone speed limits, and school bus safety laws can create a safer environment for child pedestrians.

Peer pressure also emerges during this period. Children need to be encouraged to develop a sense of their own identity and locus of control and taught strategies for dealing with inappropriate peer pressure or behavior. Health care professionals should address these issues with parents and encourage them to discuss these issues with their child. By discussing these issues openly, the health care professional is modeling safe behavior and is encouraging the parent and child to communicate.

Bullying

Bullying is a social phenomenon of childhood in which a larger or more powerful child repeatedly attacks (physically or emotionally) a smaller or weaker child.[30,31] (For more information on this topic, see the Promoting Mental Health theme.) Children can be effectively identified as bullies, victims, or bystanders. Effective bullying prevention programs have been demonstrated for use in the schools, and all rely on direct measures by school administration and the mobilization of bystanders to protect the victims and identify bullying behavior as socially intolerable. Physician counseling of individual patients

The health care professional should encourage parents to know the child's activities, daily whereabouts, and friends. Good communication between parent and child is essential to the child's safety.

begins with the recognition of bullying as a cause of psychosomatic complaints and may include both individual counseling and referral of parents to effective anti-bullying resources.[32] Bullies, themselves, are at high risk of long-term adverse consequences and often need behavioral counseling.

Play, Sports, and Physical Activity

Physical activities play an important role in the child's life during this age. Participation in team and individual sports consumes considerable amounts of time in the child's life. Although the overall health effect is usually very positive, children need to learn and follow safety rules for their protection and the protection of others. (For more information on this topic, see the Promoting Physical Activity theme.) Parents also should be encouraged to model safe behaviors, such as wearing seat belts and bicycle helmets. Children should follow traffic rules and safety guides concerning bicycle riding, skating, skiing, and other similar activities. The use of protective gear, such as helmets, eye protection, mouth and wrist guards, and life jackets or personal protective devices, is not negotiable and should be used at all times by everyone.

> Health care professionals can recognize and encourage the protective factors in youth as a strategy to promote safety and reduce injuries.

Promoting Safety and Injury Prevention: Adolescence—11 to 21 Years

In caring for the adolescent patient, the approach to injury prevention shifts from parental control to the adolescent herself. Health care professionals should direct anticipatory guidance directly to the adolescent and encourage behaviors that promote safety. Injury and violence are major causes of morbidity and mortality among adolescents. Although the leading causes of death of 11- to 21-year-olds vary by race and age, the top 3 causes are consistently vehicular injury, homicide, and suicide.[7] Although serious injuries and death are more common among

boys, violence among girls also may be increasing. Dropping out of school, using drugs, and getting in physical fights place adolescents at higher risk of severe injury or death.[58] Protective factors, such as connectedness with school and adults, are associated with reduced violence in youth.[26] Health care professionals can recognize and encourage the protective factors in youth as a strategy to promote safety and reduce injuries.

Driving

Learning to drive is a rite of passage for many adolescents and is a reflection of their growing independence and maturity. Adapted equipment and special driving techniques make it possible for many youth with special health care needs to drive. Health care professionals should encourage parents to be initially involved with their adolescent's driver's education by doing practice driving sessions together and by establishing rules that foster safe, responsible driving behaviors. Parents should continue to monitor their child's driving skills and habits to ensure that safe behaviors persist. Current research suggests

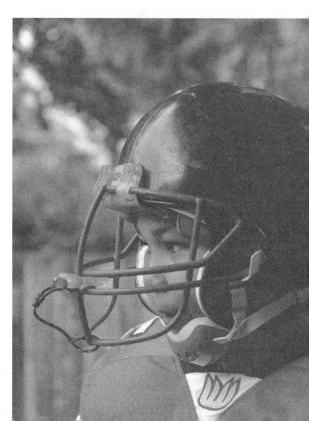

that severe motor vehicle crashes with inexperienced drivers are associated with (1) other teens in the car, (2) driving at night, and (3) distractions, such as using a cell phone, adjusting hand-held devices, such as a CD player, a personal digital assistant (PDA), or an iPod®.[59-62] Comprehensive graduated driver license programs enacted in many states have been shown to reduce fatal crashes.[63] Parents should familiarize themselves with the provisions of the Graduated Driver License law in their state, and require their adolescent to adhere to the law whether as a driver or as a passenger of a newly licensed teen driver.

Sports

Preparticipation sports physical examinations, which are directed at isolating the few adolescents for whom a sport would be dangerous, provide a unique opportunity for health care professionals to counsel adolescents and their parents on preventing sports injury and violence (eg, hazing, brawling, and foul play) and promoting general health. Generally, sports participation should be encouraged because of the physical, emotional, and social benefits.

Some medical conditions warrant a limitation in sports or require further evaluation before participating. AAP Policy Statements from the Committee on Sports Medicine and Fitness provide a more detailed review of medical issues that limit participation.[64,65] Some youth with special health care needs may have condition-specific restrictions on their activity and may require alternative or adapted activities that are safe and appropriate. If a heart murmur is innocent (eg, it does not indicate heart disease), full participation is permitted,[65] but other cardiac disorders require further evaluation. The presence of significant hypertension without heart disease or organ damage should not limit participation, but the adolescent's blood pressure should be measured at the heath care

professional's office every 2 months. Adolescents with severe hypertension should be restricted from isometric activities (eg, weight lifting) and competitive sports until their hypertension is under control and they have no end-organ damage.[64] Any temporary suspension from sports participation because of a medical condition (eg, concussion or surgery) should be reinforced by the health care professional, and children and parents should be made aware of the importance in adhering to all recommendations as to when to resume sport activities.

Health care professionals should advise adolescents to use appropriate protective gear (eg, helmets, eye protection, knee and elbow pads, life jackets or personal protective devices, mouth and wrist guards, and athletic supporter with cup) during recreational and organized sports activities and focus on overall strengthening and conditioning as well as training for their specific sport as key ways to prevent injury and maintain fitness. Performance-enhancing substances, including anabolic steroids, are an important topic for discussion, and adolescents should be urged not to use them. Health care professionals also can encourage parents to be cautious about allowing their children to participate in highly competitive sports until they are physically and emotionally mature enough, and to ensure that such programs are properly certified and staffed by qualified trainers and coaches.

Violence

Violence and exposure to violence increases the risk for homicide, aggressive behavior, and psychological sequelae, including post-traumatic stress disorders.[66-69] It has been estimated that, each year, between 3.3 and 10 million children have been exposed to intimate partner violence (IPV).[70] Childhood exposure to IPV seems to increase the likelihood of risky behaviors later in adolescence

Health care professionals should advise adolescents to use appropriate protective gear… during recreational and organized sports activities and focus on overall strengthening and conditioning as well as training for their specific sport as key ways to prevent injury and maintain fitness.

PROMOTING SAFETY AND INJURY PREVENTION

and adulthood.[71] Additionally, children who witness IPV are at increased risk for adverse behavioral and mental health issues.

Sexual and dating assaults are a leading cause of violence-related injury in adolescence.[7] Approximately 1 in 5 female high-school students report being physically and/or sexually abused by a dating partner.[72] Adolescents who report a history of experiencing dating violence are more likely to exhibit other serious risk behaviors.[72] Screening for violence exposure can identify those who need further intervention.[73] Foshee et al[74] found that *Safe Dates*, a school-based adolescent dating violence prevention program, showed promise for preventing violence among adolescents. Much of the short-term behavioral effects had disappeared at a 1-year follow-up, but effects on dating violence norms, conflict management skills, and awareness of community services for addressing dating violence were maintained.[75]

Certain youth subcultures may experience comparatively greater violence, including injury, abuse, and rape. Teens who use drugs, report having been in more than 4 fights in the past year, are failing in school, or have dropped out of school are at substantially increased risk for serious violence-related

injury.[58] Studies have found victimization, substance use, and sexual risk behaviors among gay youth to be significantly higher than among their heterosexual peers.[76] Homicide is consistently the leading cause of death for African American youth, but vehicular death is more prevalent in other ethnic groups.[7]

Gangs

The 2002 National Youth Gang Survey estimates that gangs are active in more than 2,300 cities with populations greater than 2,500.[77] The prevalence of youth gang membership varies according to the city, but is higher in larger cities and those with a history of gang activity. Risk factors for gang involvement include prior and early involvement in delinquency, especially violence and drug use; poor parent-child relations; low academic performance and attachment to school; association with peers who are delinquent; and disorganized neighborhoods with a large number of youth who are in trouble.[78,79] Health care professionals who are alert to these risk factors should screen for gang exposure. The National Youth Gang Center has resources for gang prevention, intervention, and suppression.[47,80]

Studies have found victimization, substance use, and sexual risk behaviors among gay youth to be significantly higher than among their heterosexual peers.

References

1. Gardner HG, American Academy of Pediatrics, Committee on Injury, Violence, and Poison Prevention. Office-based counseling for unintentional injury prevention. *Pediatrics*. 2007;119:202-206

2. American Academy of Pediatrics, Committee on Native American Child Health and Committee on Injury and Poison Prevention. The prevention of unintentional injury among American Indian and Alaska native children: a subject review. *Pediatrics*. 1999;104:1397-1399

3. American College of Obstetricians and Gynecologists. *Automobile Passenger Restraints for Children and Pregnant Women*. Washington, DC: American College of Obstetricians and Gynecologists; 1991. Technical bulletin no. 151

4. Elster AB, Kuznets NJ. AMA *Guidelines for Adolescent Preventive Services (GAPS)*. Baltimore, MD: Williams & Wilkins; 1994

5. American Academy of Pediatrics. *TIPP and Connected Kids on CD-ROM*. Elk Grove Village, IL: American Academy of Pediatrics; 2006

6. Widome M. *Injury Prevention and Control for Children and Youth*. 3rd ed. Elk Grove Village, IL: American Academy of Pediatrics; 1997

7. Web-based Injury Statistics Query and Reporting System (WISQARS). Fatal Injury Reports. Atlanta, GA: Centers for Disease Control and Prevention. Available at: www.cdc.gov/ncipc/wisqars/. Accessed: September 1, 2007

8. Patterson GR, DeBaryshe BD, Ramsey E. A developmental perspective on antisocial behavior. *Am Psychol*. 1989;44:329-335

9. American Academy of Pediatrics. Four steps to prepare your family for disasters. Elk Grove Village, IL: American Academy of Pediatrics; 2006. Available at: www.aap.org/terrorism/topics/TIPP_VIPP.pdf. Accessed September 13, 2007

10. Amato PR, Fowler F. Parenting practices, child adjustment, and family diversity. *J Marriage Family*. 2002;64:703-716

11. Whitlock EP, Orleans CT, Pender N, Allan J. Evaluating primary care behavioral counseling interventions: an evidence-based approach. *Am J Prev Med*. 2002;22:267-284

12. Klassen TP, MacKay JM, Moher D, Walker A, Jones AL. Community-based injury prevention interventions. *Future Child*. 2000;10:83-110

13. Mallonee S, Istre GR, Rosenberg M, et al. Surveillance and prevention of residential-fire injuries. *N Engl J Med*. 1996;335:27-31

14. Automotive Safety Program. Special Needs Transportation. Available at: www.preventinjury.org/speNeeds.asp. Accessed September 13, 2007

15. Bass JL, Christoffel KK, Widome M, et al. Childhood injury prevention counseling in primary care settings: a critical review of the literature. *Pediatrics*. 1993;92:544-550

16. DiGuiseppi C, Roberts IG. Individual-level injury prevention strategies in the clinical setting. *Future Child*. 2000;10:53-82

17. Straus MA, Sugarman DB, Giles-Sims J. Spanking by parents and subsequent antisocial behavior of children. *Arch Pediatr Adolesc Med*. 1997;151:761-767

18. Straus MA. Discipline and deviance: physical punishment of children and violence and other crimes in adulthood. *Soc Probl*. 1991;38:133-154

19. Ashton V. The relationship between attitudes toward corporal punishment and the perception and reporting of child maltreatment. *Child Abuse Negl*. 2001;25:389-399

20. Gershoff ET. Corporal punishment by parents and associated child behaviors and experiences: a meta-analytic and theoretical review. *Psychol Bull*. 2002;128:539-579

21. Straus MA. Spanking and the making of a violent society. *Pediatrics*. 1996;98:837-842

22. American Academy of Pediatrics, Committee on Psychosocial Aspects of Child and Family Health. Guidance for effective discipline. *Pediatrics*. 1998;101:723-728

23. Sege RD, Hatmaker-Flanigan E, De Vos E, Levin-Goodman R, Spivak H. Anticipatory guidance and violence prevention: results from family and pediatrician focus groups. *Pediatrics*. 2006;117:455-463

24. Wissow LS, Roter D. Toward effective discussion of discipline and corporal punishment during primary care visits: findings from studies of doctor-patient interaction. *Pediatrics*. 1994;94(4 Pt 2):587-593

25. American Academy of Pediatrics, Committee on Injury and Poison Prevention. Firearm-related injuries affecting the pediatric population. *Pediatrics*. 2000;105:888-895

26. Resnick MD, Ireland M, Borowsky I. Youth violence perpetration: what protects? What predicts? Findings from the National Longitudinal Study of Adolescent Health. *J Adolesc Health*. 2004;35:424.e1-10

27. Flay BR, Graumlich S, Segawa E, Burns JL, Holliday MY. Effects of 2 prevention programs on high-risk behaviors among African American youth: a randomized trial. *Arch Pediatr Adolesc Med*. 2004;158:377-384

28. Bell CC. Cultivating resiliency in youth. *J Adolesc Health*. 2001;29:375-381

29. Murphey DA, Lamonda KH, Carney JK, Duncan P. Relationships of a brief measure of youth assets to health-promoting and risk behaviors. *J Adolesc Health*. 2004;34:184-191

30. Olweus D. Bullying at School: *What We Know and What We Can Do*. Cambridge, MA: Blackwell Publishers; 1993

31. US Health Resources and Services Administration. Stop Bullying Now! Take A Stand. Lend A Hand. Rockville, MD: US Department of Health and Human Services; 2005. Available at: http://stopbullyingnow.hrsa.gov/index.asp?area=whatbullyingis. Accessed January 2, 2007

32. Lyznicki JM, McCaffree MA, Robinowitz CB. Childhood bullying: implications for physicians. *Am Fam Physician*. 2004;70:1723-1728

33. Kellermann AL, Rivara FP, Somes G, et al. Suicide in the home in relation to gun ownership. *N Engl J Med*. 1992;327:467-472

34. Kellermann AL, Rivara FP, Rushforth NB, et al. Gun ownership as a risk factor for homicide in the home. *N Engl J Med*. 1993;329:1084-1091

35. Kaplan MS, Geling O. Firearm suicides and homicides in the United States: regional variations and patterns of gun ownership. *Soc Sci Med*. 1998;46:1227-1233

36. Lester D. Gun availability and the use of guns for suicide and homicide in Canada. *Can J Public Health*. 2000;91:186-187

37. Miller M, Azrael D, Hemenway D. Rates of household firearm ownership and homicide across US regions and states, 1988-1997. *Am J Public Health*. 2002;92:1988-1993

38. Miller M, Azrael D, Hemenway D. Firearm availability and unintentional firearm deaths. *Accid Anal Prev*. 2001;33:477-484

39. Grossman DC, Mueller BA, Riedy C, et al. Gun storage practices and risk of youth suicide and unintentional firearm injuries. *JAMA*. 2005;293:707-714

40. Jackman GA, Farah MM, Kellermann AL, Simon HK. Seeing is believing: what do boys do when they find a real gun? *Pediatrics*. 2001;107:1247-1250

41. Hayes DN, Sege R. FiGHTS: a preliminary screening tool for adolescent firearms-carrying. *Ann Emerg Med*. 2003;42:798-807

42. Senturia YD, Christoffel KK, Donovan M. Gun storage patterns in US homes with children. A pediatric practice-based survey. Pediatric Practice Research Group. *Arch Pediatr Adolesc Med*. 1996;150:265-269

43. Brent DA, Perper JA, Allman CJ, Moritz GM, Wartella ME, Zelenak JP. The presence and accessibility of firearms in the homes of adolescent suicides. A case-control study. *JAMA*. 1991;266:2989-2995

44. Prothrow-Stith D, Spivak HR. *Murder is No Accident: Understanding and Preventing Youth Violence in America*. San Francisco, CA: Jossey-Bass; 2004

45. Kogan MD, Schuster MA, Yu SM, et al. Routine assessment of family and community health risks: parent views and what they receive. *Pediatrics*. 2004;113:1934-1943

46. Trowbridge MJ, Sege RD, Olson L, O'Connor K, Flaherty E, Spivak H. Intentional injury management and prevention in pediatric practice: results from 1998 and 2003 American Academy of Pediatrics Periodic Surveys. *Pediatrics*. 2005;116:996-1000

47. American Academy of Pediatrics, Task Force on Violence. The role of the pediatrician in youth violence prevention in clinical practice and at the community level. *Pediatrics*. 1999;103:173-181

48. McDonald EM, Solomon B, Shields W, et al. Evaluation of kiosk-based tailoring to promote household safety behaviors in an urban pediatric primary care practice. *Patient Educ Couns*. 2005;58:168-181

49. Spivak H, Sege R, Flanigan E, Licenziato V. *Connected Kids: Safe, Strong, Secure Clinical Guide*. Elk Grove Village, IL American Academy of Pediatrics; 2006

50. DiGuiseppi CG, Rivara FP, Koepsell TD, Polissar L. Bicycle helmet use by children. Evaluation of a community-wide helmet campaign. *JAMA*. 1989;262:2256-2261

51. American Academy of Pediatrics, Task Force on Sudden Infant Death Syndrome. The changing concept of sudden infant death syndrome: diagnostic coding shifts, controversies regarding the sleeping environment, and new variables to consider in reducing risk. *Pediatrics*. 2005;116:1245-1255

52. Tremblay RE, Nagin DS, Seguin JR, et al. Physical aggression during early childhood: trajectories and predictors. *Pediatrics*. 2004;114:e43-e50

53. American Academy of Pediatrics, Committee on Public Education. Children, adolescents, and television. *Pediatrics*. 2001;107:423-426

54. Embry DD, Flannery DJ, Vazsonyi AT, Powell KE, Atha H. Peacebuilders: a theoretically driven, school-based model for early violence prevention. *Am J Prev Med*. 1996;12:91-100

55. Embry DD. The Good Behavior Game: a best practice candidate as a universal behavioral vaccine. *Clin Child Fam Psychol Rev*. 2002;5:273-297

56. The Multisite Violence Prevention Project. The multisite violence prevention project: background and overview. *Am J Prev Med*. 2004;26:3-11

57. Howard BJ, Broughton DD, American Academy of Pediatrics, Committee on Psychosocial Aspects of Child and Family Health. The pediatrician's role in the prevention of missing children. *Pediatrics*. 2004;114:1100-1105

58. Sege R, Stringham P, Short S, Griffith J. Ten years after: examination of adolescent screening questions that predict future violence-related injury. *J Adolesc Health*. 1999;24:395-402

59. Chen LH, Baker SP, Li G. Graduated driver licensing programs and fatal crashes of 16-year-old drivers: a national evaluation. *Pediatrics*. 2006;118:56-62

60. Redelmeier DA, Tibshirani RJ. Association between cellular-telephone calls and motor vehicle collisions. *N Engl J Med*. 1997;336:453-458

61. Stutts JC, Reinfurt DW, Rodgman EA. The role of driver distraction in crashes: an analysis of 1995-1999 Crashworthiness Data System Data. *Annu Proc Assoc Adv Automot Med*. 2001;45:287-301

62. Strayer DL, Drews FA, Johnston WA. Cell phone-induced failures of visual attention during simulated driving. *J Exp Psychol Appl*. 2003;9:23-32

63. Williams AF, Preusser DF. Night driving restrictions for youthful drivers: a literature review and commentary. *J Public Health Policy*. 1997;18:334-345

PROMOTING SAFETY AND INJURY PREVENTION

64. American Academy of Pediatrics, Committee on Sports Medicine and Fitness. Athletic participation by children and adolescents who have systemic hypertension. *Pediatrics*. 1997;99:637-638

65. American Academy of Pediatrics, Committee on Sports Medicine and Fitness. Medical conditions affecting sports participation. *Pediatrics*. 2001;107:1205-1209

66. Giaconia RM, Reinherz HZ, Silverman AB, Pakiz B, Frost AK, Cohen E. Traumas and posttraumatic stress disorder in a community population of older adolescents. *J Am Acad Child Adolesc Psychiatry*. 1995;34:1369-1380

67. Horowitz K, Weine S, Jekel J. PTSD symptoms in urban adolescent girls: compounded community trauma. *J Am Acad Child Adolesc Psychiatry*. 1995;34:1353-1361

68. Jenkins EJ, Bell CC. Adolescent violence: can it be curbed? *Adolesc Med*. 1992;3:71-86

69. Pynoos RS, Nader K. Psychological first aid and treatment approach to children exposed to community violence: research implications. *J Traumatic Stress*. 1988;1:445-473

70. Fantuzzo JW, Mohr WK. Prevalence and effects of child exposure to domestic violence. *Future Child*. 1999;9:21-32

71. Bair-Merritt MH, Blackstone M, Feudtner C. Physical health outcomes of childhood exposure to intimate partner violence: a systematic review. *Pediatrics*. 2006;117:e278-e290

72. Silverman JG, Raj A, Mucci LA, Hathaway JE. Dating violence against adolescent girls and associated substance use, unhealthy weight control, sexual risk behavior, pregnancy, and suicidality. *JAMA*. 2001;286:572-579

73. Wordes M, Nunez M, National Council on Crime and Delinquency and the National Center for Victims of Crime. *Our Vulnerable Teenagers: Their Victimization, Its Consequences, and Directions for Prevention and Intervention*. Oakland, CA: National Council on Crime and Delinquency and the National Center for Victims of Crime; 2002

74. Foshee VA, Bauman KE, Arriaga XB, Helms RW, Koch GG, Linder GF. An evaluation of Safe Dates, an adolescent dating violence prevention program. *Am J Public Health*. 1998;88:45-50

75. Foshee VA, Bauman KE, Greene WF, Koch GG, Linder GF, MacDougall JE. The Safe Dates program: 1-year follow-up results. *Am J Public Health*. 2000;90:1619-1622

76. Bontempo DE, D'Augelli AR. Effects of at-school victimization and sexual orientation on lesbian, gay, or bisexual youths' health risk behavior. *J Adolesc Health*. 2002;30:364-374

77. Egley A, Major AK. *Highlights of the 2002 National Youth Gang Survey*. Washington, DC: US Department of Justice, Office of Juvenile Justice and Delinquency Prevention; 2004

78. Hill KG, Lui C, Hawkins JD. *Early Precursors of Gang Membership: A Study of Seattle Youth*. Washington, DC: US Department of Justice, Office of Juvenile Justice and Delinquency Prevention; 2001

79. Thornberry TP. *Gangs and Delinquency in Developmental Perspective*. New York, NY: Cambridge University Press; 2003

80. US Department of Justice, Office of Juvenile Justice and Delinquency Prevention. *A Guide to Assessing Your Community's Youth Gang Problem*. Tallahassee, FL: Institution for Intergovernmental Research; 2002. Available at: www.iir.com/nygc/assessment/assessment.pdf. Accessed September 13, 2007

PROMOTING SAFETY AND INJURY PREVENTION

Promoting Community Relationships and Resources

Theme 10

INTRODUCTION

Beyond the traditional primary care that is essential for all children, families also may benefit from a broad range of community-based services, such as family support; housing, employment, and social services; educational services; mental health services; substance abuse treatment; language assistance; respite care; recreation opportunities; and services for children and youth with special health care needs. Referring a child, youth, or family for community services and support is, therefore, a common interaction of a health care professional with the community. These services, coupled with primary care provided in a medical home,[1] constitute a community-based system of care and are critical to promoting family well-being.

Promoting community relationships involves more than just knowing enough about local providers and agencies to make referrals, however. Individuals and families are formed by the communities in which they live, whether those communities are defined by race, ethnicity, socioeconomics, or lifestyle. Learning about these communities and understanding their cultures are key to making successful links between families and the services they need and to promoting the health and well-being of children and families.

Comprehensive health supervision also involves the recognition that the health of children and families are shaped to a significant degree by their environments, as well as by their individual choices. Health care professionals can promote the public health of community residents through a variety of consultation and advocacy activities that are carried out in partnership with groups and organizations that serve the community, such as schools, parks and recreation agencies, businesses, and faith groups. They also can encourage families and children, especially adolescents, to become active in community endeavors to improve the health of their communities.

Roles for the Health Care Professional in Promoting Community Relationships

In developing a community-based system of care for their patients and families, health care professionals can pursue a number of options to increase their understanding of the community, strengthen relationships with community organizations and service providers, and foster positive health-promoting change at the community level.

Learn About the Community and Collaborate With Community Partners

Building a knowledge base of the resources in the community and collaborating with community agencies to identify and manage referrals is a natural way for office practices or clinics to expand their outreach into the community. These efforts will help promote community health services and allow the practice or clinic to address the special needs of a child, adolescent, or family. Many practices and clinics work with community partners to develop a confidential tracking system and produce an accessible, comprehensive, central record with pertinent information about the child and the services received.

Developing community partnerships and collaborating effectively can present challenges, however. The community-based system of services can be complex and difficult to navigate. Each organization or agency may offer a wide array of services, and each has unique criteria for enrollment and service provision that can present barriers. Even in small communities, developing new partners and maintaining existing relationships require commitment and effort, especially when relationships are first being established.

Box 1 lists common community resources that provide needed services for families and that can be sources of valuable community partnerships for health care professionals.

In addition to serving the needs of individual patients, health care professionals can consult with early care and education professionals and help with policy development on topics such as behavior problems, nutrition, and infectious diseases.[2] Preliminary evidence

Building a knowledge base of the resources in the community and collaborating with community agencies to identify and manage referrals is a natural way for office practices or clinics to expand their outreach into the community.

indicates that health consultation in early child care settings has positive effects on health policy, health practices, immunizations, and children's access to health care.[3-5]

Health care professionals also can provide consultation on other important issues in child care, such as physical space, staffing ratios, and staff training.[6] National organizations, such as the American Academy of Pediatrics, American Public Health Association, National Association for the Education of Young Children, Child Welfare League of America, and Zero to Three, have developed standards and voluntary systems of accreditation that are often higher than state licensing regulations. These can provide useful guidance to health care professionals.

Recognize the Special Needs of Certain Groups

Although most families benefit from community services at one time or another, several population groups may require a wider range of services or longer-term services.

RECENT IMMIGRANTS AND THOSE WITH LIMITED PROFICIENCY IN ENGLISH

Communities must acknowledge the barriers that vulnerable families who are recent immigrants or have limited English proficiency face, and find support that is culturally and linguistically competent. Organizations that have the capacity and knowledge to address the needs and preferences of vulnerable families and that represent families can play particularly important roles in these efforts.

Health care professionals also must be sensitive to the tremendous fear of exposure among immigrant families who are undocumented. This fear often makes them reluctant to request care or seek services. Health care professionals and cultural brokers (individuals from the culture who can act as linguistic interpreters and liaisons between the family and the health care professional) can work together to effectively address health and mental health issues from both community and cultural perspectives.[7,8]

Health care professionals also should be familiar with state and national organizations that can provide support or further referrals for recent immigrant families with children. Such organizations can be especially useful to parents who have limited English proficiency,

families who have literacy problems, and families who live in rural areas, tribal native lands, or other isolated communities. Nurturing and supporting families who have newly arrived and are adjusting to a new culture promotes optimal family functioning and child health outcomes.

BOX 1
Local Community Resources
Health
- Title V Services for Children and Youth with Special Health Care Needs
- State Children's Health Insurance Program (SCHIP)
- Local Child and Family Health Plus providers
- Medical specialty care
- Public health nursing
- Medical assistance programs
- Home care
- Respite care
- Mental health resources
- Substance abuse treatment
- Environmental health units
- Health literacy resources
- Physical activity resources

Development
- Head Start and Early Head Start
- Early intervention programs
- Early education and child care programs
- School-based or school-linked programs
- Recreation programs
- Playgroups

Family Support
- US Department of Agriculture's Special Supplemental Nutrition Program for Women, Infants, and Children (WIC)
- Social service agencies and child protection services
- Parenting programs/support groups
- Faith-based organizations
- Home visiting services
- Domestic violence resources
- Bereavement and related supports (due to sudden infant death syndrome, sudden unexpected infant death, or other causes of infant and child fatality)
- Food banks
- Child care resource and referral agencies
- Child care health consultants
- "Parents Helping Parents" organizations for children with special health care needs

Adult Assistance
- Adult education and literacy resources
- Job training resources
- Adult education for English language instruction
- Legal Aid
- Immigration services
- Racial- and ethnic-specific support and community development organizations
- Volunteering opportunities

PROMOTING COMMUNITY
RELATIONSHIPS AND RESOURCES

CHILDREN AND YOUTH WITH SPECIAL HEALTH CARE NEEDS

Families of children and youth with special health care needs often need strong support from their communities, and many states have organized systems that can offer links among parents for individual guidance and support. In recognizing that families of children with special needs can help each other, parents also have become advocates, consultants, educators of child health care professionals, and members of diagnostic, treatment, or hospital planning teams.

Health care professionals should educate themselves about the community resources that serve and advocate for children and youth with special health care needs, and should identify ways to link families with these important community resources. Organizations in which parents help other parents (eg, Family Voices) and consumer-directed organizations (eg, independent living centers) can provide remarkable support to families.

Encourage Informal Support

For many families, informal support is as important as receiving specific services. Informal communications with friends, relatives, or support groups can provide advice, encouragement, praise, emotional support, practical assistance, and respite for parents. These interactions help parents understand the common ground they share with other families. They are especially important to some groups, such as families of children with special health care needs and recent immigrants.

Learning about parents' support networks, encouraging families to maintain these important connections, and, if necessary, linking them with other culturally and linguistically appropriate social supports all can be part of the care provided by health care professionals. When a family is isolated from the community or needs specific kinds of support, the health care professional and office staff can help locate appropriate local resources, relevant literature, and suitable Internet resources.

Consult and Advocate

Just as community resources can supplement the services of the medical home, health care professionals can work with the community to improve the quality of health care and enhance community services. Many of the health problems that children and families face today (eg, obesity, mental illness, bullying or violence, or intentional and unintentional injuries) are influenced by environmental and community factors. Creating change at the community level can, therefore, have a positive impact on the health of many. Health care professionals can become agents for health-promoting community change through a variety of consultation and advocacy activities. Advocacy demonstrates strong concern and often links to action in the community, legislative, and policy arenas.[9] (For more information on this topic, see the Promoting Family Support Theme.)

Success in these activities, however, requires partnerships and close working relationships with the groups that are most directly affected and their communities.

> Health care professionals should educate themselves about the community resources that serve and advocate for children and youth with special health care needs, and should identify ways to link families with these important community resources.

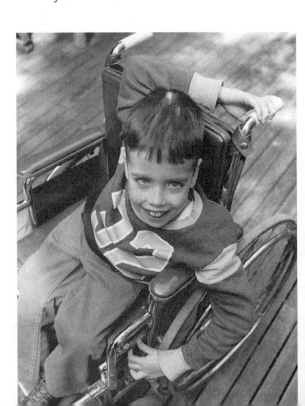

Health care professionals can partner with others to:

- Conduct a community needs and assets assessment to elucidate the strengths of the community, the opportunities for successful collaboration among community partners, and the effect on health outcomes of health and social risks that are particular to that community.
- Compile a matrix of existing services and identify service gaps.
- Develop a strategic or community improvement plan.
- Provide health consultation to a community program.
- Advocate for improved health and safety practices.
- Educate policy makers about other ways health care professionals can contribute.
- Advocate for approaches and resources that contribute to efforts to eliminate racial, ethnic, and mental health disparities.
- Assist families of low health literacy to understand and act upon health information.

A promising strategy in community assessment has been developed by Kretzmann and McKnight.[10] The Asset-Based Community Development (ABCD) approach involves using epidemiologic, demographic, economic, and other data to identify community problems, and then balancing those problems against an inventory of the skills and talents of the community members. The result is a "Community Assets Map" that describes individual talent as well as contributions by formal and informal associations (eg, faith groups or knitting circles). The American Academy of Pediatrics *Community-based Resident Projects Toolkit* describes this concept for health care professionals.[11] This approach could help address and reduce health disparities in the communities, an important objective of *Healthy People 2010*.

Other prime venues for health care professional consultation and advocacy are settings and organizations where children spend time (eg, child care programs, schools, and youth programs). Schools, early education and care settings, camps, sports teams, clubs, and faith-based groups can benefit from a partnership with a health care professional as a participant or leader. The ability to build consensus among parents, professionals, and other community members in these settings so as to address health issues that affect children requires that health care professionals be collaborative leaders with problem-solving skills[12] and knowledge of nonmedical topics, such as:

- Policy development and legal issues (eg, Americans with Disabilities Act)
- Economic and community development (eg, housing issues, employment, and business practices)
- Best practices in education, early intervention, and social and emotional health
- Community systems
- Use of public health and other data
- Communication skills
- Cultural contexts of communities

Child health care professionals often will be asked to advocate for different community programs and interventions. One important criterion is the demonstrated effectiveness. It may be helpful to consult the Centers for Disease Control and Prevention (CDC) *Guide to Community Preventive Services*, which lists effective programs and approaches.[13] Some of these recommendations, with particular implication for children and youth, are:

- Oral health
  - Community water fluoridation
  - School-based pit and fissure sealant development programs
- Social environment
  - Comprehensive center-based early childhood education development programs for low-income children

The ability to build consensus among parents, professionals, and other community members in these settings so as to address health issues that affect children requires that health care professionals be collaborative leaders with problem-solving skills and knowledge of nonmedical topics...

- Tobacco
  - Increases in the unit price for tobacco
- Motor vehicles
  - Safety belt laws
  - Child safety seat laws
- Physical activity
  - School-based physical education

Promoting Community Relationships and Resources: Infancy—Birth to 11 Months

Early brain and child development research unequivocally demonstrates that human development is powerfully affected by contextual surroundings and experiences.[14] Children's physical and emotional health and their social and cognitive functioning are strongly influenced by the one-on-one care they receive and by how well their family functions as a unit. Children achieve the best outcomes when they have nurturing, responsive caregivers and live with parents who respect and support one another, who have adequate social and financial resources, and who are actively engaged in the upbringing of their children. Parents who have adequate resources and support are better able to be responsive, gentle, and consistent with their infants. Parents with inadequate resources may have to devote significant time to meeting the basic needs of their family. This situation can make it challenging for them to be physically and psychologically available to their infant.

Connecting with groups that address issues, such as community or domestic violence, inadequate or unsafe housing, environmental hazards, poverty, substance abuse, or unemployment, is vitally important to ensure that families can meet their basic needs. Home visiting services from lactation specialists, hospitals, public health departments, and community resource centers can be important resources for families with infants.

Many families struggle to provide the high-quality early experiences that are necessary for a child's emotional well-being and social competence. Whether parents are home full-time with their children or work outside the home (eg, full- or part-time jobs, multiple jobs, or seasonal work or farmwork), they need access to sound advice and support that is relevant to their situation. Finding high-quality child care can be challenging to all families, especially those who work multiple shifts or very long hours. By increasing their involvement in existing parent education, family support, and child care programs, health care professionals can help their patients have positive and nurturing early experiences as well as raise the quality of care for all young children in their community.

Promoting Community Relationships and Resources: Early Childhood—1 to 4 Years

In 2005, 61% of children from birth through age 6 (and not in kindergarten) spent time in nonparental child care.[15] Many of these children start in such programs as infants. Health care professionals should view early education and child care programs as access points for ensuring that children have medical homes. Early care and education professionals and other colleagues with expertise in early childhood development and mental health can conduct important growth, development, and social and emotional screenings, and can help child health professionals' link families to community resources that can help children and families receive needed services at an early age.

Health care professionals often help families assess the quality of child care for their young children. Their advice and guidance on the transition from home to child care can be invaluable to families. This is especially true for families of children and youth with special health care needs, for whom medication administration and technology are 2 of the most common areas of concern.[16] Early intervention programs and respite care are additional community services that can provide support and resources for parents.

Health care professionals often help families assess the quality of child care for their young children. Their advice and guidance on the transition from home to child care can be invaluable to families.

PROMOTING COMMUNITY RELATIONSHIPS AND RESOURCES

Promoting Community Relationships and Resources: Middle Childhood—5 to 10 Years

During the middle childhood years, children become increasingly aware of the outside world and its opportunities, challenges, and fun. Communities play an essential role in promoting development and socialization and provide opportunities to explore the wider world as parents begin to relinquish some control and children demonstrate increased independence in their daily life activities. Participation in organized activities, including team sports, Scouts programs, religious groups, and organized lessons, such as dance or music, fosters independence during the middle childhood years. Health care professionals can help families find the right balance between participating in enriching activities and ensuring sufficient "down time" and family time. For families who have children and youth with special health care needs, relinquishing control and promoting the child's independence can require special considerations and adaptations that are specific to the child's individual needs.

The middle childhood years are characterized by children's need to develop friendships and participate in peer groups. These needs are met in the broad community as children begin to discern where they fit in their family, school class, and neighborhood. Providing safe and supervised recreational programs and activities for children and youth is an important community role. Communities should be encouraged to adapt programs that promote socialization and opportunities for children and youth with special health care needs. Health care professionals can advocate for safe, well-equipped facilities for children and families in neighborhoods and communities where these resources are currently absent or sparse.

School is the most important community organization for children and their families in the elementary and middle-school years. Schools are mandated to help children

achieve success with learning, a key developmental task for all children, including those with special health care needs. Children need to be as healthy as possible to learn well, and school health programs have many components to support this goal. Box 2 presents 8 critical components of a coordinated school health program, as identified by the CDC.[17]

> **BOX 2**
> **Components of a Coordinated School Health Program[17]**
> - Health education
> - Health services
> - Counseling and psychological and social services
> - Physical education
> - Nutrition services
> - Healthy school environment
> - Health promotion for staff
> - Family/community involvement

A "Healthy School Team" is composed of school professionals, parents, students, and community members who work together to improve the health outcomes for the children and youth in their schools by promoting a high-quality coordinated school health program.[18] In addition to service on, or relating to, such a committee, health care professionals can consider membership on a school board. This participation can help health care professionals improve their knowledge and understanding of their patients' community. It also gives the health care professional an opportunity to promote and advance the global understanding of the solid link between good health and learning, as well as highlight the importance of health considerations in the board's fiscal decisions.

A "Healthy School Team" is composed of school professionals, parents, students, and community members who work together to improve the health outcomes for the children and youth in their schools by promoting a high-quality coordinated school health program.

Health care professionals should ask about adolescents' "connectedness" to family, school, and community to gain valuable insights into the challenges and opportunities that exist for the physical and emotional well-being of their patients.

Promoting Community Relationships and Resources: Adolescence—11 to 21 Years

In the 1980s, the Search Institute, a social science research group, developed a framework of developmental assets. These assets described 40 positive factors in young people, families, and communities that promote healthy development.[19] Research demonstrates a correlation of a greater number of assets in the lives of youth with decreased reports of risk-taking behavior. Among these assets, those related to support, boundaries and expectations, constructive use of time, and commitment to learning have a particularly robust research base.[20]

Community contributions that enhance the adolescent's sense of being a needed, valued, and responsible member of the community firmly fit within the assets that support this stage of a young person's development.[21] Data from The National Longitudinal Study of Adolescent Health also show that "connectedness" to parents and schools protects adolescents from health risk behaviors and prepares them for comfortable relationships in the future.[22]

Health care professionals should ask about adolescents' "connectedness" to family, school, and community to gain valuable insights into the challenges and opportunities that exist for the physical and emotional well-being of their patients.[21] For youth with special health care needs and their families, a particular focus on their developmental assets and community relationships helps balance the attention that is needed to coordinate complex services, medications, and ongoing evaluation.

The asset model reinforces interactions and social involvement that promote health. Safe, supervised recreational programs and facilities, opportunities to pursue meaningful work and community service activities, and access to training programs for adolescents are examples of community assets that promote healthy development. Some communities have enacted health supervision measures, including regulating the sale and use of alcohol, cigarettes, and guns; mandating safety belt and helmet use; and instituting a graduated driver's license. Because communities differ, health care professionals should ask young people about their knowledge of opportunities and services in their community and encourage adolescents to abide by community laws and safe social practices.

Health care professionals who care for homeless youth or those in substitute care (eg, juvenile justice and the foster care system) must understand the legal protections, policies, and services that are available at the community and state levels. These youth have an increased incidence of both physical and mental health needs, such as post-traumatic stress disorder and substance abuse. Health care professionals should be advocates for high-quality, integrated services that foster young people's strengths and help them achieve long-term goals. Because these youth do not always have the support and guidance of a responsible adult who really cares about them, their success depends on the advocacy of many health care professionals, nonmedical professionals, and community members working with them and on their behalf.

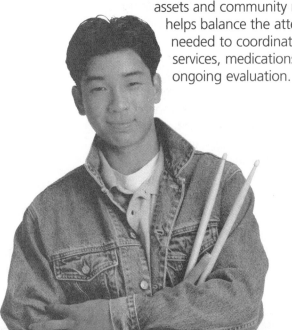

References

1. American Academy of Pediatrics, Medical Home Initiatives for Children With Special Health Care Needs Project Advisory Committee. The medical home. *Pediatrics*. 2002;110(1 Pt 1):184-186
2. American Academy of Pediatrics, American Public Health Association, National Resource Center for Health and Safety in Child Care. *Caring for Our Children: National Health and Safety Performance Standards: Guidelines for Out-of-Home Child Care*. 2nd ed. Elk Grove Village, IL: American Academy of Pediatrics; 2002
3. Cianciolo S, Trueblood-Noll R, Allingham P. Health consultation in early childhood settings. *Young Child*. 2004;59:56-61
4. Kotch JB. Child Care Health Consultation: The Quality Enhancement Project for Infants and Toddlers (QEP) Evaluation. Paper presented at the Child Care Special Interest Group, American Academy of Pediatrics National Conference and Exhibition; May 2, 2004; San Francisco, CA
5. Healthy Child Care America. American Academy of Pediatrics Web site. Child Care Health Consultation. Available at: www.healthychildcare.org/CCHC.cfm. Accessed May 16, 2007
6. American Academy of Pediatrics, Committee on Early Childhood, Adoption, and Dependent Care. Quality early education and child care from birth to kindergarten. *Pediatrics*. 2006;115:187-191
7. Buehler J. Nursing in rural Native American communities. *Nurs Clin North Am*. 1993;28:211-217
8. Dunn AM. Culture competence and the primary care provider. *J Pediatr Health Care*. 2002;16:105-111
9. Rushton FE, American Academy of Pediatrics, Committee on Community Health Services. The pediatrician's role in community pediatrics. *Pediatrics*. 2005;115:1092-1094
10. Kretzmann JP, McKnight J. *Building Communities from the Inside Out. A Path Toward Finding and Mobilizing a Community's Assets*. Chicago, IL: ACTA Publications; 1993
11. Gold A. Asset-Based Community Development (ABCD). In: *Community Pediatrics Training Initiative. Community-based Resident Projects Toolkit: A Guide to Partnering with Communities to Improve Child Health Care*. Elk Grove Village, IL: American Academy of Pediatrics; 2005:18-23
12. Garfunkel LC, Sidelinger DE, Rezet B, Blaschke GS, Risko W. Achieving consensus on competency in community pediatrics. *Pediatrics*. 2005;115(4 Suppl):1167-1171
13. Task Force on Community Preventive Services. The Guide to Community Preventive Services: *What Works to Promote Health?* New York, NY: Oxford University Press; 2005
14. Shoakoff JP, Phillips DA, eds. *From Neurons to Neighborhoods: The Science of Early Childhood Development*. Washington, DC: National Academy Press; 2000
15. Federal Interagency Forum on Child and Family Statistics. Washington, DC: US Government printing office; 2005. Available at: http://www.childstats.gov/americaschildren/tables/fam3.a. Accessed July 23, 2007
16. American Academy of Pediatrics. *The Pediatrician's Role in Promoting Health and Safety in Child Care*. Elk Grove Village, IL: American Academy of Pediatrics; 2001
17. National Center for Chronic Disease Prevention and Health Promotion. Healthy Youth. Coordinated School Health Program. Centers for Disease Control and Prevention Web site. Available at: http://www.cdc.gov/HealthyYouth/CSHP/. Accessed March 1, 2006
18. Fetro JV. Implementing coordinated school health programs in local schools. In: Marx E, Wooley SF, Northrop D, eds. *Health Is Academic: A Guide to Coordinated School Health Programs*. New York, NY: Teachers College Press; 1998:15-42
19. Developmental Assets Search Institute Web site. Available at: http://www.search-institute.org/assets/. Accessed May 16, 2007
20. Scales P, Leffert N, Lerner RM. *Developmental Assets: A Synthesis of the Scientific Research on Adolescent Development*: Minneapolis, MN: Search Institute; 1999
21. American Academy of Pediatrics, The Injury Prevention Program. *Connected Kids: Safe, Strong, Secure Clinical Guide*. Elk Grove Village, IL: American Academy of Pediatrics; 2006. Available at: www.aap.org/connectedkids/samples. Accessed September 10, 2007
22. Resnick MD, Bearman PS, Blum RW, et al. Protecting adolescents from harm. Findings from the National Longitudinal Study on Adolescent Health. *JAMA*. 1997;278:823-832

Introduction to the Bright Futures Visits

Health supervision visits are an important opportunity to assess the health and function of a family and child. The *Bright Futures Guidelines* exist "to improve the health and well-being of all children" by improving a practice's clinical health promotion and disease prevention efforts and the organizational processes necessary to meet this goal.

Many texts and guidelines for the care of children discuss what should be done in the visit. This edition of the *Bright Futures Guidelines* provides an up-to-date and concise summary of the "what to do" in primary care practice today, with an expanded focus on the "how to do" of health care delivery.

We describe the visit content in terms of 4 components: disease detection, disease prevention, health promotion, and anticipatory guidance. Each is a large task; the aggregate is a remarkable task. Certainly, no health care professional has the time to take these *Bright Futures Guidelines* and do every possible intervention discussed for a particular age visit. How, then, can health care professionals choose what is most important for one child and family at this time in this community? Experienced health care professionals often say that a visit is made up of many "to dos": things we **must** do, things we **need** to do, and things we **want** to do.

Families bring an agenda, and we **must** address these needs in the visit if we are to be successful. An overlap generally exists between what the family needs us to discuss and what we feel is important to discuss; thus, creating a shared agenda for the visit is valuable. Helping parents enumerate their concerns and questions is an efficient and effective way of establishing this shared agenda. Using a tool such as a parent/patient questionnaire also can enhance the visit efficiency by identifying concerns at the beginning of the visit.

Certainly, we **need** to do things for which evidence of effectiveness exists. We also may **need** to provide other services that we consider essential to that particular child's health and well-being as defined by professional guidelines, community protocol, or other representations of expert opinion.

What about the things that we **want** to do? We bring a personal view to health based on our training and experience, our knowledge of our unique community and its needs, and our desires to comply with guidelines from the American Academy of Pediatrics (AAP), American Academy of Family Physicians (AAFP), National Association of Pediatric Nurse Practitioners (NAPNAP), the American Academy of Pediatric Dentistry (AAPD), the American Dietetic Association (ADA), or others. Often, the interventions we **want** to include relate to disease prevention and health promotion. Elucidation and enumeration of a child and family's strengths is an important undertaking and a good example of what many experienced health care professionals **want** to do.

This sounds like a pretty big task and an extremely long visit, unless a health care professional tailors the visit and possible interventions to **one** child and family in the community. Not everything needs to be done at every visit. Rather, examinations, screening, and anticipatory guidance may be covered over a sequence of visits during an age range. The time frame for providing health supervision is not just one visit. Actually, it occurs over a child's development and may be provided by a variety of health care professionals in a variety of settings.

The following sections explore these ideas in further detail through a discussion of the content of the health supervision visit, the timing of the visit, and the structure of the visit. We also recognize both the importance and relative paucity of evidence supporting many components of the visit, and describe how supporting evidence is represented in the Guidelines.

The Content of the Visit

The value of a health supervision visit to the child and family in terms of measured outcomes is related to its content and effectiveness. Arguably, a visit is of value if one important task is done very well. Alternatively, a visit that seeks to do many things, and does them all poorly, would be judged ineffective. It follows that the most valuable visit includes as many appropriate interventions as possible, if they can be done effectively. Therefore, the task of the health care professional is to determine which interventions are the most important and how to accomplish them properly.

A visit is composed of many potential interventions or health care professional activities with the patient. Interventions include obtaining a medical history, administering questionnaires or screening tools, performing a physical examination, entering into discussion, and providing anticipatory guidance.

Some interventions, such as assessing growth and development, occur at most or all visits. In these Guidelines, we also propose promoting a healthy weight and assessing mental health and emotional well-being as universal interventions.

But how do we capture the elements of disease prevention and health promotion that are important to an individual child? And, when we find these elements, how are the best interventions chosen so that the best outcomes can be sought?

Many health care professionals see **one** child health visit as **one** encounter, a view encouraged by third-party payers and promulgated by many educators. It is one visit, which, in an ideal world, is focused and uninterrupted. Unlike sick care visits, which aim to remedy a certain malady, the health supervision visit seeks many unique outcomes, often related only in their shared goal of the child's health. Multiple desired outcomes inevitably drive many separate interventions within the one encounter of the visit. Would it not be better conceptualized as a visit of multiple encounters?

This question can be answered by considering 4 activities—disease detection, disease prevention, health promotion, and anticipatory guidance—of the health supervision encounter. Disease detection is the easiest to describe. Every professional in child health care has been trained in the disease model, in the care of children who are sick. However, the desired outcomes of the health supervision visit are broader than just detecting disease and they involve very different actions in the same encounter. Failure to recognize their inherent incongruence will lead to incongruent practice, with frustrations and compromised outcomes. The tone and content of disease detection should be remarkably different from that employed in discussing health-promoting behaviors.

Disease Detection

Child health care professionals generally report 2 techniques of disease detection over time—surveillance and screening. Dworkin discussed surveillance and screening in the context of child development and defined developmental surveillance as "a flexible, continuous process whereby knowledgeable professionals perform skilled observations of children during the provision of health care. The components of developmental surveillance include eliciting and attending to parental concerns, obtaining a relevant developmental history, making accurate and informative observations of children, and sharing opinions and concerns with other relevant professionals."[1] Screening, on the other hand, is a formal process that employs a standardized tool to detect a particular disease state. Surveillance for anemia in a 1-year-old child, for example, involves dietary history, family history, and knowledge of socioeconomic risk factors. Screening for anemia is a hemoglobin or hematocrit screening. Both surveillance and screening are essential elements of the disease-detection functions of the health supervision visit.

Screening and surveillance determine how the characteristics of an individual child compare with characteristics of other children. Through ongoing assessment, the developmental trajectory of an individual child can be plotted and compared, just as height and weight are plotted and compared. This edition of the *Bright Futures Guidelines* will broaden the health care professional's detection skills by including or recommending appropriate screening and assessment tools according to a child's age or clinical presentation. Screening tools alone, however, are not sufficient. Health care professionals should couple screening with careful attention to parental concerns and insights (particularly during crucial developmental stages). This is particularly important for families who may have a child or youth with special health care needs, as this combination of screening and careful attention is more likely to successfully identify these special health care needs early and allow the health care professional to provide quality follow-up and intervention.

Surveillance and screening for developmental disorders has been reviewed.[2]

Traditionally, health care professionals have used surveillance to assess development based on knowledge of the child over time and knowledge of child development milestones. It is held to be useful, but is certainly dependent on the health care professional, and has been shown to detect less than 30% of problems. Screening at select times, using a structured developmental assessment tool, increases the identification rate with sensitivities and specificities of 90% or higher.[2]

The standard of care dictates that visits should include a complete physical examination. The authors of this edition of the *Bright Futures Guidelines* agree. However, experienced health care professionals will simultaneously champion the complete examination based on their discovery of a previously asymptomatic neuroblastoma or murmur of aortic stenosis and point out the rarity of detecting significant pathology. Although the burden of suffering of these disease processes may be great, health analysts correctly question the cost effectiveness of this approach to disease detection: many normals must be assessed to detect one abnormal. So, we ask, "Does this standard of care represent the best care?" Despite the doubts regarding cost effectiveness, we conclude that, in current practice in the care of children and adolescents, the complete physical examination does comprise "best care."

Disease Prevention

The second essential action of the child health encounter—disease prevention—may include both primary prevention activities applied to a whole population and secondary prevention activities aimed at patients with specific risk factors. The recommendation that all infants be placed on their back for sleep to reduce the risk of Sudden Infant Death Syndrome is an example of a successful primary prevention. "Back to Sleep," like immunizations, is an essential disease prevention activity for the care of the infant younger than 6 months. Bright Futures can assist the child and adolescent health care professional to individualize additional disease prevention strategies to the community and to the specific family and patient.

The *Bright Futures Guidelines* is an appropriate compendium of both primary and secondary prevention topics, again noted by age and stage of development; but a compendium such as ours cannot, by itself, drive an encounter. Where evidence exists for specific disease prevention activities at a particular age, it has been incorporated into the guidance for that encounter. In addition, clinical guidelines may be used to assist the health care professional in choosing appropriate activities. The Bright Futures Expert Panels have used clinical guidelines and other sources of evidence to feature 5 Priorities for each visit as particularly high in value to the clinical visit for health care professionals to consider. (For more information on this topic, see the Rationale and Evidence chapter.)

Health Promotion

Health promotion activities constitute the third action of the encounter. These actions distinguish health supervision from other work that health care professionals do with children and families. Other encounters with the health care system focus on disease detection and, often, on disease prevention; but, it is health promotion activities that focus the visit on **wellness.**

Health promotion activities add new opportunities to the encounter. They shift the focus from disease to assets and strengths, on what the family does well and how health care professionals can help them do even better. The skilled health care professional uses these strengths to help the family build assets. This is an opportunity to broach important safety topics, help the family address relationship issues, access community services, and engage with the extended family, school, neighborhood, and faith communities.

Anticipatory Guidance

Brazelton described the process of anticipatory guidance as one in which child health care professionals assess emerging issues that a child and family face and give advice that is developmentally consistent.[3] For anticipatory guidance to be effective, it must be **timely** (ie, delivered at the right age), **appropriate** to the child and family in their community, and **relevant,** so that key recommendations are adopted by the family. Again, the health care professional must prioritize and select; but how? The Bright Futures system of care provides techniques to assist the health care professional in designing effective and time-efficient child health supervision interventions. An extensive collection of sample questions and anticipatory guidance highlighted by the Bright Futures Expert Panels are included.

The Timing of the Visit

Health supervision visits usually are scheduled as a longer encounter than a sick call visit. Data from a survey of pediatricians found that the average length of a preventive care visit, including all care by all personnel, ranges from 28 to 30 minutes, depending on the age of the patient. Pediatricians personally spend an average of 17 to 20 minutes with patients/parents, depending on the patient's age.[4] The complexity of family questions is often a determinant in visit duration, as are the needs of the child that are anticipated before the visit or detected during the visit. The pressures of practice cost and the day's queue of patients may limit the time available.

Experienced health care professionals see the visit as an opportunity, but most also report a genuine tension as they seek to accomplish so much in so little time.

Resolving this tension is important to the success of the visit and is key to family and health care professional satisfaction. This edition of the *Bright Futures Guidelines* provides solutions to improve clinical and organizational processes in health supervision care. Using the Bright Futures materials, committed health care professionals who work with office or clinic staff can create effective encounters that meet their goals of disease detection, disease prevention, health promotion, and anticipatory guidance.

For purposes of discussion, as well as practice efficiency, we chose 15 to 18 minutes as the target time for the face-to-face encounter of the health care professional and the patient. This time does not include screening time for the patient, which may include parent questionnaires, developmental screenings, and professional nursing time with the patient. Consequently, the patient's time of encounter will exceed that of the health care professionals.

Green, Palfrey, and colleagues emphasized the need for time management in health promotion activities,[5] and this issue also is discussed in the *Bright Futures Pocket Guide*. To maximize the time available for health promotion in the visit, they urge that the health care professional clarify the goals for the visit, identify family needs, prioritize shared goals with the family for the visit, and consider other ways to address issues that cannot be covered in the visit.

The Structure of the Visit: 2 Models for Health Supervision

Each visit includes multiple tests or examinations. Growth, development, and sensory functions (vision and hearing) always will be considered. Certain disease states, such as lead poisoning and anemia, will be specifically considered at some encounters, but not all, yet may be suspected or uncovered in the process of the general disease detection activity. Additionally, time must be allotted for

health promotion. To carry out this work during the valuable face-to-face time with the child and family, health care professionals often use the Subjective, Objective, Assessment, and Plan (SOAP) model or the Guidelines for Adolescent Preventive Services[6] (GAPS) model, 2 familiar and useful constructs for health supervision. The Bright Futures Visit is a new model for health supervision that health care professionals may adopt as an alternative or enhanced approach to SOAP or GAPS. Experienced health care professionals will note close similarities between the Bright Futures Visit approach and GAPS. Bright Futures is indebted to the American Medical Association and the authors of GAPS[6] for their important contribution to our work.

The SOAP Model

In the SOAP model, the health care professional obtains and analyzes the patient's **S**ubjective history along with **O**bjective findings of the physical examination and tests. An **A**ssessment is made and a **P**lan is developed to address any positive finding.[7] The subjective information can be obtained by an electronic or paper questionnaire. The HEEADSSS (Home, Education/Employment, Eating, Activities, Drugs [including smoking and alcohol use], Sexuality, Suicide/Depression, and Safety) assessment can be incorporated into the subjective category to provide information about how well school-aged children and adolescent youth are functioning in key life areas.[8] As shown in the following list, the categories under "Subjective" are consistent with the Bright Futures Health Promotion Themes.

As outlined by Polisky et al, in *SOAP for Pediatrics*,[9]

Subjective
- Open-ended question that solicit concerns and questions
- Developmental surveillance

- Nutrition, physical activity, and sleep
- Home, school, mental health, and strengths
- Safety, substances, and puberty

Objective
- Body mass index (BMI), vision, hearing, and other screening test results
- Physical examination

Assessment
- Well child
- Normal physical and emotional development

Plan
- Anticipatory guidance
- Immunizations

Individual and family strengths also can be highlighted in the Subjective assessment. If a problem is identified in any of these areas, it is listed under Assessment with a separate plan for action. If a need for a behavior change is identified, shared decision-making strategies are suggested. Motivational interviewing has been demonstrated to help adolescents and adults change their substance abuse behavior.[10] Prochaska's stages of change also contribute to the health care professional's knowledge in this area.[11]

The Gaps Model

The GAPS model, developed by Art Elster, MD, Missy Fleming, PhD, and colleagues, is a particularly effective method for health supervision because it prioritizes essential secondary prevention activities.[6] Originally applied to adolescent health promotion, the GAPS technique is readily applicable to disease detection in all age groups. The following schema shows how health care professionals can apply the GAPS model.

THE GAPS MODEL: GROWTH AND DEVELOPMENT, AGE-SPECIFIC RISK FACTORS
1. **G**ather information.
- Take history from child or parent.
  - Bright Futures parent or adolescent questionnaire
  - GAPS Trigger Questionnaire

- Assess strengths.
  - Measurements
    - Height
    - Weight
    - Head circumference
    - BMI
  - Physical examination
  - Screening tools
    - Parents' Evaluation of Developmental Status[12] (PEDS)
    - Ages & Stages Questionnaires®[13] (ASQ)
    - Family psychosocial screen[14]

Is there an abnormality?
No: Advance to health promotion activities.
Possibly: Advance to Step 2: **A**ssess further.

2. **A**ssess further.
- Developmental screening assessment
- Hearing or vision testing
- Laboratory tests (eg, hemoglobin [Hgb] or lead)

What do the results indicate?

3. **P**roblem Identification.
- Probably normal
- Uncertain
- Abnormal

What should I do next?

4. **S**olutions.
- Reassure and acknowledge child and family strengths; advance to health promotion activities.
- Plan follow-up.
- Refer to specialist for further evaluation.

One important application of the GAPS model to Bright Futures is its powerful improvement to the effectiveness of the screening physical examination. Although the GAPS model uses the same screening tool of the physical examination for all ages, this approach emphasizes key elements of the physical examination for each age and stage of development, which helps health care professionals focus on the unique needs of, for example, a 3-year-old versus a 13-year-old. The GAPS model is an easily implemented and highly effective technique of sorting through the many possible clinical elements for any health supervision encounter so that the work of the visit can be focused on the individual child and family. Further assessment is specific and patient driven. Use of a properly designed questionnaire, such as the Bright Futures parent or adolescent questionnaires, analyzed with a technique such as GAPS, helps the visit more effectively address the specific needs of an individual family and child. This addresses the question: How do we determine what we **should** do in the visit from what we **could** do, and of what we **could** do, what **can** we do?

Employing Evidence

Satisfactory studies on preventive health issues in children are uncommon. Few studies have evaluated effectiveness of components of the physical examination, for example. Absent evidence does not demonstrate a lack of usefulness, however. The lack of evidence of effectiveness most often simply reflects the lack of study. This edition of the *Bright Futures Guidelines* relies on a range of sources to ensure that relevant evidence and expert opinion is included in the construct of every Bright Futures encounter. (For more information on this topic, see the Rationale and Evidence chapter.)

Components of the Bright Futures Visit

The Bright Futures Expert Panels and Project Advisory Committee view the relationship of parents and pediatric health care professionals as a partnership, consistent with the "medical home" philosophy. The *Bright Futures Guidelines* support the care of children and youth in their families, in their personal cultures, and in their community.

Bright Futures practitioners recognize the importance of a family's strengths in caring for their children. We seek to identify strengths in each encounter, and move the focus of the health supervision visit away from the disease detection model toward a strength-based approach to health promotion and disease prevention. Each visit is an essential opportunity to help a family enhance its assets and health.

Over time, this emphasis on family strength assessment and asset development broadens to include the strengths and assets of the child. This supports the child's essential developmental task of developing autonomy, competence, self-efficacy, and the ability to form healthy relationships. We wish the child to see his own strengths and use them to make good health and safety decisions. We seek to reward the child's accomplishments, rather than admonish mistakes, in his development toward autonomy.

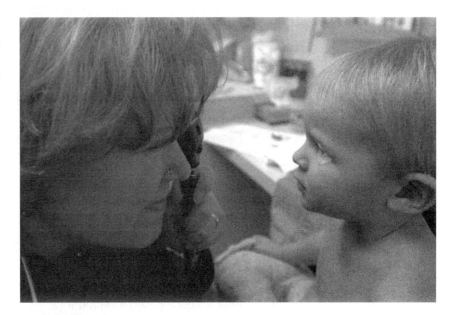

The remainder of this section describes the health supervision visit as presented in the *Bright Futures Guidelines* and illustrated in Table 1.

A. Context

For each visit, the Bright Futures Expert Panels begin with a description of children at the age of the visit, their developmental milieu, their family development, and their environment. This information reminds health care professionals of key developmental tasks and milestones for that age. Contextual discussions describe expected growth and development over time and set the stage for the priorities and tasks that follow. It is intended to assist the practitioner in focusing on the unique qualities of a child this age, as opposed to their near-age peers.

TABLE 1
Bright Futures Visit Outline, Using a Strength-based Approach
A. Context
B. Priorities for the Visit
• The first priority is to attend to the concerns of the parents.
• The Bright Futures Expert Panel has given priority to 5 additional topics for discussion in each visit.
C. Health Supervision
C1. History
C2. Observation of Parent-Child Interaction
C3. Surveillance of Development
C4. Physical Examination
• Assessment of Growth
– Younger than 2 years: Weight, length, head circumference, and weight-for-length
– Older than 2 years: Weight, height, and BMI
• Listing of particular components of the examination that are important for the child at each age visit
C5. Screening
• Universal Screening
• Selective Screening
– Risk Assessment
– Action if Risk Assessment is positive
C6. Immunizations
C7. Other Practice-based Interventions
D. Anticipatory Guidance
• Information for the health care professional
• Health promotion questions for the 5 priorities for the visit
• Anticipatory guidance for the parent and child

B. Priorities for the Visit

For the visit to be successful, the needs and agenda of the family must be addressed. Thus, the Bright Futures Expert Panels note that the first priority is to attend to the concerns of the parents.

Each Bright Futures Expert Panel has enumerated 5 additional priorities for each visit. These priorities and their component elements assist the practitioner to focus the visit on the most important priorities for a child this age. The priorities are drawn from available evidence, relevant expert opinion, and the rich conversation of Expert Panel members. They are offered as a representation of current practice in the care for children of each age. Knowing the evidence for an intervention strengthens the health care professional's knowledge of child health supervision and assists in setting priorities and managing time, but it must be remembered that, even though evidence regarding health supervision activities is sparse, a lack of evidence does not imply lower priority, lack of value, or irrelevance.

C. Health Supervision

C1. HISTORY
In each Bright Futures Visit, the History component begins with the following guidance:

- "Interval history may be obtained according to the concerns of the family and the health care professional's preference or style of practice, or by using a [AGE-SPECIFIC] Visit parent questionnaire."

The importance and utility of history in the health supervision visit was considered in the discussion of the SOAP and GAPS models in the previous section. History that is relevant to the age-specific health supervision encounter is determined to assess strengths, accomplish surveillance, and enhance the health care professional's understanding of

the child and family and to guide their work together.

The Bright Futures Expert Panels also suggest questions that can encourage an in-depth discussion about certain priorities for this visit.

C2. OBSERVATION OF PARENT-CHILD INTERACTION
Health supervision activities begin with observation of the parent-child interaction. Often accomplished without formal thought, this assessment is a starting point for the work of the visit.

C3. SURVEILLANCE OF DEVELOPMENT
Developmental surveillance occurs with each clinical encounter with the child and adolescent, and these observations are central to health supervision for children. Surveillance is the observation over time by experienced eyes of a child's acquisition of *developmental milestones.* To assist health care professionals in their observations, each Bright Futures Visit includes a rich discussion of developmental nuance for that age.

As children grow older, the *"developmental tasks* of childhood and adolescence" assume a central position in this assessment. One definitive list of developmental tasks does not exist, but the Bright Futures Adolescent Expert Panel has included connection to family and peers, competence, self-efficacy, autonomy, and empathy as important components of healthy development in adolescents. The foundation for these developmental tasks of adolescence is found in early and middle childhood.

Formal screening for developmental progress occurs in the Screening portion of the Bright Futures Visit. (See C5. Screening.) Developmental Screening employs a normed developmental screening assessment tool of known sensitivity and specificity. Structured developmental screening is recommended at the 9 Month, 18 Month, 2 Year, and $2\frac{1}{2}$ Year Visits.[2] Targeted screening is performed when indicated by the comprehensive history or findings of surveillance and the physical examination.

C4. PHYSICAL EXAMINATION

The physical examination is the cornerstone of any pediatric evaluation. It is the one portion of the evaluation that only a licensed child health care professional can perform. Molded by a thoughtful acquisition of medical history, a complete physical examination is included as part of every visit. The physical examination must be comprehensive, yet also focus on specific assessments that are appropriate to the child's or adolescent's age, developmental attainment, and needs, which are discerned from the patient history. This portion of each Bright Futures Visit opens with the following guidance:

- "A complete physical examination is included as part of every health supervision visit."

In the context of a complete physical examination, the experienced health care professional incorporates certain specific components that are necessary to the examination of a child of a specific age or stage of development. To set this stage, the following statement also is made in each visit:

- "When performing a physical examination, the health care professional's attention is directed to the following components of the examination that are important for a child this age:"

No evidence-based data exist to indicate that a complete physical examination dramatically improves health care outcomes. However, evidence does demonstrate the importance of key elements of the complete physical examination at different ages. (For more information on this topic, see the Rationale and Evidence chapter.) In addition, there are numerous reasons why the examination may be in the best interests of the child and family. Most important is the possibility that a silent or subtle illness could

be identified. Furthermore, the examination provides an opportunity for the child health care professional to model respect for the child, to educate both the child and the parents about the child and her body and growth, and to acknowledge the child's individuality.

The majority of children in the United States are healthy and have normal physical examinations, although exceptions may be found more commonly among children in poverty, some immigrant children, children with special health care needs, and others. Regardless of health status, for all children, each year's examination will be different, will demonstrate growth and maturation, and will provide the opportunity for discussion of the physical changes associated with healthy development.

The yearly physical examination should be unhurried, with adequate uninterrupted time set aside for questions and discussion by parents and the child. Ensuring privacy can help the parents and the child address a variety of issues in a comfortable and non-pressured setting. Beginning in middle childhood and by adolescence, the rules of privacy and confidentiality must be developed and reviewed for the child and family (Box 1). Children are

---

BOX 1
Privacy, Confidentiality, and the Health Visit

Practices may want to establish formal confidentiality policies. Parents are important participants in these policies. A sample confidentiality statement addressed to youth could look like this:

"Our discussions with you are private. We hope you will feel free to talk openly with us about yourself and your health. Information is not shared with other people without your permission unless we are concerned that someone is in danger."*

*This confidentiality statement is used with permission from Jack Mayer, MD, MPH, Rainbow Pediatrics, Middlebury, VT.

reminded that we want them to begin to make good health decisions, that good decisions require good information, and that our questions are aimed at really understanding them. Children and adolescents are always encouraged to discuss any concerns with their parents, the adults who know them best and, in most families, the people who can best help them find answers and solve problems. But, if young patients prefer to discuss concerns privately with their health care professional, they should be supported and allowed to do so.

The practice's or clinic's policies regarding privacy should be shared and discussed with parents and children by the 7 or 8 Year Visit. At this time, it is appropriate to offer the option of part of the visit without the parent present. Most health care professionals will always excuse the parent from part of the visit by the 12 Year Visit. It is useful to frame confidentiality and privacy as part of the child's increasing self-reliance.

The physical examination always should include an assessment of growth.

- Younger than 2 years: Weight, length, head circumference, and weight-for-length
- Older than 2 years: Weight, height, and BMI[15]

Most health care professionals no longer measure chest circumference. Measurements should be plotted on Centers for Disease Control and Prevention (CDC) growth and BMI-for-age charts, looking for appropriate changes over time. Deviations from normed percentiles require further investigation or anticipatory guidance. Certain immigrant children may not fit the CDC norms, but the growth charts can be used to determine growth patterns.

Children and youth with special health care needs have, or are at risk of, chronic physical, developmental, behavioral, or emotional conditions, including genetic or chromosomal disorders (Box 2). Their growth may be further affected by illness, medication use, congenital anomalies, and impaired motor skills. Assessment of growth is a key component of care for children with special health care needs, and use of CDC growth charts, especially weight and height charts, for early detection of growth trends is important. The CDC also has evaluated reference growth charts for some children with special health care needs, including trisomy 21, achondroplasia, Prader-Willi syndrome, Turner syndrome, and Williams syndrome. Use of these specialized charts may be considered for affected children. Important limitations of these charts are the small sample sizes on which these charts are based, the lack of BMI data, and the risk of underestimating the child's growth potential. It is recommended that these charts be used in conjunction with the standard-reference CDC growth and BMI-for-age charts. The child's growth then can be assessed against that of the general population of children and can be monitored more accurately for inadequate growth or overweight. These CDC charts and guidance regarding their use is available at http://www.cdc.gov/growthcharts/.[16]

Body mass index should be calculated at each visit beginning at age 2 or 3 years, when the measurement of height replaces the measurement of length. (For more information on this topic, see the Promoting Healthy Weight theme.) At earlier visits, when length is measured, the weight-for-length should be plotted on the standard growth chart. Body mass index charting can improve recognition of an underweight or overweight problem, prompt health care professional concerns, and enhance guidance about techniques to promote a healthy weight (Box 3).[17] Enlisting the help of parents in recognizing and addressing a tendency toward overweight is recommended.

At this time, studies do not demonstrate that addressing overweight in younger

BOX 2

Children and Youth With Special Health Care Needs

The care of children and youth with special health care needs requires a dual approach consisting of both (1) screening and ongoing assessment to identify the special health care needs and (2) health supervision and anticipatory guidance.

The first task of a Bright Futures visit is to identify children with special health care needs. Ongoing surveillance over sequential Bright Futures visits, careful attention to parental concerns, and screening allow practitioners to find and diagnose these children. Screening may be structured and generalized to be applicable for all children or it can be specific to address concerns in one child.

The second task emphasizes that children and youth with special health care needs are, of course, children, and they have health care needs like all their peers. Their special health care needs, while important, do not negate their needs for health supervision, identification of strengths, and anticipatory guidance. Immunizations, nutrition and physical activity, screening for vision and hearing, school adjustment, and vehicle or gun safety are only a few of the topics that are important to the health of every child and youth. Sufficient time and attention to identifying and reinforcing youth strengths and their healthy emotional development are key. Through ongoing assessment, the developmental trajectory of an individual child can be plotted and compared, just as height and weight are plotted and compared, and the process of providing care is normalized.

Children and youth with special health care needs can present unique challenges, which often require extended visit time. Subspecialists often are involved in the care of the child or adolescent. The primary health care professional serves as the coordinating hub, but, more importantly, ensures that the focus of care is on the child as a whole, in her family and community, and not simply a child in a disease category. Thus, the primary care visit is used not only for the physical examination but also for discussion of the subspecialists' information and recommendations. Availability and access to needed subspecialty pediatric services vary by community, which affects the scope and intensity of direct care services provided to children and youth with special health care needs and their families by the primary health care professional. The "medical home" approach affords varying levels of shared care between primary care clinicians and subspecialty consultants.

The primary health care professional has a pivotal role in coordinating care for all children and adolescents whether or not they have special health care needs. Subspecialty care provided outside the primary care setting needs to be integrated into the overall health and developmental care plans for the child as a means of ensuring proper follow-up care, appropriate surveillance of the child, and necessary coordination of services for the child and family. It is important to link results of recommended screening and assessments performed by consultants, subspecialists, and allied health care providers to a child's medical home. Integrating all this information is a key role for the generalist as it sustains the parent-clinician partnership that is essential to the care of children with unique medical and developmental challenges.[18]

Child and adolescent health care professionals, who couple clinical observation with careful attention to parental concerns and insights, particularly during crucial developmental stages, competently serve children and youth with special health care needs. The Bright Futures visits support that goal.

BOX 3
Interpreting BMI

Growth Indicator	Anthropometric Indices	Percentile Cutoff
Underweight	Low BMI for age and gender	<5th percentile
Normal	Normal BMI for age and gender	≥5th percentile but <85th percentile
Overweight	High BMI for age and gender	≥85th percentile but <95th percentile
Obese	High BMI for age and gender	≥95th percentile

patients is effective in reducing adult overweight or its consequences.[19] Nonetheless, some populations, such as Native Americans, Mexican Americans, Asian and Pacific Islanders, and non-Hispanic blacks, are at a greater risk of developing overweight than whites. Following BMI curves in these groups may offer long-term benefits.

C5. SCREENING
- Universal Screening
- Selective Screening
  - Risk Assessment
  - Action if Risk Assessment is positive

Recommended screening occurs at each Bright Futures visit. Certain screening is *universal*—it is applied to each child at that visit. Other screening is selective and occurs only if a risk assessment is positive. For example, 1-year-old children are *universally* screened for lead poisoning in most states, but only those children with parental concern are *selectively* screened with a hearing test. Where specific screening tools or tests are indicated, they are noted in the visit.

Screening recommendations were developed by the Expert Panels, the Bright Futures Users' Panel, and other experts, based on the child's age and stage and the visit priorities and derived from the Recommendations for Preventive Pediatric Health Care.[20] Screening tasks were chosen based on available evidence or on expert opinion statements from the Maternal and Child Health Bureau, CDC, AAP, AAFP, NAPNAP, and others. Broad consultation was obtained to achieve consensus.

C6. IMMUNIZATIONS
Assessing the completeness of a child's or adolescent's immunizations is a key element of preventive health services. The value of immunizations in avoiding preventable diseases and disease complications is an important discussion for providers to have with parents.

Bright Futures uses the following sources for up-to-date immunization schedules:

- The CDC National Immunization Program, http://www.cdc.gov/vaccines[21]
- American Academy of Pediatrics *Red Book*, http://www.aapredbook.org[22]

Both sources include professionals' and parents' guides, address evidence behind immunizations, and discuss myths regarding immunization. The CDC National Immunization Information Hotline, http://www.vaccines.ashastd.org (telephone: 800-CDC-INFO) is an additional source of useful information.[23]

See the Recommendations for Preventive Pediatric Health Care in Appendix C.

C7. OTHER PRACTICE-BASED INTERVENTIONS

Two interventions have demonstrated important findings that could affect the health care professional's decisions about what to incorporate in their practice setting.

When health care professionals promote literacy according to the Reach Out and Read (ROR) model, especially to low-income children, studies have demonstrated an effect on parental reports of behavior, beliefs, and attitudes toward reading as well as improvements in language scores.[24,25] Components of the ROR model include anticipatory guidance about the importance of reading, volunteers reading aloud in the waiting rooms, and distribution of developmentally and culturally appropriate books at health supervision visits of children aged 6 months to 5 years.

The Healthy Steps for Young Children program employs practice-based Healthy Step specialists and has shown positive outcomes in parent behavior (less severe discipline) and quality and use of care.[26] Components of the Healthy Steps program include office and home visits, ideas for telephone contact, and special materials keyed to each health supervision visit for young children.

D. Anticipatory Guidance

The Bright Futures Expert Panels have provided extensive detail for anticipatory guidance activities. The breadth of the guidance that a practitioner **could** do does not address what really **can** be done in the context of one visit. Thus, for each visit, anticipatory guidance activities are presented in several ways, including information for health care professionals, sample questions, discussion points, and suggested guidance for parents, children, and youth.

For each visit, anticipatory guidance is organized by the visit's 5 priorities and their component elements (eg, school readiness is a priority for the 4 Year Visit; its component elements are structured learning experiences, opportunities to socialize with other children, fears, and friends). Within each component element of a priority, the anticipatory guidance begins with a brief note for the health care professional. These notes provide a developmental context for the sample questions and guidance that follow, and they may highlight aspects of a topic that are of particular importance for discussion. The sample questions and anticipatory guidance points provide a possible script for discussion and help frame a relevant conversation with the family and child. Though some questions are framed as Ask the Parent, the term "parent" encompasses all types of caregivers who care for and raise children. Health care professionals are encouraged to adjust and enhance the questions and guidance as needed.

Examining Children and Adolescents at Each Stage: Useful Information to Make the Visit Go Smoothly

Infancy

The health care professional should examine the infant in front of the parents so that the parents can ask questions and the health care professional can comment on the physical findings. This is a wonderful opportunity to evaluate parent-infant interactions. During the examination, the health care professional can reinforce positive interactions between infant and parents as well as provide guidance for dealing with upcoming changes in infant development. The neurodevelopmental assessment is an ideal opportunity to discuss developmental milestones. The health care professional can incorporate anticipatory guidance regarding developmental stimulation and injury prevention in a developmental context.

The health care professional can speak about sounds, light, touch (both light and firm), body movement, and position (proprioceptive and vestibular input), while stressing that every baby is unique. The parents need

TABLE 2		

Calming Techniques to Improve Physical Examination Accuracy in 1- to 4-Year-Old Children

Preparation: Read stories about health checkups or health visits before the appointment.

Parent contact: The child sits or lies in the parent's lap or is held chest-to-chest by the parent.

Distraction:

Auditory: Gentle, relaxed, reassuring constant banter from the examiner or parent; singing or music; or nonsense buzzing noises or whispering.

Manual: The child holds a tongue blade in each hand or feels the stethoscope head, holds jingling keys, or brings dolls or toys to the appointment.

Visual: The otoscope is shown to the child while lighting the examiner's palm, then the child's, before the ear examination; or the examiner puts the otoscope into his or her own ear declaring, "See! It's okay! Just a flashlight. Do you have a flashlight at home?"

Demonstration: A doll or stuffed animal is examined before the patient, or the child's shoe is "listened" to with the stethoscope before listening to the patient.

Recruitment: Request the child's help in holding the stethoscope head or tongue blade; "blowing out" the otoscope light; or while listening to the chest, asking the child to blow on a piece of tissue held in front of the mouth to encourage deep breathing.

Comfort measures:

Avoidance of fear-inducing actions: avoid direct looks into the eyes of a young toddler until the eyes are examined; delay invasive portions of the examination (eg, otoscopy) until last; or examine toes or fingers first.

Pleasant office surroundings: books, toys, and pictures or drawings on the walls.

to understand the individual aspects of their baby, which will enable them to comfort and support his development.[27] Approaching the baby's development this way helps parents recognize those very important qualities of the caretaking environment. Demonstrating ways to interact with the infant helps give parents a sense of confidence in making changes to best fit their infant.

Early Childhood

Successfully accomplishing an accurate physical examination of a young child requires both skill and art. An ordered approach to the child as a whole and to each individual organ system reduces the likelihood of missing a problem. Younger children need close contact with a parent to reduce anxiety and ease performance of the examination, whereas older children may take the lead in guiding the health care professional through the examination. Table 2 summarizes some calming techniques to improve cooperation in 1- to 4-year-old children.

Middle Childhood

Middle childhood includes many important milestones for children—learning to read and write, development of important relationships outside the family with friends and teachers, and, for some, the onset of puberty. This is a period of time when lifelong habits that can influence health promotion and disease prevention become established.

The identification of learning barriers and mental health problems are important issues in this age group. Close monitoring of physical health and development are essential for preventive care and the early identification of neurodevelopmental and mental health problems.

In middle childhood, children are developing a growing consciousness about their bodies and may feel uncomfortable without an examination gown or a curtain around the examination table. The child's privacy should be respected.

Adolescence

Adolescence is often thought of as the healthiest age group in the human lifespan. The infectious diseases and developmental issues that constitute the majority of visits to health care professionals during the childhood years are much less common during adolescence, and the chronic illnesses of adulthood are not yet an issue for most adolescents. One exception may be adolescents who recently immigrated to the United States who may have infectious diseases or effects of poor early nutrition and health care.

Despite their relatively good health, adolescents have significant physical issues that require attention on preventive health visits. The significant growth and major hormonal changes that mark the adolescent years, for example, make it necessary to follow growth parameters, including height, weight, and sexual maturity rating,[28] to ensure that they are proceeding appropriately and to watch for the development of possible problems (eg, scoliosis, myopia, or acne) that accompany changes in growth and hormonal milieu.

Other medical issues are related to adolescent health-risk behaviors. Because 47% of adolescents are sexually active,[29] and with a pregnancy rate of 84.5 per 1,000,[30] among female adolescents aged 15 to 19 years, managing sexuality-related issues, including contraception, sexually transmitted infections (STIs), and Pap smear abnormalities, is an important component of adolescent health care. The CDC has estimated that approximately 3 million adolescents acquire an STI each year and that one half of all individuals who acquire STIs are younger than 25 years.[31] An American College of Obstetricians and Gynecologists tool kit helps health care professionals manage these issues in the practice setting.[32]

The health care professional also can help prevent the onset of diseases in adulthood, particularly cardiovascular disease and malignancies. Factors associated with the onset of cardiovascular disease in adults (eg, overweight, hypertension, hyperlipidemia, and cigarette smoking) may have antecedents in the adolescent age group. Screening for these cardiovascular risk factors is increasingly important. With rising levels of overweight and obesity in all age groups, the association between overweight and adult-onset diabetes mellitus in adolescents also has become a major concern. Appropriate Pap smear testing and counseling about sun protection and tobacco use also are important to prevent future malignancies.

References

1. Dworkin PH. Detection of behavioral, developmental, and psychosocial problems in pediatric primary care practice. *Curr Opin Pediatr*. 1993;5:531-536

2. American Academy of Pediatrics, Council on Children With Disabilities, Section on Developmental Behavioral Pediatrics, Bright Futures Steering Committee, and Medical Home Initiatives for Children With Special Needs Project Advisory Committee. Identifying infants and young children with developmental disorders in the medical home: an algorithm for developmental surveillance and screening. *Pediatrics*. 2006;118:405-420

3. Brazelton TB. Symposium on behavioral pediatrics. Anticipatory guidance. *Pediatr Clin North Am*. 1975;22:533-544

4. American Academy of Pediatrics, Division of Health Policy Research. Periodic Survey of Fellows #56. Executive Summary. Pediatricians' Provision of Preventative Care and Use of Health Supervision Guidelines. Elk Grove Village, IL: American Academy of Pediatrics; 2004

5. Green M, Palfrey JS, eds. *Bright Futures: Guidelines for Health Supervision of Infants, Children, and Adolescents*. 2nd ed. Arlington, VA: National Center for Education in Maternal and Child Health; 2002

6. American Medical Association. *Guidelines for Adolescent Preventative Services (GAPS)*. Chicago, IL: American Medical Association; 1994

7. Weed LL. Medical records that guide and teach. *N Engl J Med*. 1968;278:593-600

8. Goldenring J, Rosen D. Getting into adolescent heads: an essential update. *Contemp Pediatr*. 2004;21:64

9. Polisky M. *SOAP for Pediatrics*. Malden, MA: Blackwell Publishing Inc; 2005

10. Sindelar HA, Abrantes AM, Hart C, Lewander W, Spirito A. Motivational interviewing in pediatric practice. *Curr Probl Pediatr Adolesc Health Care*. 2004;34:322-339

11. Prochaska J, Norcross J, DiClemente C. *Changing for Good*. New York, NY: Avon Books Inc; 1994

12. Parents' Evaluation of Developmental Status (PEDS). Available at: http://www.pedstest.com/. Accessed February 25, 2007

13. Bricker D, Squires J, Mounts L, et al. *Ages & Stages Questionnaires (ASQ): A Parent-Completed, Child-Monitoring System*. 2nd ed. Baltimore, MD: Paul H. Brookes Publishing Co; 1999

14. Jellinek M, Patel BP, Froehle MC, eds. *Bright Futures in Practice: Mental Health, Volume II, Toolkit. Pediatric Intake Form*. Arlington, VA: National Center for Education in Maternal and Child Health; 2002

15. Accurately Weighing and Measuring: Technique. Available at: http://depts.washington.edu/growth/module5/text/contents.htm. Accessed April 11, 2006

16. Centers for Disease Control and Prevention. 2000 CDC Growth Charts: United States. Available at: http://www.cdc.gov/growthcharts/. Accessed July 7, 2006

17. Perrin EM, Flower KB, Ammerman AS. Body mass index charts: useful yet underused. *J Pediatr*. 2004;144:455-460

18. American Academy of Pediatrics, Medical Home Initiatives for Children With Special Health Care Needs Project Advisory Committee. The medical home. *Pediatrics*. 2002;110:184-186

19. Saunders N, Shouldice M. Health maintenance visits: a critical review. In: Feldman W, ed. *Evidence-Based Pediatrics*: Hamilton, British Columbia: Decker Inc; 2000:17-37

20. American Academy of Pediatrics, Committee on Practice and Ambulatory Medicine. Recommendations for preventive pediatric health care. *Pediatrics*. 2000;105:645-646

21. Centers for Disease Control and Prevention, National Immunization Program. Available at: http://www.cdc.gov/vaccines/. Accessed July 7, 2006

22. American Academy of Pediatrics. *Red Book: 2006 Report of the Committee on Infectious Diseases*. Pickering LK, Baker CJ, Long SS, McMillan JA, eds. 27th ed. Elk Grove Village, I: American Academy of Pediatrics; 2006.

23. National Immunizations Information Hotline. Available at: http://www.vaccines.ashastd.org. Accessed July 7, 2006

24. Weitzman CC, Roy L, Walls T, Tomlin R. More evidence for Reach Out and Read: a home-based study. *Pediatrics*. 2004;113:1248-1253

25. Needlman R, Silverstein M. Pediatric interventions to support reading aloud: how good is the evidence? *J Dev Behav Pediatr*. 2004;25:352-363

26. Minkovitz CS, Hughart N, Strobino D, et al. A practice-based intervention to enhance quality of care in the first 3 years of life: the Healthy Steps for Young Children Program. *JAMA*. 2003;290:3081-3091

27. Greenspan S, Greenspan N. First Feelings: *Milestones in the Emotional Development of Your Baby and Child*. New York, NY: Penguin Books USA Inc; 1985

28. Rosen DS. Physiologic growth and development during adolescence. *Pediatr Rev*. 2004;25:194-200

29. Centers for Disease Control and Prevention. Youth Risk Behavior Surveillance—United States, 2005. *MMWR Surveill Summ 2006*. 2006;55(SS-5):1-108

30. Hamilton BE, Martin JA, Ventura SJ. Births: preliminary data for 2005. *Natl Vital Stat Rep*. 2006;55:1-18

31. Centers for Disease Control and Prevention. *Sexually Transmitted Disease, Surveillance, 2005. Special Focus Profiles*. Atlanta, GA: Centers for Disease Control and Prevention, US Department of Health and Human Services; 2006

32. American College of Obstetricians and Gynecologists Web site. Available at: http://www.acog.org/. Accessed May 24, 2007

Rationale and Evidence

Introduction

Health supervision of an *individual* child is a complex package of services that takes place over the child's lifetime. It includes not only preventive and screening interventions that are recommended for all children, but also addresses the particular needs of that child in the context of family and community. Studying the outcomes over a child's lifetime of health supervision at this level of integration can be a daunting task.

Evidence for effectiveness was a core criterion for including, or excluding, certain interventions in child health supervision in the *Bright Futures Guidelines*. However, it probably would be more accurate to describe this edition of the Guidelines as evidence informed rather than fully evidence driven. The most salient barrier to evidence-driven health supervision is that our evidence is incomplete. For many interventions that are commonly performed in child or adolescent care, no, or few, properly constructed studies have been done that link the intervention with intended health outcomes. Absent evidence does not demonstrate a lack of usefulness, however. The lack of evidence of effectiveness most often simply reflects the lack of study. Filling in the gaps in evidence is highly desirable, and additional research is strongly encouraged.

Approach Used to Develop the Bright Futures Recommendations

The Bright Futures Steering Committee used 3 approaches to develop the guidance and recommendations that are contained in this edition of the *Bright Futures Guidelines.*

- Multidisciplinary Expert Panels were convened to write recommendations for Bright Futures visit priorities, the physical examination, anticipatory guidance, immunizations, and universal and selective screening topics for each age and stage of development. In carrying out this task, the Expert Panels were charged with examining the evidence for each recommendation, and evidence was an important consideration in the guidance they provided. However, lack of evidence was particularly problematic for the physical examination (the elements of which can be considered screening interventions) and for counseling interventions. For these components, the Expert Panels relied on an indirect approach buttressed by their considerable expertise and clinical experience.

- A Bright Futures Evidence Panel, composed of consultants who are experts in finding and evaluating evidence from clinical studies, was convened to examine studies and systematic evidence reviews and to develop a method of informing readers about the strength of the evidence.

The Evidence Panel conducted literature searches for key questions using the MEDLINE® database of the National Library of Medicine. Key themes were searched in the Medical Subject Headings (MeSH) database to determine the most appropriate search terms. Searches were limited to clinical trials, meta-analyses, and randomized controlled trials. Other limits included English language and designations for age, when appropriate. Standardized terms were used for counseling (ie, counseling, primary prevention, health promotion, health education, and patient education) and for screening (ie, mass screening and risk assessment). The Evidence Panel also used the systematic evidence reviews performed for the United States Preventive Services Task Force (USPSTF) and the Cochrane Collaboration. This approach was, by no means, exhaustive, but it did provide a sound assessment of the most relevant literature. The Evidence Panel's statements are found at the end of this chapter.

- Throughout the Guidelines development process, the Project Advisory Committee and Expert Panels consulted with individuals and organizations with expertise and experience in a wide range of topic areas. The entire Guidelines document also underwent public review twice in 2004 and once in 2006. More than 1,000 reviewers, representing national organizations concerned with infant,

child, and adolescent health and welfare, provided nearly 3,500 comments. The contributions of these reviewers provided a valuable opportunity to refine the guidelines and strengthen the scientific base for the guidance provided.

The result of these efforts is the third edition of the *Bright Futures Guidelines.* Unless a contraindication or extenuating circumstance exists, infants, children, and adolescents should receive mandated services and applicable services for which the evidence is strong. For those interventions that do not yet have supporting evidence, the health care professional who uses the *Bright Futures Guidelines* is guided by clinical experience, knowledge of the needs of the individual child, expert opinion that reflects recommendations from professional associations, and local practice.

The remainder of this chapter provides details on the evidence and science used to support the recommendations in the third edition of the *Bright Futures Guidelines.* The first section presents the rationale for certain Bright Futures recommendations. The second section presents the detailed findings of the Bright Futures Evidence Panel.

RATIONALE

The following section presents the scientific rationales used by the Expert Panels to craft Bright Futures recommendations, including some aspects of the physical examination, practice-based interventions, and universal and selective screening activities. These rationales were taken from policy statements and published reviews of the American Academy of Pediatrics (AAP) and other national organizations, and articles from the literature. Primary sources for each rationale are cited.

Physical Examination
Rationale for the Physical Examination

To help health care professionals prioritize aspects of the physical examination in the preventive services visit, health care professionals are alerted to the following USPSTF recommendations about cervical, breast, and testicular cancer screening and scoliosis screening. These recommendations do not preclude or preempt actions a health care professional may decide to take during a health supervision physical examination of a particular child.

The USPSTF strongly recommends **for:**

- Screening for cervical cancer in women who have been sexually active and have a cervix.

  Screening should begin within 3 years of onset of sexual activity or age 21, whichever comes first.[1] The USPSTF found "good evidence from multiple observational studies that screening with cervical cytology (Pap smears) reduces incidence of and mortality from cervical cancer.

  Direct evidence to determine the optimal starting and stopping age and interval for screening is limited. Indirect evidence suggests most of the benefit can be obtained by beginning screening

within 3 years of onset of sexual activity or age 21 (whichever comes first) and screening at least every 3 years). The USPSTF concludes that the benefits of screening substantially outweigh potential harms."

The USPSTF concludes that the **evidence is insufficient** to recommend for or against:

- Routine clinical breast examination (CBE) alone to screen for breast cancer[2]

  The USPSTF states that "no screening trial has examined the benefits of CBE alone (without accompanying mammography) compared to no screening, and design characteristics limit the generalizability of studies that have examined CBE. The USPSTF could not determine the benefits of CBE alone or the incremental benefit of adding CBE to mammography. The USPSTF, therefore, could not determine whether potential benefits of routine CBE outweigh the potential harms."

- Teaching or performing routine breast self-examination (BSE)

  The USPSTF "found poor evidence to determine whether BSE reduces breast cancer mortality. The USPSTF found fair evidence that BSE is associated with an increased risk for false-positive results and biopsies. Due to design limitations of published and ongoing studies of BSE, the USPSTF could not determine the balance of benefits and potential harms of BSE.".

  The American Cancer Society recommends that, for average-risk asymptomatic women in their 20s and 30s, CBE be part of a periodic health examination, preferably every 3 years.[3]

The USPSTF recommends **against:**

- Routine screening for testicular cancer.

  The USPSTF found no evidence "that screening with clinical examination or testicular self-examination is effective in reducing mortality from testicular cancer."[4] It further states that, "currently most testicular carcinomas are discovered by patients themselves…unintentionally or by self-examination," but recommends against clinician-taught self-examination as unnecessary screening.

- Routine screening of asymptomatic adolescents for idiopathic scoliosis.

  "The USPSTF did not find good evidence that screening asymptomatic adolescents detects idiopathic scoliosis at an earlier age than detection without screening."[5]

The complete physical examination remains a core element of disease detection and prevention. Health care professionals must individualize these recommendations for their patients. For example, pelvic examinations are often indicated in adolescent females for abnormal bleeding or dysmenorrhea. Breast examinations are employed to determine sexual maturity rating. In adolescent males, health care professionals perform testicular examinations for hernia, varicocele or epididymitis. The USPSTF warns that "clinicians should be aware of testicular cancer as a possible diagnosis."

The back is routinely inspected in all patients, with special attention to curvature during the adolescent growth spurt.[6] The USPSTF scoliosis screening statement notes that "clinicians should be prepared to evaluate idiopathic scoliosis when discovered incidentally."[5]

Therefore, the *Bright Futures Guidelines* recommend a complete physical examination, counseling, and screening as part of every health supervision visit.

Practice-based Intervention
Rationale for Practice-based Interventions

Two interventions have demonstrated important findings that could affect the health care professional's decisions about what to incorporate in their practice setting.

REACH OUT AND READ
When health care professionals promote literacy according to the Reach Out and Read (ROR) model, especially to low-income children, studies have demonstrated an effect on parental behavior, beliefs, and attitudes toward reading aloud, as well as improvements in the language scores of young children receiving the intervention. Components of the ROR model include anticipatory guidance about the importance of reading, volunteers reading aloud in waiting rooms, and distribution of developmentally and culturally appropriate books at health supervision visits of children ages 6 months to 5 years.[7,8]

HEALTHY STEPS
The Healthy Steps for Young Children program (http://www.healthysteps.org) employs practice-based Healthy Steps specialists and has shown positive outcomes in parent behavior (less severe discipline) and quality and use of care. Components of the Healthy Steps program include office and home visits, ideas for telephone contact, and special materials keyed to each health supervision visit.[9]

Universal Screening

Rationale for Universal Medical Screening

Medical screening occurs at each Bright Futures Visit. Screening may be universal, meaning that it is performed for every child at a particular visit. For example, developmental and autism screening at 18 months of age are universal screens. Other screening is selective, based on positive findings from a risk assessment. (See the following section, Rationale for Selective Medical Screening.)

For each universal screening test that is recommended in this edition of the *Bright Futures Guidelines,* we provide, in this chapter, a rationale table that presents the health supervision visits at which the screening should take place, the scientific statement upon which our recommendation is based, and the primary supporting reference. The scientific statements are taken directly from these supporting references. The rationale tables are linked to the Medical Screening tables that are found in each of the Bright Futures Visits. The tables in the Visits contain specific information about the screening test, including the action to be taken.

Newborn Metabolic and Hemoglobinopathy

BRIGHT FUTURES VISITS:	NEWBORN, FIRST WEEK; 1, 2 MONTH
Rationale:	Universal newborn screening is an essential public health responsibility that is critical for improving the health outcomes of affected children.
Citation:	American College of Medical Genetics, Newborn Screening Expert Group. Newborn screening: toward a uniform screening panel and system—executive summary. *Pediatrics.* 2006;117:296-307 (p 298)

Development

BRIGHT FUTURES VISITS:	9, 18 MONTH; 2½ YEAR
Rationale:	**Article Covers Ages: Birth Through 3 years** All children, most of whom will not have identifiable risks or whose development appears to be proceeding typically, should receive periodic developmental screening using a standardized test. In the absence of established risk factors or parental or provider concerns, a general developmental screen is recommended at the 9-, 18-, and 30-month visits. These recommended ages for developmental screening are suggested only as a starting point for children who appear to be developing normally; surveillance should continue throughout childhood, and screenings should be conducted anytime that concerns are raised by parents, child health professionals, or others involved in the care of the child.
Citation:	American Academy of Pediatrics, Council on Children With Disabilities, Section on Developmental Behavioral Pediatrics, Bright Futures Steering Committee and Medical Home Initiatives for Children With Special Needs Project Advisory Committee. Identifying infants and young children with developmental disorders in the medical home: an algorithm for developmental surveillance and screening. *Pediatrics.* 2006;118:405-420 (pp 409, 414)

Universal Screening

Autism

BRIGHT FUTURES VISITS:	18 MONTH, 24 MONTH
Rationale:	**Article Covers Ages: 18 to 24 months** The AAP has recommended administering autism-specific screening tool at the 18-month preventative care visit (in addition to a general developmental screening tool).
Citation:	Council on Children With Disabilities, Section on Developmental Behavioral Pediatrics, Bright Futures Steering Committee and Medical Home Initiatives for Children With Special Needs Project Advisory Committee. Identifying infants and young children with developmental disorders in the medical home: an algorithm for developmental surveillance and screening. *Pediatrics.* 2006;118:405-420
Rationale:	The policy statement recommends surveillance for developmental problems at all well-child preventative care visits and routine screening with a general screening tool at the 9-, 18-, and 30-month visits, plus screening with an autism-specific tool at the age of 18 months. ...[S]creening with an autism-specific screening tool should be repeated at the age of 24 months or at any encounter when a parent raises concern.
Citation:	Gupta VB, Hyman SL, Johnson CP, et al. Identifying children with autism early? *Pediatrics.* 2007;119:152-153

Oral Health

BRIGHT FUTURES VISITS:	6, 9 MONTH
Rationale:	**Article Covers Ages: 6 to 12 months** Referral by the primary care physician or health provider has been recommended, based on risk assessment, as early as 6 months of age, 6 months after the first tooth erupts, and no later than 12 months of age.
Citation:	American Academy of Pediatric Dentistry Council on Clinical Affairs. Policy on the dental home. In: *Oral Health Policies Reference Manual 2005-2006.* Chicago, IL: American Academy of Pediatric Dentistry; 2004:18-19. Available at: http://www.aapd.org/media/Policies_Guidelines/P_DentalHome.pdf. Accessed April 25, 2007
Citation:	Casamassimo P, Holt K, eds. *Bright Futures in Practice: Oral Health—Pocket Guide.* Washington, DC: National Maternal and Child Oral Health Resource Center; 2004

Vision

BRIGHT FUTURES VISITS:	3, 4, 5 YEAR
Rationale:	**Article Covers Ages: Preschool children** The USPSTF recommends screening to detect amblyopia, strabismus, and defects in visual acuity in children younger than age 5 years. Traditional vision testing requires a cooperative, verbal child and cannot be performed reliably until ages 3 to 4 years.
Citation:	US Preventive Services Task Force. Screening for Visual Impairment in Children Younger Than Age 5 Years: Recommendation Statement. Rockville, MD: Agency for Healthcare Research and Quality; 2004, Available at: http://www.ahrq.gov/clinic/3rduspstf/visionscr/vischrs.htm. Accessed April 25, 2007
BRIGHT FUTURES VISITS:	6, 8, 10 YEAR, AND ONCE DURING EACH PERIOD OF EARLY, MIDDLE, AND LATE ADOLESCENCE
Rationale:	**Article Covers Ages: 3 years and older** • Age appropriate visual acuity measurement • Attempt at opthalmoscopy
Citation:	American Academy of Pediatrics Committee on Practice and Ambulatory Medicine, Section on Ophthalmology, American Association of Certified Orthoptists, American Association for Pediatric Ophthalmology and Strabismus, and American Academy of Ophthalmology. Eye examination in infants, children, and young adults by pediatricians. *Pediatrics.* 2003;111:902-907 (p 902)

Hearing

BRIGHT FUTURES VISITS:	NEWBORN, FIRST WEEK; 1, 2 MONTH; 4, 5, 6, 8, 10 YEAR
Rationale:	**Article Covers Ages: Newborn and Infant** The American Academy of Pediatrics supports the statement of the Joint Committee on Infant Hearing (1994), which endorses the goal of universal detection of hearing loss in infants before 3 months of age, with appropriate intervention no later than 6 months of age. Universal detection of infant hearing loss requires universal screening of all infants.
Citation:	American Academy of Pediatrics, Task Force on Newborn and Infant Hearing. Newborn and infant hearing loss: detection and intervention. *Pediatrics.* 1999;103:527-530
Rationale:	**Article Covers Ages: Beyond Neonatal to Adolescence** The AAP promotes objective newborn hearing screening as well as periodic hearing screening for every child through adolescence.
Citation:	Cunningham M, Cox EO, American Academy of Pediatrics, Committee on Practice and Ambulatory Medicine, Section on Otolaryngology and Bronchoesophagology. Hearing assessment in infants and children: recommendations beyond neonatal screening. *Pediatrics.* 2003;111:436-440 (p436)
Citation:	American Academy of Pediatrics, Committee on Practice and Ambulatory Medicine. Recommendations for preventive pediatric health care. *Pediatrics.* 2000;105:645-646

Universal Screening

Anemia

BRIGHT FUTURES VISITS:	12 MONTH
Rationale:	**Section in Book Covers Ages through 12 months** Initial measurement of hemoglobin or hematocrit for all full-term infants between 9 and 12 months of age.
Citation:	American Academy of Pediatrics, Committee on Nutrition. Iron deficency. In: Kleinman RE, ed. *Pediatric Nutrition Handbook*. 5th ed. Elk Grove Village, IL: American Academy of Pediatrics; 2004:299-312 (p 309)

Lead

BRIGHT FUTURES VISITS:	12 MONTH, 2 YEAR (HIGH PREVALENCE AREA OR MEDICAID)
Rationale:	**Article Covers Ages: 9 to 72 months** Universal screening was recommended for children 9 to 72 months of age except in communities with sufficient data to conclude that children would not be at risk of exposure. To prevent lead poisoning, lead screening should begin at 9 to 12 months of age and be considered again at ~24 months of age when blood lead levels (BLLs) peak. In communities where universal screening is recommended, pediatricians should follow this recommendation. In communities where targeted screening is recommended, pediatricians should determine whether each young patient is at risk and screen when necessary.
Citation:	American Academy of Pediatrics, Committee on Environmental Health. Screening for elevated blood lead levels. *Pediatrics*. 1998;101:1072-1078 (p 1072, 1076)

Dyslipidemia

BRIGHT FUTURES VISITS:	OLDER ADOLESCENTS
Rationale:	**Article Covers Ages: Older Adolescents and Adults (Age 20 and above)** In all adults aged 20 years or older, a fasting lipoprotein profile (total cholesterol, LDL cholesterol, high density lipoprotein [HDL] cholesterol and triglyceride) should be obtained once every 5 years.
Citation:	Third Report of the National Cholesterol Education Program (NCEP) Expert Panel on Detection, Evaluation, and Treatment of High Blood Cholesterol in Adults (Adult Treatment Panel III) final report. *Circulation*. 2002;106:3143-3421 (p 3200)

Selective Screening
Rationale for Selective Medical Screening

Selective medical screening is performed if risk assessment is positive. For example, tuberculosis screening is performed selectively. For each selective screening test that is recommended in this edition of the *Bright Futures Guidelines,* we provide a rationale table that presents the health supervision visit at which the screening should take place, the risk assessment criteria that should be used to determine whether to conduct the screen, and the primary supporting reference from the literature (consensus, evidence informed, or evidence based). The scientific statements are taken directly from these supporting references.

The following rationale tables are linked to the Medical Screening tables found in each of the Bright Futures Visits. The tables in the Visits contain additional specific information about the screening test, including the criteria for testing and the action to be taken.

Oral Health (Dental Home)

BRIGHT FUTURES VISITS:	12, 18 MONTH; 2, 2½, 3, 6 YEAR
Rationale:	**Article Covers Ages: 6 to 12 months** Referral by the primary care physician or health provider has been recommended, based on risk assessment, as early as 6 months of age, 6 months after the first tooth erupts, and no later than 12 months of age.
Citation:	American Academy of Pediatric Dentistry, Council on Clinical Affairs. Policy on the dental home. In: *Oral Health Policies Reference Manual 2005-2006*. Chicago, IL: American Academy of Pediatric Dentistry; 2004. Available at: http://www.aapd.org/media/Policies_Guidelines/P_DentalHome.pdf. Accessed April 25, 2007
Citation:	Casamassimo P, Holt K, eds. *Bright Futures in Practice: Oral Health—Pocket Guide.* Washington, DC: National Maternal and Child Oral Health Resource Center; 2004

Oral Health (Fluoride)

BRIGHT FUTURES VISITS:	12, 18 MONTH; 2, 2½, 3, 6 YEAR
Rationale:	**Article Covers Ages: Older than 6 months** The US Preventive Services Task Force (USPSTF) recommends that primary care clinicians prescribe oral fluoride supplementation at currently recommended doses to preschool children older than 6 months of age whose primary water source is deficient in fluoride.
Citation:	US Preventive Services Task Force. Prevention of Dental Caries in Preschool Children: Recommendations and Rationale. Rockville, MD. Agency for Healthcare Research and Quality; 2004. Available at: http://www.ahrq.gov/clinic/3rduspstf/dentalchild/dentchrs.htm. Accessed April 25, 2007
Rationale:	Systemic fluoride intake via optimal fluoridation of drinking water or professionally prescribed supplements is recommended to 16 years of age or the eruption of the second permanent molars, whichever comes first.
Citation:	American Academy of Pediatric Dentistry. *Clinical Guideline on Adolescent Oral Health Care: Reference Manual.* Chicago, IL: American Academy of Pediatric Dentistry; 2005

**Selective
Screening**

Blood Pressure

BRIGHT FUTURES VISITS:	ALL VISITS OF CHILDREN YOUNGER THAN AGE 3 YEARS (THIS SCREEN BECOMES A COMPONENT OF THE ANNUAL PHYSICAL EXAMINATION AT AGE 3 YEARS.)
Rationale:	• History of prematurity, very low birth weight, or other neonatal complication requiring intensive care • Congenital heart disease (repaired or nonrepaired) • Recurrent urinary tract infections, hematuria or proteinuria • Known renal disease or urologic malformations • Family history of congenital renal disease • Solid-organ transplant • Malignancy or bone marrow transplant • Treatment with drugs known to raise blood pressure • Other systemic illnesses associated with hypertension (neurofibromatosis, tuberous sclerosis etc) • Evidence of increased elevated intracranial pressure
Citation:	National High Blood Pressure Education Program Working Group on High Blood Pressure in Children and Adolescents. The fourth report on the diagnosis, evaluation, and treatment of high blood pressure in children and adolescents. *Pediatrics.* 2004;114;555-576 (p 556)

Vision

BRIGHT FUTURES VISITS:	NEWBORN, FIRST WEEK; 1, 2, 4, 6, 9, 12, 15, 18 MONTH; 2, 2½, 7, 9; AND ADOLESCENTS (11 TO 21 YEAR VISITS)
Rationale:	**Article covers ages: All ages** Children should have an assessment for eye problems in the newborn period and then at all subsequent routine health supervision visits. These should be age-appropriate evaluations.... Infants and children at high risk of eye problems should be referred for specialized eye examination by an ophthalmologist experienced in treating children. This includes children who are very premature; those with family histories of congenital cataracts, retinoblastoma, and metabolic or genetic diseases; those who have significant developmental delay or neurologic difficulties; and those with systematic diseases associated with eye abnormalities. **Birth to age 3 years** Eye evaluation should include: • Ocular history • Vision assessment • External inspection of the eyes and lids • Ocular motility assessment • Pupil examination • Red reflex examination Ocular history: Parents observations are valuable. Questions that can be asked include: • Does your child seem to see well? • Does your child hold objects close to his or her face when trying to focus? • Do your child's eyes appear straight or do they seem to cross or drift or seem lazy? • Do your child's eyes appear unusual? • Do your child's eyelids droop or does 1 eyelid tend to close? • Have your child's eye(s) ever been injured? Relevant family histories regarding eye disorders or preschool or early childhood use of glasses in parents or siblings should be explored. **3 years and older** Above criteria, plus: • Age appropriate visual acuity measurement • Attempt at opthalmoscopy
Citation:	American Academy of Pediatrics, Committee on Practice and Ambulatory Medicine; Section on Ophthalmology, American Association of Certified Orthoptists; American Association for Pediatric Ophthalmology and Strabismus; and American Academy of Ophthalmology. Eye examination in infants, children, and young adults by pediatricians. *Pediatrics.* 2003;111:902-907 (p 902)
BRIGHT FUTURES VISITS:	7, 9 YEAR; ADOLESCENTS (11 TO 21 YEAR VISITS — WHEN UNIVERSAL SCREENING IS NOT PERFORMED)
Rationale:	**Article covers ages: 3 years and older** In addition, the following may be indicative of myopia: • Complaint that the classroom blackboard has become difficult to see • Failure to pass a school vision screening test • Holds toys or books close to the eyes • Difficulty recognizing faces at a distance • Tend to squint
Citation:	Greenwald MJ. Refractive abnormalities in childhood. *Pediatr Clin N Am.* 2003;50:197-212 (p 200-201)

Selective Screening

Hearing

BRIGHT FUTURES VISITS:	4, 6, 12, 15, 18 MONTH; 2, 2½ YEAR
Rationale:	**Article Covers Ages: Birth to age 2 years** • Caregiver concern* regarding hearing, speech, language or developmental delay • Family history* of permanent childhood hearing loss • Neonatal intensive care of >5 days, which may include extracorporeal membrane oxygenation* (ECMO) assisted ventilation, exposure to ototoxic medications (gentamycin and tobramycin) or loop diuretics (furosemide/lasix), and hyperbilirubinemia requiring exchange transfusion • In-utero infections such as cytomegalovirus,* herpes, rubella, syphilis, and toxoplasmosis • Craniofacial anomalies, including those involving the pinna, ear canal, ear tags, ear pits, and temporal bone anomalies • Physical findings such as white forelock, associated with a syndrome known to include a sensorineural or permanent conductive hearing loss • Syndromes associated with hearing loss or progressive or late onset hearing loss* such as neurofibromatosis, osteopetrosis, and Usher's syndrome. Other frequently identified syndromes include Waardenburg, Alport, Pendred, and Jervell and Lange-Nielson • Neurodegenerative disorders,* such as Hunter syndrome, or sensory motor neuropathies, such as Friedreich's ataxia and Charcot-Marie-Tooth syndrome • Culture positive postnatal infections associated with sensorineural hearing loss,* including confirmed bacterial and viral (especially herpes viruses and varicella) meningitis • Head trauma, especially basal skull/temporal bone fracture* requiring hospitalization • Chemotherapy* *Risk indicators that are marked with an asterisk are of greater concern for delayed onset hearing loss. The Joint Committee on Infant Hearing (JCIH) recognizes that an optimal surveillance and screening program within the medical home would include the following: • At each visit consistent with the AAP periodicity schedule, infants should be monitored for auditory skills, middle ear status, and developmental milestones (surveillance). Concerns during surveillance should be followed by administration of a validated global screening tool. A validated global screening tool is administered at 9, 18, and 24-30 months to all infants, or sooner, if there is physician or parental concern about hearing or language. • Infants who do not pass the speech-language portion of the global screen in the medical home or if there is caregiver concern about hearing or spoken language development should be referred immediately for further evaluation by an audiologist and a speech language pathologist for a speech and language evaluation with validated tools. • A careful assessment of middle ear status (pneumatic otoscopy and/or tympanometry) should be completed at all well-child visits, and children with persistent middle ear effusion ≥3 months should be referred for otologic evaluation.
Citation:	Joint Committee on Infant Hearing. Year 2007 position statement: principles and guidelines for early hearing detection and intervention programs. *Pediatrics.* 2007;120:898-921

Hearing (continued)

BRIGHT FUTURES VISITS:	ADOLESCENTS (11 TO 21 YEAR VISITS)
Rationale:	**Article Covers Ages: Older children and adults** • Do you have a problem hearing over the telephone? • Do you have trouble following the conversation when two or more people are talking at the same time? • Do people complain that you turn the TV volume up too high? • Do you have to strain to understand conversation? • Do you have trouble hearing in a noisy background? • Do you find yourself asking people to repeat themselves? • Do many people you talk to seem to mumble (or not speak clearly)? • Do you misunderstand what others are saying and respond inappropriately? • Do you have trouble understanding the speech of women and children? • Do people get annoyed because you misunderstand what they say?
Citation:	National Institute on Deafness and Other Communication Disorders. *Ten Ways to Recognize Hearing Loss.* Bethesda, MD: National Institute of Health; 2006. NIH Publication No 01-4913. Available at: http://www.nidcd.nih.gov/health/hearing/10ways.asp. Accessed April 25, 2007

Anemia

BRIGHT FUTURES VISITS:	4, 18 MONTH; ANNUALLY BEGINNING WITH 2 YEAR VISIT
Rationale:	**4 Month Visit** • Prematurity • Low birth weight • Use of low-iron formula or infants not receiving iron-fortified formula • Early introduction of cow milk **18 Month; 2, 3, 4, 5 Year Visits** • At risk of iron deficiency because of special health needs • Low-iron diet (eg, nonmeat diet) • Environmental factors (eg, poverty, limited access to food)
Citation:	American Academy of Pediatrics, Committee on Nutrition. Iron deficiency. In: Kleinman RE, ed. *Pediatric Nutrition Handbook.* Elk Grove Village, IL: American Academy of Pediatrics; 2004:299-312 (p 309)
Rationale:	**6 to 10 Year Visits** • Children who consume a strict vegetarian diet and are not receiving an iron supplement
Citation:	American Academy of Pediatrics, Committee on Nutrition. Iron deficiency. In: Kleinman RE, ed. *Pediatric Nutrition Handbook.* Elk Grove Village, IL: American Academy of Pediatrics; 2004:299-312 (p 310)
Rationale:	**Adolescents (11 to 21 Year Visits)** • Starting in adolescence, screen all nonpregnant women for anemia every 5 to 10 years throughout their childbearing years during routine health examinations. • Annually screen for anemia women having risk factors for iron deficiency (eg, extensive menstrual or other blood loss, low iron intake, or a previous diagnosis of iron-deficiency anemia).
Citation:	Centers for Disease Control and Prevention. Recommendations to prevent and control iron deficiency in the United States. *MMWR Recomm Rep.* 1998;47(RR-3):1-36 (p 29)

RATIONALE AND EVIDENCE

**Selective
Screening**

Lead

BRIGHT FUTURES VISITS:	6, 9 MONTH; 12 MONTH (LOW PREVALENCE, NOT ON MEDICAID); 18 MONTH; 2 YEAR (LOW PREVALENCE, NOT ON MEDICAID); 3, 4, 5, 6 YEAR
Rationale:	**Article Covers Ages: Article recommends for children 9 to 72 months** • Does your child live in or regularly visit a house or child care facility built before 1950? • Does your child live in or regularly visit a house or child care facility built before 1978 that is being or has recently been renovated or remodeled (within the last 6 months)? • Does your child have a sibling or playmate who has or did have lead poisoning?
Citation:	American Academy of Pediatrics, Committee on Environmental Health. Screening for elevated blood lead levels. *Pediatrics.* 1998;101:1072-1078 (p 1074)
Rationale:	Local practitioners should work with state, county, local health authorities to develop sensitive, customized questions appropriate to the housing and hazards encountered locally.
Citation:	American Academy of Pediatrics, Committee on Environmental Health. Lead exposure in children: prevention, detection, and management. *Pediatrics.* 2005;116:1036-1046 (p 1043)
Rationale:	The Centers for Disease Control and Prevention recommends blood lead testing for all refugee children who are 6 months to 16 years old upon entering the United States. Repeat BLL testing of all refugee children who are 6 months to 6 years of age, 3 to 6 months after they are placed in permanent residences, should be considered a "medical necessity," regardless of initial test results.
Citation:	Centers for Disease Control and Prevention. CDC Lead Poisoning Prevention and Treatment Recommendations for Refugee Children. In: *Lead Poisoning Prevention in Newly Arrived Refugee Children: Tool Kit.* Atlanta, GA: Centers for Disease Control and Prevention; 2006

Tuberculosis

BRIGHT FUTURES VISITS:	1, 6, 12, 18 MONTH; ANNUALLY BEGINNING AT THE 2 YEAR VISIT
Rationale:	**Article Covers Ages: All ages** Children who should have annual Tuberculin Skin Test: • Children infected with HIV • Incarcerated adolescents Validated Questions for Determining Risk of Latent Tuberculosis Infection in Children in the United States • Has a family member or contact had tuberculosis disease? • Has a family member had a positive tuberculin skin test? • Was your child born in a high-risk country (countries other than the United States, Canada, Australia, New Zealand, or Western European countries)? • Has your child traveled (had contact with resident populations) to a high-risk country for more than 1 week?
Citation:	American Academy of Pediatrics. Tuberculosis. In: Pickering LK, Baker CJ, Long SS, McMillan JA, eds. *Red Book: 2006 Report of the Committee on Infectious Diseases.* 27th ed. Elk Grove Village, IL: American Academy of Pediatrics; 2006:678-698 (p 683-684)

Dyslipidemia

BRIGHT FUTURES VISITS:	2, 4, 6, 8, 10 YEAR; ADOLESCENTS (11 TO 21 YEAR VISITS — WHEN UNIVERSAL SCREENING IS NOT PERFORMED)

Rationale:	**Article Covers Ages: 2 to 18 years**
	
	• Screen children and adolescents whose parents or grandparents, at ≤55 years of age, underwent diagnostic coronary arteriography and were found to have coronary atherosclerosis. This includes those who have undergone balloon angioplasty or coronary artery bypass surgery.
	
	• Screen children and adolescents whose parents or grandparents, at ≤55 years of age, had a documented myocardial infarction, angina pectoris, peripheral vascular disease, cerebrovascular disease, or sudden cardiac death.
	
	• Screen the offspring of a parent with an elevated blood cholesterol level (240 mg/dL or higher).
	
	• For children and adolescents whose parental history is unobtainable, particularly for those with other risk factors, physicians may choose to measure cholesterol levels to identify those in need of nutritional and medical advice.
	
	• Optional cholesterol testing by participating physicians may be appropriate for children who are judged to be at a higher risk for coronary heart disease independent of family history. For example, adolescents who smoke, consume excessive of saturated fats and cholesterol, or are overweight.
	
	• Other risk factors that contribute to earlier onset of coronary heart disease:
	  • Family history of premature coronary heart disease, cerebrovascular disease, or occlusive peripheral vascular disease (definite onset before age of 55 years in siblings, parent, or sibling of parent)
	  • Cigarette smoking
	  • Elevated blood pressure
	  • Diabetes mellitus
	  • Physical inactivity

Citation:	American Academy of Pediatrics, Committee on Nutrition. Cholesterol in childhood. *Pediatrics.* 1998;101:141-147 (p 143-145)

Rationale:	**Article Covers Ages: 2 to 18 years**
	
	The Expert Committee recommends that the following laboratory tests be considered in the evaluation of a child identified as overweight or obese:
	  • If the BMI for age and sex is 85th to 94th percentile (overweight) with no risk factors: fasting lipid profile (FLP)
	  • If the BMI for age and sex is 85th to 94th with risk factors in history or physical exam obtain in addition: aspartate aminotransferase (AST) and alanine aminotransferase (ALT), fasting glucose
	  • If the BMI for age and sex is greater than the 95th percentile (obese), even in the absence of risk factors: AST, ALT, plus blood urea nitrogen (BUN) and creatinine

Citation:	The Expert Committee Recommendations on the assessment, prevention, and treatment of child and adolescent overweight and obesity. Supplement to *Pediatrics.* In press

**Selective
Screening**

Chlamydia

BRIGHT FUTURES VISITS:	ADOLESCENTS (11 TO 21 YEAR VISITS), IF SEXUALLY ACTIVE
Rationale:	**Article Covers Age: Sexually active youth** The USPSTF strongly recommends that clinicians routinely screen all sexually active women aged 25 years or younger, and other asymptomatic women at increased risk for infection, for chlamydial infection.
Citation:	US Preventive Services Task Force. *Screening for Chlamydial Infection: Recommendations and Rationale.* Rockville MD: Agency for Healthcare Research and Quality; 2001. Available at: http://www.ahrq.gov/clinic/ajpmsuppl/chlarr.htm. Accessed April 25, 2007 (Article originally in *Am J Prev Med.* 2001;20:90-94)
Rationale:	Sexually active adolescent females should be tested at least annually for chlamydia infection during preventative health care visits and gynecologic examinations, even if no symptoms are present and even if barrier contraception is reported. Screening of young adult women 20 to 24 years of age also is recommended.
Citation:	American Academy of Pediatrics. Chlamydia trachomatis. *Red Book: 2006 Report of the Committee on Infectious Diseases.* Pickering LK, Baker CJ, Long SS, McMillan JA, eds. 27th ed. Elk Grove Village, IL: American Academy of Pediatrics; 2006:252-257

Gonorrhea

BRIGHT FUTURES VISITS:	ADOLESCENTS (11 TO 21 YEAR VISITS), IF SEXUALLY ACTIVE
Rationale:	**Age: Sexually active youth** The USPSTF recommends that clinicians screen all sexually active women, including those who are pregnant, for gonorrhea infection if they are at increased risk for infection (that is, if they are young or have other individual or population risk factors).
Citation:	US Preventive Services Task Force. *Screening for Gonorrhea: Recommendation Statement.* Rockville, MD: Agency for Healthcare Research and Quality; 2005. AHRQ Publication No 05-0579-A. Available at: http://www.ahrq.gov/clinic/uspstf05/gonorrhea/gonrs.htm. Accessed April 25, 2007

Human Immunodeficiency Virus Testing

BRIGHT FUTURES VISITS:	ADOLESCENTS (11 TO 21 YEAR VISITS), IF SEXUALLY ACTIVE

Rationale:	**Article Covers Age: Sexually active youth**
	
	• Past or present injection drug users
	• Men who have had sex with men
	• Men and women having unprotected sex with multiple partners
	• Men and women who exchange sex for money or drugs or have sex partners who do
	• Past or present sex partners were HIV-infected, bisexual or injection drug users
	• Persons being treated for sexually transmitted diseases (STDs)
	• Persons who request an HIV test despite reporting no individual risk factors
	• Persons who report no individual risk factors but are seen in high-risk or high-prevalence clinical settings
	    • High-risk settings include STD clinics, correctional facilities, homeless shelters, tuberculosis clinics, clinics serving men who have sex with men, and adolescent health clinics with a high prevalence of STDs
	    • High-prevalence settings are defined by the Centers for Disease Control and Prevention (CDC) as those known to have a 1% or greater prevalence of infection among the patient population being served

Citation:	US Preventive Services Task Force. *Screening for HIV: Recommendation Statement.* Rockville, MD: Agency for Healthcare Research and Quality; 2005. AHRQ Publication No 05-0580-A. Available at: http://www.ahrq.gov/clinic/uspstf05/hiv/hivrs.htm. Accessed April 25, 2007
Citation:	US Preventive Services Task Force. *Screening for HIV: Recommendation Statement.* Rockville, MD: Agency for Healthcare Research and Quality; 2005. AHRQ Publication No 05-0580-A. Available at: http://www.ahrq.gov/clinic/uspstf05/hiv/hivrs.htm. Accessed April 25, 2007
Rationale:	**Article Covers Ages: 13 to Adult** In all health-care settings, screening for HIV infection should be performed routinely for all patients aged 13-64 years. Health-care providers should initiate screening unless prevalence of undiagnosed HIV infection in their patients has been documented to be <1 per 1,000 patients screened, at which point such screening is no longer warranted. HIV screening should be discussed with all adolescents and encouraged for those who are sexually active. Providing information regarding HIV infection, HIV testing, HIV transmission, and implications of infection should be regarded as an essential component of the anticipatory guidance provided to all adolescents as part of primary care.
Citation:	Centers for Disease Control and Prevention. Revised recommendations for HIV testing of adults, adolescents, and pregnant women in health-care settings. *MMWR Recomm Rep.* 2006;55(RR-14):1-17

Syphilis Infection

BRIGHT FUTURES VISITS:	ADOLESCENTS (11 TO 21 YEAR VISITS), IF SEXUALLY ACTIVE
Rationale:	**Article Covers Age: Sexually active youth** • Men who have sex with men and engage in high-risk sexual behavior • Commercial sex workers • Persons who exchange sex for drugs • Those in adult correctional facilities
Citation:	US Preventive Services Task Force. *Screening for Syphilis Infection: Recommendation Statement.* Rockville, MD: Agency for Healthcare Research and Quality; 2005. Available at: http://www.ahrq.gov/clinic/3rduspstf/syphilis/syphilrs.htm. Accessed April 25, 2007

Selective Screening

Cervical Dysplasia

BRIGHT FUTURES VISITS:	ADOLESCENTS (11 TO 21 YEAR VISITS), IF SEXUALLY ACTIVE OR AGE 21
Rationale:	**Ages: Sexually active youth, within 3 years of onset of sexual activity** • The USPSTF strongly recommends screening for cervical cancer in women who have been sexually active and have a cervix. • The optimal age to begin screening is unknown. Data on natural history of HPV infection and the incidence of high-grade lesions and cervical cancer suggest that screening can safely be delayed until 3 years after onset of sexual activity or until age 21, whichever comes first. Although there is little value in screening women who have never been sexually active, many US organizations recommend routine screening by age 18 or 21 for all women, based on the generally high prevalence of sexual activity by that age in the U.S. and concerns that clinicians may not always obtain accurate sexual histories.
Citation:	US Preventive Services Task Force. *Screening for Cervical Cancer: Recommendations and Rationale.* Rockville, MD: Agency for Healthcare Research and Quality; 2003. AHRQ Publication No 03-515A. Available at: http://www.ahrq.gov/clinic/3rduspstf/cervcan/cervcanrr.htm. Accessed April 25, 2007

Alcohol or Drug Use

BRIGHT FUTURES VISITS:	ADOLESCENTS (11 TO 21 YEAR VISITS)
Rationale:	Have you ever had an alcoholic drink? Have you ever used marijuana or any other drug to get high?
Citation:	Levy S. Knight JR. Office management of substance use. *Adolesc Health Update.* 2003;15:1-11

References

1. US Preventive Services Task Force. *Screening for Cervical Cancer: Recommendations and Rationale.* Rockville, MD: Agency for Healthcare Research and Quality; 2003. Available at: www.ahrq.gov/clinic/3rduspstf/cervcan/cervcanrr.htm. Accessed September 13, 2007
2. US Preventive Services Task Force. *Screening for Breast Cancer: Recommendations and Rationale.* Rockville, MD: Agency for Healthcare Research and Quality; 2002. Available at: www.ahrq.gov/clinic/3rduspstf/breastcancer/brcanrr.htm. Accessed September 13, 2007
3. Smith RA, Saslow D, Sawyer KA, et al. American Cancer Society guidelines for breast cancer screening: update 2003. *CA Cancer J Clin.* 2003;53:141-169
4. US Preventive Services Task Force. *Screening for Testicular Cancer: Recommendation Statement.* Rockville, MD: Agency for Healthcare Research and Quality; 2004. Available at: www.ahrq.gov/clinic/3rduspstf/testicular/testiculrs.pdf. Accessed September 13, 2007
5. US Preventive Services Task Force. *Screening for Idiopathic Scoliosis in Adolescents: Recommendation Statement.* Rockville, MD: Agency for Healthcare Research and Quality; 2004. Avaialble at: www.ahrq.gov/clinic/3rduspstf/scoliosis/scoliors.pdf. Accessed September 13, 2007
6. Stewart DG, Skaggs DL. Consultation with the specialist: adolescent idiopathic scoliosis. *Pediatr Rev.* 2006;27:299-306
7. Needlman R, Silverstein M. Pediatric interventions to support reading aloud: how good is the evidence? *J Dev Behav Pediatr.* 2004;25:352-363
8. Weitzman CC, Roy L, Walls T, Tomlin R. More evidence for Reach Out and Read: a home-based study. *Pediatrics.* 2004;113:1248-1253
9. Minkovitz CS, Hughart N, Strobino D, et al. A practice-based intervention to enhance quality of care in the first 3 years of life: the healthy steps for young children program. *JAMA.* 2003;290:3081-3091

RATIONALE AND EVIDENCE

Bright FUTURES

EVIDENCE

Detailed Findings of the Bright Futures Evidence Panel

The following section presents the statements written by the Evidence Panel. These statements summarize the current status of evidence from clinical studies, meta-analyses, and randomized controlled trials regarding screening and counseling interventions that are covered in the *Bright Futures Guidelines*. The physical examination is reviewed first, followed by topics included in the medical screening tables. The final portion covers screening and counseling topics, organized by Bright Futures Themes.

The Physical Examination

Physical examination, including growth monitoring and developmental examination, traditionally has been considered an important part of the health supervision visit, perhaps the most basic screening procedure in health care. It is important to note that "screening" applies to patients who are not seeking help for a specific problem—if a parent or patient voices a concern, the evaluation of that concern becomes a diagnostic process and is no longer considered screening. The price of false-negative and false-positive findings in screening has often been underestimated. At the end of the visit, if the health care provider notes no abnormalities, parents and patients are reassured that nothing is wrong. If the provider has missed an abnormality, parents, when they notice it, may assume it is unimportant and fail to seek care because of false reassurance. If, on the other hand, the provider notes a concern, the previously healthy child is immediately considered less healthy, even if the concern turns out to be a false alarm. Further harm from false-positive findings may occur if follow-up testing is expensive or invasive, or if treatment is instituted for "disease" that is clinically unimportant (ie, it never would have affected the child's overall health). Evidence that any screening procedure is beneficial is thus very important, but, in the case of the physical examination, frustratingly elusive.

The best evidence would come from clinical trials of the physical examination, as a whole or in parts, with outcomes that are important to patients and parents. Few such studies are available. Most studies address isolated aspects of the physical examination, and are done from the perspective of a specific condition, such as growth failure, scoliosis, or speech delay, rather than from the perspective of the general examination. It is difficult to evaluate the usefulness of a screening test when the condition or conditions that are the target of screening are not specified. We found no trials evaluating the yield of repeated physical examination over the duration of well child care. One large trial[1] (n = 9712) of 1 versus 2 newborn examinations showed no difference in the use of health care resources between the 2 groups.

Aspects of repeated examination, including growth monitoring, routine blood pressure measurement, and screening for signs of physical and sexual abuse have not been rigorously evaluated, and concerns have been raised that false positive screening examinations for child abuse may cause significant harm. It is important to note that the physical examination and developmental evaluation may have uses other than screening for specific abnormalities; most importantly, the opportunity to reassure and educate parents and patients about the range of normal findings. Parents or patients may talk more readily or be reminded of concerns during the examination, so performing the examination might enhance communication and encourage a closer relationship with the health care provider. No studies have specifically evaluated these potential benefits of routine physical examination. Some aspects of the physical examination are mandated by payers (such as some state Medicaid requirements of a

RATIONALE AND EVIDENCE

standardized, validated, developmental-behavioral/mental health screening at all well child visits) or used to assess the quality of health care providers.

Medical Screening

NEWBORN METABOLIC AND HEMOGLOBINOPATHY

The evidence for newborn screening and metabolic screening was not evaluated because it is mandated by state laws.

DEVELOPMENTAL SCREENING (SPEECH AND LANGUAGE)

There is evidence of benefit from treatment of speech and language delay, such as improved speech and language.[2] However, no successful screening strategy for use in primary care has been identified.

SCREENING FOR SPEECH AND LANGUAGE DELAY IN PRESCHOOL-AGED CHILDREN

The USPSTF concluded that there is insufficient evidence to recommend for or against routine use of brief, formal screening instruments in primary care to detect speech and language delay in children up to 5 years of age. Specifically, the task force found that, although interventions for delayed speech and language appear effective (at least in the short term), there is insufficient evidence that formal screening in primary care would add to this effectiveness.[3]

ORAL HEALTH

No controlled trials were found that examined accuracy by the primary care clinician in identifying children who displayed one or more risk indicators for oral disease, other than identification of caries.

VISION SCREENING OF PRESCHOOL CHILDREN

Treatment for amblyopia, strabismus, and refractive error is effective. A randomized controlled trial (RCT)[4] of intensive screening (versus usual care) of children 0 to 3 years of age demonstrated improved vision at school age. Screening tests have reasonable accuracy. No high-quality evidence was found regarding vision screening for adolescents.

The USPSTF recommends **for** vision screening in children from birth to age 5 years.[5]

SCREENING FOR VISUAL IMPAIRMENT IN CHILDREN YOUNGER THAN 5 YEARS

The USPSTF recommended screening to detect amblyopia, strabismus, and defects in visual acuity in children younger than 5 years.[5] Specifically, the USPSTF found fair evidence that screening tests have reasonable accuracy in identifying strabismus, amblyopia, and refractive error in children with these conditions, and that treatment of strabismus and amblyopia can improve visual acuity and reduce long-term amblyopia.

HEARING

There is good evidence[6] that newborn hearing screening leads to earlier identification and treatment of infants with hearing loss. However, evidence to determine whether earlier treatment resulting from screening leads to clinically important improvement in speech and language skills at age 3 years or beyond is inconclusive. Newborn hearing screening is mandated in most states. No controlled trials were found regarding hearing screening for older children or adolescents.

ANEMIA

Screening for anemia has limited accuracy in defining iron-deficiency anemia. Treatment of iron-deficiency anemia shows improvement in iron deficiency, but not in developmental outcomes.[7] There is evidence of harm[8] due to increased incidence of iron poisoning when iron-containing medications are kept in the home. No controlled trials were found regarding screening adolescents for anemia.

LEAD

Controlled trials demonstrate no neurodevelopmental benefit from interventions to decrease blood lead levels in asymptomatic children.[9] However, benefit may accrue to future children living in an environment where lead abatement has been done.

RATIONALE AND EVIDENCE

TUBERCULOSIS

There is no evidence of benefit or harm from screening asymptomatic children and adolescents for tuberculosis. Questionnaires that address contact with a tuberculosis case, birth in or travel to endemic areas, regular contact with high-risk adults, and human immunodeficiency virus infection in the child have been shown to have adequate sensitivity and specificity when compared with a positive tuberculosis skin test.[10]

LIPID SCREENING/CHOLESTEROL

No controlled trials of cholesterol screening in children or adolescents were found. One large RCT of dietary counseling (Special Turku Coronary Risk Factor Intervention Project [STRIP]) in infancy has shown no evidence of harm at repeated evaluations through age 10 years, although power is low to detect most potential harms.[11] One case-control study[12] showed behavioral and psychological abnormalities among 4- to 17-year-olds who were evaluated shortly after learning of high cholesterol on screening.

SEXUALLY TRANSMITTED INFECTIONS

The USPSTF found that routine sexually transmitted infection screening for low-risk women and men (including adolescents) do not result in improved outcomes. A benefit of screening for chlamydia, gonorrhea, human immunodeficiency virus (HIV), and syphilis has been found for women at high risk, and for men at high risk for HIV and syphilis. Benefit to the infant has been found for screening all pregnant women for syphilis, HIV, and hepatitis B, and for screening pregnant women at increased risk for chlamydia, gonorrhea, syphilis, HIV, and hepatitis B.

At this time, the USPSTF recommends for chlamydia screening in sexually active females.[13]

CERVICAL DYSPLASIA

The USPSTF found good evidence from multiple observational studies that screening with cervical cytology (Pap smears) reduces incidence of, and mortality from, cervical cancer.[14] Direct evidence to determine the optimal starting and stopping age and interval for screening is limited. Indirect evidence suggests most of the benefit can be obtained by beginning screening within 3 years of onset of sexual activity or age 21 years (whichever comes first) and screening at least every 3 years.

The USPSTF recommends **for** cervical dysplasia screening within 3 years of the onset of sexual activity.[15]

Screening and Counseling

PROMOTING FAMILY SUPPORT

Screening for Family Social Support
Evidence demonstrates mixed results of screening for psychosocial support for the mother antenatally through adolescence. Nurse home visits during the first 2 years of a child's life, especially among women with few psychological resources, demonstrate benefits to both maternal health and child's well-being many years after the intervention has ended.[16]

Screening for Parental Concerns
No controlled trials were identified regarding screening for parental concerns.

Counseling About Pregnancy Spacing
Studies regarding pregnancy planning demonstrate mixed results. Findings vary based on the target population (adolescents, women with limited resources, pregnant women) and the type of intervention implemented (health education, nurse home visit, paraprofessional home visitation). Women with limited psychosocial resources who received home visitation by a nurse demonstrated decreased rates of future pregnancy and increased intervals between pregnancies.[16]

PROMOTING CHILD DEVELOPMENT

Effects of Early Intervention Services
The Healthy Steps for Young Children Program is a practice-based intervention to enhance quality of care in the first 3 years

RATIONALE AND EVIDENCE

of life.[17] Positive, sustained effects of home visits have been demonstrated in 4-year follow-up results of a randomized trial. Nurse-visited families showed more benefit than paraprofessional-visited families, but both had effect demonstrable 2 years following the cessation of the program, especially if mothers had "low levels of psychologic resources."[18]

Counseling About Appropriate Discipline Methods

Evidence[17] demonstrates that, in a pediatric care setting, the use of a developmental specialist and developmental services among families with children from 0 to 3 years of age can decrease the odds of families that use severe discipline (eg, slapping the face or hitting with an object).

Infant Massage for Promoting Growth and Development of Preterm and/or Low Birth Weight Infants

Evidence that massage for preterm infants positively impacts developmental outcomes is weak.[19]

Media-based Behavioral Treatments for Behavioral Problems in Children

Eleven studies, which included 943 participants, were reviewed. Across these studies, media-based therapies for behavioral disorders had moderate, but variable, effects, and should likely be considered more as adjunctive therapy.[20]

Early Skin-to-Skin Contact for Mothers and Healthy Newborns

Although the quality of the studies varies, early skin-to-skin contact appears to have some benefit relative to breastfeeding outcomes and infant crying.[21]

Office-based Literacy Intervention

A randomized controlled trial has demonstrated that a primary care ROR program led to an increase in home-reading activities as measured by self-report.[22,23] While nonexperimental studies support improved language acquisition among ROR participants, no RCTs have been published with language acquisition as an outcome.

PROMOTING MENTAL HEALTH

Screening for and Counseling About Alcohol Use

The USPSTF concludes that the evidence is insufficient to recommend for or against screening and behavioral counseling interventions to prevent or reduce alcohol misuse by adolescents in primary care settings.[24]

Screening for and Counseling About Tobacco Use

The USPSTF found limited evidence that screening and counseling children and adolescents in the primary care setting are effective in either preventing initiation or promoting cessation of tobacco use. As a result, the USPSTF could not determine the balance of benefits and harms of tobacco prevention or cessation interventions in the clinical setting for children or adolescents.[25]

Screening for and Counseling About Substance Misuse and Abuse

Substance abuse or misuse is broadly defined to include alcohol, illicit drugs, body image-changing substances (anabolic steroids or laxatives), and prescription medications. Chemical detection is the most valid method for screening, but tests may not exist for all available types of substances. Behavioral counseling can include brief, motivational, or intensive counseling.

The evidence is mixed regarding the benefit of screening for substance abuse/misuse, depending on the substance and target population. For adolescents, counseling regarding alcohol use has been associated with reported increased alcohol consumption.[26] As part of a larger risk reduction intervention among 13- to 16-year-olds and their parents, intensive counseling demonstrated decreased use of illicit drugs, while no change in alcohol use was reported.[27]

No studies were found that addressed the effectiveness of screening for substance abuse/misuse in the primary care setting. In the school setting, mandatory drug testing among athletes decreased the use of body image-changing substances and illicit drugs, but was associated with increased risk factors that are known to be associated with drug misuse.[28]

Counseling About Body Image
No controlled trials were found regarding the effectiveness of discussing healthy body image.

Exercise to Improve Self-esteem in Children and Young People
Results suggest that exercise has positive short-term effects on self-esteem; however, it is noted that the conclusions are based on low-quality studies.[29]

PROMOTING HEALTHY WEIGHT
Screening for Nutritional Intake in Primary Care
No studies were found regarding the outcomes of screening for infant, child, or adolescent nutritional intake in primary care.

Monitoring and Counseling About Infant Feeding Adequacy
There are no controlled trials that indicated whether physician monitoring of infant feeding resulted in improved outcomes. There are no controlled trials that indicated whether physician counseling regarding feeding frequency improved infant outcomes.

Counseling About Limiting Juice and Sweetened Beverages
No controlled trials were found regarding the outcomes of parental or patient counseling to limit intake of juice or sweetened beverages.

Counseling Parents About Watching TV During Meals
No clinical trials were found regarding counseling about eating while watching television.

PROMOTING HEALTHY NUTRITION
Counseling About Infant Feeding in General
There are no controlled trials that indicated whether physician nutritional counseling regarding infant feeding improves infant outcomes.

Counseling About Breastfeeding
A systematic review suggests that physician counseling can be effective as one part of a larger intervention to increase breastfeeding rates.[30] The USPSTF found fair evidence that programs that combine breastfeeding education with behaviorally oriented counseling are associated with increased rates of breastfeeding initiation and its continuation for up to 3 months, although effects beyond 3 months are uncertain. Effective programs generally involved at least 1 extended session, followed structured protocols, and included practical, behavioral skills training and problem solving, in addition to didactic instruction.[31] One controlled trial indicated that use of pacifiers does not affect breastfeeding duration.[32] One small RCT demonstrated improved bone mineralization and vitamin D levels in breastfeeding infants for whom vitamin D was prescribed.[33]

Counseling About Formula Preparation
There are no controlled trials that indicated whether physician counseling regarding formula preparation resulted in improved infant outcomes. There are no controlled trials of counseling to promote use of iron-fortified formula.

Counseling About Infant Stooling and Voiding Patterns
There are no controlled trials that indicated whether physician counseling regarding infant stooling and voiding patterns improved infant outcomes.

RATIONALE AND EVIDENCE

Counseling About Introduction of Complementary Foods

No controlled trials were found on counseling regarding introduction of complementary foods. There is one systematic review[34] that suggests that early solid feeding may increase the risk of eczema. However, there is no study that supports an association between early solid feeding and other allergic conditions.

Counseling Parents and Children About Type of Nutritional Intake

Several controlled trials indicate that physician nutritional counseling regarding type of nutritional intake, as part of a larger intervention (ie, with counseling from other health professionals, or with additional educational support), improved pediatric outcomes.[35,36]

PROMOTING PHYSICAL ACTIVITY

Counseling About Obesity Prevention and Treatment

A 2005 Cochrane Review[37] studied the effectiveness of interventions that were designed to prevent obesity in childhood through diet, physical activity, and/or lifestyle and social support. The majority of studies were school- or community-based and primarily employed only short-term follow-up. The Cochrane Review concluded that studies that focused on combining dietary and physical activity approaches did not significantly improve BMI or showed a very small effect; however, nearly all studies did show some improvement in diet or physical activity.

The 2006 USPSTF Report on Screening and Interventions for Overweight in Children and Adolescents[38] found "insufficient evidence for the effectiveness of behavioral counseling or other preventive interventions with overweight children and adolescents that can be conducted in primary care settings or to which primary care clinicians can make referrals."

PROMOTING ORAL HEALTH

Monitoring Maternal Oral Health

No controlled trials were found that indicated whether monitoring maternal oral health, either prenatal or in the neonatal period, affects the child's oral health.

Counseling About Preventing Dental Caries

No controlled trials were found that assessed the effectiveness of primary care-supplied counseling interventions (eg, about bottle propping or pacifier use) in preventing dental caries or improving other oral health outcomes.

Counseling About Tooth Eruption

No controlled trials were found that assessed the effectiveness of primary care-supplied counseling on tooth eruption.

Fluoride to Prevent Dental Caries

There is one systematic review of the literature that suggests that combination treatments that involve fluoride (eg, tooth brushing, professional tooth cleaning, varnish, and sealant) have a preventive effect on caries in children and adolescents.[39] No studies were found that examine the effectiveness of risk-assessment tools or physician screening for risk for low fluoride exposure.

Counseling About Brushing/Flossing Teeth

No controlled trials were found that indicated whether advising parents to brush/floss their children's teeth improves outcomes.

PROMOTING HEALTHY SEXUAL DEVELOPMENT AND SEXUALITY

Screening for Condom Use Among Sexually Active Adolescents

No controlled trials examined the effectiveness of physician counseling regarding condom use.

Screening for Sexual Activity

There are several controlled trials that suggested minimal effect of brief, office-based counseling targeted to adolescent and adult

RATIONALE AND EVIDENCE

populations resulting in decreased incidence of STDs.[40-43]

Counseling Adolescents About Pregnancy Prevention

A systematic review of primary prevention programs found that adolescents who received health education demonstrated no increase in use of contraception. Adolescents who received abstinence-only education had increased rates of pregnancy.[44]

Counseling About Sexual Development/ Puberty

No studies were found that examined the effectiveness of counseling regarding puberty.

Counseling About Sexual Behavior

No studies were found regarding the effectiveness of counseling adolescents in the primary care setting about sexual behavior.

Counseling About Alcohol

No evidence was found to support the effectiveness of counseling adolescents in the primary care setting about alcohol misuse.

PROMOTING SAFETY AND INJURY PREVENTION

General Statement

Approaches to injury prevention often involve multifaceted interventions (educational, environmental, and regulatory) as well as cross over multiple settings (primary care settings, community, and school). Furthermore, the strategy needed for a specific injury hazard varies depending on the age of the individual (infant vs adolescent), the target of the counseling (individual or family), and the type of injury (burns vs motor vehicle injuries).

Evidence demonstrates that behavioral counseling can increase the use (self-reported or observed) of safety equipment as well as decrease hazardous environments, especially when the counseling is intensive and repetitive. Fewer studies evaluate the impact of behavioral counseling on injuries. Those

addressing home-based safety devices demonstrate no impact on injury incidence compared to controls.

Counseling About Passenger Safety

There is evidence to support the benefit of counseling and demonstrating the use of child safety seats. While controlled trials in community settings demonstrate that education and distribution of booster seats increases use, no studies were found that addressed counseling for booster seats in the primary care setting. Controlled trials targeting safety belt use demonstrated no effect in the primary care setting.[45]

Counseling to Discourage Driving Under the Influence of Alcohol

No controlled trials were found that address the effectiveness of counseling in the primary care setting about the risk of drinking and driving or riding in a motor vehicle.

Counseling About Using Smoke Detectors

Behavioral counseling demonstrates increased ownership of smoke detectors.[46] No trials were found linking the reduction of fire-related injuries with smoke detectors.

Counseling About Using Carbon Monoxide Detector/Alarms

No controlled trials were found that address the effectiveness of counseling regarding the use of carbon monoxide detector/alarms.

Counseling About Safe Water Temperature

Evidence supports the benefit of behavioral counseling in reducing hot-water temperatures. Studies also demonstrate the accuracy of parents' self-report.[47]

No studies were found demonstrating reducing this burn hazard with injury incidence.

Counseling About Preventing Firearm Injury

A randomized trial demonstrated[48] no benefit of counseling in the primary care setting regarding gun ownership, safe storage, or removal of firearms.

Counseling About Crib Safety
No controlled trials were found that address the effectiveness of counseling in the primary care setting regarding crib safety.

Counseling About Sunburn Protection
No controlled trials were found that address the effectiveness of counseling in the primary care setting regarding the prevention of sunburn injury.

Screening for, and Counseling About, Preventing Domestic Violence/Child Abuse
A systematic review under the auspices of the USPSTF found no studies identifying accurate screening tools to identify family violence among children or women in the primary care setting. The role of case findings was not addressed. Evidence was found to support the benefit of interventions when abuse was identified. Controlled trials of home visitation demonstrate benefits in the reduction of child abuse, but these interventions were conducted outside the primary care setting.[49,50]

Counseling About Using Bicycle Helmets
Studies report conflicting results regarding the benefit of counseling for bicycle helmet use depending on the target age group. One study demonstrated that counseling increased helmet use among fourth to ninth graders, while another study found no benefit among 11- to 24-year-olds. Multifaceted community-based interventions do demonstrate an increase in helmet use.[51-53]

Counseling About Preventing Sudden Infant Death Syndrome
The "Back to Sleep" campaign, initiated in the 1990s, has been associated with a significant decrease in the proportion of infants sleeping in the prone position, as well as a decreased incidence of SIDS.[54] One study that evaluated the impact of a multifaceted risk reduction education program that included health care professional advice along with other strategies and targeted predominately black urban communities demonstrated a decrease in the proportion of families who reported placing infants in the prone position.[55]

Counseling About Swimming Pool Safety
Epidemiologic studies support the effectiveness of pool fencing in the prevention of drowning. Fences that surround the pool are superior to fences that use the property as part of the enclosure. No studies were found that address the effectiveness of counseling in the primary care setting regarding pool fences.[56]

Counseling for Smoking Cessation
Multiple interventions are used for smoking cessation. These included counseling that can be brief, motivational, or intensive. The education and counseling can be provided in person, via the phone, or on the Internet. Studies demonstrate that the benefit of smoking cessation interventions depend on the target audience (caregiver vs youth) and the modality used.[25]

Studies that demonstrate increased cessation among parents or teenagers involve intensive counseling and result in only short-term impact (less than 1 year).[57] A Cochrane systematic review concluded that brief interventions effective for adults are not effective for caregivers in a pediatric setting. Rather, in this setting, intensive counseling is needed to increase caregiver smoking cessation.[58]

PROMOTING COMMUNITY RELATIONSHIPS AND RESOURCES
Surveying the evidence base for preventive health services delivered in the community is beyond the scope of this edition. Excellent information is, however, available in the *Guide to Community Preventive Services* (the *Guide*), which can be found at www.thecommunityguide.org. The Guide represents the findings of the Task Force on

Community Preventive Services, an independent group of experts convened by the Centers for Disease Control and Prevention to make recommendations about interventions to promote community health. The Task Force on Community Preventive Services works in parallel with the USPSTF, which is convened by the Agency for Healthcare Research and Quality and considers the evidence for clinical preventive services. The Guide is updated regularly, and new topics are added as they are considered. Topics that are covered by the Guide, as of early September 2006, include alcohol, cancer, diabetes, mental health, motor vehicle, nutrition, obesity, oral health, physical activity, pregnancy, sexual behavior, social environment, substance abuse, tobacco, vaccines, violence, and worksite. Clinicians are encouraged to take advantage of the information in the guide when making decisions for referral purposes about the likely effectiveness of a particular type of community-based intervention and in their advocacy efforts.[59]

References

1. Glazener CMA, Ramsay CR, Campbell MK, et al. Neonatal examination and screening trial (NEST): a randomised, controlled, switchback trial of alternative policies for low risk infants. *BMJ*. 1999;318:627-632

2. Nelson HD, Nygren P, Walker M, Panoscha R. Screening for speech and language delay in preschool children: systematic evidence review for the US Preventive Services Task Force. *Pediatrics*. 2006;117(2):e298-e319. Available at: http://pediatrics.aappublications.org/cgi/content/full/117/2/e298. Accessed August 2, 2007

3. Nelson HD, Nygren P, Walker M, Panoscha R. *Screening for Speech and Language Delay in Preschool Children: Evidence Synthesis Review No. 41*. Rockville, MD: Agency for Healthcare Research and Quality; Prepared by the Oregon Health and Science University Evidence-based Practice Center; 2006. Available at: http://www.ahrq.gov/downloads/pub/prevent/pdfser/speechsyn.pdf. Accessed April 25, 2007

4. Williams C, Northstone K, Harrad RA, Sparrow JM, Harvey I, ALSPAC Study Team. Amblyopia treatment outcomes after screening before or at age 3 years: follow up from randomised trial. *BMJ*. 2002;324:1549

5. US Preventive Services Task Force. *Screening for Visual Impairment in Children Younger than Age 5 Years: Recommendation Statement*. Rockville, MD: Agency for Healthcare Research and Quality; 2004. Available at: www.ahrq.gov/clinic/3rduspstf/visionscr/vischrs.pdf. Accessed September 13, 2007

6. Helfand H, Thompson D, Davis R, et al. *Newborn Hearing Screening: A Summary of the Evidence for the U.S. Preventive Services Task Force*. Rockville, MD: Agency for Healthcare Research and Quality; 2001. Available at: www.ahrq.gov/clinic/3rduspstf/newbornscreen/newbornsum1.htm. Accessed September 13, 2007

7. Martins S, Logan S, Gilbert R. Iron therapy for improving psychomotor development and cognitive function in children under the age of three with iron deficiency anaemia. *Cochrane Database Syst Rev*. 2001;(2):CD001444

8. US Preventive Services Task Force. *Screening for Iron Deficiency Anemia—Including Iron Supplementation for Children and Pregnant Women: Recommendation Statement*. Rockville, MD: Agency for Healthcare Research and Quality; 2006

9. Rischitelli G, Nygren P, Bougatsos C, Freeman M, Helfand M. Screening for elevated lead levels in childhood and pregnancy: updated summary of evidence for the US Preventive Services Task Force. *Pediatrics*. 2006;118(6):e1867-1895. Available at: http://pediatrics.aappublications.org/cgi/content/full/118/6/e1867. Accessed August 2, 2007

10. Ozuah PO, Ozuah TP, Stein REK, Burton W, Mulvihill M. Evaluation of a risk assessment questionnaire used to target tuberculin skin testing in children. *JAMA*. 2001;285:451-453

11. Talvia S, Lagstrom H, Rasanen M, et al. A randomized intervention since infancy to reduce intake of saturated fat: calorie (energy) and nutrient intakes up to the age of 10 years in the special Turku Coronary Risk Factor Intervention Project. *Arch Pediatr Adolesc Med*. 2004;158:41-47

12. Rosenberg E, Lamping DL, Joseph L, Pless IB, Franco ED. Cholesterol screening of children at high risk: behavioural and psychological effects. *Can Med Assoc J*. 1997;156:489-496

13. US Preventive Services Task Force. Screening for chlamydial infection: recommendations and rationale. *Am J Prev Med*. 2001;20(3 Suppl):90-94

14. US Department of Health and Human Services, Agency for Healthcare Research and Quality. *Screening for Cervical Cancer: Systematic Evidence Review*. Research Triangle Park, NC: Research Triangle Institute–University of North Carolina; 2002

15. US Preventive Services Task Force. *Screening for Cervical Cancer: Recommendations and Rationale*. Rockville, MD: Agency for Healthcare Research and Quality; 2003

16. Olds DL, Robinson J, Pettitt L, et al. Effects of home visits by paraprofessionals and by nurses: age 4 follow-up results of a randomized trial. *Pediatrics*. 2004;114:1560-1568

17. Minkovitz CS, Hughart N, Strobino D, et al. A practice-based intervention to enhance quality of care in the first 3 years of life: the Healthy Steps for Young Children Program. *JAMA*. 2003;290:3081-1091

18. Olds DL. Robinson J, Pettitt L, et al. Effects of home visits by paraprofessionals and by nurses: age 4 follow-up results of a randomized trial. *Pediatrics*. 2004;114:1560-1568. Comment in: *Evid Based Nurs*. 2005;8(3):75 and *Pediatrics*. 2005;115 (4):1113; author reply 1113-1114

19. Vickers A, Ohlsson A, Lacy JB, Horsley A. Massage for promoting growth and development of preterm and/or low birth-weight infants. *Cochrane Database Syst Rev*. 2004;(2):CD000390

20. Montgomery P, Bjornstad G, Dennis J. Media-based behavioural treatments for behavioural problems in children. *Cochrane Database Syst Rev*. 2006;(1):CD002206

21. Moore ER, Anderson G, Bergman N. Early skin-to-skin contact for mothers and their healthy newborn infants. *Cochrane Database Syst Rev*. 2007:CD003519

22. Needlman R, Silverstein M. Pediatric interventions to support reading aloud: how good is the evidence? *J Dev Behav Pediatr*. 2004;25:352-363

23. Weitzman CC, Roy L, Walls T, Tomlin R. More evidence for Reach Out and Read: a home-based study. 2004;113:1248-1253

24. US Preventive Services Task Force. *Screening and Behavioral Counseling Interventions in Primary Care to Reduce Alcohol Misuse: Recommendation Statement*. Ann Intern Med. 2004;140:554-556

25. US Preventive Services Task Force. *Counseling to Prevent Tobacco Use and Tobacco-Caused Disease: Recommendations Statement*. Rockville, MD: Agency for Healthcare Research and Quality; 2003

26. Stevens MM, Olson AL, Gaffney CA, Tosteson TD, Mott LA, Starr P. A Pediatric, practice-based, randomized trial of drinking and smoking prevention and bicycle helmet, gun, and seatbelt safety promotion. *Pediatrics*. 2002;109:490-497

Bright FUTURES

27. Foxcroft DR, Ireland D, Lowe G, Breen R. Primary prevention for alcohol misuse in young people. *Cochrane Database Syst Rev.* 2002;(3):CD003024

28. Goldberg L, Elliot DL, MacKinnon DP, et al. Drug testing athletes to prevent substance abuse: background and pilot study results of the SATURN (Student Athlete Testing Using Random Notification) Study. *J Adolesc Health.* 2003;32:16-25

29. Ekeland E, Heian F, Hagen K, Abbott J, Nordheim L. Exercise to improve self-esteem in children and young people. *Cochrane Database Syst Rev.* 2004;(1):CD003683

30. Dyson L, McCormick F, Renfrew M. Interventions for promoting the initiation of breastfeeding. *Cochrane Database Syst Rev.* 2005;(2):CD001688

31. US Preventive Services Task Force. Behavioral Interventions to Promote Breastfeeding: Recommendations and Rationale. Rockville, MD: Agency for Healthcare Research and Quality; 2003

32. Kramer MS, Barr RG, Dagenais S, et al. Pacifier use, early weaning, and cry/fuss behavior: a randomized controlled trial. JAMA. 2001;286:322-326

33. Greer FR, Searcy JE, Levin RS, Steichen JJ, Asch PS, Tsang RC. Bone mineral content and serum 25-hydroxyvitamin D concentration in breast-fed infants with and without supplemental vitamin D. *J Pediatr.* 1981;98:696-701

34. Tarini BA, Carroll AE, Sox CM, Christakis DA. Systematic review of the relationship between early introduction of solid foods to infants and the development of allergic disease. *Arch Pediatr Adolesc Med.* 2006;160:502-507

35. Patrick K, Sallis JF, Prochaska JJ, et al. A multicomponent program for nutrition and physical activity change in primary care: PACE+ for adolescents. *Arch Pediatr Adolesc Med.* 2001;155:940-946

36. Saarilehto S, Lapinleimu H, Keskinen S, Helenius H, Simell O. Body satisfaction in 8-year-old children after long-term dietary counseling in a prospective randomized atherosclerosis prevention trial. *Arch Pediatr Adolesc Med.* 2003;157:753-758

37. Summerbell CD, Waters E, Edmunds LD, Kelly S, Brown T, Campbell KJ. Interventions for preventing obesity in children. *Cochrane Database Syst Rev* 2005;(3):CD001871

38. US Preventive Services Task Force. *Screening and Interventions for Overweight in Children and Adolescents: Recommendation Statement.* Rockville, MD: Agency for Healthcare Research and Quality; 2005

39. Axelsson S, Soder B, Nordenram G, et al. Effect of combined caries-preventive methods: a systematic review of controlled clinical trials. *Acto Odontol Scand.* 2004;62:163-169

40. Yamada J, DiCenso A, Feldman L, et al. *A Systematic Review of the Effectiveness of Primary Prevention Programs to Prevent Sexually Transmitted Diseases in Adolescents.* Hamilton, Ontario: Ontario Ministry of Health, Public health Branch; 1999

41. Kim N, Stanton B, Li X, Dickersin K, Galbraith J. Effectiveness of the 40 adolescent AIDS-risk reduction interventions: a quantitative review. *J Adolesc Health.* 1997;20:204-215

42. Boekeloo BO, Schamus LA, Simmens SJ, Cheng TL, O'Connor K, D'Angelo LJ. A STD/HIV prevention trial among adolescents in managed care. *Pediatrics.* 1999;103:107-115

43. Kamb ML, Fishbein M, Douglas JM Jr, et al. Efficacy of risk-reduction counseling to prevent human immunodeficiency virus and sexually transmitted diseases: a randomized controlled trial. JAMA. 1998;280:1161-1167

44. Bennett SE, Assefi NP. School-based teenage pregnancy prevention programs: a systematic review of randomized controlled trials. *J Adolesc Health.* 2005;36:72-81

45. Williams SB, Whitlock EP, Edgerton EA, Smith PR, Beil TL. *Counseling about proper use of motor vehicle occupant restraints and avoidance of alcohol use while driving: a systematic evidence review for the US Preventive Services Task Force.* Ann Intern Med. 2007;147:194-206

46. Clamp M, Kendrick D. A randomised controlled trial of general practitioner safety advice for families with children under 5 years. *BMJ.* 1998;316:1576-1579

47. King WJ, Klassen TP, LeBlanc J, et al. The effectiveness of a home visit to prevent childhood injury. *Pediatrics.* 2001;108:382-388

48. Grossman DC, Cummings P, Koepsell TD, et al. Firearm safety counseling in primary care pediatrics: a randomized, controlled trial. *Pediatrics.* 2000;106:22-26

49. Nygren P, Nelson HD, Klein J. Screening children for family violence: a review of the evidence for the US Preventive Services Task Force. *Ann Fam Med.* 2004;2:161-169

50. Nelson HD, Nygren P, McInerney Y, Klein J. Screening women and elderly adults for family and intimate partner violence: a review of the evidence for the US Preventive Services Task Force. *Ann Intern Med.* 2004;140:387-396

51. Cushman R, James W, Waclawik H. Physicians promoting bicycle helmets for children: a randomized trial. *Am J Public Health.* 1991;81:1044-1046

52. Leverence RR, Martinez M, Whisler S, et al. Does office-based counseling of adolescents and young adults improve self-reported safety habits? A randomized controlled effectiveness trial. *J Adolesc Health.* 2005;36:523-528

53. Thompson DC, Rivara FP, Thompson RS. Effectiveness of bicycle safety helmets in preventing head injuries. A case-control study. JAMA. 1996;276:1968-1973

54. Willinger M, Ko C-W, Hoffman HJ, Kessler RC, Corwin MJ. Factors associated with caregivers' choice of infant sleep position, 1994-1998: the National Infant Sleep Position Study. JAMA. 2000;283:2135-2142

55. Rasinski KA, Kuby A, Bzdusek SA, Silvestri JM, Weese-Mayer DE. Effect of a sudden infant death syndrome risk reduction education program on risk factor compliance and information sources in primarily black urban communities. *Pediatrics.* 2003;111(4):e347-e354. Available at: http://pediatrics.aappublications.org/cgi/content/full/111/4/e347. Accessed August 2, 2007

RATIONALE AND EVIDENCE

249

56. Thompson DC, Rivara FP. Pool fencing for preventing drowning in children. *Cochrane Database Syst Rev*. 1998;(1):CD001047

57. Lipkus IM, McBride CM, Pollak KI, Schwartz-Bloom RD, Tilson E, Bloom PN. A randomized trial comparing the effects of self-help materials and proactive telephone counseling on teen smoking cessation. *Health Psychol*. 2004;23:397-406

58. Roseby R, Waters E, Polnay A, Campbell R, Webster P, Spencer N. Family and carer smoking control programmes for reducing children's exposure to environmental tobacco smoke. *Cochrane Database Syst Rev*. 2002;(3):CD001746

59. Ockene JK, Edgerton EA, Teutsch SM, et al. Integrating evidence-based clinical and community strategies to improve health. *Am J Prev Med*. 2007;32:244-252

Acronyms Used in the *Bright Futures* Health Supervision Visits

ACRONYM	DEFINITION
AAP	American Academy of Pediatrics
ACOG	American College of Obstetricians and Gynecologists
ADHD	Attention-Deficit/Hyperactivity Disorder
ACIP	Advisory Committee on Immunization Practices
ATV	All-Terrain vehicle
BMI	Body mass index
CD	Compact disc
CDC	Centers for Disease Control and Prevention
CMV	Cytomegalovirus
CPR	Cardiopulmonary resuscitation
CPSC	Consumer Product Safety Commission
DVD	Digital Versatile Disc
FAE	Fetal Alcohol Effects
FAS	Fetal Alcohol Syndrome
G6PD	Glucose-6-phosphate dehydrogenase deficiency
hCG	Human chorionic gonadotropin
HIV	human immunodeficiency virus
IDEA	Individuals with Disabilities Education Act
IEP	Individualized Education Program
IU	International units
JPMA	Juvenile Products Manufacturers Association
MCHB	Maternal and Child Health Bureau
MTHFR	5,10-methylenetetrahydrofolate reductase
NICU	Neonatal intensive care unit
OTC	Over-the-counter
SIDS	Sudden Infant Death Syndrome
SMR	Sexual maturity rating
SPF	Sun protection factor
STI	Sexually transmitted infection
TB	Tuberculosis
TV	Television
UDP-GT	Uridine Diphosphate-Glucuronosyl Transferase
UL	Underwriters Laboratories
USDA	United States Department of Agriculture
WIC	The Special Supplemental Nutrition Program for Women, Infants, and Children

Infancy

Prenatal to 11 Months

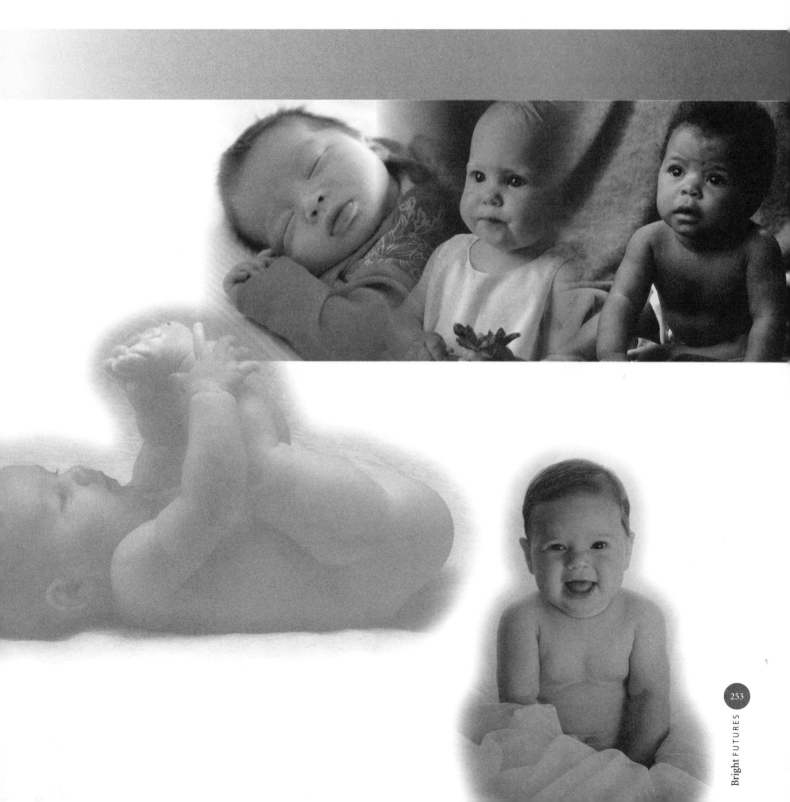

Health Supervision: Prenatal Visit

CONTEXT

A prenatal visit is recommended for all expectant families as an important first step in establishing a child's medical home. Some parents use this opportunity to select a health care professional, and this first visit is about establishing a relationship. It provides an opportunity to introduce parents to the practice, gather basic information, provide guidance, identify high-risk situations, and promote parenting skills.[1,2] The prenatal visit is especially valuable for first pregnancies, single parents, families with high-risk pregnancies, pregnancy complications, multiple pregnancies, parents who anticipate health problems for the newborn, parents who have experienced a perinatal or infant death, and parents who are planning to adopt a child.

Optimally, the prenatal visit entails a full office visit during which the expectant parents have the opportunity to meet with the health care professional. Among issues for discussion are the newborn metabolic and hearing screenings, the anticipated timing of the newborn's discharge from the nursery, typical health care concerns for a newborn during the first week of life, newborn behaviors, practice guidelines, and the typical course of health supervision during the first year. During the prenatal visit, the parents and health care professionals also discuss the importance of a healthy diet for fetal development; identify any unique dietary concerns for the family, including the use of herbal or complementary products; and discuss the plan for infant feeding after birth. Breastfeeding promotion is a key aspect of this visit,

in particular for expectant mothers who have not yet decided on a feeding method or who are unsure about the benefits or their ability to successfully breastfeed. The benefits of breastfeeding for the mother and baby can be emphasized, and parental questions or concerns about breastfeeding and breast milk can be addressed.

During the prenatal visit, the health care professional also is able to learn about the family constellation, the family's genetic history and health beliefs, the mother's health and wellness, including her mental health, life stressors, and support systems, and the couple's developmental adaptation to becoming parents. This visit also provides an opportunity to assess the family's preparations for the newborn's homecoming and potential safety concerns, identify potential resource needs, and determine the availability of support for the family at home and within the community.

The health care professional should reach out to the prospective parents, emphasizing the importance of each parent's role in the health, development, and nurturing of the child, and encouraging both parents and other important caregivers to attend subsequent health supervision visits if possible.

Before their baby's birth, many parents do not meet their baby's health care professional in a full prenatal office visit. However, a practice may use alternative strategies to obtain information, such as group prenatal visits, a prenatal/family history completed by the parents, or telephone contact, once the parents have decided to use the practice for their primary care and medical home.

PRIORITIES FOR THE VISIT

The first priority is to attend to the concerns of the parents. In addition, the Bright Futures Infancy Expert Panel has given priority to the following topics for discussion in this visit:

■ Family resources (family support systems, transition home [assistance after discharge], family resources, use of community resources)
■ Parental (maternal) well-being (physical, mental, and oral health; nutritional status; medication use; pregnancy risks)
■ Breastfeeding decision (breastfeeding plans, breastfeeding concerns [past experiences, prescription or nonprescription medications/drugs, family support of breastfeeding], breastfeeding support systems, financial resources for infant feeding)
■ Safety (car safety seats, pets, alcohol/substance use [fetal effects, driving], environmental health risks [smoking, lead, mold], guns, fire/burns [water heater setting, smoke detectors], carbon monoxide detectors/alarms)
■ Newborn care (introduction to the practice, illness prevention, sleep [back to sleep, crib safety, sleep location], newborn health risks [hand washing, outings])

HEALTH SUPERVISION

History

Interval history may be obtained according to the concerns of the family and the health care professional's preference or style of practice. The following questions can encourage in-depth discussion:

■ How has your pregnancy gone so far? What are similarities and differences from what you expected? From previous pregnancies? Did you have a prenatal ultrasound and were any problems noted?
■ What questions do you or other family members have about your baby after you deliver? Are there any concerns about the health of your baby?
■ What have you heard about the purpose/intent of routine child health care? Immunizations?
■ What do you think might be the most delightful aspect of being a parent? What do you think might be the most challenging aspect of being a parent?

Observation of Parent-Child Interaction

During the visit, the health care professional should observe:

■ Who asks questions and who provides responses to questions? (Observe parent with partner, other children, other family members accompanying mother.)
■ Verbal and nonverbal behaviors/communication among family members indicating support, understanding, or differences of opinion/conflicts.

Surveillance of Development

What have you heard about what newborns can do at birth? What would you like to know about what newborns can do at birth?

SOCIAL-EMOTIONAL

- Newborns are able to smell (especially breast milk), hear their parents' voices, see about 7 to 8 inches (eg, they can see their parent's face when being held), and respond to different types of touch (soothing touch and alerting touch).

COMMUNICATIVE

- Newborns communicate through crying and through behaviors such as facial expressions, body movements, and movement of their arms and legs. Initially, these behaviors may seem random, but, gradually, it will be possible to understand this early nonverbal language.

COGNITIVE

- Newborns learn to anticipate and trust their world through their parents' consistent and predictable caregiving (eg, through feeding and sleep patterns).

PHYSICAL DEVELOPMENT

- For the first months of life, newborns learn to live in a world that is very different from the womb. In the womb, they had a dark environment and felt swaying movements when their mother walked. They were used to a small space where their movements were restricted and they heard the constant swishing sounds of the placenta and their mother's heartbeat. During the first month of life, learning to suck, swallow, and breathe while eating, learning some pattern of sleeping, and learning to control their movements are all important steps in their physical development.

Physical Examination

Not applicable

Screening

Discuss the purpose and importance of the newborn screening tests (metabolic screening and hearing screening) that will be done in the hospital before the baby is discharged. Explain that the hospital, state health department, and the health care professional provide the results of these tests and follow up if any problems exist.

Inquire about prenatal screening (eg, HIV).

Immunizations

Discuss routine initiation of immunizations, including state-specific recommendations for immunization before discharge.

Consult the CDC/ACIP or AAP Web sites for the current immunization schedule.
CDC National Immunization Program (NIP): http://www.cdc.gov/vaccines
American Academy of Pediatrics *Red Book*: http://www.aapredbook.org

ANTICIPATORY GUIDANCE

The following sample questions, which address the Infancy Expert Panel's Anticipatory Guidance Priorities, are intended to be used selectively to invite discussion, gather information, address the needs and concerns of the family, and build partnerships. Use of the questions may vary from visit to visit and from family to family. Questions can be modified to match the health care professional's communication style. The accompanying anticipatory guidance for the family should be geared to questions, issues, or concerns for that particular child and family.

FAMILY RESOURCES

Family support systems, transition home (assistance after discharge), family resources, use of community resources

Inquire about other children and older family members, family routines, and relationships. Anticipatory guidance regarding the infant's health and safety will vary, based on the specific cultural traditions of the family.

SAMPLE QUESTIONS:
Tell me about yourself and your family. Are there other children in your home? How old are they?

ANTICIPATORY GUIDANCE:
- Parents need a support network, whether with friends or family members or through community programs.
- The information you share with me about your family traditions and your sources of support and assistance will help my professional relationship with you and your family and help us in medical decision making.
- After the baby is born and, over time, you'll find yourself weighing information from your family, friends, or the Internet with information from me and other health care professionals and your own beliefs. I can help you find a balance that is comfortable for you and that ensures the health of your baby.

Obtaining a 3-generation family health history is an important component of the prenatal visit. This will provide information about family members with learning disabilities, hearing loss, inheritable conditions, physical or psychiatric conditions, or mental retardation that may be critical to understanding the family and potential future problems in the newborn.

A family's health beliefs and use of any complementary and alternative health practices need to be examined and, if safe, considered for incorporation into the child's health care plan.

SAMPLE QUESTIONS:
Are there any special family health concerns that I should know about to better care for your baby and family? What health practices do you follow to keep your family healthy? Where do you get information when you have questions about health issues or caring for a child? How do you prefer to receive information?

ANTICIPATORY GUIDANCE:

- Knowing the health of all your family gives me additional information about your baby's health needs.
- Recognizing your family values, health beliefs, health practices, and learning styles will allow me to better answer your questions about the care of your baby.

Discuss with the mother her support systems at home.

SAMPLE QUESTIONS:

Who will be helping you take care of the baby and you when you go home from the hospital? How will you respond to your other children's needs? Are you working outside the home or attending school now? Who do you go to for help when you need a hand? Do you have friends or relatives that you can call on for help? Who are they? Do they live near you? How are decisions made in your family? Is there anyone that you rely on to help you with decisions? Is there anyone that you want me to include in our discussions about the baby?

ANTICIPATORY GUIDANCE:

- It is hard to provide care to several children at once, especially knowing and understanding the unique needs of each child.
- Understanding age-related aspects of care and strategies to meet these needs will be an important part of helping you meet the needs of your children.

Suggest community resources that help with finding quality child care, accessing transportation or getting a car safety seat, or addressing issues such as financial concerns, inadequate resources to cover health care expenses, inadequate or unsafe housing, limited food resources, parental inexperience, or lack of social support.

SAMPLE QUESTIONS:

Tell me about your living situation. Do you have:
- *Enough heat, hot water, and electricity?*
- *Appliances that work?*
- *Problems with bugs, rodents, peeling paint or plaster, or mold or dampness?*

How are your resources for caring for your baby? Do you have:
- *Enough knowledge to feel comfortable in caring for your baby?*
- *Health insurance?*
- *Enough money for food, clothing, diapers, and child care?*

ANTICIPATORY GUIDANCE:

- Community agencies are available to help you with concerns about your living situation. Public health agencies are often the best place to start because they work with all types of community agencies and family needs. Think about contacting them for help.

PARENTAL (MATERNAL) WELL-BEING

Physical, mental, and oral health; nutritional status; medication use; pregnancy risks

Mothers should be reminded about the importance of taking a prenatal vitamin, as it contains folic acid in an amount sufficient to protect against neural tube defects, as well as the importance of a balanced diet. Mothers at increased risk of having babies with neural tube defects and other birth defects, and women with a variant of the MTHFR gene (this variant increases the risk of neural tube birth defects), should discuss the optimal dose with their obstetric care professionals.

Each year, about 1 in 12 pregnant women are battered by their intimate partner. Homicide is the leading cause of death for pregnant and recently pregnant women. When inquiring, avoid asking about "abuse" or "domestic violence." Instead, use descriptive terms, such as hit, kicked, shoved, choked, and threatened. Provide information on the impact of domestic violence on the fetus and children and the community resources that provide assistance. Recommend resources and support groups.

Reinforce compliance with recommended prenatal care and encourage the mother to share her concerns with her obstetrician or other health care professional. If the patient is a pregnant teen or new to the practice and seeking care for another child, reinforcing the importance of early and appropriate prenatal care may be necessary if she is not receiving prenatal care. If she has not already been tested for HIV during this pregnancy or if she does not know her HIV status, encourage her to seek counseling for HIV testing.

SAMPLE QUESTIONS:

How has your pregnancy been going? What have you been doing to keep yourself and your baby healthy during your pregnancy?

Do you always feel safe with your partner? Has your partner or ex-partner ever hit, kicked, or shoved you or physically hurt you in any way? Has he or she ever threatened to hurt you or someone close to you? Do you have any questions about your safety at home? What will you do if you feel afraid? Do you have a plan? Would you like information on where to go or who to contact if you ever need help?

Are you aware of your HIV status?

ANTICIPATORY GUIDANCE:

- It is important to maintain your own health by going to all your prenatal care appointments, getting enough sleep, regular activity, and exercise, as well as eating a healthy diet with an appropriate weight gain. It also is important to maintain good oral health care and to make sure that you get regular dental checkups.
- One way that I and other health care professionals can help you if your partner is hitting or threatening you is to support you and provide information about local resources that can help you.

■ All mothers should know their HIV status because early treatment for themselves, and particularly for their baby, is so important. At this time, HIV testing is voluntary for the mother, but, in some locations, it may be mandatory for your baby if your status is unknown. If you do not know your status already, we recommend that you get tested, because proper treatment before, during, and after delivery can protect your baby from transmission.

SAMPLE QUESTIONS:

Are you taking any medicines or vitamins at the present time? Are you using any prescription or OTC medications or pain relievers? Have you used any health remedies or special herbs or teas to improve your health since you have been pregnant? Is there anything that you used to take but stopped using when you learned that you were pregnant?

ANTICIPATORY GUIDANCE:

■ To understand how it may affect your baby, it is important to know what OTC medication or herbal product you are taking.

Discuss the parents' feelings about the pregnancy and gauge whether disagreements or conflicts in the parents' relationship are likely to be a problem. Suggest community sources of help if appropriate.

SAMPLE QUESTIONS:

How do you feel about your pregnancy? What has been the most exciting aspect? What has been the hardest part? Pregnancy can be a stressful time for expectant families; do you have any specific worries? How have you been feeling physically and emotionally? Is this a good time for you to be pregnant? How does your family feel about it? Is it a wanted pregnancy by the mother? By the father? Is your pregnancy a source of marital discord? Was abortion or adoption ever considered? If this is not a wanted pregnancy, what are the reasons (eg, wrong timing, feeling that it deprives an older sibling, mother-father marital problems, financial concerns, housing concerns, mother's wish to go back to school or work, never wanted children, insecurity about parenting)?
What works in your family for communicating with each other, making decisions, managing stress, or handling emotions?

ANTICIPATORY GUIDANCE:

■ Availability and use of social (family and friends) and community support are important considerations in the first few days after you get home with your new baby.

■ If you and your partner disagree a lot or have many conflicts, consider contacting community resources that can help you work out these difficulties. It is important to work on resolving differences or conflicts because of the stress it may cause. Resolving these problems also can help you be emotionally ready for the baby's birth.

■ If you would like, I can suggest readings, relationship classes, or adult classes that may be helpful. Pregnancy is a time of personal growth and learning about yourself and your partner. Programs for this type of support are available in most communities.

BREASTFEEDING DECISION

Breastfeeding plans, breastfeeding concerns (past experiences, prescription or nonprescription medications/drugs, family support of breastfeeding) breastfeeding support systems, financial resources for infant feeding

Feeding guidance will be based on the mother's plan for feeding her baby (ie, breastfeeding, formula feeding, or a combination of both) and any perceived barriers or contraindications to breastfeeding. The prenatal visit is a perfect opportunity to address any concerns parents have about breastfeeding their newborn, provide information, and dispel any myths the parents may have heard. A woman's knowledge about newborn feeding is significantly linked with a decision to breastfeed. The major reasons women report for choosing not to breastfeed include lack of information about the benefits of breastfeeding, returning to work, restrictions on breastfeeding at work, embarrassment, fear of feeling tied down, and family influences. Maternal history of breast surgery or implants or past breastfeeding concerns may need in-depth discussions, and a lactation consultant may be a resource to provide support and answer these questions.

Mothers with a strong family history of allergies need to understand that their babies may benefit from breastfeeding through the first year of life.

Mothers who are considering combining breastfeeding and formula-feeding should be counseled to wait until lactation is well established (usually 2 to 4 weeks) before introducing formula. Discuss the benefits of exclusive breastfeeding and breastfeeding duration.

Ultimately, the decision is up to the mother (parents), and the health care professional should respect the decision and also allow for the mother to change her mind by the time the baby arrives.

SAMPLE QUESTIONS:
What are your plans for feeding your baby? What have you heard about breastfeeding? Do you have questions about breastfeeding that I can answer for you? What kinds of experiences have you had feeding babies? Did you breastfeed your other children? How did that go? Do you have concerns about these experiences that we should talk about if they will affect the new baby? Do you have any concerns about having support for breastfeeding, privacy, having enough breast milk, or changes in your body? Have you had any breast surgery? Do you or does anyone in your family have a history of food allergy or intolerance? Have you attended any classes that taught you how to nurse your baby? Do you know anyone who breastfeeds her baby? Did any of your family or friends breastfeed? Would you be able to get help from them as you are learning to breastfeed? Will they support your decision?

ANTICIPATORY GUIDANCE:
- Successful breastfeeding begins with knowledge and information about breastfeeding. Prenatal classes through local hospitals can be very helpful for new parents. In addition, many communities have lactation consultants and nurses who are available to assist with breastfeeding. Having these resources available helps you be comfortable with breastfeeding and can help you get off to a good start.

- Begin breastfeeding as soon as possible after the baby is born. Start in the delivery room if you can.
- Breastfeeding exclusively for about the first 6 months of life, and then combining it with solid foods from 6 to 12 months of age and for as long after that as you and the baby want, provides the best nutrition and supports the best possible growth and development.

Share information about the known effects for an expectant mother of any drugs, medications, or herbal or traditional health remedies. If the mother is planning on breastfeeding, provide information about the safety of continued medication or herbal use while breastfeeding. (Many herbal teas contain ephedra and other substances that may be harmful to the baby.)

The mother also should consult with her obstetrician or other health care professional about any OTC medications or herbal/traditional products that she is using.

SAMPLE QUESTIONS:

Are you taking any prescribed or OTC medications now or have you taken any in the past? Have you used any special or traditional health remedies to improve your health since you have been pregnant? Do you drink alcohol, any special teas, or take any herbs? Is there anything that you were taking but stopped using when you learned that you were pregnant?

ANTICIPATORY GUIDANCE:

- Because some medications, herbs, or, especially, alcohol can be passed into breast milk, it is important to know what these might be so that you can be advised appropriately when you are breastfeeding.

Most mothers are able to successfully breastfeed their babies. Babies with conditions that make breastfeeding challenging may still be breastfed and benefit greatly from appropriate breastfeeding consultation and close monitoring. Babies who have a very low birth weight or have special health care needs particularly benefit from expressed breast milk if they are unable to breastfeed from their mother.

Describe actions the other parent or caregiver can take to support breastfeeding, including cuddling, bathing, and diapering the baby. Family members, significant others, or friends should be included in breastfeeding education. Share options for engaging family members in the care of both the mother and baby. Provide information about community resources if the mother does not have an adequate, positive family and friend support network.

Emphasize the need for a follow-up visit within 48 hours of discharge at the health care professional's office, with someone who is knowledgeable about breastfeeding, to check on the baby's feeding, weight, and how the mother is doing and whether she has any questions or concerns. Other options for breastfeeding follow-up may include a visit by a home health nurse, if this is covered by insurance, or by a public health nurse. Provide parents with specific information about who they may contact with questions. Encourage parents with phrases such as, "From our discussion, it seems you are going to do very well with breastfeeding."

SAMPLE QUESTION:
Do you know how to contact support groups or lactation consultants?

ANTICIPATORY GUIDANCE:
- **Resources for help with breastfeeding are available through the hospital, lactation consultants, and some public health programs.**

For babies who are unable to breastfeed or tolerate expressed breast milk (classic galactosemia), or parents who choose not to breastfeed, parents need to understand that iron-fortified formula is the recommended alternative for feeding the baby during the first year of life.

Families need to understand the rationale for iron fortification, that iron-fortified formulas are well tolerated, and that studies show that iron-fortified formulas do not cause constipation. They also need to understand the importance of formula selection to best meet their baby's needs, and why changes in the types of formulas should be guided by the baby's health care professional, along with the parent.

Encourage parents to discuss choice of formula and any proposed changes in formula with their pediatric health care professional. Review steps for preparing formula and reinforce the need to carefully read the directions on the cans. Mixing directions differ among powdered formulas. Provide written information about the importance of food safety with formula, including heating and cleaning bottles and nipples.

SAMPLE QUESTIONS:
What have you read or heard about the different infant formulas (eg, iron-fortified, soy, lactose-free, and others)? Would you like some guidance about choosing an appropriate formula for your baby? How do you plan to prepare the formula? What have you heard about formula safety? Do you have any other questions about formula feeding?

ANTICIPATORY GUIDANCE:
- **If you are unable to breastfeed or choose not to breastfeed your baby, iron-fortified formula is the recommended substitute for breast milk for feeding your full-term baby during the first year of life.**

Parents may need referrals about resources for community food or nutrition assistance programs for which they are eligible (eg, Commodity Supplemental Food Program, Food Stamp Program, or WIC), and housing or transportation if needed. WIC provides nutritious foods for children, foods for mothers who breastfeed, nutrition education, and referrals to health and other social services. Mothers who choose to breastfeed can receive breast pumps or breastfeeding supplies and support through peer counselors. WIC continues to provide food after delivery to mothers who breastfeed.

SAMPLE QUESTIONS:
Are you concerned about having enough money to buy food or infant formula? Would you be interested in resources that would help you afford to care for you and your baby?

ANTICIPATORY GUIDANCE:

■ Programs and resources are available to help you and your baby. You may be eligible for food, nutrition, and/or housing or transportation assistance programs. Several food programs, such as the Commodity Supplemental Food Program and the Food Stamp Program, can help you. If you are breastfeeding and eligible for WIC, you can get nutritious food for yourself and support from peer counselors.

SAFETY

Car safety seats, pets, alcohol/substance use (fetal effects, driving), environmental health risks (smoking, lead, mold), guns, fire/burns (water heater setting, smoke detectors), carbon monoxide detectors/alarms

The type of transportation the family uses will determine counseling about car safety seats. Many families rely on other family members or friends for transportation and may not be familiar with car safety seat information. The family members' use of safety belts will help determine their level of knowledge about the need for a car safety seat for their child. The family must obtain a car safety seat and learn how to install it properly before the birth, so this visit is a good opportunity to review this information.

Special considerations should be made for evaluating newborns with special health care needs to determine the safest method of transportation at hospital discharge. Newborns with documented oxygen desaturation, apnea, or bradycardia when in a semi-upright position should travel in a supine or prone position, using an alternative safety device. If an apnea monitor is prescribed, it should be used during travel. The monitor and any additional equipment in the car should be secured to prevent it from becoming a projectile in a collision. The newborn should be properly positioned in the car safety seat, and rolled towels or diapers may be used for postural support. The newborn should be visible to an adult passenger, either directly or through the rearview mirror. A mirror that attaches to the car safety seat or vehicle seat should not be used because it can become a projectile in a crash.

The parents' own safe driving behaviors (including using safety belts at all times and not driving under the influence of alcohol or drugs) are important to the health of their children. The use of safety belts during pregnancy is especially critical.

Questions about proper installation should be referred to a certified Child Passenger Safety Technician in the community.
Child Safety Seat Inspection Station Locator: www.seatcheck.org
Toll-free Number: 866-SEATCHECK (866-732-8243)

Child Safety Seat Inspection Station Locator: www.seatcheck.org. Toll-free Number: 866-SEATCHECK (866-732-8243).

SAMPLE QUESTIONS:
Does everyone in the family use a safety belt every time they ride in the car?
What type of car safety seat do you have for the baby? Have you tried installing it?

ANTICIPATORY GUIDANCE:

- Using a safety belt during pregnancy is the best way to protect you and your unborn baby, even if your vehicle has an air bag. Wear the lap belt across your hips/pelvis and below your belly; place the shoulder belt across your chest between your breasts and away from your neck; and move your seat as far away from the steering wheel as you can.
- Make sure you bring your newborn home from the hospital in an infant-only car safety seat, or a convertible car safety seat without an armrest or shield, as these provide the best protection for newborns. Both are installed rear facing in the back seat of the vehicle.
- Even if you do not own a vehicle, you should still have a car safety seat for your child and know how to install it when you are riding in a taxi or in someone else's vehicle.
- Learn how the harnesses are adjusted and how to install the seat in your vehicle. You can get help from a local certified Child Passenger Safety Technician.
- Never put a rear-facing car safety seat in the front seat of a vehicle that has a passenger air bag, because air bags deploy with great force against a car safety seat and cause serious injury or death.

Pet guidance is based on the specific animals in the home (eg, domestic and exotic birds, cats, dogs, reptiles, or monkeys). Discussion points may include the need for maintaining physical separation of the pet from the child, introducing the pet to the new baby, avoiding contact with animal waste, the importance of hand washing, and limiting indoor air contamination with animal dander or waste products.

SAMPLE QUESTIONS:
Do you have any pets at home or do you handle any animals? If you have handled cats, have you ever been tested for antibodies to toxoplasmosis?

ANTICIPATORY GUIDANCE:

- Pets may be dangerous for infants and young children. Learn about the risks that may occur with your pets and determine the best method of protecting your baby.
- Talk to your own health care professional about getting tested for toxoplasmosis.

If the mother acknowledges alcohol use during pregnancy, discuss the concerns of both FAE and FAS to the developing fetus. Both FAE and FAS impair a child's lifetime ability to function mentally, physically, and socially. Fetal alcohol exposure, including the timing during the pregnancy, quantity, and duration, is important to document for future diagnosis of FAE or FAS. The pregnant woman should be advised to stop drinking and referred for additional counseling if needed.

If the mother acknowledges drug or alcohol use, also discuss state- and hospital-specific policies related to Child Protection referrals and practices related to child custody.

Based on the newborn's clinical findings at birth and state-specific policy, the newborn will need referral to either the state Child Find or Early Intervention Program after birth.

Referrals to community social service agencies and drug treatment programs can be provided if the mother is not already linked to these services.

SAMPLE QUESTIONS:

How much alcohol did you use before you knew you were pregnant? When did you find out you were pregnant? How much alcohol have you used since then? Do you, or does anyone you ride with, ever drive after having a drink? Does your partner use alcohol? What kind and for how long? Have you or your partner used any drugs either before or during the pregnancy? What kind and for how long?

ANTICIPATORY GUIDANCE:

- The reason we are concerned about a pregnant mother's use of alcohol or drugs is because of the effects on the baby's mental, physical, and social development. We know that a mother's alcohol or drug use affects her unborn baby and we have no way to know whether any alcohol is safe. Therefore, our recommendation is that women not drink alcohol while they are pregnant. If you are drinking alcohol, we encourage you to stop.
- If you need help with alcohol or drug use, some community agencies help women during their pregnancy as well as after their baby arrives so that they can safely care for their baby and themselves.

Smoking cessation national triage: 1-800-QUITNOW

Address how smoking affects the baby, including increasing the risk of low birth weight, preterm delivery, premature rupture of the membranes, placental abruption, SIDS, asthma, acute otitis media and middle ear effusion, and respiratory infections. Provide smoking cessation strategies and make specific referrals. Consider the safety of various treatments during pregnancy for patients who are committed to smoking cessation.

1-800-QUITNOW is a national telephone triage and support service that is routed to local resources. Health care professionals also may investigate what is available in their own communities, through their hospitals and health departments and through Internet-based resources such as the American Cancer Society (www.cancer.org) or the American Lung Association (www.lungusa.org).

SAMPLE QUESTIONS:

Have you smoked during this pregnancy? Does anyone else in your home smoke? Have you thought about cutting down now that you are pregnant? Have you been able to cut down the daily number of cigarettes? Do you know where to get help with stopping smoking?

ANTICIPATORY GUIDANCE:

- A smoke-free environment, in your car, home, and other places where your baby spends time, is important. Smoking affects the baby by increasing the risk of SIDS, asthma, ear infections, and respiratory infections.

Explain the risks of dampness, mold, and lead and discuss strategies for minimizing these risks.

SAMPLE QUESTION:
Some homes may have health risks that may affect your baby. Are you aware of any health concerns in your family related to your home due to dampness, mold, or lead?

ANTICIPATORY GUIDANCE:
- Molds are often found in homes that have leaking water or dampness that does not dry out, such as in showers or humidifiers that have not been regularly cleaned. It is important to keep such areas as clean and as dry as possible. Cleaning includes using a solution of 1 part bleach and 4 parts water and allowing the area to dry overnight. If the area cannot be cleaned, it is important to remove the materials to prevent the release of spores that can cause illnesses.
- Lead can be found in the paint of older homes (built before 1978), pottery and pewter, folk medicines, insecticides, industry, and hobbies, as well as other sources. Lead is toxic and it is important to be aware of any sources of lead in your home to prevent lead exposure for your family.

The hottest water temperature at the faucet should be no higher than 120°F.

Discuss gun safety in the home and the danger to family members and children. Homicide and suicide are more common in homes in which guns are kept. The AAP recommends that guns be removed from the places children live and play, and that, if it is necessary to keep a gun, it should be stored unloaded and locked, with the ammunition locked separately from the gun.

SAMPLE QUESTIONS:
Do you keep guns at home? Are they unloaded and locked? Is the ammunition locked and stored separately? Are there guns in the homes where you visit, such as the homes of grandparents, other relatives, or friends?

ANTICIPATORY GUIDANCE:
- Homicide and suicide are more common in homes that have guns. The best way to keep your child safe from injury or death from guns is to never have a gun in the home.
- If it is necessary to keep a gun in your home or if the homes of people you visit have guns, they should be stored unloaded and locked, with the ammunition locked separately from the gun.

Discuss other home safety precautions with parents.

SAMPLE QUESTION:
What home safety precautions have you taken for newborns and children?

ANTICIPATORY GUIDANCE:
- To protect your child from tap water scalds, the hottest temperature at the faucet should be no higher than 120°F. In many cases, you can adjust your water heater.

- Milk and formula should not be heated in the microwave because they can heat unevenly, causing pockets of liquid that are hot enough to scald your baby's mouth.
- Make sure you have a working smoke detector on every level of your home, especially in the furnace and sleeping areas. Test the detectors every month. It's best to use smoke detectors that use long-life batteries, but, if you don't, change the batteries at least once a year. Plan several escape routes from the house and conduct home fire drills.
- Install a carbon monoxide detector/alarm, certified by UL, in the hallway near every separate sleeping area of the home.

NEWBORN CARE

Introduction to the practice, illness prevention, sleep (back to sleep, crib safety, sleep location), newborn health risks (hand washing, outings)

Practice guidelines for newborn care during the postnatal period should be provided in writing to parents. This information includes the need for follow-up visits within 48 hours of discharge, and phone numbers in case there are any particular concerns (eg, jaundice, first time breast-feeding mother or concerns about infant's intake or feeding skills, or infant prematurity [35- to 37-weeks' gestation]). Information about the practice policies for after-hours and weekend routines and when parents should be concerned and contact the baby's health care professional usually are included as well.

First-time parents may need detailed information about typical early care and supply needs for the newborn. Mothers who have had a cesarean-section delivery may have additional information and referral needs. Home health care or public health nursing referrals for post-discharge assessment and supportive care may be appropriate.

Discussion of issues around circumcision would be appropriate at this time, but must be handled in a culturally sensitive manner. The parents' decision may be based on family and cultural beliefs. Information also should be provided regarding types of circumcision as well as used for babies who are not circumcised.

Culturally sensitive information should be provided about what is known about safe-sleep environments for babies. Room sharing is recommended, with the baby in a separate, but nearby, sleep space. Bed sharing (sleeping in the same bed as the parents) is not recommended. A supine position ("back to sleep") is best for babies, including premature infants, because of the reduction of SIDS. Prone sleep may be appropriate in only a few circumstances, such as for babies with certain craniofacial problems, like Pierre Robin Sequence, or babies with significant gastroesophageal reflux. These babies may require home cardiorespiratory monitoring because of risks of respiratory compromise.

Common beliefs and concerns expressed by families as justification for not placing their babies to sleep in the supine position include the fear of infant choking/aspiration, perceived uncomfortable/less peaceful sleep, concern about a flat occiput and hair loss, and family beliefs about appropriate infant sleep patterns, position, and sleep location.

Parents need strategies about how to advise relatives, friends, and child care providers to do the same. A consistent message about "back to sleep" provides family members with the best information when they ask about side sleeping.

SAMPLE QUESTION:
Do you have questions about the baby's care after the delivery?

ANTICIPATORY GUIDANCE:
- If your family is new to the practice, we will give you written information about the practice, such as names and background of the health care professionals, staff, appointment scheduling, and urgent and emergency access information.

SAMPLE QUESTIONS:
What have you heard about how babies should sleep? Where will your baby sleep? How about at naptime?

ANTICIPATORY GUIDANCE:
- To reduce the risk of SIDS, it is best to always have your baby sleep on her back.
- It is also a good idea if your baby sleeps in your room in her own crib (not in your bed).
- Choose a crib with slats that are no more than $2\frac{3}{8}$ inches (60 mm) apart and with a mattress the same size as the crib. A crib should be certified by the JPMA.
- If you choose a mesh playpen or portable crib, the weave should have openings less than $\frac{1}{4}$ inch (6 mm). Never leave your baby in a mesh playpen with the drop-side down.

Remind all family members or guests to wash their hands before handling the baby. Remind the family to protect the baby from anyone with colds or Illnesses, especially for the first couple of months.

Provide recommendations for outings to faith-based activities, restaurants, and closed quarters during the first 2 months and/or during flu season.

SAMPLE QUESTIONS:
What other suggestions have you heard about that will keep your baby healthy? How do you plan to protect your baby from getting infections?

ANTICIPATORY GUIDANCE:
- Wash your hands frequently with soap and water or a non-water antiseptic, especially after diaper changes and before feeding the baby.
- For the first few weeks, it is important to limit the baby's exposure to people with colds or to large groups where there may be people with illnesses.
- Breastfeeding also is known to provide protection and reduce the frequency of illnesses in babies.

Health Supervision: Newborn Visit

CONTEXT

Tremendous excitement accompanies the birth of a baby, but new parents also often feel overwhelmed and fatigued. During the typically short postpartum hospital stay, mothers must attempt to recover from the birth and get to know their newborns while getting visits from elated family and friends and interruptions from hospital personnel. During this time, the mother needs to become comfortable with feeding and caring for her newborn while beginning her own recovery.

Ideally, the parents have met or spoken with the health care professional for a prenatal visit, but, for many, the newborn visit is the first opportunity for the parents and health care professional to meet. The number of visits in the immediate newborn period will depend on the mode of delivery and the presence of maternal or neonatal complications. The duration of each visit also will vary, based upon the specific needs of the baby and family. Prior parental experience with newborns, the newborn's health status, and the presence of social support influence the parents' responses and guide the health care professional's interactions with the family. New parents always ask one question first: "Is our baby OK?" Once they hear that their baby is healthy, the parents want to learn how to care for him, establish a good

schedule, recover physically and emotionally from the birth, and go home to begin their new adventure.

Examining the newborn in the mother's room within the first 24 hours of life gives the health care professional an important opportunity to demonstrate the newborn's abilities, observe the parents' interactions with the baby, and model behaviors that engage and support the newborn during this transition time. The health care professional can elicit the newborn's response to voices and other forms of stimulation, such as noises in the room, touch, light, movement, being undressed, and being comforted. If this visit also is the first meeting the health care professional has with the mother, questions from the prenatal visit may need to be incorporated to gain a more comprehensive understanding of the family's values and beliefs, strengths, resources, and needs.

This interaction with the family gives the health care professional the chance to build the health supervision partnership with the family. Answering questions and addressing concerns during this visit will reassure parents and lessen the anxiety they may be feeling about taking their baby home. Knowing that the health care professional will be available after they leave the hospital will add to the parents' comfort and confidence as they embark on this new phase of their lives.

PRIORITIES FOR THE VISIT

The first priority is to attend to the concerns of the parents. In addition, the Bright Futures Infancy Expert Panel has given priority to the following topics for discussion in this visit:

- Family readiness (family support, maternal wellness, transition, sibling relationships, family resources)
- Infant behaviors (infant capabilities, parent-child relationship, sleep [location, position, crib safety], sleep/wake states [calming])
- Feeding (feeding initiation, hunger/satiation cues, hydration/jaundice, feeding strategies [holding, burping], feeding guidance [breastfeeding, formula])
- Safety (car safety seats, tobacco smoke, falls, home safety [review of priority items if no prenatal visit was conducted])
- Routine baby care (infant supplies, skin care, illness prevention, introduction to practice/early intervention referrals)

HEALTH SUPERVISION

History

Interval history may be obtained according to the concerns of the family and the health care professional's preference or style of practice. After congratulating the parents on the birth of their new baby, asking the following questions can encourage in-depth discussion:

- How are you feeling? How was the delivery?
- Have you named the baby yet?
- How have things been going with the baby? *(Use the baby's name if it is given.)*
- What questions do you have about your baby? Do you have any concerns about taking care of your baby?

History of Labor and Delivery

Prenatal history

- Preterm labor, premature rupture of the membranes, pregnancy complications, abnormal ultrasound findings
- Maternal conditions potentially affecting the infant's health—preexisting maternal health conditions, gestational diabetes, hypertensive disorders of pregnancy, special dietary restrictions, infections (group B streptococcus, chorioamnionitis, urinary tract infection, HIV, hepatitis B, sexually transmitted infections, toxoplasmosis, CMV)
- Maternal medication, tobacco, alcohol, other drugs, complementary medicine

Delivery

- Mode of delivery—vaginal versus cesarean section, breech presentation, instrumentation (forceps, vacuum)
- Medications used—terbutaline, magnesium sulfate, pitocin, demerol, antenatal steroids, antibiotics

- Anesthesia used—epidural, spinal, general
- Use of episiotomy (degree) or lacerations
- Duration of labor, length of delivery, indication(s) for delivery/induction
- Complications of labor and delivery—fever, infection, bleeding, HELLP Syndrome, toxemia

Infant at Delivery
Delivery history
- Fetal distress—heart-rate tracing abnormalities, decreased movement, meconium-stained fluid, oligohydramnios or polyhydramnios, mode of delivery
- Complications—intrauterine growth restriction (IUGR), large baby, maternal hypertensive disease, diabetes, infection, withdrawal from substance use or abuse, intrapartum anesthesia/analgesia or other medical condition affecting the fetus or newborn (eg, antenatal diagnosis of hydronephrosis), birth trauma
- Gestational age, birth weight, and Apgar score
- Newborn transition problems—respiratory distress, cyanosis, hypoglycemia, poor feeding, temperature instability, jitteriness
- Administration of vitamin K and eye prophylaxis

Neonatal Course
Information obtained about the postnatal course for the mother and infant will influence further interactions, assessments, and recommendations for the care of the child and mother. This information includes underlying maternal health, including the level of maternal discomfort and pain medication use, affect on and interaction with baby, perspectives on breastfeeding, attempts at breastfeeding, and perceived success with breastfeeding.

Neonatal history
- Maternal syphilis serology, group B streptococcus and hepatitis B status, and possibly HIV and TB status, depending on each state's public health law requirements.
- Maternal blood type, Rh factor.
- Infant blood type and direct Coombs test.
- Vital signs (temperature, respirations, heart rate, blood sugar [if at risk]).
- Weight loss/gain.
- Feeding history—breastfeeding LATCH Scores, frequency, duration.
- Sleep pattern—ease of awakening, duration of sleep cycles.
- Elimination pattern—meconium, number of wet diapers.
- Evidence of jaundice—blood group incompatibility, prematurity, racial background, recommendations for follow-up after discharge.
- Presence of a major anomaly or 3 or more minor anomalies, a combination of major and minor anomalies, or a recognized pattern or distribution of anomalies suggesting a need for genetic evaluation.
- Newborn metabolic and hearing screening.
- The family members' cultural beliefs relating to illness and disability and their reaction to screening, particularly if the screening is mandatory. Screening requirements may violate some cultural and religious beliefs. If the family's religious or cultural beliefs include acceptance of disabilities or illness, pursuit of some types of interventions may not fit family values.

Observation of Parent-Child Interaction

During the visit, the health care professional should observe:
- Do the parents recognize and respond to the baby's needs?
- Are they comfortable when feeding, holding, or caring for the baby?
- Do they have visitors or any other signs of a support network?

Surveillance of Development

Do you have any specific concerns about your baby's development, learning, or behavior?

SOCIAL-EMOTIONAL
- Has periods of wakefulness
- Responsive to parental voice and touch

COMMUNICATIVE
- Able to be calmed when picked up

COGNITIVE
- Looks at parents when awake

PHYSICAL DEVELOPMENT
- Moves in response to visual or auditory stimuli

Physical Examination

A complete physical examination is included as part of every health supervision visit.

When performing a physical examination, the health care professional's attention is directed to the following components of the examination that are important for a child this age:

- **Measure and plot (adjust for gestational age, as indicated):**
  - Length
  - Weight
  - Head circumference
- **Plot:**
  - Weight-for-length
- **General observations:**
  - Assess alertness and if in any apparent distress
  - Observe for congenital anomalies
- **Skin**
  - Note skin lesions or jaundice
- **Head**
  - Observe shape (sutures, molding), size, fontanelles
  - Note any signs of birth trauma
- **Eyes**
  - Perform inspection of eyes and eyelids
  - Assess ocular mobility
  - Examine pupils for opacification and red reflexes

- **Ears**
  - Observe shape and position of pinnae, patency of auditory canals, presence of pits or tags
- **Nose**
  - Observe for patency, septal deviation
- **Mouth**
  - Note clefts of lip or palate
  - Note presence of natal teeth
  - Note short frenulum
- **Heart**
  - Observe rate, rhythm, heart sounds, murmurs
  - Palpate femoral pulses
- **Abdomen**
  - Examine umbilical cord and cord vessels
- **Genitalia/rectum**
  - Determine that testes are descended; observe for penile anomalies
  - Determine patency of anus
- **Musculoskeletal**
  - Note any deformities of the back and spine
  - Note any foot abnormalities
- **Developmental hip dysplasia**
  - Perform Ortolani and Barlow maneuvers
- **Neurologic**
  - Detect primitive reflexes
  - Observe symmetry of extremity movement
  - Observe muscle tone

Screening

UNIVERSAL SCREENING	ACTION
Metabolic and hemoglobinopathy	Conduct screening as required by the state. Know the conditions that are screened for in your state.
Hearing	All newborns should receive an initial hearing screening before being discharged from the hospital. If this is not possible, a screening should be completed within the first month of life.

SELECTIVE SCREENING	RISK ASSESSMENT*	ACTION IF RA +
Blood pressure	Children with specific risk conditions	Blood pressure
Vision	Abnormal fundoscopic examination	Ophthalmology referral

*See the Rationale and Evidence chapter for the criteria on which risk screening questions are based.

Immunizations

Consult the CDC/ACIP or AAP Web sites for the current immunization schedule.
CDC National Immunization Program (NIP): http://www.cdc.gov/vaccines
American Academy of Pediatrics *Red Book*: http://www.aapredbook.org

Review state requirements for Hepatitis B immunization.

ANTICIPATORY GUIDANCE

The following sample questions, which address the Infancy Expert Panel's Anticipatory Guidance Priorities, are intended to be used selectively to invite discussion, gather information, address the needs and concerns of the family, and build partnerships. Use of the questions may vary from visit to visit and from family to family. Questions can be modified to match the health care professional's communication style. The accompanying anticipatory guidance for the family should be geared to questions, issues, or concerns for that particular child and family.

FAMILY READINESS

Family support, maternal wellness, transition, sibling relationships, family resources

The newborn period is a time of great adjustment and change for parents. Discuss and provide suggestions about making life easier during the first week at home. Parents need support and help from their family, friends, and community. Not only is it important to assess the newborn's status but also to listen and observe for concerns the parents may have in obtaining adequate support during the transition period right after the birth that would indicate the need for a referral to home care services. It also is important to provide contact information for parenting classes, support groups, community resources, or social services to help parents care for their baby and reduce feelings of isolation.

Many parents feel overwhelmed by a new baby. Knowing appropriate coping strategies can prevent parents from harming their baby when they feel tired, overwhelmed, or frustrated.

SAMPLE QUESTIONS:

Do you have family and friends you can call who are willing and able to help you and your baby when you have a question or need help, or in case of an emergency? How accessible are these people? Are they able to help you care for the baby? Are they able to help with transportation? Is there someone you can leave the baby with? Are you getting the support (medical, physical, emotional, financial) you need?

ANTICIPATORY GUIDANCE:

- It's important to have people you can turn to when you need help with the baby. Consider talking with family members or friends and making arrangements with them so that they can be prepared to help if needed. These people usually are willing to help, but may need specific instructions on ways they can be most helpful.

SAMPLE QUESTIONS:

What makes you get upset with your baby? What do you do when you get upset?

ANTICIPATORY GUIDANCE:

- All parents get upset at least sometimes. When you have these feelings, put the baby down in a safe place, like a crib or cradle. It helps if you have somebody to call or ask for help when you feel upset.
- Never yell at, hit, or shake your baby.

SAMPLE QUESTIONS:

When you go home, what are your plans to help you get the rest you need and get back into your usual routines? How do you think your baby will change your lives? Will you be able to take time for yourself, individually and as a couple?

ANTICIPATORY GUIDANCE:

- You'll probably want to spend most of your time and attention on the new baby, but don't forget to take time for yourself alone and for you and your partner. Nurturing yourself will help you stay healthy and happy for your baby.
- Here are a few suggestions about making life easier the first week at home:
  - Tell family and friends about needing family time, as well as what they can do to really help.
  - Set up ideas for organization that will make outings a little easier.
  - Identify the activities that are more difficult for you to do (such as grocery shopping, laundry, vacuuming) now that you are a new mom.
- Many mothers feel tired or overwhelmed in the first weeks at home. They also may experience some "baby blues" for a short time. These feelings should not continue, however. If you find that you are continuing to feel very tired, overwhelmed, or blue, you need to let your partner, your health care professional, and/or me know so that we can get the resources to help you.

Parent concerns about sibling reactions to meeting the baby are best guided based on the siblings' developmental ages and responses. Behavior regression and jealousy sometimes occur with an older sibling.

SAMPLE QUESTION:

What do your other children think about the new baby?

ANTICIPATORY GUIDANCE:

- To help your older children adjust to the new baby and still feel wanted and loved, ask for their help in caring for the baby. Make sure not to ask them to do anything beyond their capability. Do not leave the baby unsupervised with young or inexperienced brothers or sisters.
- Spend individual time every day with your other children doing things they like to do.

Parents in difficult living situations or with limited resources will have concerns about their ability to care for their newborn. Provide information and referrals, as needed, for community resources that help with finding quality child care, accessing transportation or getting a car safety seat, or addressing issues such as financial concerns, inadequate or unsafe housing, or limited food resources. Provide information on the impact of domestic violence on children and on community resources that provide assistance.

If the baby has special health care needs, provide information and referral to the local public health nursing services for MCHB Title V Information (Health Care Program for Children with Special Needs) and the local Early Intervention Program agency, often referred to as IDEA. These 2 programs will be able to assist in connecting families to many community resources.

SAMPLE QUESTIONS:
Tell me about your living situation.
Do you have:
- *Enough heat, hot water, and electricity?*
- *Appliances that work?*
- *Problems with bugs, rodents, peeling paint or plaster, or mold or dampness?*
How are your resources for caring for your baby? Do you have:
- *Enough knowledge to feel comfortable in caring for your baby?*
- *Health insurance?*
- *Enough money for food, clothing, diapers, and child care?*
Do you have a trusted source of child care?
Do you know where to go for help if your partner is hitting or threatening you?

ANTICIPATORY GUIDANCE:
- Resources for parent education and/or parent support groups are available to help you learn about your developing baby.
- Community agencies are available to assist you with concerns about your living situation. Public health agencies are often the best place to start because they work with all types of community agencies and family needs. You may consider contacting them for help.
- Social, faith-based, cultural, volunteer, and recreational organizations or programs are available in the community to help support new families.
- If your baby has special health care needs, your local public health department is required by law to provide services for you and your baby. Contact the department for help and information about community resources.

INFANT BEHAVIORS

Infant capabilities, parent-child relationship, sleep (location, position, crib safety), sleep/wake states (calming)

Encourage parents to learn about their baby's temperament and how it affects the way he relates to the world. Demonstrate the newborn's skills and his competence and readiness to respond to his parents. Demonstrate the parents' capabilities as they handle and care for their newborn to reinforce their sense of competence. Because families from some cultures may be uncomfortable with publicly praising the newborn because of concerns about this bringing on harm, it may be best to note these skills in a neutral way until ascertaining the parents' feelings about this issue.

SAMPLE QUESTIONS:
How do you think your baby sees, hears, and reacts to you? What do you do to calm your baby? What do you do if that does not work?

ANTICIPATORY GUIDANCE:

- Your baby already is beginning to know you. See how he brightens when he hears your voice? He shows you that he likes it when you hold him, feed him, and talk to him. You will soon learn what your baby is trying to tell you when he cries, looks at you, turns away, or smiles.

- As you try to console your baby, you will begin to recognize that he may not always be consolable. Actions such as stroking your baby's head or gentle, repetitive rocking may help you calm him. Your baby's head is fragile. It is very important to never shake your baby because of the damage this can cause to his head.

- If you are breastfeeding, wait to introduce a pacifier until your baby is 1 month old to ensure that breastfeeding is firmly established.

Creating more nurturing routines and promoting child and family development and parental well-being are benefits of tactile contact and stimulation. This exchange is a special way of enhancing the attachment experience for parents and baby, just as breastfeeding does for mother and baby. First-time parents and young parents gain self-confidence and become more proficient in their nurturing abilities through this exchange.

SAMPLE QUESTION:

What do you do to help the baby feel safe and comfortable?

ANTICIPATORY GUIDANCE:

- Make touching your baby (caressing, massaging, holding, carrying, and rocking) an important part of all the everyday care activities of feeding, diapering, bathing, and bedtime. This physical contact helps your baby feel secure and understand that he is loved and cared for. It is a special way for you and your partner to develop a strong attachment to your baby and it will help you grow together as a family.

- Physical contact also offers important health and developmental benefits if your baby was premature or has special health care needs. It can enhance his sleep, help him regulate his sleep and wake times, and foster the parent-baby attachment that may have been delayed or disrupted because of prolonged or repeated hospitalizations.

Families' beliefs and cultural traditions will have a significant impact on where and how the baby sleeps, and whether they or other caregivers follow the "back to sleep" message. Counsel parents about sleep location, sleep position ("back to sleep"), and cribs.

SAMPLE QUESTIONS:

Where will your baby be sleeping once you get home? What have you heard about bed sharing or room sharing? What have you heard about the relationship of the use of pacifiers and breastfeeding and SIDS? What type of bassinet or portable crib will you be using?

ANTICIPATORY GUIDANCE:

- Always put your baby down to sleep on his back, not on his tummy or side. Ask your relatives and caregivers also to put your baby "back to sleep." Experts also recommend that your baby sleep in your room in his own crib (not in your bed). If you breastfeed or bottle-feed your baby in your bed, return him to his own crib or bassinet when you both are ready to go back to sleep.
- Do not use loose, soft bedding (blankets, comforters, sheepskins, quilts, pillows, pillow-like bumper pads) or soft toys in the baby's crib, because they are associated with an increased risk of SIDS. Thin blankets can be used to swaddle the baby, or in a crib if the blankets are tucked in under the crib mattress.
- Using a pacifier during sleep is strongly associated with a reduced risk of SIDS. Consider offering a pacifier when your baby lies down for sleep. Never reinsert the pacifier if it falls out after the baby falls asleep, and do not coat it with a sweet solution. If you are breastfeeding, wait to introduce a pacifier until your baby is 1 month old to ensure that breastfeeding is firmly established.
- The room temperature should be comfortable and the baby should be kept from getting too warm or too cold while sleeping.
- Be sure your baby's crib is safe. The slats should be no more than $2\frac{3}{8}$ inches (60 mm) apart. The mattress should be firm and fit snugly into the crib. Keep the sides of the crib raised when the baby is sleeping in it. Be sure the crib is certified by the JPMA.
- If you use a mesh playpen or portable crib, the weave should have small openings less than $\frac{1}{4}$ inch (6 mm). Never leave your baby in a mesh playpen or crib with the drop-side down.

FEEDING

Feeding initiation, hunger/satiation cues, hydration/jaundice, feeding strategies (holding, burping), feeding guidance (breastfeeding, formula)

General Guidance on Feeding

Parents find great enjoyment and satisfaction in feeding their newborn. It is a time the newborn is awake and alert, looking intently at her parent. Most parents gauge their early parenting ability with their success in feeding their baby. Therefore, providing guidance, assurance, and early assistance with any feeding concerns is a critical element of the newborn visit.

Many newborns and mothers find early feeding a challenge because of difficulties in waking the newborn and the newborn's immature organization for sucking, swallowing, and breathing.

Newborns, including breastfed and/or premature newborns with jaundice, may be difficult to wake, resulting in greater difficulty with feedings. Close supervision and counseling are needed to assist parents in ensuring their newborn awakens for feedings to ensure adequate hydration. Feeding difficulty also may be one of the first signs of neurologic problems and should always be evaluated.

Mothers of newborns with special health care needs particularly need support and specialized assistance with feeding and nutrition. Referral for dietary support and familiarity with special techniques for specific conditions may be helpful.

Observing breastfeeding or formula feeding often provides insight into the newborn's neuromotor abilities and the parent-newborn interaction. This examination is of value for all infants, but especially for infants who experience feeding difficulties, or if there is concern about the parent-newborn interaction. The mother's comfort in feeding the newborn, eye contact between the mother and newborn, the mother's interaction with the newborn, the mother's and newborn's responses to distractions in the environment, and the newborn's ability to suck can be assessed with observation.

Before talking with the mother about how feedings are going, it is advisable to determine the weight difference from birth, type of feedings, frequency, duration, wet diapers, and stools to provide the mother with specific indications that the feedings are going well and to identify any possible concerns.

SAMPLE QUESTIONS:
How is feeding going? What questions or concerns do you have about feeding? How often does your baby feed? How long does it generally take for a feeding? How does the baby behave during a feeding? Pulls away, arches back, is irritable, or calm? Has your baby received any other fluids from a bottle? How does the baby behave after feedings? Satisfied baby look, still rooting, anxious? How do you know whether your baby is hungry? How do you know if she has had enough to eat? What is the longest time your baby has slept at one time?

ANTICIPATORY GUIDANCE:
- Breastfeeding exclusively during the first 4 to 6 months of life provides ideal nutrition and supports the best possible growth and development. For mothers who are unable to breastfeed their baby or who choose not to breastfeed, iron-fortified formula is the recommended substitute for breast milk for feeding the full-term infant during the first year of life.
- You should feed your baby when she is hungry. A baby's usual signs of hunger include putting her hand to her mouth, sucking, rooting, pre-cry facial grimaces, and fussing. Crying is a late sign of hunger. You can avoid crying by responding to the baby's more subtle cues. Once a baby is crying, feeding may become more difficult, especially with breastfeeding, as crying interferes with latching on.
- In the first days of life, your baby should be encouraged to breastfeed about 8 to 12 times in 24 hours to help the mature breast milk come in.
- At about 3 to 4 days after birth, babies go through a "feeding frenzy" where they want to eat every 1 to 2 hours. This is when they begin to make up for the weight loss that happens right after birth. As your milk supply comes in, you will provide enough breast milk to meet your baby's needs.
- At about 1 week of age, your baby should settle into a more typical breastfeeding routine of every 2 to 3 hours in the daytime, and every 3 hours at night with one longer 4- to 5-hour stretch between feedings. At this time, your baby will be nursing at least 8 to 12 times in 24 hours.

- Feed your baby until she seems full. Signs of fullness are turning the head away from nipple, closing the mouth, and relaxed hands. If she is sleeping more than 4 hours at a time, she should be awakened for feeding during the first 2 weeks. Keeping her close by (rooming in) while in the hospital and at home will make it easier for you to recognize the early feeding cues.
- A newborn is often very sleepy after delivery, especially if the mother had medication for delivery or if the baby is jaundiced. She may need gentle stimulation (such as rocking, patting, or stroking) and time to come to an alert state for feeding. These movements also are helpful for consoling your baby.
- Healthy babies do not require extra water, as breast milk or formula (when properly prepared) are adequate to meet the newborn's fluid needs.

SAMPLE QUESTION:
How many wet diapers and stools does your baby have each day?

ANTICIPATORY GUIDANCE:
- Your baby should have about 6 to 8 wet diapers in 24 hours after your milk comes in. She may have stools as frequently as one per feeding or she may go for a number of days without a stool. If you are breastfeeding, your baby's stools will be loose. This is normal and is not diarrhea.

SAMPLE QUESTION:
How easy is it to burp your baby during or after a feeding?

ANTICIPATORY GUIDANCE:
- Burp your baby at natural breaks (eg, midway through or after a feeding) by gently rubbing or patting her back while holding her against your shoulder and chest or supporting her in a sitting position on your lap.

New mothers need to take care of their baby and themselves. This includes making sure they have adequate resources to feed themselves and their baby. WIC provides nutritious foods for children, foods for mothers who exclusively breastfeed their babies, nutrition education, and referrals to health and other social services.

SAMPLE QUESTION:
How much rest are you getting?

ANTICIPATORY GUIDANCE:
- If you are not getting enough sleep because of pain related to the birth or to breastfeeding (eg, engorged breasts or nipple soreness), ask your obstetrician to suggest an OTC medication to help you, and get help from a lactation professional to make sure your baby is latching on correctly.

SAMPLE QUESTION:
Are you concerned about having enough money to buy food or infant formula?

ANTICIPATORY GUIDANCE:

- Programs and resources are available to help you and your baby. You may be eligible for food, nutrition, and/or housing or transportation assistance programs. Several food programs, such as the Commodity Supplemental Food Program and the Food Stamp Program, can help you. If you are breastfeeding and eligible for WIC, you can get nutritious food for yourself and support from peer counselors.

Guidance on Breastfeeding

Explore cultural beliefs and family beliefs, sources of advice for the family, and past experience with breastfeeding. Some cultures believe that colostrum is harmful to the baby and that breastfeeding should not begin until the full milk has come in. Educate the parents about the health benefits of colostrum, but respect cultural beliefs.

It is important to get the breastfeeding mother off to a good start by assessing her plans, making sure she is eating right and taking vitamins, and that there are no contraindications to breastfeeding. Very few contraindications to breastfeeding exist, and most need to be considered on a case-by-case basis. Breastfeeding is contraindicated for a baby with classic galactosemia. Additional contraindications include HIV-positive status (see the CDC Web site [www.cdc.gov] for most current recommendations), substance abuse, TB (only until treatment is initiated and the mother is no longer infectious), herpetic lesions localized to the breast, and chemotherapy or other contraindicated drugs.

SAMPLE QUESTIONS:
How is breastfeeding going for you and your baby? Have you had any problems with your breasts or nipples (eg, tenderness, swelling, or pain)?

ANTICIPATORY GUIDANCE:

- Breastfeeding should not hurt, and pain is a warning sign that something is not right. You may experience nipple tenderness at first, but this should be mild. Anything other than mild tenderness should be evaluated.

SAMPLE QUESTION:
What vitamin or mineral supplements do you take or plan to take?

ANTICIPATORY GUIDANCE:

- You should continue to take your prenatal vitamin or a multivitamin every day. If you are vegetarian, make sure the supplement contains iron, zinc, and vitamin B_{12}. If you are vegan, it is essential that the supplement contains vitamin B_{12}.

SAMPLE QUESTIONS:
What drugs or medications do you use (eg, herbs; prescription, OTC, homeopathic, or street drugs)? Do you drink wine, beer, or other alcoholic beverages? Do you know your HIV status?

ANTICIPATORY GUIDANCE:

- Most medications are compatible with breastfeeding but should be checked on an individual basis.

- Because alcohol is passed into the breast milk, it is important for mothers to avoid alcohol for 2 to 3 hours before breastfeeding or during breastfeeding. This also means that, because newborns breastfeed so frequently (every 2 to 3 hours), a mother most likely will have to avoid alcohol during the first several months of her baby's life.
- If you do not know your HIV status, it is a good idea to get tested because, if you are HIV positive, it is possible to prevent transmission of the virus to your baby.

Guidance on Formula Feeding

If a woman cannot or chooses not to breastfeed, iron-fortified formula is the recommended substitute for feeding the full-term infant for the first year of life. Although formula feeding may be considered easier for parents, information regarding formula preparation, formula safety, infant holding, and burping should be provided to ensure safe and appropriate formula feeding.

A newborn who is growing appropriately will average 20 oz of formula per day.

SAMPLE QUESTIONS:
What formula are you planning to use? How often does your baby eat? How much does your baby take at a feeding?

ANTICIPATORY GUIDANCE:
- Prepare 2 oz of infant formula every 2 to 3 hours at first, and then provide more if your baby still seems hungry.
- As your baby's appetite increases over time, you will need to prepare and offer larger quantities of formula.

SAMPLE QUESTION:
What information do you have about preparing formula and formula safety?

ANTICIPATORY GUIDANCE:
- Carefully read the instructions on the formula container. It will give you important information about how to prepare the formula and store it safely. Talk with me or another health care professional if you have any questions about how to prepare formula or before switching to a different brand or kind of formula.

SAMPLE QUESTION:
How does your baby like to be held when you feed her?

ANTICIPATORY GUIDANCE:
- It is important for you to always hold your baby close when feeding, in a semi-upright position, so that you are able to sense her behavioral cues of hunger, being full, comfort, and distress. Hold your baby so you can look into her eyes during feeding.
- When you feed your baby with a bottle, do not prop the bottle in her mouth. Propping increases the risk that she may choke, get an ear infection, and

develop early childhood caries. Holding your baby in your arms and holding the bottle for her gives you a wonderful opportunity for warm and loving interaction with her.

SAMPLE QUESTION:

How easy is it to burp your baby during or after a feeding?

ANTICIPATORY GUIDANCE:

- Burp your baby at natural breaks (eg, midway through or after a feeding) by gently rubbing or patting her back while holding her against your shoulder and chest or supporting her in a sitting position on your lap.

SAFETY

Car safety seats, tobacco smoke, falls, home safety (review of priority items if no prenatal visit was conducted)

Reinforce the use of a rear-facing car safety seat to transport the newborn home. If no prenatal visit was conducted, review general safety for newborns, including exposure to smoking and falls.

Infants with special needs need special consideration for safe transportation. Refer parents to a local, specially trained child passenger safety technician for assistance with special positioning and restraint devices (www.preventinjury.org).

Questions about proper installation should be referred to a certified Child Passenger Safety Technician in the community.
Child Safety Seat Inspection Station Locator: www.seatcheck.org
Toll-free Number: 866-SEATCHECK (866-732-8243)

Child Safety Seat Inspection Station Locator: www.seatcheck.org. Toll-free Number: 866-SEATCHECK (866-732-8243).

SAMPLE QUESTIONS:

How are you taking the baby home? (Note: If they are taking a taxi or if someone is picking them up, discuss car safety seat issues within that context.) *What questions do you have about using your car safety seat?*

ANTICIPATORY GUIDANCE:

- A rear-facing car safety seat should always be used to transport your baby in all vehicles, including taxis and cars owned by friends or other family members.
- Never put your baby's car safety seat in the front seat of a vehicle with a passenger air bag. Air bags deploy with great force against a car safety seat and cause serious injury or death.
- The car safety seat should be positioned at the recommended angle so that your baby's head does not fall forward. Bring your car safety seat into the hospital, and staff can help you adjust the harness so it fits correctly.
- The back seat is the safest place for children to ride.
- Your baby needs to remain in his car safety seat at all times during travel. If he becomes fussy or needs to nurse, stop the vehicle and remove him from the car safety seat to attend to his needs. Strap him safely back into his seat before traveling again.

- Keeping the harnesses buckled snugly whenever he is in the car safety seat will help prevent falls out of the seat and strangulation on the harnesses. Car safety seats should be used only for travel and not for positioning outside the vehicle.
- Babies with special needs, such as premature babies or babies in casts need special consideration for safe transportation.
- Your own safe-driving behaviors are important to the health of your children. Always use a safety belt and do not drive under the influence of alcohol or drugs.

SAMPLE QUESTIONS:

Does anyone in your home smoke? What about other family members or close friends?

ANTICIPATORY GUIDANCE:

- It is very important for your baby's health that your home, vehicle, and other places the baby stays are smoke-free.

SAMPLE QUESTION:

What changes have you made in your home to ensure your baby's safety?

ANTICIPATORY GUIDANCE:

- Always keep one hand on your baby when changing diapers or clothing on a changing table, couch, or bed to prevent her from falling.

ROUTINE BABY CARE

Infant supplies, skin care, illness prevention, introduction to practice/early intervention referrals

Discuss newborn supplies and safety precautions. Most babies use 8 to 12 diapers a day, or a diaper before and/or after each feeding. Often, this is not a supply or expense that parents anticipate. Thus, this information may be helpful in their decision to use disposable versus cloth diapers. Parents are often counseled by family members on cultural and family beliefs about skin care. Listening to parents' plans for skin care provides information about how to approach skin-care counseling.

Because parents are fearful of touching the "soft spot," they hesitate to wash the baby's scalp. Demonstrating washing the scalp during an examination and reinforcing the need for frequent scalp washing will assure the parents and help prevent "cradle cap."

Counsel parents on the decision to circumcise their baby boy. Their decision may be based on their family and cultural beliefs. Provide information about types of circumcision as well as issues for babies who are not circumcised.

Parents/caregivers need to know about the possibility of some female vaginal bleeding in female infants as a result of maternal hormones.

Newborns with recognizable diagnoses or prematurity should be referred for early intervention services, as required or provided by specific state eligibility guidelines, so that families may receive the support and be connected to the community services they need.

SAMPLE QUESTIONS:

What questions do you have about your baby's skin care? Is there any special care or treatment you or your family provides to the umbilical cord?

ANTICIPATORY GUIDANCE:

- A newborn baby's skin is sensitive. Using fragrance-free soaps and lotions for bathing and fragrance-free detergents for washing clothing will reduce the likelihood of rashes. In addition, oils and heavy lotions tend to clog pores and increase the likelihood of rashes. For areas of dry skin, such as creases and feet, moisturizing lotions are recommended. Powders are not recommended because of the possibility of inhalation and possible respiratory problems.

- Also, because your baby's skin is sensitive, do not expose her to direct sunlight. Sunscreens are not recommended. As much as possible, keep your baby out of the sun. If she has to be in the sun, use a sunscreen made for children. For babies younger than 6 months, sunscreen may be used on small areas of the body, such as the face and backs of the hands, if adequate clothing and shade are not available.

- Your baby's skin may not need to be washed with soap daily. However, "cradle cap" can be prevented with frequent washing of the scalp.

- To prevent diaper rash, clean your baby after wet diapers or stools and change her diaper frequently. For some babies, diaper creams or ointments may be helpful, but good cleaning and air drying before replacing the diaper are best.

- Current cord care recommendations include "air drying," by keeping the diaper below the cord until the cord falls off (about 10 to 14 days). There may be some slight bleeding for a day or 2 after the cord falls off. Belly bands and alcohol on the cord are not recommended. Call our office if there is a bad smell, redness, or fluid from the cord area.

SAMPLE QUESTIONS:

What suggestions have you heard about things you can do to keep your baby healthy? How do you plan to protect your baby from getting infections?

ANTICIPATORY GUIDANCE:

- One of the most important steps in keeping your baby healthy is to wash your hands frequently with soap and water or a non-water antiseptic, always after diaper changes and before feeding your baby. You also should ask all family members and guests to wash their hands before handling the baby.

- Newborns are susceptible to illnesses in the first few months of life and need to be protected from anyone with colds or other illnesses. Outings to faith-based activities, restaurants, and movies should be considered carefully and avoided during cold and flu season.

- As long as you wash your hands before breastfeeding, you can continue to breastfeed through most illnesses that you or your baby have.

Practices usually have a written brochure for parents that:
- Introduces all of the practice staff
- Explains the appointment procedures and after-hours and emergency call procedures
- Discusses health supervision versus sick child visits, the purpose of developmental screening, considerations for children with special health care needs, and newborn behaviors
- Provides information about community resources and instructions on when to call the office

SAMPLE QUESTION:
What additional questions do you have about when to call the office and how we can work with you to ensure your baby's health and well-being?

ANTICIPATORY GUIDANCE:
- To help you remember what we've just talked about, here's a brochure that provides much of the same information.

Health Supervision: First Week Visit

CONTEXT

Families need a clear plan, tailored to their individual needs, for continuing care of the newborn. Early discharge at 48 hours or less after delivery has become the standard of care following the normal vaginal birth of a healthy, full-term newborn (38- to 42-weeks' gestation).[3] Existing medical information about the physical and psychosocial needs of newborns and mothers indicate that clinical evaluation is warranted within 3 to 5 days of birth. The most important criterion for discharge at 48 hours or less is a full-term singleton baby at 38- to 42-weeks' gestation. However, late preterm newborns (at 35- to 37-weeks' gestation) are increasingly being discharged within this limited window of time, further emphasizing the importance of early follow-up care for this subset of newborns.

In the past, the timing of the initial follow-up visit after nursery discharge varied by patient, locale, and community. Many communities have continued the longstanding practice of scheduling the initial newborn visit following nursery discharge for 2 weeks of age. This arose during the era when newborns were kept in the hospital for 5 to 7 days, and it has not been systematically studied to evaluate its efficacy and safety in the care of young newborns. Current recommendations for timing the initial continuing care visit are based on the known health risks for a newborn during the first week of life—jaundice, feeding difficulties, hydration problems, excessive weight loss, sepsis, and detection of significant congenital malformations

that are not apparent on the initial examinations but become symptomatic during the first weeks of life.[4] A follow-up visit should, therefore, occur within 3 to 5 days after birth and within 48 to 72 hours after discharge.[5] The recommendation for babies delivered by cesarean section and whose hospital stay is 96 hours or longer is for a first office visit up to a week after discharge. The exact timing of this visit depends on the specific issues, health concerns, and needs of the baby and mother.

Potential risks to consider at the First Week Visit include prematurity, hyperbilirubinemia due to blood group incompatibility, other causes of hemolytic anemia in the newborn, bruising, cephalohematoma, newborns of diabetic mothers, newborns of Asian descent, as well as newborns with breastfeeding problems or oral defects affecting feeding.

Appropriate specialty referral or consultation must be arranged promptly for babies with special health care needs. Mothers and families who have experienced a perinatal complication need extra attention. They may experience depression, anxiety, guilt, loss of control, reduced satisfaction with the birth experience, and even loss of self-esteem. Family members may need extra support to resolve their feelings and additional time to understand their newborn's condition and appreciate their newborn's unique characteristics and strengths rather than only the special needs.

Ethnicity influences a newborn's risk of significant hyperbilirubinemia. Recent studies report higher risk in Asian and American

Indian newborns than in whites or Hispanics, with newborns of black mothers having the lowest risk for hyperbilirubinemia during the first 5 days of life.[6] In Asians, a common DNA sequence variant causes an amino acid change in the UDP-GT protein, which contributes to the pathophysiology of newborn jaundice.[7] Genetic polymorphisms in UDP-GT and transporter gene variants are responsible for severe hyperbilirubinemia in Asian newborns.[7,8] Asian newborns of mixed race are at lower risk than newborns whose both parents are Asian.[9] X-linked recessive G6PD deficiency also occurs more frequently among Greek, African American, Southeast Asian, Italian, and Sephardic Jewish male newborns than among newborns of other races and ethnicities.[10] It is important to recognize the increasing number of newborns of mixed race and the potential difficulty in determining hyperbilirubinemia risk based solely on perceived maternal race/ethnicity.[6]

Despite recommendations and evidence supporting the utility of follow-up care within the first week of life for newborns discharged within 48 hours of birth, the majority of these newborns are not receiving timely continuing care.[11] Early follow-up care may not be feasible in some rural communities, and compliance may be poor in indigent populations among families who do not have a previously established medical home.[12] Health care professionals will need to use a variety of approaches (both office-based and home visits conducted by a hospital home care program, public health nurse, or community outreach worker) to ensure follow-up care within the first week of life.

PRIORITIES FOR THE VISIT

The first priority is to attend to the concerns of the parents. In addition, the Bright Futures Infancy Expert Panel has given priority to the following topics for discussion in this visit:

- Parental (maternal) well-being (health and depression, family stress, uninvited advice, parent roles)
- Newborn transition (daily routines, sleep [location, position, crib safety], state modulation [calming], parent-child relationship, early developmental referrals)
- Nutritional adequacy (feeding success [weight gain], feeding strategies [holding, burping], hydration/jaundice, hunger/satiation cues, feeding guidance [breastfeeding, formula])
- Safety (car safety seats, tobacco smoke, hot liquids [water temperature])
- Newborn care (when to call [temperature taking], emergency readiness [CPR], illness prevention [hand washing, outings], skin care [sun exposure])

HEALTH SUPERVISION

History

Interval history may be obtained according to the concerns of the family and the health care professional's preference or style of practice. The following questions can encourage in-depth discussion:

- **General Questions**
  - Tell me how things are going for your baby.
  - What questions or concerns do you have at this time?

- **Newborn**
  - How have things been going since you got home from the hospital?
  - What has been easier or harder than you expected?

- **Family**
  - How are things going for you and your family?
  - Have there been any major changes in your family?

Observation of Parent-Child Interaction

During the visit, the health care professional should observe:

- Do the parents and newborn respond to each other (gazing, talking, smiling, holding, cuddling, comforting, showing affection)?
- Do the parents appear content, happy, depressed, tearful, angry, anxious, fatigued, overwhelmed, or uncomfortable?
- Are the parents aware of, responsive to, and effective in responding to the newborn's distress?
- Do the parents appear confident in holding, comforting, feeding, and understanding the newborn's cues or behaviors?

- What are the parents' and newborn's interactions around comforting, dressing/changing diapers, and feeding?
- Are both parents present and do they support each other or show signs of disagreement?

Surveillance of Development

Do you have any specific concerns about your baby's development, learning, or behavior?

SOCIAL-EMOTIONAL
- Is able to sustain periods of wakefulness for feeding
- Will gradually become able to establish longer stretch of sleep (4 to 5 hours at night)
- Has indefinite regard of surroundings

COMMUNICATIVE
- Turns and calms to parent's voice
- Communicates needs through his behaviors
- Has an undifferentiated cry

COGNITIVE
- Is able to fix briefly on faces or objects
- Follows face to midline

PHYSICAL DEVELOPMENT
- Is able to suck, swallow, and breathe
- Shows strong primitive reflexes (suck, rooting, palmer grasp, stepping, Moro reflex, tonic neck reflex)
- Is able to lift head briefly when in the prone position

Physical Examination

A complete physical examination is included as part of every health supervision visit.

When performing a physical examination, the health care professional's attention is directed to the following components of the examination that are important for a child this age:

- **Measure and plot (adjust for gestational age, as indicated):**
  - Length
  - Weight
  - Head circumference
- **Plot:**
  - Weight-for-length
- **Skin**
  - Inspect for rashes or jaundice
- **Head**
  - Note any dysmorphic features

- **Eyes**
  - Inspect eyes and eyelids
  - Assess ocular mobility
  - Examine pupils for opacification and red reflexes
  - Assess for dacryocystitis
- **Heart**
  - Ascult for murmurs
  - Palpate femoral pulses
- **Abdomen**
  - Inspect umbilical cord and cord vessels
- **Musculoskeletal**
  - Perform Ortolani and Barlow maneuvers
- **Neurologic**
  - Note posture, tone, activity level, symmetry of movement, and state regulation

Screening

UNIVERSAL SCREENING	ACTION	
Metabolic and hemoglobinopathy	If not done previously (eg, newborn delivered at home or discharged from NICU), conduct screening as required by the state.[†]	
Hearing	If not done at birth (eg, newborn delivered at home or discharged from the NICU), screening should be completed within the first month of life.[‡]	
	Regardless of screening results, a family history of hearing loss or conditions associated with hearing impairment should be obtained, as well as identification of any risk factors for progressive hearing loss to inform ongoing surveillance of hearing and communication skill development.	

SELECTIVE SCREENING	RISK ASSESSMENT[*]	ACTION IF RA' +
Blood pressure	Children with specific risk conditions or change in risk	Blood pressure
Vision	Abnormal fundoscopic examination or prematurity with risk conditions	Ophthalmology referral

[†]If completed, review results of the state newborn metabolic screening test. Unavailable or pending results must be obtained immediately. If there are any abnormal results, ensure that appropriate retesting has been performed and/or referrals are made to appropriate subspecialists, if required. State newborn screening programs are available for assistance with referrals to appropriate resources.

[‡]Any newborn who does not pass the initial screen or any subsequent rescreen should be referred for a diagnostic audiologic assessment, and any newborn with a definitive diagnosis should be referred to the state Early Intervention Program.

[*]See the Rationale and Evidence chapter for the criteria on which risk screening questions are based.

Immunizations

Consult the CDC/ACIP or AAP Web sites for the current immunization schedule.
CDC National Immunization Program (NIP): http://www.cdc.gov/vaccines
American Academy of Pediatrics *Red Book*: http://www.aapredbook.org

Consider **influenza vaccine** for caregivers of infants younger than 6 months.

ANTICIPATORY GUIDANCE

The following sample questions, which address the Infancy Expert Panel's Anticipatory Guidance Priorities, are intended to be used selectively to invite discussion, gather information, address the needs and concerns of the family, and build partnerships. Use of the questions may vary from visit to visit and from family to family. Questions can be modified to match the health care professional's communication style. The accompanying anticipatory guidance for the family should be geared to questions, issues, or concerns for that particular child and family.

PARENTAL (MATERNAL) WELL-BEING

Health and depression, family stress, uninvited advice, parent roles

The first weeks with a new baby are a stressful time of transitions in which parents and other family members must learn how to care for the baby and adjust to new roles. New mothers also must focus on their physical recovery from the birth. Counsel the new parents on this transitional time and provide strategies for settling into a routine. Differentiate between short-term "baby blues" and postpartum depression, and counsel or refer as appropriate.

Review expectations, perspectives, and satisfaction with parenthood, how well any siblings and the extended family are functioning, and stressors, such as return to work/school or the inability to return to work/school, competing family needs, or loss of social and/or financial support. Provide guidance, referrals, and help in connecting with community resources as needed.

SAMPLE QUESTIONS:

How is the adjustment to the new baby going? How is your partner helping with the baby? Are there any times you feel sad, hopeless, or overwhelmed? Are you sleeping too much or too little? Are you having trouble focusing, remembering, or making decisions? Have you had feelings of worthlessness or guilt? Do you have any physical symptoms (headache, chest pain, palpitations)? At times, do you feel uninterested in the baby?

ANTICIPATORY GUIDANCE:

- The first week home is a time of transitions. It is normal for you to feel uncertain, overwhelmed, and very tired at times. As you and your baby get to know each other, it gets much better!
- Making sure to rest and sleep when the baby sleeps is one way to help you maintain your sense of well-being. Another is to let your partner and other family members do things for you and participate in the care of the baby by holding, bathing, changing, dressing, and calming her.
- Many new mothers experience the "baby blues." These feelings usually go away after a week or 2. If the feelings are overwhelming or last for a long time, this could be a sign of something more serious. Let's talk about it and make sure you get the help you need.

SAMPLE QUESTIONS:

How are your other children coping with the new baby? Is that difficult for you? Are any specific things especially stressful for you, such as meeting basic needs (housing, food, clothing, heat, phone, and electricity), or your relationship with your partner or other family members or friends?

ANTICIPATORY GUIDANCE:

- Your other children need special time with you and your partner. Make time to play and read with them. Acknowledge your older children's possible negative feelings and regression. Consider letting your other children help take care of the baby, if they have reached a level of development and maturity where they can do so without harming the baby.
- Maintaining routines as much as possible can help reduce stress.
- One way to deal with unwanted advice from family and friends is to acknowledge their concerns and desire to help and then change the subject to something you do agree on. Trying to justify your desire to follow the recommendations of your health care professional may only lead to a long and futile conversation.

NEWBORN TRANSITION

Daily routines, sleep (location, position, crib safety), state modulation (calming), parent-child relationship, early developmental referrals

Evidence of ambivalence or stress due to the home situation or the care of the newborn may require referrals to community support systems, such as public health nursing, home care, or other community agencies.

If the parents express no desire for a schedule or usual routine, if they impose a rigid schedule, if the newborn sleeps all the time or never sleeps, or the newborn is irritable, difficult to console, difficult to feed, or fed less than 8 to 12 feedings in 24 hours, additional counseling is needed.

Newborns with rapid state changes from sleep or drowsiness to crying, or newborns whose parents are concerned with excessive crying, may need additional counseling.

SAMPLE QUESTIONS:

How has the baby been adjusting since you got home? What is your baby's daily routine/schedule for sleep and feeding? Where does he sleep? Is he able to establish uninterrupted sleep? Is he able to come to an alert state for feeding?

ANTICIPATORY GUIDANCE:

- At this age, newborns usually lack a day/night schedule and sleep for a longer stretch during the day. Your baby will need help from you and other caregivers to develop sleep and feeding routines.
- Putting your baby down to sleep in the same place every time and establishing a regular routine for feeding and sleeping will help him get on a schedule and will help him sleep at night.

A family's beliefs and cultural traditions will have a significant impact on where and how the baby sleeps, and whether the family or other caregivers follow the "back to sleep" message. Counsel parents about sleep location, sleep position ("back to sleep"), and cribs.

SAMPLE QUESTION:
Where is your baby sleeping for naps and at nighttime?

ANTICIPATORY GUIDANCE:
- We now understand that "back to sleep" is safest for babies. Therefore, always put your baby down to sleep on his back, not his tummy or side. We also know that the use of loose, soft bedding (blankets, comforters, sheepskins, quilts, pillows, pillow-like bumper pads), or soft toys is dangerous because they are associated with a higher risk of SIDS.
- We understand that most parents want their baby to sleep close to them in the early months at home, and, certainly, having the baby sleep in the same room as the parent in the early months is much easier for breastfeeding. Concern for the newborn's safety occurs, however, when a baby sleeps in the same bed as the parents, and the parents are very tired and may not know the baby is there. Put your baby to sleep in your room, but in his own crib.
- Make sure that your baby's crib has slats that are no more than $2\frac{3}{8}$ inches (60 mm) apart; the mattress should be firm and fit snugly into the crib. Keep the sides raised when your baby is sleeping in it.
- The room temperature should be comfortable and the baby should be kept from getting too warm or too cold while sleeping.

SAMPLE QUESTION:
What have you found works to wake up your baby for feedings or to calm him for sleep?

ANTICIPATORY GUIDANCE:
- A newborn is often very sleepy after delivery because of jaundice or because of medications you received. For your baby to feed consistently through the day and night, he may need help waking up for feedings. Use a variety of stimulating actions, such as rocking, patting, stroking, diaper changes, and undressing, to help him come to an alert state for feeding.
- Other types of actions, such as stroking your baby's head or gentle repetitive rocking, help put your baby to sleep and are useful for consoling him.

NUTRITIONAL ADEQUACY

Feeding success (weight gain), feeding strategies (holding, burping), hydration/ jaundice, hunger/satiation cues, feeding guidance (breastfeeding, formula)

General Guidance on Feeding

One of the first tasks for parents during their newborn's first week is learning when and how much their baby needs either for breastfeeding or formula. The first-week visit usually provides parents with reassurance that their baby has returned to her birth weight or is gaining weight and thus getting the appropriate feedings. Newborns with jaundice may be more difficult to awaken, resulting in greater difficulty with feedings, especially breastfeeding. Close supervision and counseling is needed to assist parents in ensuring that their newborn awakens for feedings to ensure adequate hydration.

Providing parents with guidance to recognize their baby's signals for both hunger and satiation will help them provide an appropriate feeding amount and frequency, as well as avoid overfeeding.

Counseling may be needed to discuss benefits of holding the baby during feedings. It also may be advisable to actually observe the newborn feeding because some newborns with reflux will arch their back and pull away from the parent, leaving the parent with the impression that the newborn does not like the breast milk, formula, or being held. This is an important cue that the family needs additional counseling and assistance. Consider mentioning the need to delay introduction of complementary foods until after 6 months of age. If the family is having difficulty obtaining sufficient formula or nutritious food, provide information about WIC and local community food programs.

SAMPLE QUESTIONS:
How is feeding going? How are you feeding your baby? How does your baby like to be held when you feed her? How easy is it to burp your baby during or after feedings?

ANTICIPATORY GUIDANCE:
- If you are bottle-feeding, do not prop the bottle, as this puts your baby at risk of choking, ear infections, and early childhood caries. Holding your baby close while you feed her gives you the opportunity for warm and loving interaction with her.
- Babies usually burp at natural breaks (eg, midway through or after a feeding). Help her burp by gently rubbing or patting her back while holding her against your shoulder and chest or supporting her in a sitting position on your lap.

SAMPLE QUESTIONS:
Are you comfortable that your baby is getting enough to eat? How many wet diapers and stools does your baby have each day?

ANTICIPATORY GUIDANCE:
- Your baby is getting enough milk if she has 6 to 8 wet cloth diapers (5 or 6 disposable diapers) and 3 or 4 stools per day and is gaining weight appropriately.
- Breastfed newborns usually have loose, frequent stools. After several weeks, the number of bowel movements may decrease. Breastfed babies who are 6 weeks old and older may have stools as infrequently as every 3 days.
- Healthy babies do not require extra water, as breast milk and formula (when properly prepared) are adequate to meet the newborn's fluid needs.

SAMPLE QUESTIONS:
How do you know if your baby is hungry? How do you know if she has had enough to eat?

ANTICIPATORY GUIDANCE:

- A baby's usual signs of hunger include putting her hand to her mouth, sucking, rooting, facial grimaces, and fussing. Crying is a late sign of hunger.
- You can tell she's full because she will turn her head away from the breast or bottle, close her mouth, or relax her arms and hands.

Guidance on Breastfeeding

New mothers should make sure that they continue to receive an appropriate diet and extra fluids. They also should get the sleep they need. Supportive partners, family, and friends can provide invaluable help for the new mother by taking care of her and the rest of the household to allow her to concentrate on the care of her newborn. A health care or lactation professional can provide information and support to address positioning for the mother's comfort and to prevent or minimize sore nipples, breast infection, and improper latching on. If a baby is not gaining weight or is not wetting her diaper 6 to 8 times per day, discuss with parents the quantity, frequency, and duration of feeding and closely monitor the newborn's feedings and weight until weight gain is satisfactory. Mothers who breastfeed their babies can receive from WIC breast pumps, breast shells, or nursing supplements to help support the initiation of breastfeeding.

A newborn who has a parent with a food allergy and/or a sibling with a significant allergy also may be at risk of allergies. Mothers who breastfeed should be careful to avoid their own allergens.

SAMPLE QUESTIONS:

How is breastfeeding going for you and your baby? How often does your baby nurse? How long do feedings last? In what ways is breastfeeding different now from when you were last here? Does it seem like your baby is breastfeeding more often or for longer periods of time, compared to the first couple of days? How can you tell whether your baby is satisfied at the breast? What concerns do you have about breastfeeding? Is nursing uncomfortable or do you have sore nipples? Are you continuing to take prenatal vitamins? What OTC or prescription medications are you taking? What questions do you have about any condition that might prevent you from breastfeeding? Are you offering the baby breast milk in a bottle? Are you using a pacifier? Will you be able to breastfeed your baby if you return to work or school?

ANTICIPATORY GUIDANCE:

- Exclusive breastfeeding continues to be the ideal source of nutrition for at least the first 4 to 6 months of life.
- At about 1 week of age, your baby should settle into a more typical breastfeeding routine of every 2 to 3 hours in the daytime, and every 3 hours at night, with one longer 4- to 5-hour stretch between feedings, for a total of 8 to 12 feedings in 24 hours.
- You can help your baby by paying attention to her sleep cycles in the day. When she comes to a drowsy state, change her diaper and wake her for a feeding about every 2 to 3 hours. Doing this with your baby is called "state modulation," and it helps your family and the baby develop a routine around feeding and sleep.

- If you are breastfeeding, wait until your baby is 1 month old before giving her a pacifier.
- Breastfeeding is often a challenge for mothers, whether or not they have breastfed before. Every baby is different and "catches on" a little differently. That is why lactation consultants are available to give you consultation, education, and support as you and your baby are beginning to breastfeed. I can give you contact information for a lactation consultant.

Guidance on Formula Feeding

A newborn who is growing appropriately will average 20 oz of formula per day with a range of 16 to 24 oz per day. Formula preparation and formula safety information is needed for parents, especially the length of time over which formula from one feeding can be offered to the newborn. Parents also need to know why it is important to seek professional guidance before changing to a different formula.

SAMPLE QUESTIONS:

Do you have any concerns about formula? What concerns do you have about cost, nutrient content, and differences across brands? What questions do you have about preparing formula and storing it safely?

ANTICIPATORY GUIDANCE:

- Make sure to always use iron-fortified formula. At first, give your baby 2 oz of prepared formula every 2 to 3 hours. Give her more if she still seems hungry. As she grows and her appetite increases, you will need to prepare larger amounts.
- Because formula is expensive, you may be hesitant to throw away any that is left in the bottle. For food safety reasons, if your baby has not taken all of the formula at one feeding and you plan to continue using it, you should put it back in the refrigerator. Do not mix this formula with new formula. If the formula has been heated and has been out of the refrigerator for 1 hour or more, discard it.
- If you are thinking about switching brands of formula, talk to me first.

SAFETY

Car safety seats, tobacco smoke, hot liquids (water temperature)

Parents should not place their baby's car safety seat in the front seat of a vehicle with a passenger air bag because the air bags deploy with great force against a car safety seat and cause serious injury or death.

Counsel parents that their own safe driving behaviors (including using safety belts at all times and not driving under the influence of alcohol or drugs) are important to the health of their children.

Infants with special needs need special consideration for safe transportation. Refer parents to a local, specially trained child passenger safety technician for assistance with special positioning and restraint devices (www.preventinjury.org).

Questions about proper installation should be referred to a certified Child Passenger Safety Technician in the community.
Child Safety Seat Inspection Station Locator: www.seatcheck.org
Toll-free Number: 866-SEATCHECK (866-732-8243)

SAMPLE QUESTIONS:
Is your baby fastened securely in a rear-facing car safety seat in the back seat every time he rides in a vehicle? Do you have any problems using your baby's car safety seat?

ANTICIPATORY GUIDANCE:
- A rear-facing car safety seat that is properly secured in the back seat is the best place for your baby to ride in a vehicle.
- The harnesses should be snug and the car safety seat should be positioned at the recommended angle so that the baby's head does not fall forward. Babies with special needs, such as premature babies or babies in casts, need special consideration for safe transportation.
- Your baby needs to stay in his car safety seat at all times during travel. If he becomes fussy or needs to nurse, stop the vehicle and take him out of the car safety seat to attend to his needs. Strap him safely back into his seat before traveling again.
- Car safety seats should be used only for travel (not for positioning outside the vehicle). Keep the harnesses snug whenever your baby is in the car safety seat. This will help prevent falls out of the seat and strangulation on the harnesses.

Child Safety Seat Inspection Station Locator: www.seatcheck.org. Toll-free Number: 866-SEATCHECK (866-732-8243).

Discuss other strategies parents can use to keep their baby safe.

SAMPLE QUESTION:
What other things are you doing to keep your baby safe and healthy?

ANTICIPATORY GUIDANCE:
- If you smoke, try to cut down or quit. Make your home and vehicle smoke-free zones (smoke only outside the home and car).
- Do not drink hot liquids while holding the baby.
- To protect your child from tap water scalds, the hottest temperature at the faucet should be no higher than 120°F. In many cases, you can adjust your water heater. Before bathing the baby, always test the water temperature with your wrist to make sure it is not too hot.

NEWBORN CARE

When to call (temperature taking), emergency readiness (CPR), illness prevention (hand washing, outings), skin care (sun exposure)

It may take some time for parents of newborns to develop confidence in their ability to care for their baby. They may welcome guidance about issues such as knowing when to call the practice, knowing how to determine and prevent illness in their baby, and how to handle emergencies.

Newborns with recognizable diagnosis or prematurity should be referred for early intervention services so that families may receive the support and be connected to the community services they need.

SAMPLE QUESTIONS:
What type of thermometer do you have? Do you know how to use it?

ANTICIPATORY GUIDANCE:
- You may have been given an ear thermometer as a baby gift, but do not take your baby's temperature by ear or mouth until she is 4 years old. Taking your baby's temperature rectally is preferred. A rectal temperature of 100.4°F/38.0°C is considered a fever.

SAMPLE QUESTION:
Do you know what to do in an emergency or if you have concerns or questions about your baby?

ANTICIPATORY GUIDANCE:
- Here are some emergency preparedness strategies:
  - Complete an American Heart Association or American Red Cross First Aid or Infant CPR program.
  - Have a family first-aid kit.
  - Make a list of the local emergency telephone numbers, including the Poison Control Center (1-800-222-1222), and post it at every telephone.
- Have a family emergency preparedness plan and become familiar with your community's plan.

Poison Control Center (1-800-222-1222)

SAMPLE QUESTIONS:
What questions do you have about:
- *Going out with your baby?*
- *Going to public places, such as faith-based activities?*
- *What to tell visitors about handling your baby?*

ANTICIPATORY GUIDANCE:
- To protect your baby in the first month of life, do not let her be handled by many people. Avoid crowded places, overdressing, and exposure to very hot or cold temperatures.
- Make sure to wash your hands often, especially after diaper changes and before feeding the baby.

- As much as possible, keep your baby out of the sun. If she has to be in the sun, use a sunscreen made for children. For babies younger than 6 months, sunscreen may be used on small areas of the body, such as the face and backs of the hands, if adequate clothing and shade are not available.
- Your baby may get a skin rash. Rashes are normal and happen between 4 and 8 weeks. Let me know if you have any questions or concerns.

Health Supervision: 1 Month Visit

CONTEXT

Within the first month, parents become increasingly attuned to their baby as they learn to interpret the meanings of their baby's cues and how their caregiving responses to the baby's behaviors may influence his behaviors. Through their growing understanding of their newborn, parents learn strategies to support the baby's emerging personality and self-regulation. The primary focus of parents' caregiving relates to feedings, sleep and wake patterns, elimination, and assimilation into the family.

The frequency of visits during the first 2 months of life will depend on the baby's health status and the family's needs. Babies who were premature or sick at birth, those entering foster care or adoptive families, those with special health or developmental needs, and first-time or anxious parents likely will need more frequent visits. In addition to offering counseling and reassurance to the parents, the health care professional may need to arrange referrals for comprehensive evaluation and management of the infant's problems and for community-based family support services. As coordinator of the infant's medical home, the health care professional will ascertain and assist the family in ensuring that appropriate linkages are in place for any needed subspecialty medical or surgical care and early intervention services.

The 1 Month Visit encompasses routine health surveillance; response to parental concerns; and encouragement, support, and practical guidance about the infant's growth and nutrition, development, and transition to a consistent sleep and wake pattern. For the infant born prematurely or with a health condition that makes feeding a challenge, additional attention will need to be directed toward feeding skills, the adequacy of nutrient and caloric intake, and infant growth. The results of newborn metabolic/genetic and hearing screening tests should be reviewed and repeat testing, as required, should be arranged or completed. Risk factors requiring future testing should be documented. If the mother will be returning to work or school in the near future, guidance regarding the selection of safe child care may be provided. Counseling to reduce the risk of injury in the home,[13] and anticipatory guidance to address nighttime awakening and crying problems,[14] both of which have been demonstrated to be efficacious, are additional appropriate topics for the 1 Month Visit.

Families experiencing adjustment difficulties, and mothers manifesting postpartum psychological symptoms, will require close involvement and interaction with the health care professional and may need referral to resources to support their material or emotional needs.

PRIORITIES FOR THE VISIT

The first priority is to attend to the concerns of the parents. In addition, the Bright Futures Infancy Expert Panel has given priority to the following topics for discussion in this visit:

- Parental (maternal) well-being (health [maternal postpartum checkup, depression, substance abuse], return to work/school [breastfeeding plans, child care])
- Family adjustment (family resources, family support, parent roles, domestic violence, community resources)
- Infant adjustment (sleep/wake schedule, sleep position [back to sleep, location, crib safety], state modulation [crying, consoling, shaken baby], developmental changes [bored baby, tummy time], early developmental referrals)
- Feeding routines (feeding frequency [growth spurts], feeding choices [types of foods/ fluids], hunger cues, feeding strategies [holding, burping], pacifier use [cleanliness], feeding guidance [breast feeding, formula])
- Safety (car safety seats, toys with loops and strings, falls, tobacco smoke)

HEALTH SUPERVISION

History

Interval history may be obtained according to the concerns of the family and the health care professional's preference or style of practice. The following questions can encourage in-depth discussion:

- Tell me how things are going for your baby.
- What are your baby's routine and schedule like now?
- What are some of your best and most difficult times of day with the baby?
- Have you been feeling tired or blue?
- Have you and your partner had some time for yourselves?
- Who helps you with the baby and your other children? Who watches the baby for you? Do you have any conflicts with that person(s) about what is safe and healthy for the baby?

Observation of Parent-Child Interaction

During the visit, the health care professional should observe:

- Do the parents appear content, happy, depressed, tearful, angry, anxious, fatigued, overwhelmed, or uncomfortable?
- Do the parents appear uncertain or nervous (eg, partner is uninvolved, parents lack awareness about questions)?
- How do the parent and infant interact around feeding/eating?
- How do they respond to one another (eg, affectionate, comfortable, distant, anxious)?

If both parents are present:
- How do they each interact, care for, and respond to the infant's cues?
- Do they individually express an awareness and understanding of their infant and their infant's health and developmental needs?
- Do they appear to be comfortable with each other and with the infant?

Surveillance of Development

Do you have any specific concerns about your baby's development, learning, or behavior?

SOCIAL-EMOTIONAL
- Is responsive to calming actions when upset

COMMUNICATIVE
- Is able to follow parents with his eyes
- Recognizes the parents' voices

COGNITIVE
- Has started to smile

PHYSICAL DEVELOPMENT
- Is able to lift his head when on his tummy

Physical Examination

A complete physical examination is included as part of every health supervision visit.

When performing a physical examination, the health care professional's attention is directed to the following components of the examination that are important for a child this age:

- **Measure and plot (adjust for gestational age, as indicated):**
  - Length
  - Weight
  - Head circumference
- **Plot:**
  - Weight-for-length
- **Head**
  - Note positional skull deformities

- **Eyes**
  - Examine for red reflexes
  - Ensure eyes are of equivalent color, intensity, and clarity
  - Observe for opacities or clouding of cornea
- **Heart**
  - Ascult for heart murmurs
  - Palpate femoral pulses
- **Abdomen**
  - Search for abdominal masses
  - Note healing of the umbilicus
- **Musculoskeletal**
  - Perform Ortolani and Barlow maneuvers
- **Neurologic**
  - Assess tone and neurodevelopmental status, including attentiveness to visual and auditory stimuli

Screening

UNIVERSAL SCREENING	ACTION	
Metabolic and hemoglobinopathy	If not done previously (eg, baby delivered at home, or discharged from the NICU), conduct screening as required by the state.[†]	
Hearing	If not done at birth (eg, baby delivered at home, or discharged from the NICU), screening should be completed within the first month of life.[‡]	

SELECTIVE SCREENING	RISK ASSESSMENT*	ACTION IF RA +
Blood pressure	Children with specific risk conditions or change in risk	Blood pressure
Vision	Parental concern or abnormal fundoscopic examination or prematurity with risk conditions	Ophthalmology referral
Tuberculosis	+ on risk screening questions	Tuberculin skin test

[†]Verify documentation of newborn metabolic screening results, appropriate rescreening, and needed follow-up.

[‡]Positive screenings should be followed up with a diagnostic audiologic assessment, and an infant with a definitive diagnosis should be referred to the state Early Intervention Program.

*See the Rationale and Evidence chapter for the criteria on which risk screening questions are based.

Immunizations

Consult the CDC/ACIP or AAP Web sites for the current immunization schedule.
CDC National Immunization Program (NIP): http://www.cdc.gov/vaccines
American Academy of Pediatrics *Red Book*: http://www.aapredbook.org

Consider **influenza vaccine** for caregivers of infants younger than 6 months.

ANTICIPATORY GUIDANCE

The following sample questions, which address the Infancy Expert Panel's Anticipatory Guidance Priorities, are intended to be used selectively to invite discussion, gather information, address the needs and concerns of the family, and build partnerships. Use of the questions may vary from visit to visit and from family to family. Questions can be modified to match the health care professional's communication style. The accompanying anticipatory guidance for the family should be geared to questions, issues, or concerns for that particular child and family.

PARENTAL (MATERNAL) WELL-BEING

Health (maternal postpartum checkup, depression, substance abuse), return to work/school (breastfeeding plans, child care)

Discuss the mother's postpartum physical and emotional health and provide information about her needs during this period. Any suggestion of depression should trigger screening questions for increased drug and alcohol use. Explore issues of substance abuse (with legal and illegal drugs) as self-medication of mood. As needed, refer the mother to her obstetrician or other health care professional and appropriate community-based mental health services.

Mothers who are planning on returning to work have many feelings about leaving their babies and need assistance in finding high-quality child care and in determining how to continue breastfeeding.

SAMPLE QUESTIONS:
What have you heard from your obstetrician or other health care professional about resuming your normal daily activities after delivery? When is your postpartum checkup? How are you managing any pain or discomfort from delivery or breastfeeding?

ANTICIPATORY GUIDANCE:
- Typically, a 6-week postpartum checkup should be scheduled to discuss how you are feeling and make any arrangement you wish about birth control. Sometimes, moms are so tired they forget or just don't make their post-partum appointment.
- If you are still feeling discomfort from the delivery or with breastfeeding, you should talk with your obstetrician or health care professional.

SAMPLE QUESTIONS:
What are some of your best, and most difficult, times of day with the baby? How are your spirits? Have you been feeling sad, blue, or hopeless since the delivery? Are you still interested in activities you used to enjoy? Do you find that you are drinking, using herbs, or taking drugs to help make you feel better (less depressed, less anxious, less frustrated, calmer)?

ANTICIPATORY GUIDANCE:

■ Many mothers feel tired or overwhelmed in the first weeks at home. They also may experience some "baby blues" for a short time. These feelings should not continue, however. If you find that you are still feeling very tired or overwhelmed, or you are using alcohol or drugs to feel better, let your partner, your health care professional, and/or your baby's health care professional know so that you can get the help you need.

SAMPLE QUESTIONS:

How do you feel about returning to work or school? Do you wonder about how returning to work or school may affect your relationship with your baby? How it may affect breastfeeding? Have you spoken with your employer about continuing to breastfeed when you return to work? Have you made arrangements for child care?

ANTICIPATORY GUIDANCE:

■ Returning to work is often a hard thing to do. Finding a good child care arrangement that you trust will help you feel better about this decision. There are helpful resources and written guides as well as community resources available to assist you in selecting the right child care for you and your child.

■ I also can give you advice and resources that can help you identify child care and help you continue breastfeeding after you go back to work/school.

FAMILY ADJUSTMENT

Family resources, family support, parent roles, domestic violence, community resources

A new mother needs strategies to help her juggle her multiple responsibilities, and support from her partner and other family members so that she can adequately take care of herself and her baby. Help parents understand the importance of asking for help when they need it. Fathers also may feel intense role strain when their natural family support system is not available to them. In many cultures, the grandmother or other female relative provides for, or supervises the care of, the young infant. Immigrant families may not have this resource available to them.

Suggest community resources that help with finding quality child care, accessing transportation, or getting a car safety seat, or addressing issues such as financial concerns, inadequate resources to cover health care expenses, inadequate or unsafe housing, limited food resources, parental inexperience, or lack of social support.

For mothers or caregivers who have a limited support network, community services and resources may be able to help the family.

Support family connection to the community through social, faith-based, cultural, volunteer, and recreational organizations or programs.

If the baby has special health care needs, provide information and referral to the local public health nursing services for MCHB Title V Information (Health Care Program for Children with Special Needs) and the local Early Intervention Program agency, often referred to as IDEA. These 2 programs will be able to assist in connecting families to many community resources.

Families need issue-specific guidance on ways to support their other children's emotional and developmental needs, as well as strategies to help their children adjust to the new baby's presence in the home. This is particularly important if the infant is premature or has other special health and developmental care needs, or if this is a multiple birth.

SAMPLE QUESTIONS:
Tell me about your living situation. Do you have:
- *Enough heat, hot water, and electricity?*
- *Appliances that work?*
- *Problems with bugs, rodents, peeling paint or plaster, or mold or dampness?*
How are your resources for caring for your baby? Do you have:
- *Enough knowledge to feel comfortable in caring for your baby?*
- *Health insurance?*
- *Enough money for food, clothing, diapers, and child care?*

ANTICIPATORY GUIDANCE:
- **If you have problems with your living situation, consider contacting community services for help.**

Families who are living with others (eg, their elders, those who are helping them from being homeless, or teen parents living with their parents) may have little control over their environment and caregiver roles and responsibilities. For some families, gender roles may preclude women from asking men for help. In a culturally sensitive way, health care professionals need to develop strategies with parents and the family about how to support the mother's needs.

SAMPLE QUESTIONS:
How are you finding taking care of yourself and the baby? Are you able to find time for your other children? Who helps you with the baby? Is your partner able to help care for the baby or with things around the house? How are your other children reacting to the baby? Have you observed any behavior changes, jealousy, or anything that concerns you? How are you handling this?

ANTICIPATORY GUIDANCE:
- **Finding time for yourself can be a challenge. Talking with your partner and problem solving together will help your partner feel involved and identify ways to help you. It also may be important to have someone to talk with if you feel isolated and alone.**
- **Please let us know if this is happening so that we can provide you with community contacts that can assist you.**

Provide information about the impact of domestic violence on children and about community resources that provide assistance. Recommend resources for parent education and/or parent support groups.

SAMPLE QUESTIONS:

Do you always feel safe in your home? Has your partner or ex-partner ever hit, kicked, or shoved you, or physically hurt you or the baby? Are you scared that you and/or other caretakers may hurt the baby? Do you have any questions about your safety at home? What will you do if you feel afraid? Do you have a plan? Would you like information on where to go or who to contact if you ever need help?

ANTICIPATORY GUIDANCE:

- One way that I and other health care professionals can help you if your partner is hitting or threatening you is to support you and provide information about local resources that can help you.

The health care professional should clearly explain the office practice plan for telephone triage, after-hours calls, and same-day illness appointments. Parents should specifically know early illness signs and symptoms and when to call the health care professional. Parents should be encouraged to call about any change in the infant's activity, appearance, or behavior that makes them uncomfortable.

It is also helpful if the health care professional has a list of strategies and resources to share with families who do not have telephone service in their home or whose communities may not have ready access to public telephones.

Culturally based practices to prevent illness, such as tying amulets or strings and any other related safety issues, are important to discuss.

SAMPLE QUESTIONS:

Do you know what to do in an emergency? Do you have a list of emergency numbers? Depending on the family, it may be appropriate to ask: *Do you know when to call the health care professional? What type of thermometer do you have? Are you comfortable using it and knowing when to call the office if your child has a temperature? Do you know when and where to go to an emergency department? Do you have access to a telephone for emergencies?*

ANTICIPATORY GUIDANCE:

- I encourage you to complete an American Heart Association or American Red Cross First Aid or infant CPR program.
- You also should learn what to do if your baby begins to choke.
- Make sure you have a first-aid kit, know the local emergency telephone numbers, and be aware of concerns that might require a 911 call.
- Familiarity with disaster preparedness measures is also important.
- A rectal temperature of 100.4°F/38.°C is considered a fever. Use of a rectal digital thermometer is preferred. Do not take the baby's temperature by mouth until he is 4 years old.
- Wash your hands with soap and water often, or use a non-water antiseptic, especially after diaper changes and before feeding the baby.

INFANT ADJUSTMENT

Sleep/wake schedule, sleep position (back to sleep, location, crib safety), state modulation (crying, consoling, shaken baby), developmental changes (bored baby, tummy time), early developmental referrals

Discuss the infant's cues for sleep and ways for parents to help the infant develop a regular sleep pattern. Note that infant irritability may be due to lack of sleep. Consider an intervention if the infant sleeps all the time, never sleeps, is irritable, is difficult to console, or is difficult to feed.

Address the risks of bed sharing with a caregiver and with other children, and appropriate cautions regarding bed and bedding type tobacco, alcohol, or substance use by the caregiver. At the same time, health care professionals should be sensitive to parents' cultural traditions and beliefs about infant sleep and sleep location.

Parents or caregivers may have concerns about the infant's comfort and restfulness in the supine sleep position and a comfortable room temperature for the baby. The health care professional can provide suggestions about how to keep the infant from getting too warm or too cold while sleeping.

SAMPLE QUESTION:
How is your baby sleeping?

ANTICIPATORY GUIDANCE:
- Many babies are unable to develop a regular sleep/wake pattern on their own and need your help. Providing a consistent and predictable routine for your baby will help her learn to develop a regular sleep/wake pattern.
- Putting the baby in her crib either awake or drowsy, not in a deep sleep, will help her make the transition from being awake to asleep in the crib. This will avoid problems with night waking later on because, when she wakes up, she will be in a familiar place.
- Do not use loose, soft bedding (blankets, comforters, sheepskins, quilts, pillows, pillow-like bumper pads) or soft toys in the baby's crib because they are associated with an increased risk of SIDS.
- The room temperature should be comfortable and the baby should be kept from getting too warm or too cold while sleeping.

SAMPLE QUESTIONS:
Where does your baby sleep now? What have you heard about "back to sleep and prone to play"?

ANTICIPATORY GUIDANCE:
- Always put your baby down to sleep on her back, not her tummy or side. Ask your relatives and caregivers to also put your baby "back to sleep."
- Experts recommend that your baby sleep in your room in her own crib (not in your bed). If you breastfeed or bottle-feed your baby in your bed, return her to her own crib or bassinet when you both are ready to go back to sleep.

- Be sure your baby's crib is safe. The slats should be no more than $2\frac{3}{8}$ inches (60 mm) apart. The mattress should be firm and fit snugly into the crib. Keep the sides of the crib raised when your baby is in the crib.
- If you use a mesh playpen or portable crib, the weave should have small openings less than $\frac{1}{4}$ inch (6 mm). Never leave your baby in a mesh playpen or crib with the drop-side down.

SAMPLE QUESTION:

Have you tried to give your baby a pacifier?

ANTICIPATORY GUIDANCE:

- Using a pacifier during sleep is strongly associated with a reduced risk of SIDS. After your baby is about 1 month old, consider offering a pacifier when she lies down for sleep. Never reinsert the pacifier if it falls out after the baby falls asleep and do not coat it with a sweet solution.

Offer strategies to support the infant's state regulation and behavioral maturation, including ways to engage the infant and console and calm her. This is particularly important if the infant is premature or exhibits signs of easily being over-stimulated or overwhelmed or if the baby is difficult to engage. Encourage parents to learn about their baby's temperament and how it affects the way she relates to the world.

If the intensity, frequency, duration, and constancy of the infant's crying is intense, it should be evaluated. Discuss with parents strategies to manage their infant and her responses. Concerns about infant attachment or parent-infant interaction should prompt the health care professional to refer the family to community parenting and support programs. If concerns about infant development are evident, consider referral to the local Early Intervention Program agency, often referred to as IDEA.

Counsel parents about how fragile an infant's head is and how it is important to protect an infant from shaking. Parents should be counseled to ensure that other caregivers also recognize the infant's vulnerabilities and understand how important it is to avoid shaking a baby, and that, if the baby cannot be consoled, they need to call for help.

If parents are feeling stressed or if they are having difficulty getting along together, they need referral to an appropriate mental health care professional.

Parents/caregivers can be encouraged to seek support from their natural support network for respite. Not all families will have this resource accessible to them. Health care professionals can give parents the telephone numbers for community resources that can help.

SAMPLE QUESTIONS:

Tell me how you know what your baby wants. What is your baby's cry like? Are the cries different at different times? What do you think they mean? How much is your baby crying? How often? What seems to help? What do you do when you get frustrated with your baby? What are some of the ways you have found to calm your baby when she is crying? What do you do if they don't work? Who is helping you at home? Who helps care for the baby or with other home activities?

ANTICIPATORY GUIDANCE:

- A young infant cannot be "spoiled" by holding, cuddling, and rocking her, or by talking and singing to her. Responding quickly to your baby's cry will not spoil her, but it will teach her that she will be cared for. It is important to respond to your baby's crying now because it actually will decrease clingy behavior later on, which is commonly associated with the term, "spoiled child."
- Many babies have fussy periods in the late afternoon or evening. Strategies to calm a fussy infant include being there with her, talking, patting or stroking, bundling or containing, holding, and rocking her, and letting her suck. Sometimes it is hard to console a fussy or crying baby, no matter what you do.
- An infant's developmental progress toward self-consoling includes putting her hands to her mouth or sucking on her fingers, thumb, and pacifier (used appropriately).
- Holding a baby in a front carrier or sling may decrease crying, but these may not be safe for infants who are premature or have neuromuscular or neurologic problems.
- All new parents feel overwhelmed, frustrated, exhausted, or angry occasionally. If all else fails, you can try putting the baby in her crib, making certain she is safe, closing the door, and checking on her every few minutes. Never, ever, shake your baby, because it could cause permanent brain damage. If you ever feel that you need help because your baby is crying so much, contact community resources that can help you.

SAMPLE QUESTION:
Tell me what happens with you and the baby when she is alert and awake.

ANTICIPATORY GUIDANCE:

- Spending time playing and talking during quiet, alert states helps strengthen the parent-child bond by building a trusting relationship.
- Babies need "tummy time" to develop head control and to get used to being on their stomach. This time is important because it stimulates muscle development and can help prevent the development of a flat area on the back of the head. During these times, place your baby in a position where she can see around the room and you can talk and interact with her even while doing other chores.

FEEDING ROUTINES

Feeding frequency (growth spurts), feeding choices (types of foods/fluids), hunger cues, feeding strategies (holding, burping); pacifier use (cleanliness), feeding guidance (breastfeeding, formula)

General Guidance on Feeding
Feeding strategies and information depends on whether the mother is breastfeeding or formula-feeding her baby, or both.

An infant who cries inconsolably for several hours a day and passes a lot of gas may have colic or reflux.

Parents may give their infants OTC medications or herbal products (eg, teas, digestive aids, or sleep or discomfort remedies), some of which may be harmful to the infant. Discussion about use of these products should be conducted within the family's cultural context, recognizing that, for many families, these are important practices believed to protect the child's health and well-being.

Discuss contraindications to breastfeeding as warranted.

SAMPLE QUESTIONS:
How is feeding going? What are you feeding your baby at this time? How often are you feeding your baby during the day? During the night? Tell me about all foods and fluids you are offering the baby. Has anyone given the baby cereal or other food?

ANTICIPATORY GUIDANCE:
- Mothers who exclusively breastfeed provide ideal nutrition for their babies for about the first 6 months of life. For infants who are not breastfeeding, iron-fortified formula is the recommended substitute.
- Feed your baby when he shows signs of hunger, usually 8 to 12 times in 24 hours. Babies should not be overfed.
- Do not offer your baby food other than breast milk or formula until he is developmentally ready (around the middle of his first year).
- Healthy babies do not require extra water. Breast milk and formula (when properly prepared) are adequate to meet your baby's fluid needs. Juice is not recommended in the first 6 months of life.
- Infants often go through growth spurts between 6 and 8 weeks of age and significantly increase their milk intake during that time.

SAMPLE QUESTIONS:
How do you know if your baby is hungry? How do you know if he has had enough to eat?

ANTICIPATORY GUIDANCE:
- Signs of fullness are turning the head away from nipple, closing the mouth, and showing interest in things other than eating.

SAMPLE QUESTIONS:
How do you hold your baby when you feed him? Do you ever prop the bottle to feed or put your baby to bed with the bottle?

ANTICIPATORY GUIDANCE:
- When feeding your baby, always hold him in your arms in a partly upright position. This will prevent him from choking and will allow you to look into his eyes during feedings. Feeding is a wonderful opportunity for warm and loving interaction with your baby.
- As infants grow, they are more easily distracted during feeding and may need gentle repetitive stimulation (eg, rocking, patting, stroking, and a quiet, dimly lit environment).

- Do not prop a bottle in your baby's mouth or put him to bed with a bottle containing juice, milk, or other sugary liquid. Propping and putting him to bed with a bottle increases the risk of choking and developing early dental caries (tooth decay).

SAMPLE QUESTION:
How easily does your baby burp during or after a feeding?

ANTICIPATORY GUIDANCE:
- Burp your baby at natural breaks (eg, midway through or after a feeding) by gently rubbing or patting his back while holding him against your shoulder and chest or supporting him in a sitting position on your lap.

SAMPLE QUESTION:
How many wet diapers and stools does your baby have each day?

ANTICIPATORY GUIDANCE:
- Your baby is getting enough milk if he has 6 to 8 wet cloth diapers (5 or 6 disposable diapers) and 3 or 4 stools per day and is gaining weight appropriately. The number of bowel movements may decrease and, by 6 weeks, breastfed infants may have stools as infrequently as every 3 days.

SAMPLE QUESTIONS:
Are you giving your baby any supplements, herbs, or vitamins? What vitamin or mineral supplements do you take or plan to take? Are you taking any herbs or drinking any special teas? What medications do you use (eg, prescription, OTC, homeopathic, herbs, or street drugs)?

ANTICIPATORY GUIDANCE:
- Most medications are compatible with breastfeeding, but check them out individually with me or your other health care professionals.
- For formula-fed infants, vitamin supplements are not needed if the formula is iron fortified and the baby is consuming an adequate volume of formula for appropriate growth.

Guidance on Breastfeeding

Mothers who breastfeed should receive 400 µg of folate or folic acid daily by taking a daily prenatal vitamin or a multivitamin in addition to eating a nutritious diet. Vegetarian mothers will need a daily vitamin/mineral supplement containing iron, zinc, and vitamin B_{12}. It is essential that strict vegan mothers who eat no animal products take a daily vitamin B_{12} supplement. Suggest that the mother contact her own health care professional with any questions or concerns about supplements.

Vitamin D (400 IU) supplements are recommended for breastfed infants beginning between 2 weeks and 2 months.

Breastfed premature infants should begin an iron supplement (2 mg/kg/d) by 2 months, and consideration should be given to a phosphate supplement to avoid rickets.

SAMPLE QUESTIONS:

How is breastfeeding going for you and your baby? Are you breastfeeding exclusively? If not, what else is the baby getting? Do you need any help with breastfeeding? Does it seem as though your baby is breastfeeding more often or for longer periods of time? In what ways is breastfeeding different now from when you were last here? How can you tell if your baby is satisfied at the breast?

ANTICIPATORY GUIDANCE:

- Exclusive breastfeeding continues to be the baby's best source of nutrition during the first 4 to 6 months of life.
- You can be reassured about your baby's weight gain by reviewing the growth chart.

SAMPLE QUESTION:

What vitamin or mineral supplements do you take or plan to take?

ANTICIPATORY GUIDANCE:

- Continue to take a daily prenatal vitamin or a multivitamin, in addition to eating a nutritious diet.

SAMPLE QUESTION:

Has your baby received breast milk or other fluids from a bottle?

ANTICIPATORY GUIDANCE:

- Avoid using any artificial nipples (pacifiers, bottles) and supplements (unless medically indicated) until breastfeeding is well established. For most infants, this occurs around 4 to 6 weeks. Some babies may never use pacifiers or bottles.
- If you wish to introduce a bottle to your breastfeeding baby, pick a time when he is not overly hungry or full. Have someone other than you offer the bottle. Allow the baby to explore the bottle's nipple and take it in his mouth. Experiment with different bottle nipples and flow rates. Once you find a nipple that works well for your baby, it is important to stay with that type so that he can get used to a consistent flow of milk. Over time, as his suck becomes stronger, he may need a nipple with a slower flow rate.

Guidance on Formula Feeding

Proper preparation, heating, and storage of infant formula should be reinforced. If there is evidence of inadequate formula availability to meet the infant's needs, appropriate referrals to WIC and other community resources should be provided.

A 1-month-old girl will average 24 oz of formula daily and a 1-month-old boy will average 27 oz of formula daily. Infants may, however, range from 20 to 31 oz of formula daily.

SAMPLE QUESTIONS:

How is formula feeding going for you and your baby? What formula do you use? Is the formula iron fortified? How often does your baby feed? How much does your baby take at a feeding? Have you offered your baby anything other than formula? What concerns do you have about the formula (cost, preparation, nutrient content)?

ANTICIPATORY GUIDANCE:

- You will need to prepare and offer more infant formula as your baby's appetite increases and he goes through growth spurts.

SAFETY

Car safety seats, toys with loops and strings, falls, tobacco smoke

Parents should not place their baby's car safety seat in the front seat of a vehicle with a passenger air bag because the air bags deploy with great force against a car safety seat and cause serious injury or death.

Counsel parents that their own safe driving behaviors (including using safety belts at all times and not driving under the influence of alcohol or drugs) are important to the health of their children.

Infants with special needs need special consideration for safe transportation. Refer parents to a local, specially trained child passenger safety technician for assistance with special positioning and restraint devices (www.preventinjury.org).

Questions about proper installation should be referred to a certified Child Passenger Safety Technician in the community.
Child Safety Seat Inspection Station Locator: www.seatcheck.org
Toll-free Number: 866-SEATCHECK (866-732-8243)

Child Safety Seat Inspection Station Locator: www.seatcheck.org. Toll-free Number: 866-SEATCHECK (866-732-8243).

SAMPLE QUESTION:

Are you having any problems using the baby's car safety seat?

ANTICIPATORY GUIDANCE:

- A rear-facing car safety seat should always be used to transport your baby in all vehicles, including taxis and cars owned by friends or other family members.
- Never place your baby's car safety seat in the front seat of a vehicle with a passenger air bag because air bags deploy with great force against a car safety seat and cause serious injury and death.
- Your baby needs to remain in the car safety seat at all times during travel. If she becomes fussy or needs to nurse, stop the car and remove her from the car safety seat to attend to her needs. Strap her safely back into her seat before traveling again.
- The back seat is the safest place for children to ride.

■ Your own safe driving behaviors are important to the health of your children. Use a safety belt at all times and do not drive after using alcohol or drugs.

Discuss other strategies that parents can use to keep their baby safe.

SAMPLE QUESTION:
What other suggestions have you heard that will keep your baby safe?

ANTICIPATORY GUIDANCE:
■ Always keep one hand on your baby when changing diapers or clothing on a changing table, couch, or bed, especially as she begins to roll over. Falls are the most frequent reason for emergency room visits for injury.
■ Bracelets, toys with loops, or string cords should be kept away from your baby, and string or necklaces should never be around her neck. Dangling electrical, telephone, window blind, or drapery cords should be far from her reach.

Discuss the risks to the infant of smoking. Encourage parents who are quitting, and provide information about smoking cessation strategies and resources for those who are considering quitting.

SAMPLE QUESTION:
Does anyone who lives in or visits the home smoke?

ANTICIPATORY GUIDANCE:
■ It is very important for your baby's health that your home, vehicle, and other places the baby stays are smoke-free. Smoking can increase your baby's risk of SIDS, asthma, ear infections, and respiratory infections.

Health Supervision: 2 Month Visit

CONTEXT

By 2 months after birth, parents and their baby are communicating with each other. The parent/caregiver and baby can gain each other's attention and respond to each other's cues. The baby looks into his parents' eyes, smiles, coos, and vocalizes reciprocally. He is attentive to his parents' voices, and reacts with enjoyment when his senses are stimulated with pleasant sights, sounds, and touch. The infant's responses to his parents when they cuddle him or talk and sing to him provide important feedback that helps the parents feel pleasure and competence. Likewise, the parents' prompt responses to his cries and other more subtle cues help teach him cause and effect and, most importantly, trust.

Typically, parents have settled into their new roles, learning how to divide the tasks of caring for their baby, themselves, and the needs of the family. They may still feel tired and express a desire for rest. Other relatives and members of the support network feel a connection to the baby, and the parents are comfortable with them holding or caring for the baby.

The baby can now hold his head upright for brief periods of time while he is being held. His weight, length, and head circumference should increase along his predicted growth curve. Parents appreciate the health care professional's review of early milestone development because it helps them understand and anticipate the resolution of newborn reflexes. The Moro reflex, reflex grasp, and tonic neck reflexes disappear before purposeful motor skills emerge. Opportunities for motor activity when the baby is awake, such as "tummy time," should be encouraged because they promote head control and appropriate gross motor development.

By this age, if the parents have been using a consistent and predictable routine for the baby, the baby should have established a fairly regular feeding and sleeping schedule. Frequent feedings are still normal for the breastfed baby. The formula-fed baby may need to be fed less frequently. As the baby is able to consolidate longer sleep cycles, a nighttime sleep cycle of 4 to 5 hours may be expected. As a result, night feedings may occur less frequently.

Parents need to be counseled on delaying the introduction of complementary foods until the middle of the first year of the baby's life and when the baby shows definite signs of readiness. These signs include increasing volume of breast milk or formula consumed, weight gain, and continuing physical development. Although it is a common belief, adding cereal to the diet will not increase the hours of sleep at night. Rather, the frequency and duration of feedings, regular naptimes, and active playtimes are more likely to encourage a consolidation of nighttime sleep cycles and longer sleep duration.

As the infant and family settle into a routine, parents begin to resume more of their previous activities and routines, reengage with other family members and friends, and return to school or work. Siblings and other members of the family can be encouraged to participate in the baby's care, fostering their involvement and connection to the baby. Ideally, parents make plans to spend adult time together. Single parents may choose to spend time on outside interests and relationships. It also is important that other children in the family have some time alone with their parents for activities they enjoy. Parents can encourage responsible siblings to participate in the care of the baby to help them feel a valued connection with their little sibling. Arranging for quality, affordable child care is an important priority.

The mother's health (both physical and emotional) will determine her emotional and physical availability to care for her infant. Thus, she should consider talking with her partner and health care professional about completing her postpartum checkup and making family-planning arrangements.

At this visit, it is important for the health care professional to review infant safety measures, including appropriate sleep position and sleep practices, because families and other caregivers may have modified the recommended safe-sleeping measures due to perceived infant or caregiver needs. For example, the parents or other caregivers may feel that the infant's sleep is less comfortable or that spitting up poses a choking threat if the infant is on his back. It is important to ask the parents whether their caregiving practices or preferences differ from recommended practices. In addition, consideration must be given to the family's environment and living circumstances, as some aspects of the child's caregiving may not be under the control of the parent or primary caregiver. Health care professionals must be sensitive to cultural practices, gender roles, parental age, functional abilities, and financial independence of the parents.

PRIORITIES FOR THE VISIT

The first priority is to attend to the concerns of the parents. In addition, the Bright Futures Infancy Expert Panel has given priority to the following topics for discussion in this visit:

- Parental (maternal) well-being (health [maternal postpartum checkup and resumption of activities, depression], parent roles and responsibilities, family support, sibling relationships)
- Infant behavior (parent-child relationship, daily routines, sleep [location, position, crib safety], developmental changes, physical activity [tummy time, rolling over, diminishing newborn reflexes], communication and calming)
- Infant-family synchrony (parent-infant separation [return to work/school], child care)
- Nutritional adequacy (feeding routine, feeding choices [delaying complementary foods, herbs/vitamins/supplements], hunger/satiation cues, feeding strategies [holding, burping], feeding guidance [breastfeeding, formula])
- Safety (car safety seats, water temperature [hot liquids], choking, tobacco smoke, drowning, falls [rolling over])

HEALTH SUPERVISION

History

Interval history may be obtained according to the concerns of the family and the health care professional's preference or style of practice. The following questions can encourage in-depth discussion:

- How are you?
- How have things been going in your family?
- How is your baby doing?
- What concerns or questions do you have about your baby?

Observation of Parent-Child Interaction

During the visit, the health care professional should observe:

- How responsive are the parents and the infant to each other (eg, gazing, talking, smiling, holding, cuddling, comforting, and showing affection)?
- How do the parents appear (eg, content, happy, depressed, tearful, angry, anxious, fatigued, overwhelmed, or uncomfortable)?
- Are the parents aware of, responsive to, and effective in responding to the infant's distress?
- Are the parents comfortable and confident with the infant?
- What are the parent-infant interactions around feeding/eating, comforting, and responding to infant cues?
- Do the parent and partner support each other or show signs of disagreement?

Surveillance of Development

Do you have any specific concerns about your baby's development, learning, or behavior?

SOCIAL-EMOTIONAL
- Attempts to look at parent
- Smiles
- Is able to console and comfort self (brings hands to midline and mouth)

COMMUNICATIVE
- Begins to demonstrate differentiated types of crying (hunger, discomfort, fatigue)
- Coos
- Has clearer behaviors to indicate needs for food, sleep, play, comforting

COGNITIVE
- Indicates boredom (crying/fussiness) when no changes in activity occur

PHYSICAL DEVELOPMENT
- Is able to hold up head and begins to push up in prone position
- Has consistent head control in supported sitting position
- Shows symmetrical movements of head, arms, and legs
- Shows diminishing newborn reflexes

Physical Examination

A complete physical examination is included as part of every health supervision visit.

When performing a physical examination, the health care professional's attention is directed to the following components of the examination that are important for a child this age:

- **Measure and plot:**
  - Length
  - Weight
  - Head circumference
- **Plot:**
  - Weight-for-length
- **Skin**
  - Inspect for rashes or bruising

- **Head**
  - Palpate fontanelles
- **Eyes**
  - Inspect eyes and eyelids
  - Assess ocular mobility
  - Examine pupils for opacification and red reflexes
- **Heart**
  - Ascult for murmurs
  - Palpate femoral pulses
- **Musculoskeletal**
  - Perform Ortolani and Barlow maneuvers
  - Inspect for torticollis
- **Neurologic**
  - Evaluate tone, strength, and symmetry of movements

Screening

UNIVERSAL SCREENING	ACTION	
Metabolic and Hemoglobinopathy	If not done previously, verify documentation of newborn metabolic screening results, appropriate rescreening, and needed follow-up.	
Hearing	If not done previously, verify documentation of newborn hearing screening results and appropriate rescreening.[†]	
SELECTIVE SCREENING	RISK ASSESSMENT[*]	ACTION IF RA +
Blood Pressure	Children with specific risk conditions or change in risk	Blood pressure
Vision	Parental concern or abnormal fundoscopic examination or prematurity with risk conditions	Ophthalmology referral

[†]Positive screenings should be followed up with a diagnostic audiologic assessment, and an infant with a definitive diagnosis should be referred to the state Early Intervention Program.

[*]See the Rationale and Evidence chapter for the criteria on which risk screening questions are based.

Immunizations

Consult the CDC/ACIP or AAP Web sites for the current immunization schedule.
CDC National Immunization Program (NIP): http://www.cdc.gov/vaccines
American Academy of Pediatrics *Red Book*: http://www.aapredbook.org

Consider **influenza vaccine** for caregivers of infants younger than 6 months.

ANTICIPATORY GUIDANCE

The following sample questions, which address the Infancy Expert Panel's Anticipatory Guidance Priorities, are intended to be used selectively to invite discussion, gather information, address the needs and concerns of the family, and build partnerships. Use of the questions may vary from visit to visit and from family to family. Questions can be modified to match the health care professional's communication style. The accompanying anticipatory guidance for the family should be geared to questions, issues, or concerns for that particular child and family.

PARENTAL (MATERNAL) WELL-BEING

Health (maternal postpartum checkup and resumption of activities, depression), parent roles and responsibilities, family support, sibling relationships

Discuss the mother's perspective of her own health and steps she is taking to care for herself. Mothers at this stage may feel sad, exhausted, frustrated, discouraged, or disappointed in their ability to care for their infant. Health care professionals should take into account economic pressures on the family, the need for the mother to return to work quickly, the need to care for other children, and neighborhood issues, such as safety and lack of sidewalks and recreational space. Provide phone numbers and contact information if the mother expresses any concerns about taking care of herself, and provide follow-up to ensure that she is able to access these resources.

SAMPLE QUESTIONS:
To both parents: How are you feeling?
To the mother: Have you had a postpartum checkup? Did you discuss family planning arrangements at this checkup? With your partner? What have you heard from your obstetrician about resuming your normal daily activities after delivery?

ANTICIPATORY GUIDANCE:
■ Because your role as parents requires both physical and emotional energy, you must take care of yourselves so you can care for your baby.

SAMPLE QUESTIONS:
What help do you have with the baby? Are you getting enough rest? Have you been out of the house without the baby? Who takes care of the baby when you go out? How does your baby handle this separation? Do you have the opportunity to spend time with other parents and babies?

ANTICIPATORY GUIDANCE:
■ It is important to take time for yourself as well as time with your partner. Your baby has a strong need to be with you. This need is stronger for some babies than for others. Let me know if you would like some suggestions for how to arrange time away from the baby or ideas for creative ways to spend time with your partner that do not compromise your baby's needs (such as activities when the infant is sleeping).

- It is important for you to identify ways to keep in contact with your friends and family members so that you do not become socially isolated.

SAMPLE QUESTIONS:

How are your other children? Are you able to spend time with each of them individually?

ANTICIPATORY GUIDANCE:

- One of the ways that you can meet the needs of your other children is by appropriately engaging them in the care of the baby. Having them bring supplies and hold the baby's hand are 2 ways they can help. Giving them a "baby/doll" of their own to hold, feed, and diaper is important. So is setting aside regular one-on-one time with your other children to read, talk, and do things together.

INFANT BEHAVIOR

Parent-child relationship, daily routines, sleep (location, position, crib safety), developmental changes, physical activity (tummy time, rolling over, diminishing newborn reflexes), communication and calming

The parents are beginning to experience some of the joys of their baby's behavior, such as an emerging smile, longer periods of alertness, and responsiveness. Parent uncertainty or nervousness, an uninvolved partner, or a statement that caring for the baby is "work" without relaxed or pleasant moments, requires further exploration and counseling, as does a lack of parental involvement as shown by a lack of questions about the baby and his development, or a demeanor of sadness, withdrawal, or anger.

SAMPLE QUESTIONS:

What do you and your partner enjoy most about your baby? What are some of your best times of day with him? What are you enjoying about caring for your baby? What is challenging about caring for your baby?

ANTICIPATORY GUIDANCE:

- At 2 months, your baby is beginning be alert and awake for longer stretches of time. He also will begin to respond more actively to you now by smiling and babbling. Make the most of this new development by cuddling, talking, and playing with your baby.
- It is important to know that a young infant cannot be "spoiled" by holding, cuddling, and rocking him, or by talking and singing to him. Spending time playing and talking during quiet, alert states helps strengthen the parent-child relationship by building trust between you and your baby.

325

A consistent, predictable sleep/wake pattern should be encouraged so that the infant can anticipate sleep and learn to sleep on his own, which means being placed in his crib in a drowsy state. Counseling may be needed for parents with no desire for schedule, no usual routine, or strict adherence to a restrictive feeding schedule. Parents with atypical and inconsistent sleeping patterns, and parents of infants with difficulty developing consistent sleep patterns, irritability, difficulty consoling, or difficulty with feeding also may need additional counseling because these problems all may be related to poor sleep patterns.

SAMPLE QUESTION:
What is your baby's sleep/wake schedule?

ANTICIPATORY GUIDANCE:
- Your baby is still developing regular sleep patterns. Help him by paying attention to his cues for sleep and by sticking to a regular schedule for naps and nighttime sleep. Infant irritability usually is due to lack of sleep.
- By this point, you may be waiting for your baby to sleep through the night. Infants usually have one long stretch of sleep during a 24-hour period. Many babies have this stretch of sleep during the daytime. You may need to help him move it to nighttime hours. More frequent feedings during the daytime will help him have a longer, 4- to 5-hour sleep stretch during the night.

It is recommended that the infant sleep in a separate, but proximate, sleep environment. The infant should sleep in a crib, bassinet, or cradle in the same room as the parents. Infants should not share a bed with parents or any other caregivers or children.

SAMPLE QUESTIONS:
Where does your baby sleep? What position does your baby sleep in? Is your baby having any difficulty sleeping on his back?

ANTICIPATORY GUIDANCE:
- Don't forget, to reduce the risk of SIDS, "back to sleep and prone to play." Make sure that any others who put your baby down to sleep follow "back to sleep" as well.
- A separate but nearby sleep environment is recommended. Babies should sleep in their parents' room, but not in their parents' bed.
- The room temperature should be kept comfortable; make sure the baby doesn't get too warm or cold while sleeping.
- Your baby's crib should have slats that are no more than $2\frac{3}{8}$ inches (60 mm) apart and with a mattress the same size as the crib. A crib should be certified by the JPMA. Keep the sides raised when your baby is sleeping in it.
- If you choose a mesh playpen or portable crib, the weave should have openings less than $\frac{1}{4}$ inch (6 mm). Never leave the baby in a mesh playpen with the drop-side down.

While observing the infant in prone position, discuss the importance of tummy time in the baby's daily activities. During the physical examination, demonstrate how the infant will try to grasp objects held close to his hand and learn to put his hands in his mouth, which aids in self-consoling.

SAMPLE QUESTION:

Physical activity is important for all of us, even young children. How is your baby moving about now?

ANTICIPATORY GUIDANCE:

■ When babies are awake, they enjoy looking around their environment and moving their bodies. One of the first skills babies must learn is holding their head up. One of the ways babies learn to do this is through "tummy time." Although babies need to sleep on their backs, we want to encourage them to play on their tummies. Having them lie on their father's chest and look up into his face is a good activity in the first month. Tummy time also can help prevent the development of a flat area on the back of the head.

Assist the parents in becoming attuned to their infant's ability to handle stimulation and movement, and how best to incorporate activity into their infant's daily routine. Resources for parents to learn infant massage can be provided if parents are interested.

SAMPLE QUESTIONS:

What sounds does your baby make? Does the baby startle or respond to sounds and voices? Does he look at you and watch you as you move your face when you talk? What do you think your baby is feeling and trying to tell you? How does it make you feel? How do you know what your baby wants? Have you noticed any differences in your baby's cries? How would you describe your baby's personality? How does he respond to you? Is it easy or hard to know what he wants? What does your baby do with his hands? What are you enjoying about caring for your baby? What is challenging about caring for your baby?

ANTICIPATORY GUIDANCE:

■ Responding to your baby's sounds by making sounds, too, and by showing your face as you talk, encourages him to "talk back," especially during dressing, bathing, feeding, playing, and walking. This kind of "turn taking" is a foundation of language and conversation. Singing and talking during these typical daily routines also encourages language, as does reading aloud, looking at books, and talking about the pictures. Gradually, your baby will increase the variety and frequency of the sounds he makes as well as how he responds to sounds, especially his parents' voices.

■ It is important to understand and recognize your infant's early temperament and personality so that you know how to adjust to meet his needs. As you learn about his temperament and the way he processes sensory stimulation (ie, whether he is active, quiet, sensitive, demanding, or easily distracted), you will be better able to understand how it affects the way your baby relates to the world.

327

- Getting in tune with your baby's likes and dislikes also can help you feel comfortable and confident in your abilities as a parent. Infant massage is a helpful way for you to understand what your baby likes or dislikes. It can help you calm and relax him, and it enhances your baby's ability to go to sleep easily. Infant massage also offers important health and developmental benefits for premature infants and babies with special health care needs. It helps them sleep, regulate, and organize their waking and sleeping patterns, and promotes muscle tone and infant movement.

Parents may need strategies that will help them find ways to console their baby, and they need to be counseled about how fragile an infant's head is. Helping parents understand that, by responding quickly to their infant's crying, they are teaching the infant to trust that he will be cared for. It will not spoil the infant, as many parents believe.

Putting their hands to their mouth and sucking is an important self-comforting strategy used by infants, and it is an important step in self-regulation. Explain that this strategy helps infants with the earliest feelings of competence and mastery.

If the baby is very irritable, parents need to find a way to avoid frustration. They need to be cautioned to never shake their baby or leave the baby where this could happen, because it causes severe, permanent brain damage. Provide telephone numbers for local community resources that can help parents.

SAMPLE QUESTIONS:

How much is your baby crying? How often? What are some of the ways you have found to calm your baby when he is crying? What do you do if that does not work? Do you ever feel that you and/or other caretakers may hurt the baby? What makes you feel that way? How do you handle the feeling?

ANTICIPATORY GUIDANCE:

- Spending time playing and talking to your baby during the quiet, alert times during the day supports his continuing brain development. Many babies have fussy periods in the late afternoon or evening. These are normal. There are many possible strategies for calming your baby, including just being there with him, talking, patting or stroking, bundling or containing, holding, and rocking. Other calming strategies include caressing or dancing with your infant, walking with him in a carriage or stroller, and going on car rides. Some babies can be very difficult to calm no matter what you do.
- At this age, your baby is developing the ability to put his hands to his mouth, suck on his fingers or his thumb, or use a pacifier. This is one of the ways your baby will learn to calm himself, and it is normal, age-appropriate behavior. He will use these methods until he is able to use other self-calming strategies.

■ Never, ever, shake your baby, because it could cause permanent brain damage. If you ever feel that you need help because your baby is crying so much, contact your health care professional who can, if appropriate, refer you to community resources that can help you and give you appropriate calming techniques.

INFANT-FAMILY SYNCHRONY

Parent-infant separation (return to work/school), child care

At this time, parents may need to return to work or school and should make plans for quality, affordable child care. Parents may benefit from guidance in finding child care and ensuring that caregivers are providing developmental stimulation as well as physical care.

SAMPLE QUESTIONS:
What have you done about locating someone for child care when you return to work or school, need to run errands, or go out with family? Are you comfortable with these arrangements?

ANTICIPATORY GUIDANCE:
■ We can give you suggestions for finding good child care, if you wish. Standards for child care exist. You should look for licensed child care centers and family child care centers that meet specific criteria. It is important to visit and spend time in any setting where you will be leaving your baby to make sure you know how it operates.
■ You can expect a good child care provider to have good infection control practices in place and to give you a daily activity report about your baby's feedings, sleep, play, and elimination.

Concerns about leaving the baby may conflict with the need to support the family or pursue career goals. Separation usually is hard, and the parent may feel guilty and will need to be able to trust or receive support from family members and the child care provider. Changes in routine and separation also may be hard on the infant, and parents may find it helpful to spend extra time comforting the infant during the transition.

SAMPLE QUESTION:
How do you feel now about leaving your baby with someone else?

ANTICIPATORY GUIDANCE:
■ It is not uncommon for mothers to have strong feelings about leaving their baby. Knowing that your baby is with someone you trust and who will take good care of her is a very important first step.

NUTRITIONAL ADEQUACY

Feeding routine, feeding choices (delaying complementary foods, herbs/vitamins/supplements), hunger/satiation cues, feeding strategies (holding, burping), feeding guidance (breastfeeding, formula)

General Guidance on Feeding

Changing infant cues for hunger and satiation, as well as the 3- to 4-month growth spurt, significantly increase nutritional needs, thus increasing the frequency of feedings.

SAMPLE QUESTIONS:
How is your baby's feeding going? Tell me about all the foods and fluids you are offering your baby. What questions or concerns do you have about feeding?

ANTICIPATORY GUIDANCE:
- Exclusive breastfeeding for the first 4 to 6 months of life provides ideal nutrition and supports the best possible growth and development. If you are still breastfeeding, congratulations!
- If your baby is not breastfed, iron-fortified formula is the recommended substitute during the first year of life.
- Do not give your baby food other than breast milk or formula until he is developmentally ready (around the middle of his first year).
- Usually, healthy babies do not require extra water. On very hot days with no air conditioning or when there is excess water loss due to sweating, fever, or diarrhea, babies will benefit from some extra water. Breast milk and formula (when properly prepared) are adequate to meet the baby's fluid needs. Juice is not recommended in the first 6 months of life.

SAMPLE QUESTIONS:
How do you know if your baby is hungry? How do you know if he has had enough to eat? How easily does your baby burp during or after a feeding?

ANTICIPATORY GUIDANCE:
- Breastfed and formula-fed infants have different needs for the frequency of feeding, although both formula and breast milk provide all the nutrition that infants need until about 6 months of age.
- To prevent overfeeding, which often leads to more frequent spit-ups, recognize your baby's individual signs of hunger and fullness. An infant's stomach is still small; therefore, your baby still needs to eat every 2 to 4 hours, even during the night. Hopefully, your baby will have one longer stretch at night of 4 to 5 hours without feeding.
- Burp your baby at natural breaks (eg, midway through or after a feeding) by gently rubbing or patting his back while holding him against your shoulder and chest or supporting him in a sitting position on your lap.

Guidance on Breastfeeding

Explain that, as infants grow, they are more easily distracted during feeding and may need gentle repetitive stimulation (eg, rocking, patting, or stroking). The infant may need a quiet environment, perhaps with low lighting and without other people present. Feeding times offer a wonderful opportunity for social interaction between the infant and the mother.

Counsel mothers on safe storage of breast milk.

SAMPLE QUESTIONS:

How is breastfeeding going for you and your baby? Is your baby breastfeeding exclusively? If not, what else is the baby getting? Do you need any help with breastfeeding? Does it seem like your baby is breastfeeding more often or for longer periods of time? In what ways is breastfeeding different now from when you were last here? How can you tell if your baby is satisfied at the breast?

ANTICIPATORY GUIDANCE:

- Breastfed infants continue to need about 8 to 12 feedings in 24 hours. They may feed more frequently when they go through growth spurts. By 3 months of age, breastfed infants generally will be feeding every 2 to 3 hours. If your baby is receiving frequent feedings during the day and continuing to receive between 6 and 12 feedings in 24 hours, he may have one longer stretch of 4 to 5 hours at night between feedings.

SAMPLE QUESTIONS:

Are you planning to return to work or school? If so, will you express your breast milk? Does your school or workplace have a place where you can pump your milk in privacy? How will you store your milk? How long will you keep it?

ANTICIPATORY GUIDANCE:

- Consider how to plan your activities and schedules to make things easier when you are home with your baby. Storing breast milk properly is very important. If you are interested, I can give you written guidelines to help you make sure your stored breast milk remains safe for your baby.
- I can help you with strategies to support breast-milk production if you will be away from the baby for extended periods.

Guidance on Formula Feeding

If parents feel they do not have time to hold the bottle, review the importance of the feeding relationship and the benefits of holding the infant during feeding, as well as the risks of propping the bottle. Parents also may need to be reminded not to put the baby to bed with a bottle.

The usual amount of formula for a 2-month-old infant in 24 hours is about 26 to 28 oz with a range of 21 to 32 oz.

SAMPLE QUESTIONS:

How is formula feeding going for you and your baby? What formula do you use? Is the formula fortified with iron? How often does your baby feed? How much does your baby drink at a feeding? Have you offered your baby anything other than formula? What questions or concerns do you have about the formula (cost, preparation, nutrient content)? Has your baby received breast milk or other fluids from a bottle?

ANTICIPATORY GUIDANCE:

- Babies who receive formula usually will feed every 3 to 4 hours, with one longer stretch at night of up to 5 or 6 hours at night between feedings. Overall, a 2-month-old baby still needs about 6 to 8 feedings in 24 hours.
- When feeding your baby, always hold him in your arms in a partly upright position. This will prevent him from choking and will allow you to look into his eyes during feedings. Feeding is a wonderful opportunity for warm and loving interaction with your baby.

SAMPLE QUESTIONS:

How do you hold your baby when you feed him? Do you ever prop the bottle to feed or put your baby to bed with the bottle?

ANTICIPATORY GUIDANCE:

- Do not prop a bottle in your baby's mouth or put him to bed with a bottle containing juice, milk, or other sugary liquid. Propping and putting him to bed with a bottle increases the risk of choking and developing early dental caries (tooth decay).

Child Safety Seat Inspection Station Locator: www.seatcheck.org. Toll-free Number: 866-SEATCHECK (866-732-8243).

SAFETY

Car safety seats, water temperature (hot liquids), choking, tobacco smoke, drowning, falls (rolling over)

Review car safety seat guidelines with the parents.

Counsel parents that their own safe driving behaviors (including using safety belts at all times and not driving under the influence of alcohol or drugs) are important to the health of their children.

Questions about proper installation should be referred to a certified Child Passenger Safety Technician in the community.
Child Safety Seat Inspection Station Locator: www.seatcheck.org
Toll-free Number: 866-SEATCHECK (866-732-8243)

SAMPLE QUESTION:
Do you have any questions about using your car safety seat?

ANTICIPATORY GUIDANCE:
- A rear-facing car safety seat that is properly secured in the back seat should always be used to transport your baby in all vehicles, including taxis and cars owned by friends or other family members.
- Never place your baby's car safety seat in the front seat of a vehicle with a passenger air bag because air bags deploy with great force against a car safety seat and cause serious injury and death.
- Your own safe driving behaviors are important to the health of your children. Use a safety belt at all times and do not drive after using alcohol or drugs.

Exposure to tobacco smoke is related to increased risk of otitis, respiratory infections, asthma, and hospitalization.

Discuss the importance of not leaving the baby alone in a tub of water, even when using a bath ring or seat, even for a second, or in high places, such as changing tables, beds, sofas, or chairs.

SAMPLE QUESTION:
What other things are you doing to keep your baby safe and healthy?

ANTICIPATORY GUIDANCE:
- Do not drink hot liquids while holding the baby.
- To protect your child from tap water scalds, the hottest temperature at the faucet should be no higher than 120°F. In many cases, you can adjust your water heater. Before bathing the baby, always test the water temperature with your wrist to make sure it is not too hot.
- Never leave your baby alone in a tub of water. A bath seat or bath ring is not a safety device and is not a substitute for adult supervision.
- Your baby's environment should continue to be free of tobacco smoke. Consider your home and vehicle as nonsmoking zones.
- Leaving the baby on a changing table, couch, infant seat, or bed becomes increasingly dangerous because of your baby's ability to roll or push off. Her legs are getting stronger now that her newborn reflexes that prevent rolling over are gradually fading away. Get in the habit of always keeping one hand on the baby when changing diapers or clothing on a changing table, couch, or bed, especially as she begins to roll over.
- Remember to keep all small objects, especially sibling's toys, away from your baby, who will soon be learning to reach and put things in her mouth. Keep away plastic bags, which can block the airway, and latex balloons, which can cause choking, from your child.

Health Supervision: 4 Month Visit

CONTEXT

The relationship between parents and their 4-month-old baby is pleasurable and rewarding. The baby's ability to smile, coo, and laugh encourages his parents to talk and play with him. Clear and predictable cues from the infant are met with appropriate and predictable responses from his parents, promoting mutual trust. During this period, the infant masters early motor, language, and social skills by interacting with those who care for him.

The infant's fussiness should begin to decrease as the infant develops self-consoling skills and improved self-regulation. If crying is still a concern, parents need additional specific strategies for calming their baby. Evaluation of the infant's temperament and parent temperament may be needed to help the parents understand the importance of these strategies.

Responding to the sights and sounds around him, the 4-month-old baby raises his body from a prone position with his arms and holds his head steady. He may be so interested in his world that he sometimes refuses to settle down to eat. He may stop feeding from the breast or bottle after just a minute or 2 to check out what else is happening in the room. Parents may need to feed him in a quiet, darkened room for the next few weeks.

Over the next 2 months, the baby may be developmentally ready to start eating complementary foods. However, continuing exclusive breastfeeding until 6 months has many benefits for the infant, including accelerated neuromotor development; decreased risk of infections, especially diarrhea; decreased risk of developing allergies; decreased risk of ear infections; and decreased health risks from contaminated foods. Exclusive breastfeeding has benefits for the mother as well, including a longer delay in the return of fertility, a more rapid weight loss, and assistance in maintaining her milk supply.

As key social and motor abilities become apparent at 4 months, the infant who appears to have a delay in achieving these skills may benefit from a formal developmental assessment. If developmental delays are found, exploring their origin and making referrals for early intervention will be important.

Most employed mothers will have returned to work by the time their infant is 4 months old, and it is important that child care arrangements work for both the infant and the family. An irritable child who cries frequently or does not sleep through the night may clash temperamentally with a family that values regularity and tranquility. Family problems, such as inadequate finances, few social supports, or low parental self-esteem, may impair the parents' ability to nurture. It is important that parents seek help when they feel sad, discouraged, depressed, overwhelmed, or inadequate. Parents who have the support they need can be warmly rewarded by their interactions with their 4-month-old infant.

PRIORITIES FOR THE VISIT

The first priority is to attend to the concerns of the parents. In addition, the Bright Futures Infancy Expert Panel has given priority to the following topics for discussion in this visit:

- Family functioning (parent roles/responsibilities, parental responses to infant, child care providers [number, quality])
- Infant development (consistent daily routines, sleep [crib safety, sleep location], parent-child relationship [play, tummy time], infant self-regulation [social development, infant self-calming])
- Nutrition adequacy and growth (feeding success, weight gain, feeding choices [complementary foods, food allergies], feeding guidance [breastfeeding, formula])
- Oral health (maternal oral health care, use of clean pacifier, teething/drooling, avoidance of bottle in bed)
- Safety (car safety seats, falls, walkers, lead poisoning, drowning, water temperature [hot liquids], burns, choking)

HEALTH SUPERVISION

History

Interval history may be obtained according to the concerns of the family and the health care professional's preference or style of practice. The following questions can encourage in-depth discussion:

- How are you?
- How are things going in your family?
- Tell me how things are going for your baby.
- What questions or concerns do you have about your baby?
- How are you enjoying your baby now? What are the challenges?

Observation of Parent-Child Interaction

During the visit, the health care professional should observe:

- Are parents and the infant interested in and responsive to each other (eg, gazing, talking, smiling, holding, cuddling)?
- Do the parents provide comforting actions when the infant cries?
- Are the parents attentive to their infant during the examination?
- Do the parents and infant demonstrate a reciprocal engagement around feeding/eating?
- Do the parents respond to the infant's cues and how does the infant respond to the parents?

Surveillance of Development

Do you have any specific concerns about your baby's development, learning, or behavior?

SOCIAL-EMOTIONAL
- Smiles spontaneously
- Elicits social interactions
- Shows solidified self-consolation skills

COMMUNICATIVE
- Cries in a differentiated manner to express hunger, fatigue, pain
- Babbles more expressively and spontaneously

COGNITIVE
- Responds to affection, changes in environment
- Indicates pleasure and displeasure

PHYSICAL DEVELOPMENT
- Pushes chest up to elbows
- Has good head control
- Demonstrates symmetrical movements of arms and legs
- Begins to roll and reach for objects

Physical Examination

A complete physical examination is included as part of every health supervision visit.

When performing a physical examination, the health care professional's attention is directed to the following components of the examination that are important for a child this age:

- ■ **Measure and plot:**
  - Length
  - Weight
  - Head circumference
- ■ **Plot:**
  - Weight-for-length
- ■ **Skin**
  - Inspect for rashes and bruising

- ■ **Head**
  - Palpate for positional skull deformities
- ■ **Eyes**
  - Assess ocular mobility for lateral gaze
  - Examine pupils for opacification and red reflexes
- ■ **Heart**
  - Ascult for heart murmurs
  - Palpate femoral pulses
- ■ **Musculoskeletal**
  - Assess for developmental hip dysplasia by examining for abduction
- ■ **Neurologic**
  - Evaluate tone, strength, and symmetry of movements

Screening

UNIVERSAL SCREENING	ACTION	
None		
SELECTIVE SCREENING	RISK ASSESSMENT*	ACTION IF RA +
Blood pressure	Children with specific risk conditions or change in risk	Blood pressure
Vision	Parental concern or abnormal fundoscopic examination or abnormal alignment of eyes	Ophthalmology referral
Hearing	+ on risk screening questions	Referral for diagnostic audiologic assessment
Anemia	Pre-term and low birth weight infants and those not on iron-fortified formula	Hemoglobin or hematocrit
*See the Rationale and Evidence chapter for the criteria on which risk screening questions are based.		

Immunizations

Consult the CDC/ACIP or AAP Web sites for the current immunization schedule.
CDC National Immunization Program (NIP): http://www.cdc.gov/vaccines
American Academy of Pediatrics *Red Book*: http://www.aapredbook.org

Consider **influenza vaccine** for caregivers of infants younger than 6 months.

ANTICIPATORY GUIDANCE

The following sample questions, which address the Infancy Expert Panel's Anticipatory Guidance Priorities, are intended to be used selectively to invite discussion, gather information, address the needs and concerns of the family, and build partnerships. Use of the questions may vary from visit to visit and from family to family. Questions can be modified to match the health care professional's communication style. The accompanying anticipatory guidance for the family should be geared to questions, issues, or concerns for that particular child and family.

FAMILY FUNCTIONING

Parent roles/responsibilities, parental responses to infant, child care providers (number, quality)

Usually by the time their infant is 4 months old, parents truly are enjoying their role as parents and beginning to gain confidence in their ability to care for their infant. For those parents who are juggling work or school and child care and parenting, they may be less likely to find this time as enjoyable and may begin to feel the stress of their many responsibilities.

SAMPLE QUESTIONS:

What do you do when problems really get to you? Who do you turn to at times like that? How are you and your partner getting along together? Have you and your partner been getting out without the baby? Who helps you care for your infant? How are your other children doing? Do you spend time with each of them individually?

ANTICIPATORY GUIDANCE:

- Stay in touch with friends and family members. It will help you avoid social isolation.
- Talk to me or another health care professional if you and your partner are in conflict.
- Take some time for yourself and spend some individual time with your partner.
- Make sure you meet the needs of your other children by spending time with them each day doing things they like to do. Help them enjoy the baby by appropriately engaging them in the care of the baby, such as by bringing you supplies or holding the baby's hand.

SAMPLE QUESTION:

What do you think your baby is trying to tell you when she cries, looks at you, turns away, or smiles?

ANTICIPATORY GUIDANCE:

- As you begin to understand and recognize your infant's early temperament and personality, you also will begin to feel more comfortable in knowing how to adjust your responses to meet her needs. This also will help your baby better understand how she relates to the world.

- Infant massage may be a helpful way for you to understand what your baby likes or dislikes. It can help you calm and relax her, and it helps your baby go to sleep easily. Getting in tune with your baby's likes and dislikes can help you feel more comfortable and confident in your abilities as a parent. Infant massage also offers important health and developmental benefits for premature infants and babies with special health care needs, as long as you pay close attention to your baby's cues and when she needs a break or to stop. It helps babies sleep, regulate, and organize their state, and promotes muscle tone and infant movement.
- It is important to know that an infant cannot be "spoiled" by holding, cuddling, and rocking her, and by talking and singing to her. Spending time playing and talking with your baby helps to strengthen the parent-child relationship by building trust between you and your baby.

Parents need help in identifying and evaluating their child care options. Provide written material or contact information for community resources that are available to assist parents in identifying family home care or child care centers that meet their requirements.

Parents of children with special needs often will have significant difficulty locating child care resources and, therefore, may particularly benefit from being connected to local public health resources as well as contacts through the local Early Intervention Program agency, often referred to as IDEA. These contacts can help with developmental concerns and also for links to other community resources.

SAMPLE QUESTIONS:
Have you returned to work or school, or do you plan to do so? What are your child care arrangements? Who takes care of the baby when you go out?

ANTICIPATORY GUIDANCE:
- If you are returning to work, talk with me or another health care professional about child care arrangements and your feelings about leaving your baby.
- Choose babysitters and caregivers who are mature, trained, responsible, and recommended by someone you trust.
- Encourage your partner to participate in the care of the baby.

INFANT DEVELOPMENT

Consistent daily routines, sleep (crib safety, sleep location), parent-child relationship (play, tummy time), infant self-regulation (social development, infant self-calming)

To receive adequate calories, most 4-month-old babies continue to wake at night for feeding. Parents often see the infant not "sleeping through the night" as a problem and they want solutions. This visit is a good time to explore the importance of a consistent daily routine and its impact on sleep, typical sleep patterns, ways to establish a good sleep routine, and the overall relationship between feeding, sleep, and play activities. Also, it may be important to clarify "sleeping through the night." Some parents may expect an infant to sleep 12 hours at night, where actually having a longer stretch of sleep for 5 to 6 hours would be more typical.

Parents who describe infants with inconsistent and unpredictable behaviors, or parents who are unable to depict their baby's schedule, may need additional monitoring and intervention.

Discuss difficulties integrating the routines of the infant with that of scheduling demands of older siblings and family members. Monitor atypical sleep/wake patterns, night awakenings, and inconsistent stooling patterns. Provide intervention for excessive sleep or wakefulness and lack of consistent, predictable daily routines.

SAMPLE QUESTIONS:
What type of daily routine do you have for your baby? How long is your baby sleeping at night? Do you have a bedtime routine for your baby?

ANTICIPATORY GUIDANCE:
- An established daily routine for feedings and naps and a bedtime routine is a good idea because they will help establish eventual longer sleeping stretches at night.
- It also is important to help your baby learn to put himself to sleep by placing him in his crib when he is drowsy, talking gently to him, and even patting him to sleep.
- Continuing to provide regular structure and routines for the baby will increase his sense of security.

Remind parents of the continuing importance of "back to sleep, prone to play."

SAMPLE QUESTIONS:
Do you have any difficulty getting your baby to sleep on his back? Have you discussed with your child care provider the importance of back sleeping?

ANTICIPATORY GUIDANCE:
- Your baby should continue to sleep on his back to reduce the risk of SIDS, and relatives and child care providers should be reminded to follow the same practice.
- To reduce the risk of suffocation, do not use loose, soft bedding (blankets, quilts, sheepskins, comforters, pillows, and pillow-like bumper pads) or soft toys.
- Be sure your baby's crib is safe both at home and at the babysitter's home. The slats should be no more than $2\frac{3}{8}$ inches (60 mm) apart. The mattress should be firm and fit snugly into the crib. Keep the sides of the crib raised when your baby is in the crib.
- Lower the crib mattress before the baby can sit up by himself.

■ If you choose a mesh playpen or portable crib, the weave should have openings less than $\frac{1}{4}$ inch (6 mm). Never leave the baby in a mesh playpen with the drop-side down.

As parents learn about their infant through observing his behaviors, they are able to respond appropriately to his ever-changing needs. Helping parents have "watchful wonder" about their baby's behaviors allows them to discover the uniqueness of their baby's own temperament and sensory processing, and how it affects the way he relates to the world. To demonstrate this "watchful wondering," during the physical examination, describe the infant's behaviors and responses to being handled and engaged in play. This can lead to a discussion about what is developmentally appropriate and, if needed, when and how it is appropriate to redirect the infant's behavior.

SAMPLE QUESTIONS:
Tell me about your baby? What do you like best about your baby? What does your partner enjoy most about your baby?

ANTICIPATORY GUIDANCE:
■ Babies use their behaviors to communicate their likes and dislikes. Each baby has a unique way of communicating. By watching your baby closely, and how he responds to you and the world around him, you become the expert on your baby and the best way to meet his needs.

Counsel parents on the steps in development that are likely to occur during the next 2 months, based on the baby's current development and how the daily physical activities of the baby encourage normal development.

Encourage parents to use both active and quiet playtime. Discuss alternatives to infants watching TV. Discourage any television or video viewing for children younger than 2 years.

Health care professionals can use the physical examination to demonstrate the integration of the newborn reflexes and emergence of the protective reflexes, and discuss what these reflexes, plus the infant's head control and sitting with support, mean in terms of the infant's ability to roll over and sit. As the infant improves his ability to move on his own, parents must begin to use extra caution about protecting him from rolling off the bed or couch or changing table. During the physical examination, demonstrate the protective reflexes, if emerging.

SAMPLE QUESTIONS:
What are some of your baby's new achievements? What are some of your baby's favorite activities? Favorite toys? How is your baby getting around now? How is "tummy time" working for your baby? How have you been able to fit together your physical activities with the baby?

ANTICIPATORY GUIDANCE:

- Use both quiet and active playtime with your baby. Quiet playtime activities include reading or singing to your baby or sitting together outside in the park. For active playtime activities, give your baby age-appropriate toys to play with, such as a floor play gym so that, when he is placed on his back, he can reach for the toys or kick them with his feet. Another choice is a colorful blanket, a mirror, or toys for him to look at when he is on his tummy. Make sure your baby has safe opportunities to explore his environment.

Babies who are described as excessively active or extremely quiet should be monitored. Management assistance is extremely important for parents who are sad or unhappy, or who rarely sleep. Consider referring parents for mental health evaluation and treatment.

SAMPLE QUESTIONS:

How would you describe your baby's personality? How does your baby act around other people? Is he responsive or withdrawn with family members?

ANTICIPATORY GUIDANCE:

- Babies at 4 months find that interacting with their parents is their favorite activity. Their emerging social play and interaction can be a delight but also frustrating for parents who are balancing other responsibilities. Understanding ways to engage your baby in activities, if even for a short time, will help provide some time to accomplish your other responsibilities.

Four-month-old babies still will have fussy times, and parents need to have a variety of strategies to calm their infant. Setting up a variety of play activities so that the infant can be moved easily from one to the other is often helpful in adjusting for the infant's increasing awake time and short attention span. As they try to console their baby, sometimes unsuccessfully, parents begin to recognize that their baby may not always be consolable. Discuss additional strategies for calming the infant when this occurs.

SAMPLE QUESTIONS:

What do you do to calm your baby? What do you do if that does not work? Do you ever feel that you and/or other caretakers may hurt the baby? What will you do if you feel this way? Do you have a plan? How do you handle the feeling?

ANTICIPATORY GUIDANCE:

- If your baby is being very fussy and you have checked that he is fed, clean, and safe and you are beginning to get upset and frustrated, put the baby in his crib and give yourself a break—make a cup of tea or call a friend. Babies cry a lot at this age; it gets better as they get older. Crying won't hurt your baby. If this happens consistently, though, call me for advice.

NUTRITION ADEQUACY AND GROWTH

Feeding success, weight gain, feeding choices (complementary foods, food allergies), feeding guidance (breastfeeding, formula)

General Guidance on Feeding

At 4 months, feeding can be one of the most enjoyable experiences for parents, and both parents often share in this responsibility. Babies continue to gain about $\frac{1}{2}$ pound a week, or 2 pounds a month. Their feedings may become less frequent, with 6 to 10 feedings in 24 hours. Only one parent might be present at this visit and a complete feeding history may not be available. This is particularly true if the infant is in child care. If there are concerns with feeding, irritability, or weight gain, it may be advisable to have the parents work together with the child care provider to complete a 24-hour or 3-day diet history that can be reviewed for nutritional adequacy. A referral can be made to a dietitian, if needed.

SAMPLE QUESTIONS:

How is feeding going? What questions or concerns do you have about feeding? Tell me about what you are feeding your baby. How often are you feeding your baby? How much does your baby take at a feeding? About how long does a feeding last? Are you feeding your baby any foods besides breast milk or formula?

ANTICIPATORY GUIDANCE:

- Exclusive breastfeeding provides the ideal source of nutrition for all infants during first 4 to 6 months of life. For those infants who are not breastfed, iron-fortified formula is the recommended substitute.

Parents continue to need reassurance that their infant is getting enough to eat when feeding patterns change because of a temporary increase in the frequency of feedings due to growth spurts. Discuss the meaning of the growth chart and the relationship between the infant's birth weight and current weight and length.

As babies learn that they can put their hands in their mouth for chewing and sucking, they use this technique to calm themselves. Some parents think this means their baby is still hungry and they use it as a rationale for starting complementary foods. Cereal can be introduced between 4 to 6 months of age, and parents need guidance about introducing complementary foods when their baby is developmentally ready.

Parents also should be counseled on the appropriate use of supplements, herbs, and vitamins. Supplements that should be considered include:

Breastfed infants
- Vitamin D (400 IU) supplements are recommended beginning between 2 weeks and 2 months.

Formula-fed infants
• Vitamin supplements are not needed if the formula is iron fortified and the baby is consuming an adequate volume of formula for appropriate growth.

Preterm or low birth weight infants
• Preterm or low birth weight infants may become iron deficient at an early age and need iron supplements. Breastfed premature infants should begin an iron supplement (2 mg/kg/d) by 2 months and consideration should be given to a phosphate supplement to avoid rickets.

SAMPLE QUESTION:
Have you thought about when you will begin to give your baby solids?

ANTICIPATORY GUIDANCE:
■ Normal gain in fat mass is higher in infancy than at any other age, and a healthy infant may appear chubby even when her growth is normal. This normal gain gives your baby energy reserves when she is ill. The growth chart shows the weight of your baby along her growth curve in relation to her length, and this is the best indicator of her appropriate weight.
■ Foods associated with lifelong sensitization (peanuts, tree nuts, fish, and shellfish) should not be introduced until after 1 year or even later.
■ Adding complementary foods (also called solids) is very individualized. There is no evidence that adding cereal helps babies sleep through the night. Between 4 and 6 months of age, the baby will be ready to begin eating solid foods. One of the signs that she is ready to eat solids is the fading of the tongue thrust reflex (pushing food out of the mouth). Another sign is that the baby can raise her tongue to move pureed food to the back of the mouth and, as she sees a spoon approach, she opens her mouth in anticipation of the next bite. At this stage, your baby sits with arm support and has good head and neck control so she can indicate a desire for food by opening her mouth and leaning forward. She can tell you she is full or doesn't want food by leaning back and turning away.

SAMPLE QUESTIONS:
Are you giving your baby any supplements, herbs, or vitamins? Do you take any supplements, herbs, vitamins, or medications?

ANTICIPATORY GUIDANCE:
■ It is important to tell me about any supplements, herbs, or vitamins you may be giving your baby. This information will help me give you the best care and advice. Although most of the time these supplements do no harm, I should know about them if there is ever an incompatibility with other medications or treatments your child might receive.
■ Most medications are compatible with breastfeeding but should be checked on an individual basis.

Guidance on Breastfeeding

Commend mothers who are still breastfeeding. Reinforce that exclusive breastfeeding is the ideal source of nutrition for the first 4 to 6 months and that breastfeeding should be continued for as long as the mother and child want.

Discuss how demand for more frequent breastfeeding is usually related to an infant's growth spurt and is nature's way of increasing breast milk supply. If an increased demand continues for a few days, is not affected by increased breastfeeding, and is unrelated to illness, teething, or changes in routine, it may be a sign that the breastfed infant is ready for complementary foods.

Counsel mothers on safe storage of breast milk.

SAMPLE QUESTIONS:

How is breastfeeding going for you and your baby? In what ways is breastfeeding different now from when you were last here? How often does your baby breastfeed? Does it seem as though your baby is breastfeeding more often or for longer periods of time? How can you tell whether your baby is satisfied at the breast? Has your baby received breast milk or other fluids from a bottle? How are you storing pumped breast milk?

ANTICIPATORY GUIDANCE:

- Congratulations for continuing to breastfeed your baby! It is not unusual for babies to go through growth spurts during the first year of life and, whenever this occurs, your baby will begin to breastfeed more frequently, and often at night. This is nature's way of increasing your milk supply. This is a temporary situation and it does not indicate that your baby is not getting enough to eat.
- Storing breast milk properly is very important. If you are interested, I can give you written guidelines to help you make sure your stored breast milk remains safe for your baby.

Guidance on Formula Feeding

Discuss with parents that, as the infant's appetite increases and she grows, they will need to continue to prepare and offer a little more infant formula. Instruct parents to feed the infant when she is hungry (usually 8 to 12 times in 24 hours).

Discuss with parents that formula is the most important nutrition for the infant. Other foods or drinks are not advised unless recommended by the health care professional.

The usual amount of formula for a 4-month-old infant in 24 hours is about 30 to 32 oz of formula per day, with a range of 26 to 36 oz.

SAMPLE QUESTIONS:

How is feeding going? What formula are you using now? Is the formula fortified with iron? Have you tried other formulas? How often does your baby feed? How much at a feeding? How much in 24 hours? How does your baby show she is hungry or full? Has your baby begun to put her hands around the bottle? Are you still holding your baby for feedings? What questions or concerns do you have about the formula (cost, preparation, nutrient content)? Have you offered your baby anything other than formula?

ANTICIPATORY GUIDANCE:

- Your baby is now able to clearly show when she is hungry or full. It also is not unusual for her to want different amounts of formula at different times of the day (she may take more at a morning feeding than at a noon feeding). It is important to respond to your baby's behaviors for feeding to avoid overfeeding (spitting up) or underfeeding. Holding your baby during feeding also helps you understand the meaning of your baby's behaviors. This will help you meet her needs and reduce fussiness. It will even help with her learning as she watches you and listens to your voice.
- It is important to hold your baby for all bottle-feedings to reduce the risks of choking and to ensure that your baby gets enough of the formula. To reduce the risk of developing dental caries, do not prop the bottle.
- As your baby begins to drink larger amounts of formula, you may want to contact community resources, like WIC, which can provide formula for your baby.

ORAL HEALTH

Maternal oral health care, use of clean pacifier, teething/drooling, avoidance of bottle in bed

Most parents are not aware that their own oral health has an impact on their baby's eventual dental health. Therefore, it is important to discuss this with parents.

SAMPLE QUESTIONS:

When was your last dental checkup? What is your daily dental care routine?

ANTICIPATORY GUIDANCE:

- Sharing spoons and cleaning a dropped pacifier in your mouth may increase the growth of bacteria in your baby's mouth and increase the risk that he will develop dental decay when his teeth come in.
- To protect your child's eventual dental health, it is important for you to maintain good dental health. Because you may be the source of caries-promoting bacteria for your baby, it is important you visit the dentist, reduce the amount of sugary drinks in your diet, take meticulous care of your teeth through brushing and flossing, and use a fluoridated toothpaste and/or rinse.

SAMPLE QUESTION:
Is your baby beginning to drool?

ANTICIPATORY GUIDANCE:

■ If your baby is teething, he may drool, become fussy, or put things in his mouth. A cold teething ring may help ease his discomfort. Talk with me if his symptoms persist.

SAMPLE QUESTION:
What are your plans for protecting your baby's teeth?

ANTICIPATORY GUIDANCE:

■ To avoid developing a habit that will harm your baby's teeth, do not put him to bed with a bottle containing juice, milk, or other sugary liquid. Always hold your baby for a bottle-feeding and do not prop the bottle in his mouth or allow him "graze" (drink from a bottle at will during the day).

SAFETY

Car safety seats, falls, walkers, lead poisoning, drowning, water temperature (hot liquids), burns, choking

Child Safety Seat Inspection Station Locator: www.seatcheck.org. Toll-free Number: 866-SEATCHECK (866-732-8243).

Remind parents about proper car safety seat use and the importance of putting the infant in the rear seat of the vehicle.

Remind parents that their own safe driving behaviors (including using safety belts at all times and not driving under the influence of alcohol or drugs) are important to the health of their children.

Questions about proper installation should be referred to a certified Child Passenger Safety Technician in the community.
Child Safety Seat Inspection Station Locator: www.seatcheck.org
Toll-free Number: 866-SEATCHECK (866-732-8243)

SAMPLE QUESTIONS:
Do you use a rear-facing car safety seat in the back seat every time the baby rides in a vehicle? Do you know when to change from an infant-only to a convertible car safety seat?

ANTICIPATORY GUIDANCE:

■ A baby's car safety seat must never be placed in the front seat of a vehicle with a passenger air bag. Air bags deploy with great force against a car safety seat and cause serious injury or death. Babies are best protected in the event of a crash when they are in the back seat and in a rear-facing car safety seat.

■ Keep your baby's car safety seat rear facing in the back seat of the vehicle until your baby is at least 1 year old **and** weighs at least 20 pounds. It is preferable to wait even longer, until the baby reaches the highest weight or height allowed by the manufacturer of the seat.

- Infants who reach 20 pounds or 26 to 29 inches before 1 year should use a convertible seat or infant-only seat that is approved for use rear-facing to higher weights and heights (up to 30 pounds and 32 inches for infant-only seats and up to 35 pounds and at least 36 inches for convertible seats). Your baby will be safest if she rides rear facing to the highest weight or height allowed by the manufacturer.
- The back seat is the safest place for children to ride.
- Do not start the engine until everyone is buckled in.
- Your own safe driving behaviors are important to the health of your children. Use a safety belt at all times and do not drive after using alcohol or drugs.

As their baby develops more fine and gross motor skills, it is important to review with the parents how to keep the home environment safe for their active baby. This applies to all homes where the baby spends time, including child care and grandparents' and friends' homes.

SAMPLE QUESTIONS:
Where does your baby spend awake time during the day?

ANTICIPATORY GUIDANCE:
- Always keep one hand on your baby when changing diapers or clothing on a changing table, couch, or bed, especially as she begins to roll over. Falls are the most common reason for emergency room visits for injury.
- A baby should not be left alone for even a second in a tub of water, even if using a bath ring or seat, or on high places such as changing tables, beds, sofas, or chairs.
- Infant walkers should not be used by young children at any age. They are frequently associated with falls and can slow development of motor skills in children.

SAMPLE QUESTION:
Have you made any changes in your home to help keep your baby safe?

ANTICIPATORY GUIDANCE:
- The kitchen is the most dangerous room for children. A safer place for your child while you are cooking, eating, or unable to provide your full attention is the playpen, crib, or stationary activity center, or buckled into a high chair.
- To protect your child from tap water scalds, the hottest temperature at the faucet should be no more then 120°F. In many cases, you can adjust your water heater.
- Drinking hot liquids, cooking, ironing, or smoking while holding a baby puts your baby at risk of burns.
- To prevent choking, keep small objects, sibling's toys, pieces of plastic, and latex balloons out of the baby's reach as she develops skills with reaching.

SAMPLE QUESTION:

Do you know how to assess the risk of lead poisoning in your home?

ANTICIPATORY GUIDANCE:

- Lead can be found in the paint of older homes (built before 1978), pottery and pewter, folk medicines, insecticides, industry, and hobbies, as well as other sources. Lead is toxic, and it is important to be aware of any sources of lead in your home to prevent lead exposure for your family.

Health Supervision: 6 Month Visit

CONTEXT

Parents cherish their interactions with their social 6-month-old infant, who smiles and vocalizes back at them but has not yet mastered the ability to move from one place to another. The feelings of attachment between the parents and their child create a secure emotional attachment that will help provide stability to the changing family. The major developmental markers of a 6-month-old baby are social and emotional. A 6-month-old baby likes to interact with people. He increasingly engages in reciprocal and face-to-face play and often initiates these games. From these reciprocal interactions, he develops a sense of trust and self-efficacy. His distress is less frequent than in previous weeks.

The infant also is starting to distinguish between strangers and those with whom he wants to be sociable. He usually prefers interacting with familiar adults. At 7 or 8 months, he may appear to be afraid of new people.

The 6-month-old baby can sit with support, and he smiles or babbles with a loving adult. He may have a block or toy in his hand. As he watches his hands, he can reach for objects, such as cubes, and grasp them with his fingers and thumbs. He can transfer objects between his hands and obtain small objects by raking with all his fingers. He also may mouth, shake, bang, and drop toys or other objects. The infant's language has moved beyond making razzing noises to single-consonant vocalizing. The 6-month-old produces long strings of vocalizations in play, usually during interactions with adults. He can recognize his own name. He also can stand with help and enjoys bouncing up and down in the standing position. He likes rocking back and forth on his hands and knees, in preparation for crawling forward or backward.

An infant who lies on his back, shows little interest in social interaction, avoids eye contact, and smiles and vocalizes infrequently is indicating either developmental problems or a lack of attention from his parents and other caregivers. He may need more nurturance, increased health supervision, formal developmental assessment, or other interventions.

Over the next few months, as the infant develops an increasing repertoire of motor skills for mobility, such as rolling over and crawling, parents must be vigilant about falls. The expanding world of the infant must be looked at through his eyes to make exploration as safe as possible. The infant will do more than most parents anticipate, and sooner. Toys must be sturdy and have no small parts that could be swallowed or inhaled. Baby walkers should never be used at any age. To avoid possible injury, it is never too early to secure safety gates at the top and bottom of stairs and install window guards.

Parents need to understand developmentally appropriate strategies to redirect their child's behavior when safety is threatened or inappropriate behaviors occur.

PRIORITIES FOR THE VISIT

The first priority is to attend to the concerns of the parents. In addition, the Bright Futures Infancy Expert Panel has given priority to the following topics for discussion in this visit:

- Family functioning (balancing parent roles [health care decision making, parent support systems], child care)
- Infant development (parent expectations [parents as teachers], infant developmental changes [cognitive development/learning, playtime], communication [babbling, reciprocal activities, early intervention], emerging infant independence [infant self-regulation/behavior management], sleep routine [self-calming/putting self to sleep, crib safety])
- Nutrition and feeding: adequacy/growth (feeding strategies [quantity, limits, location, responsibilities] feeding choices [complementary foods, choices of fluids/juice], feeding guidance [breastfeeding, formula])
- Oral health (fluoride, oral hygiene/soft toothbrush, avoidance of bottle in bed)
- Safety (car safety seats, burns [hot water/hot surfaces], falls [gates at stairs and no walkers], choking, poisoning, drowning)

HEALTH SUPERVISION

History

Interval history may be obtained according to the concerns of the family and the health care professional's preference or style of practice. The following questions can encourage in-depth discussion:

- How are things going for you and your family?
- What questions or concerns do you have about your baby?
- What does your partner enjoy most about your baby?
- Are there differences in your views about the baby and those of your partner?
- Have there been any major stresses or changes in your family since your last visit?

Observation of Parent-Child Interaction

During the visit, the health care professional should observe:

- Are the parents and infant responsive to one another (eg, holding, talking, smiling, providing toys for play and distraction, especially during the examination)?
- Are the parents aware of, responsive to, and effective in responding to the infant?
- Do the parents express and show comfort and confidence with their infant?
- Does the parent-infant relationship demonstrate comfort, adequate feeding/eating, and response to the infant's cues?
- Do parents appear to be happy, content, depressed, tearful, angry, anxious, fatigued, overwhelmed, or uncomfortable?
- Do the parents/partners support each other or show signs of disagreement?

Surveillance of Development,

Do you have any specific concerns about your baby's development, learning, or behavior?

SOCIAL-EMOTIONAL
- Is socially interactive with parent
- Recognizes familiar faces and is beginning to recognize whether a person is a stranger

COMMUNICATIVE
- Uses a string of vowels together (babbling "ah," "eh," "oh") and enjoys vocal turn taking
- Is beginning to recognize own name
- Will begin to use consonant sounds ("m," "b") and then combine together ("ah," "ba,") as jargon

COGNITIVE
- Continues to use visual exploration to learn about the environment but is also beginning to use oral exploration for learning

PHYSICAL DEVELOPMENT
- Rolling over and sitting allow for increasing mobility, standing and bouncing; in prone position, will gradually move into crawling position
- Rocks back and forth, often crawling backward before moving forward
- Will learn to rotate in sitting and eventually move from sitting to crawling position

Physical Examination

A complete physical examination is included as part of every health supervision visit.

When performing a physical examination, the health care professional's attention is directed to the following components of the examination that are important for a child this age:

- ■ **Measure and plot:**
  - Length
  - Weight
  - Head circumference
- ■ **Plot:**
  - Weight-for-length
- ■ **Skin**
  - Rashes; bruising

- ■ **Eyes**
  - Assess ocular mobility for lateral and horizontal gaze
  - Assess eye alignment
  - Examine pupils for opacification and red reflexes
- ■ **Heart**
  - Ascult for murmurs
  - Palpate for femoral pulses
- ■ **Musculoskeletal**
  - Assess for developmental hip dysplasia by examining for abduction
- ■ **Neurologic**
  - Evaluate tone, strength, and symmetry of movements

Screening

UNIVERSAL SCREENING	ACTION	
Oral health	Administer the oral health risk assessment	
SELECTIVE SCREENING	RISK ASSESSMENT*	ACTION IF RA +
Blood pressure	Children with specific risk conditions or change in risk	Blood pressure
Vision	Parental concern or abnormal fundoscopic examination or abnormal alignment of eyes	Ophthalmology referral
Hearing	+ on risk screening questions	Referral for diagnostic audiologic assessment
Lead	+ on risk screening questions	Lead screen
Tuberculosis	+ on risk screening questions	Tuberculin skin test

*See the Rationale and Evidence chapter for the criteria on which risk screening questions are based.

Immunizations

Consult the CDC/ACIP or AAP Web sites for the current immunization schedule.
CDC National Immunization Program (NIP): http://www.cdc.gov/vaccines
American Academy of Pediatrics *Red Book*: http://www.aapredbook.org

ANTICIPATORY GUIDANCE

The following sample questions, which address the Infancy Expert Panel's Anticipatory Guidance Priorities, are intended to be used selectively to invite discussion, gather information, address the needs and concerns of the family, and build partnerships. Use of the questions may vary from visit to visit and from family to family. Questions can be modified to match the health care professional's communication style. The accompanying anticipatory guidance for the family should be geared to questions, issues, or concerns for that particular child and family.

FAMILY FUNCTIONING

Balancing parent roles (health care decision making, parent support systems), child care

For some families, gender roles may preclude one parent from asking for help from the other. It is important to periodically review the family's living circumstances, familial relationships, and who is currently responsible for decision making and care giving to the child and family.

SAMPLE QUESTIONS:
How are you balancing your roles of partner and parent? How do you feel you are managing in meeting the needs of your family? Who are you able to go to when you need help with your family?

ANTICIPATORY GUIDANCE:
- Families who are living with others—such as elders, those who are helping them from being homeless, or teen parents living with their parents—may have little control over their environment and caregiver roles and responsibilities. If you are in this situation, it may add to the stress of your family's living situation.

As the infant becomes increasingly awake and alert and demands attention and personal contact, parents find that their responsibilities become more demanding. Mothers may find that early family support systems are actually less available now that she needs more support. Often, one family member is the decision maker about health decisions. Therefore, health care professionals should determine who should get the health information needed for health care decisions.

SAMPLE QUESTION:
Who are you able to rely on to assist you with the baby or when you are tired?

ANTICIPATORY GUIDANCE:
- When you are feeling stressed or overwhelmed, you need to be able to use the natural support network that is available to help you. If you are having difficulty doing this or are hesitant to do so, we may be able to give you additional counseling and support.

Review parents' selection of child care providers, including what they may expect from a child care provider, safeguards in place, and the importance of their infant having a consistent child care provider with regular and predictable daily routines.

SAMPLE QUESTIONS:
What are your child care arrangements? Do you have a reliable person to care for your baby when you need or want to go out? Are you satisfied with the arrangements? How many hours is your child in child care each day?

ANTICIPATORY GUIDANCE:
- It is important that you have a child care provider whom you like and trust and who gives your baby a healthy and predictable daily routine that is similar to what you provide.
- If you are at home with your infant and you are not getting out, you may want to join a playgroup or invite other mothers and babies over for a play-date.

INFANT DEVELOPMENT

Parent expectations (parents as teachers), infant developmental changes (cognitive development/learning, playtime), communication (babbling, reciprocal activities, early intervention), emerging infant independence (infant self-regulation/behavior management), sleep routine (self-calming/putting self to sleep, crib safety)

Parents' expectations about their infant's development should demonstrate evolving attachment and an understanding of their infant's desire for independence. Parents need to understand the developmental next steps that are likely to occur after each visit as well as the parent's role as a teacher and the importance of using appropriate behavioral management strategies for the child's developmental age. Infants learn about their environment through visual exploration, mouthing toys, and, eventually, imitation. Show parents examples of age-appropriate books such as "touch and feel" and other soft plastic or hardcover books that cannot be damaged by the infant's ripping or chewing.

SAMPLE QUESTIONS:
How do you think your baby is learning? Does your baby watch you as you walk around the room?

ANTICIPATORY GUIDANCE:
- Your baby's vision gradually improves during the first year of life. By 6 months, he should be able to follow you around the room with his eyes. Putting your baby in a high chair or an upright seat during awake time (as opposed to a crib), will allow him to visually explore and verbally interact with you and his brothers and sisters.

As the baby matures, parents will need to develop strategies to support their child's neuro-behavioral maturation, self-regulation, and ability to tolerate specific sensory stimuli. If developmental or behavioral concerns exist, a referral to a local Early Intervention Program, often referred to as Part C of IDEA, is appropriate to provide parents with education and counseling on strategies they may be able to implement during everyday routines that will support their child's ever-changing development.

SAMPLE QUESTIONS:

What have you noticed about changes in your baby's development and behaviors around you and other people? How does your baby adapt to new situations, such as people or places? Is he sensitive to any kind of stimulation? Does he seem to get anxious or easily upset? If yes: What things seem to trigger these reactions?

ANTICIPATORY GUIDANCE:

■ **Your baby's temperament and sensory processing and how it affects the way he relates to the world will become more evident at 6 months of age. Parents who understand their baby's temperament will respond to his needs and fussy behaviors appropriately.**

This is a time when gestural communication, joint attention, and social referencing should be established. An infant who is not pointing with an index finger and not making good eye contact should be closely followed. Encourage parents to engage in interactive, reciprocal play with their infants, as this promotes emotional security as well as language development. This playtime should not be a teaching session but rather a time to follow the infant's interests and expand the play with simple words.

SAMPLE QUESTIONS:

How does your baby communicate or tell you what he wants and needs? With gestures? Does he point? What sounds is your baby making (eg, "aa," "ee," "oo," "ba," "da")?

ANTICIPATORY GUIDANCE:

■ **Babies learn to communicate during typical daily routines, such as bedtime, naptime, baths, diaper changes, and dressing. Here are some things you can do to help your baby develop these communication skills:**
  • **Look at books and pat pictures.**
  • **Play music and sing.**
  • **Imitate vocalizations.**
  • **Read to your baby.**
  • **Play games such as "pat-a-cake," "peek-a-boo," and "so big."**

Infants who have consistent and predictable daily routines are able to develop their own self-regulation in the first year of life, which leads to better self-regulation later. Parents who are unable to provide this type of environment for their infant may need additional counseling, monitoring, and intervention.

Monitor infants who are excessively active or extremely quiet. Additional counseling and assistance for parents who are sad or unhappy or who rarely sleep or sleep more than expected, is extremely important. Infants, especially those with special health needs, such as premature infants or babies with chronic health or developmental conditions, who exhibit any stereo-typical behaviors or sensory issues may need additional assistance. Parents who are excessively anxious, or, conversely, parents who are unaware of potential dangers, also need additional assistance.

SAMPLE QUESTIONS:
What is your baby's typical day like? When does he wake up, eat, play, nap, and go to sleep for the night?

ANTICIPATORY GUIDANCE:
- As much as possible, maintain a consistent and predictable daily routine for your baby. This will help him learn how to manage his own behavior appropriately now and as he gets older.

By 6 months, some, but not all, babies are sleeping for longer stretches at night (6 to 8 hours), which parents consider "through the night." Parents need to support their infant's increasing ability to put himself to sleep initially and put himself back to sleep after awakening at night. Explore the parent's comfort with the infant sleeping in a crib in another room. If parents have concerns in this area, additional counseling and assistance may prevent later sleep problems.

Suggestions about establishing a bedtime routine, putting the infant to bed when he is awake, and other habits to discourage night waking help parents help their baby learn self-consoling. In many cultures, family sleep arrangements are viewed as a part of the parent's commitment to their children's well-being. Infant sleep patterns are often among the last traditions to change among immigrant and minority families.

Parents also may have questions about their ability to keep their infant on his back now that he has learned to roll over. Information on continuing to keep the crib safe is important in providing reassurance.

SAMPLE QUESTION:
How is your baby learning to go to sleep by himself?

ANTICIPATORY GUIDANCE:
- Placing your baby in the crib when he is drowsy but not asleep will help your baby learn that he can go to sleep on his own. Then, when he awakens at night, he will be more likely to be able to go back to sleep without your help. This approach will help both you and your baby get a good night's sleep.

- Remember to always put your baby down to sleep on his back, not his tummy or side, even though he may now roll over on his own during sleep. Ask your relatives and caregivers to also put your baby "back to sleep." Experts also recommend that your baby sleep in his own crib, not in your bed. If you breastfeed or bottle-feed your baby in your bed, return him to his own crib or bassinet when you both are ready to go back to sleep.
- Be sure your baby's crib is safe. The slats should be no more than $2\frac{3}{8}$ inches (60 mm) apart. The mattress should be firm and fit snugly into the crib. Keep the sides of the crib raised when the baby is sleeping in it. Be sure it is certified by the JPMA.
- The crib mattress should be at its lowest point before the baby begins to stand. If bumper pads are used, remove them when the baby begins to stand so that they cannot be used as steps.
- If you choose a mesh playpen or portable crib, the weave should have openings less than $\frac{1}{4}$ inch (6 mm). Never leave the baby in a mesh playpen with the drop-side down.

Even at 6 months, infants may have periods of fussiness and irritability. Parents need strategies to deal with these periods without endangering the infant. Parents always need to know that, if they have checked that the infant is fed and clean and safe, it is all right to put him in his crib and give themselves a break. Let them know that babies may cry a lot at this age and that it does get better as the infant gets older and is more able to calm himself. Sometimes, it may be necessary to allow another responsible adult to take care of the baby so that the parents can have some needed time off.

Review the importance of protecting an infant's head even though the baby has head control, and to never shake or hit an infant, as even unintentional shaking or hitting may cause brain damage.

SAMPLE QUESTIONS:
How does your baby calm himself? How much does your baby cry? What helps to calm your baby? What do you do if that does not work? Do you ever feel that you and/or other caretakers may hurt the baby because of the crying? What will you do if you feel this way? Do you have a plan? How do you handle the feeling?

ANTICIPATORY GUIDANCE:
- At 6 months, your baby may still have fussy periods. If he is clean, dry, and not hungry, his fussiness may be telling you that he is tired or bored. Regular daily naps and giving him a variety of short play activities are 2 good strategies for dealing with overtiredness and boredom.
- By 6 months, your baby will have different strategies that will allow him to begin calming himself, such as grasping safe and appropriate toys, oral exploration, and visual exploration.

NUTRITION AND FEEDING: ADEQUACY/GROWTH

Feeding strategies (quantity, limits, location, responsibilities), feeding choices (complementary foods, choices of fluids/juice), feeding guidance (breastfeeding, formula)

General Guidelines on Feeding

By reviewing the growth chart with parents at each visit, parents become aware of the importance of growth and nutrition and become partners in providing appropriate nutrition for their child. This review also will determine the need for more in-depth assessment of nutritional adequacy and anticipatory guidance about the use of nutritional supplements (eg, vitamins, herbs, alternative formulas, and foods). Infants who take longer than 35 to 45 minutes to feed should be evaluated carefully for developmental and nutritional concerns.

Significant transitions in feeding occur during the next 3 months, and parents need clear guidance about what to expect. Managing this transition includes a discussion about the cultural/extended family beliefs about introduction of solids and types and textures of foods. The concept of the division of responsibility between parent and infant with feeding is especially helpful. In this division, the parent is responsible for providing appropriate foods, and the infant is responsible for how much to eat.

SAMPLE QUESTIONS:

What questions or concerns do you have about your baby's growth and feeding? What are you feeding your baby at this time? How often are you feeding your baby? How much does your baby eat or drink? When you begin solids, where are you going to be feeding your baby? Are you feeding your baby any drinks or foods besides breast milk or formula? About how long do feedings last?

ANTICIPATORY GUIDANCE:

- In the next 6 months, it is typical for your baby's growth to slow down a little, as you can see on the growth chart.
- Breastfeeding exclusively for the first 4 to 6 months of life, and then combining it with solid foods from about 6 to 12 months of age and for as long after that as you and the baby want, provides the best nutrition and supports the best possible growth and development. For infants who are not breastfed, iron-fortified infant formula, with the addition of solid foods, is the recommended alternative through the first year of life.
- As you begin solids, it is important to feed your baby in a bouncy seat or high chair that is adjusted to make sure your baby's head, trunk, and feet are supported, so that you can look at each other. Your baby's arms also should be free, as this is her way of communicating with you. Of course, when offering the bottle, it is still very important to continue to hold your baby so that you can see each other and communicate with each other. Your baby then will be able to let you know when she is still hungry and when she is full.
- Responding appropriately to your baby's behaviors during feedings lets her know that you understand her needs so you can provide the appropriate amount of food at a feeding. Remember, you are responsible for providing a variety of nutritious foods, but she is responsible for deciding how much to eat.

Parents need specific verbal or written guidance on the introduction of complementary foods. The order in which they are introduced is not critical as long as essential nutrients are provided. For the breastfed infant, emphasize the need to include a good dietary source of iron to prevent iron deficiency.

Parents can offer store-bought and home-prepared baby food as well as soft table foods. As the infant progresses from purees to foods with more consistency, encourage parents to offer finger foods, such as soft bananas and cereal. Advise parents that infants do not need salt or sugar added to their food.

WIC can provide information and guidance on introducing complementary foods.

SAMPLE QUESTIONS:
How are you planning on introducing solid foods, such as cereal, fruits, vegetables, meats, and other foods?
- *How much does your baby eat at a time?*
- *How does your baby let you know when he likes a certain food?*
- *Does your baby have any favorite foods?*

ANTICIPATORY GUIDANCE:
- Adding complementary foods (also called solids) to your baby's diet is very individualized. There are different steps involved in transitioning from breast milk or formula at 4 to 6 months to table foods at 12 months.
- A key step is to determine when your baby is ready for solids.
  - One of the signs that a baby is ready for eating solids is the fading of the baby's tongue-thrust reflex (pushing food out of the mouth).
  - Another sign is that the baby can elevate her tongue to move pureed food to the back of her mouth and, as she sees a spoon approach, she opens her mouth in anticipation of the next bite. At this stage, your baby sits with arm support and has good head and neck control, so she can indicate a desire for food by opening her mouth and leaning forward.
  - She can tell you she's full or doesn't want food by leaning back and turning away.
- Introduce single-ingredient new foods, one at a time, and watch for adverse reactions over several days to a week.
- Good sources of iron include iron-fortified infant cereal and meats, especially red meats. One ounce (30 g) of infant cereal provides the daily iron requirement, particularly if fed with vitamin C-rich foods, such as baby fruits, which enhance iron absorption from the cereal.
- Gradually introduce other pureed or soft fruits and vegetables after your baby has accepted iron-fortified, single-grain infant cereal and/or pureed or soft meats. Offer solid food 2 to 3 times per day and let her decide how much to eat.
- As with all feeding interactions, watch your baby's verbal and nonverbal cues and respond appropriately. If a food is rejected, move on and try it again later. Don't force her to eat or finish foods.

- Repeated exposure to foods enhances acceptance of new foods by both breastfed and formula-fed infants. It may take up to 10 to 15 experiences before a new food is accepted, because of the transition to textures as well as tastes.
- Foods associated with lifelong sensitization (peanuts, tree nuts, fish, and shell-fish) should not be introduced until after 1 year or even later.

Parents can begin offering sips of breast milk, formula, or water from a small cup held by the feeder, but an infant this age is unlikely or unable to take adequate amounts of fluids and energy needs in a cup. Caution parents about the need to limit juice to 2 to 4 oz per day and to avoid the use of sweetened drinks, such as sodas and artificially flavored "fruit" drinks, which provide calories without other nutrients.

SAMPLE QUESTION:
What types of liquids/fluids is your baby getting in the bottle or cup?

ANTICIPATORY GUIDANCE:
- Give your baby only 2 to 4 oz of juice per day; it is not considered a snack or food. It is best to offer juice in a cup during snack time when she is beginning to take solids more than 3 times a day and when she is developmentally ready.

Guidance on Breastfeeding
Congratulate the mother for continuing to breastfeed.

Weaning ages vary considerably from child to child. Although breastfeeding is recommended for at least 12 months, some infants are ready to wean earlier than that. Refer mothers to breastfeeding support groups or a lactation consultant as needed for questions or concerns.

SAMPLE QUESTIONS:
How is breastfeeding going?
- *In what ways is breastfeeding different now from when you were last here?*
- *How often are you breastfeeding your baby? For how long on each breast?*
- *Does it seem like your baby is breastfeeding more often or for longer periods of time?*
- *How can you tell if your baby is satisfied at the breast?*
- *What are your plans for continuing to breastfeed?*

ANTICIPATORY GUIDANCE:
- At 6 months, breast milk with solids continue to be your baby's best source of nutrition. You should try to continue to breastfeed for the first year of your baby's life and for as long thereafter as you and your baby want to continue.

Guidance on Formula Feeding

Older infants generally consume 24 to 32 oz of formula per day with complementary food, but larger male infants (6 months old, 90th percentile for weight) may take as much as 42 oz of formula per day without complementary foods. Often, at this age, parents may consider using a less expensive formula and may need guidance based on the individual needs of the infant.

SAMPLE QUESTIONS:

How is formula feeding going?
- *What formula are you using now? Have you tried other formulas or are you thinking of using other formulas?*
- *How often does your baby feed in 24 hours and how much does she take at a feeding? Day feeding versus night feedings?*
- *Do you have any concerns about the formula (eg, cost, preparation, or nutrient content)?*

ANTICIPATORY GUIDANCE:
- Continue to feed your baby when she shows hunger cues, usually 5 to 6 times in 24 hours.
- Supplements are not needed if the formula is iron fortified and your baby is consuming an adequate volume of formula for appropriate growth.
- During the first year of life, babies continue to need iron-fortified formula if they are not breastfeeding. If the cost of the formula is a concern, programs such as WIC or other community services may be able to help you.

ORAL HEALTH

Fluoride, oral hygiene/soft toothbrush, avoidance of bottle in bed

To promote preventive dental care, counseling for parents about their infant's oral health needs to begin early. This includes parental awareness of the importance of their own dental health and modeling of brushing their teeth. The oral health risk assessment recommended by the American Academy of Pediatric Dentistry is recommended at 6 months.

SAMPLE QUESTION:

What have you thought about doing to protect your infant's teeth during this first year?

ANTICIPATORY GUIDANCE:
- The use of fluoride supplements will depend on whether your baby is breast-fed or formula fed, as well as the water source. The local health department may be a resource for information about local community fluoride levels.

SAMPLE QUESTION:

What are your plans for protecting your baby's teeth?

ANTICIPATORY GUIDANCE:

- Early dental care, with the eruption of the first tooth, means using a soft toothbrush or cloth to clean your baby's teeth with water only.

SAMPLE QUESTION:

What have you heard about giving your baby a bottle in bed?

ANTICIPATORY GUIDANCE:

- Continue to hold your baby for bottle-feeding. Do not prop the bottle or let your baby graze (drinking from a bottle at will during the day). Putting your baby to bed with a bottle containing juice, milk, or other sugary liquid will harm his teeth. If you ever do give your baby a bottle in bed, make sure it contains only plain water.

SAFETY

Car safety seats, burns (hot water/hot surfaces), falls (gates at stairs and no walkers), choking, poisoning, drowning

If parents are concerned that the child's feet are touching the vehicle seat in the rear-facing position and the child is reaching the highest weight or height allowed for use of the infant-only car safety seat, counsel them to consider switching from their infant-only seat to either a rear-facing convertible seat or an infant-only seat approved for weights greater than 22 pounds. These seats typically allow more room for the infant's legs and are designed to be used rear facing to higher weights.

Remind parents that their own safe driving behaviors (including using safety belts at all times and not driving under the influence of alcohol or drugs) are important to the health of their children.

Questions about proper installation should be referred to a certified Child Passenger Safety Technician in the community.
Child Safety Seat Inspection Station Locator: www.seatcheck.org
Toll-free Number: 866-SEATCHECK (866-732-8243)

SAMPLE QUESTION:

How well does your baby fit in his rear-facing car safety seat?

ANTICIPATORY GUIDANCE:

- A baby's car safety seat must never be placed in the front seat of a vehicle with a passenger air bag. Air bags deploy with great force against a car safety seat and cause serious injury or death. Babies are best protected in the event of a crash when they are in the back seat and in a rear-facing car safety seat.
- Keep your baby's car safety seat rear facing in the back seat of your vehicle until your baby is at least 1 year old and weighs at least 20 pounds. It is preferable to wait even longer, until the baby reaches the highest weight or height allowed by the manufacturer of the seat.

- Infants who reach 20 pounds or 26 to 29 inches before 1 year should use a convertible seat or infant-only seat that is approved for use rear facing to higher weights and heights (up to 30 pounds and 32 inches for infant-only seats and up to 35 pounds and at least 36 inches for convertible seats). Your baby will be safest if she rides rear facing to the highest weight or height allowed by the manufacturer.
- The back seat is the safest place for children to ride.
- Do not start the engine until everyone is buckled in.
- Your own safe driving behaviors are important to the health of your children. Use a safety belt at all times and do not drive after using alcohol or drugs.

If a parent has unrealistic developmental expectations or is negative about infant's new abilities (eg, "She's a little terror," or "I have to keep her in the playpen all the time"), additional counseling may be indicated, especially related to other safety issues.

SAMPLE QUESTION:
What other things are you doing to keep your baby safe and healthy?

ANTICIPATORY GUIDANCE:
- As your baby begins to crawl, it is a good idea to do a safety check of your home and the home of family or friends.
- Before bathing your baby, test the water temperature on your wrist to make sure it is not too hot. To protect your child from tap water scalds, the hottest temperature at the faucet should be no more than 120°F. In many cases, you can adjust your water heater.
- Don't leave your baby alone, for even a second, in a tub of water, even if you use a bath ring or seat, or on high places such as changing tables, beds, sofas, or chairs.
- Use appropriate barriers around space heaters, wood stoves, and kerosene heaters.
- The kitchen is the most dangerous room for children. A safer place for your child while you are cooking, eating, or unable to provide your full attention is the playpen, crib, stationary activity center, or buckled into a high chair.
- Babies at this age explore their environment by putting anything and everything into their mouths. NEVER leave small objects or latex balloons within your baby's reach.
- To prevent choking, limit "finger foods" to soft bits not much larger than a Cheerio®. Children younger than 4 years should not eat hard food like nuts or popcorn.
- Be sure to keep household products, such as cleaners, chemicals, and medicines, locked up and out of your child's sight and reach. If your child does eat something that could be poisonous, call the Poison Control Center at 1-800-222-1222 immediately. Do not make your child vomit.

Poison Control Center
(1-800-222-1222)

■ Your baby may be able to crawl as early as 6 months. Use gates on stairways and close doors to keep her out of rooms where she might get hurt.

■ Do not use a baby walker. Your baby may tip the walker over, fall out of it, or fall down the stairs and seriously injure her head. Baby walkers let children get to places where they can pull heavy objects or hot food on themselves.

Health Supervision: 9 Month Visit

CONTEXT

The 9-month-old has made some striking developmental gains and displays growing independence. He is increasingly mobile and will express explicit opinions about everything, from the foods he eats to his bedtime. These opinions often will take the form of protests. He will say "No" in his own way, from closing his mouth and shaking his head when a parent wants to feed him, to screaming when he finds himself alone. The baby also has gained a sense of "object permanence" (ie, he understands that an object or person, such as a parent, exists in spite of not being visible at the moment).

The 9-month-old's behaviors are an adaptation to his uncertainties about how the world works. Though certain that an unseen object exists, he is not yet confident that the out-of-sight object or the absent person will reappear. His protests when a parent leaves show his attachment and his ability to fear loss. His insecurity about the whereabouts of his parents may lead to night waking. Until this age, he was waking during his normal sleep cycle, but usually fell back to sleep. Now, when he awakens, he realizes that he is in a dark room without his parents. This realization generally leads to distressed crying (a behavior that causes difficulties for parents).

As a result of these developments, the parents' tasks have changed dramatically. The infant's increasing activity and protests necessitate setting limits. The parents must decide when it is important for them to say, "No."

This requires self-esteem, confidence in their role as responsible parents, and a great deal of energy. Parents also view their infant's growing independence with a sense of loss. No longer content to be held, cuddled, and coddled, the baby will now wiggle, want to be put down, and may even crawl away. This physical independence requires a heightened vigilance about safety around the house.

Recognizing and responding appropriately to infant cues associated with basic care, such as nurturing and feeding, now require complex skills. As the baby's first birthday approaches, the parents' attitudes and expectations, based in part on their own early childhood experiences, will become a significant factor. At the 9 Month Visit, it is important for the health care professional to assess the parents' attitudes and abilities to cope with their child's growing independence of body and mind. The health care professional also should provide the parents with basic skills and resources for making decisions about methods of managing their child's behavior.

At 9 months of age, infants are at the height of stranger awareness. The intensity of their responses to strangers is highly variable. Although they may have been friendly and cooperative at the previous visit, they are far more likely to become upset with the physical examination at this age. The health care professional can minimize this reaction by approaching the infant very slowly, by examining the infant in a parent's arms, by first touching the infant's shoe or leg and gradually moving to the chest, and by distracting the infant with a toy or stethoscope during the examination.

This is an appropriate age to start guidance for the parents about discipline. Discuss the difference between discipline (which involves the parent teaching appropriate behaviors) and punishment (which places emphasis only on negative behaviors). Assist parents in making their baby's environment safe rather than trying to teach their baby how to be safe. Emphasize that yelling, spanking, and hitting are ineffective punishment in changing behaviors. Also point out that, at this age, an infant is NOT capable of learning or remembering "rules."

PRIORITIES FOR THE VISIT

The first priority is to attend to the concerns of the parents. In addition, the Bright Futures Infancy Expert Panel has given priority to the following topics for discussion in this visit:

- Family adaptations (discipline [parenting expectations, consistency, behavior management], cultural beliefs about child-rearing, family functioning, domestic violence)
- Infant independence (changing sleep pattern [sleep schedule], developmental mobility [safe exploration, play], cognitive development [object permanence, separation anxiety, behavior and learning, temperament versus self-regulation, visual exploration, cause and effect], communication)
- Feeding routine (self-feeding, mealtime routines, transition to solids [table food introduction], cup drinking [plans for weaning])
- Safety (car safety seats, burns [hot stoves, heaters], window guards, drowning, poisoning [safety locks], guns)

HEALTH SUPERVISION

History

Interval history may be obtained according to the concerns of the family and the health care professional's preference or style of practice. The following questions can encourage in-depth discussion:

- How are you? How are things going in your family?
- What questions or concerns do you have today? What questions do you have about your baby's care?
- Tell me about your baby.
- What do you like best about your baby?
- What is most challenging about caring for your baby?

Observation of Parent-Child Interaction

During the visit, the health care professional should observe:

- Do the parents stimulate the infant with language and play?
- Do the parents and infant demonstrate a reciprocal engagement around feeding/eating?
- Is the infant free to move away from the parent to explore and check back with the parent visually and physically?
- Are the parents' developmental expectations appropriate?
- How do the parents respond to their infant's autonomy or independent behavior within a safe environment?

Surveillance of Development

Do you have any specific concerns about your baby's development, learning, or behavior?

SOCIAL-EMOTIONAL
- Has developed apprehension with strangers
- Seeks parent for play and comfort, and as a resource

COMMUNICATIVE
- Uses wide variety of repetitive consonants and vowel sounds
- Starts to point out objects

COGNITIVE
- Develops object permanence
- Learns interactive games, such as "peek-a-boo" and "so big"
- Looks at books and explores environment, physically and visually

PHYSICAL DEVELOPMENT
- Rapidly expands motor skills—crawls reciprocally, gets to sitting, begins to pull to stand

Physical Examination

A complete physical examination is included as part of every health supervision visit.

When performing a physical examination, the health care professional's attention is directed to the following components of the examination that are important for a child this age:

- ◼ **Measure and plot:**
  - Length
  - Weight
  - Head circumference
- ◼ **Plot:**
  - Weight-for-length
- ◼ **Head**
  - Palpate for positional skull deformities

- ◼ **Eyes**
  - Assess ocular mobility for lateral and horizontal gaze
  - Assess eye alignment
  - Examine pupils for opacification and red reflexes
- ◼ **Heart**
  - Ascult for murmurs
  - Palpate femoral pulses
- ◼ **Musculoskeletal**
  - Assess for developmental hip dysplasia by examining for abduction
- ◼ **Neurologic**
  - Evaluate tone, strength, and symmetry of movements
  - Elicit parachute reflex

Screening

UNIVERSAL SCREENING	ACTION	
Development	Structured developmental screen	
Oral health	Administer the oral health risk assessment	

SELECTIVE SCREENING	RISK ASSESSMENT*	ACTION IF RA +
Blood pressure	Children with specific risk conditions or change in risk	Blood pressure
Vision	Parental concern or abnormal fundoscopic examination or abnormal cover/uncover test	Ophthalmology referral
Hearing	+ on risk screening questions	Referral for diagnostic audiologic assessment
Lead	+ on risk screening questions	Lead screen

*See the Rationale and Evidence chapter for the criteria on which risk screening questions are based.

Immunizations

Consult the CDC/ACIP or AAP Web sites for the current immunization schedule.
CDC National Immunization Program (NIP): http://www.cdc.gov/vaccines
American Academy of Pediatrics *Red Book*: http://www.aapredbook.org

ANTICIPATORY GUIDANCE

The following sample questions, which address the Infancy Expert Panel's Anticipatory Guidance Priorities, are intended to be used selectively to invite discussion, gather information, address the needs and concerns of the family, and build partnerships. Use of the questions may vary from visit to visit and from family to family. Questions can be modified to match the health care professional's communication style. The accompanying anticipatory guidance for the family should be geared to questions, issues, or concerns for that particular child and family.

FAMILY ADAPTATIONS

Discipline (parenting expectations, consistency, behavior management), cultural beliefs about child-rearing, family functioning, domestic violence

This is an age when the entire family needs to adapt to the increasingly mobile infant. The more consistent parents are in establishing and reinforcing appropriate behavior, the easier it will be for the infant to learn what is, and is not, allowed. Providing parents with appropriate developmental expectations is an important aspect of helping parents come to an agreement on their approaches to parenting.

Discuss whether the parents have time to themselves, with each other, and with other family and friends. Social contacts and activities apart from the baby can help maintain parental well-being. Ideally, both partners are involved in health supervision visits and infant care.

SAMPLE QUESTIONS:

What are your thoughts about discipline? Do you and your partner agree on ways to manage the baby's environment to support healthy behavior? Do you and other key family members (such as mothers, mothers-in-law, and other elders) agree on ways to manage the baby's environment to support healthy behavior? Have you discussed these issues with your child care provider? How are your other children adapting to the baby as she gets older?

ANTICIPATORY GUIDANCE:

- An important aspect of discipline is teaching your child what behaviors you expect. During the first year of life, the parents' primary role is that of protector for an infant's natural curiosity. During this time, babies learn more by example from what they observe than through what their parents may say to them. Therefore, setting an example of the behaviors you expect of your child is very important.
- Using descriptions of the behavior that is desired, as often as possible (eg, saying, "Time to sit," rather than, "Don't stand," will provide better direction about the behavior that is desired).
- A critical step in establishing discipline is to limit "No" to the most important issues. One way to do this is to remove other reasons to say, "No" (such as putting dangerous or tempting objects out of reach). Then, when an important issue comes up (such as your baby going toward the stove or radiator), saying, "NO, hot, don't touch" and removing the baby will have real meaning for her.

- Because infants have a natural curiosity about objects they see their parents using but also a short attention span, distraction and replacing a forbidden object with one that is permissible are excellent strategies for managing your baby's behavior in a positive way.
- Another aspect of discipline is consistency between parents, other family members, and child care providers. It is important to discuss what behaviors are allowed and what behaviors are not allowed. Have this discussion with your partner, family members, and child care provider. Some simple rules for your child can be established, such as saying, "Don't touch," for certain objects.
- Asking siblings to help with the baby to the extent they are able will continue to meet their needs of being involved and feeling they are an important member of the family.

SAMPLE QUESTIONS:

Do you have regular time for yourself? How often do you see friends and get out of the house to do other activities?

ANTICIPATORY GUIDANCE:

- All parents need time alone and individual time with their partner.
- Staying in touch with friends and family members and participating in activities without the baby helps avoid social isolation.

SAMPLE QUESTIONS:

*Do you have someone to turn to when you need help caring for your baby?
Do you have child care? How is it going?*

ANTICIPATORY GUIDANCE:

- Choose babysitters and caregivers who are mature, trained, responsible, and recommended by someone you trust.

Children who are exposed to domestic violence are at increased risk of adverse mental and physical health outcomes. Domestic violence cannot be determined through observation, but is best identified through direct inquiry. Avoid asking about "abuse" or "domestic violence," but use descriptive terms, such as hit, kick, shove, choke, or threaten. Provide information about the impact of domestic violence on children and about community resources that provide assistance. Recommend resources for parent education and/or parent support groups.

SAMPLE QUESTIONS:

*Because violence is so common in so many people's lives, I've begun to ask about it. I don't know if this is a problem for you, but many children I see have parents who have been hurt by someone else. Some are too afraid or uncomfortable to bring it up, so I've started asking about it routinely.
Do you always feel safe in your home?*
- *Has your partner or ex-partner ever hit, kicked, or shoved you, or physically hurt you or the baby?*
- *Are you scared that you and/or other caretakers may hurt the baby?*
Do you have any questions about your safety at home? What will you do if you feel afraid? Do you have a plan? Would you like information on where to go or who to contact if you ever need help?

ANTICIPATORY GUIDANCE:
- One way that I and other health care professionals can help you if your partner is hitting or threatening you is to support you and provide information about local resources that can help you.

INFANT INDEPENDENCE

Changing sleep pattern (sleep schedule), developmental mobility (safe exploration, play), cognitive development (object permanence, separation anxiety, behavior and learning, temperament versus self-regulation, visual exploration, cause and effect), communication

The infant's increasing mobility and independence, but also his need for referencing and looking over to see that the parent is still there for protection, is an important developmental step. Parents need to understand their baby's temperament and sensory processing, and how the family can adapt to it. At around 9 months, it is not unusual for infants who have been sleeping through the night to begin to awaken.

Parents are interested in learning about screen time and alternatives to media entertainment, so reinforce alternative forms of entertainment, such as reading or playing games together or walking in the park. Parents are the target of increasing marketing of video products with unsubstantiated implications of educational value. Current data reveal that children younger than 2 years spend 48 minutes per day watching TV and videos/DVDs and playing on the computer.

During the 9 Month Visit, consider having parents complete a standardized developmental screening tool that can be used to identify any developmental concerns. This type of tool also educates parents about developmental skills that might be expected and assists them in asking questions during the visit.

SAMPLE QUESTIONS:
Have you noticed any changes in your baby's sleeping habits? Does your baby wake up during the night?

ANTICIPATORY GUIDANCE:
- This is an age when sleep routines that help your baby gradually relax and get ready for sleep are especially important. The pre-bedtime hour, before the routine begins, should be especially affectionate and nurturing. Disruptions in routine, such as vacations, visitors, or late evenings out, can significantly disturb sleep patterns. Try to avoid these disruptions if possible.
- If your baby is waking in the night, continue to just check on him and settle him back to sleep. This routine can help your baby put himself back to sleep.
- As your baby begins to stand at the crib, it is important to lower the mattress in your baby's crib to the lowest level before he learns to stand up. If bumper pads are used, remove them when the baby begins to stand so that they cannot be used as steps.

SAMPLE QUESTIONS:
How is your baby getting around now? Do you have any concerns about your baby's development or behavior?

ANTICIPATORY GUIDANCE:

- Your baby's gross motor skills (his ability to control his head and body parts and to move around) will rapidly develop during the next 3 months.
- Give your baby opportunities to safely explore. Be there with him so that he can always check to see that you are nearby.
- Sometimes, it's easy to think that your baby can do more than he's really able to do. Be realistic about his abilities at this age and set realistic, nonthreatening, enforceable limits.

SAMPLE QUESTIONS:

What have you noticed about changes in your baby's behaviors around you and other people? How does your baby adapt to new situations, people, and places?

ANTICIPATORY GUIDANCE:

- Your baby is eager to interact and play with other people as a way to develop interpersonal relationships. At the same time, be sensitive to the fact that, at this age, he will show separation anxiety from you and other important caregivers. This anxiety is a sign of his strong attachment to you.
- Pay attention to the way your baby reacts and adapts to new situations and people. These reactions reflect his personality and temperament. To the extent possible, make these situations easy on your baby (eg, if he is a quiet baby who does not like a lot of noise and bustle, explain that to a person meeting him for the first time and ask the person to greet him in a calm and soothing way).

SAMPLE QUESTIONS:

How do you think your baby is learning? How is your baby communicating with you now?

ANTICIPATORY GUIDANCE:

- Your baby's way of learning is changing from exploring with his eyes and putting things in his mouth to noticing cause and effect, imitating others, and understanding that objects he cannot see still exist.
- Help your baby develop these skills by playing with simple cause-and-effect toys. Try balls that you can roll back and forth, toy cars and trucks that he can push, and blocks that can be put into a container and dumped out. Songs with clapping and gestures and songs with finger actions will help him learn imitation. Peek-a-boo and hide-and-seek are great ways to help him understand "object permanence." It is important to use these ideas to entertain your child. Children younger than 2 years should not watch TV, DVDs, or videos, or use computer products.
- Babies now begin to use gestures such as pointing as well as vocalizations to let you know what they want. They also begin to show their preferences more clearly, such as refusing to eat certain foods by clearly turning away. It still is important to respond to your baby's efforts to communicate with you by acknowledging his preferences, yet being consistent in your expectations. Using modeling, demonstration, and simple descriptions of what behaviors you want from your baby will work much better than long sentences or a raised voice.

FEEDING ROUTINE

Self-feeding, mealtime routines, transition to solids (table food introduction), cup drinking (plans for weaning)

During the next 3 months, infants demonstrate a growing ability to feed themselves. As infants begin to want independence with self-feeding, it is increasingly important for parents to understand the division of responsibility between parent and child with regard to feeding—the parent is responsible for providing a sufficient amount and variety of nutritious foods, and the child is responsible for deciding how much to eat.

The time between the introduction of complementary foods and 9 months is a sensitive period for learning to chew. A gradual exposure to solid textures during this time may decrease the risk of feeding problems, such as rejecting certain textures, refusing to chew, or vomiting.

SAMPLE QUESTIONS:
How has feeding been going?
- *What is your baby feeding herself?*
- *What does your baby eat with her fingers?*
- *Has she used a cup?*
Has your baby received breast milk or other fluids from a bottle or cup?

ANTICIPATORY GUIDANCE:
- Try to be patient and understanding as your baby tries new foods and learns to feed herself. Removing distractions, like television, will help her stay focused on eating. Remember, it may take 10 to 15 tries before your baby will accept a new food.
- As your baby becomes more independent in feeding herself, remember that you are responsible for providing a variety of sufficient nutritious foods, but she is responsible for deciding how much to eat.
- Most 9-month-old infants can be on the same eating schedule as the family (breakfast, lunch, and dinner), plus a mid-morning, afternoon, and bedtime snack. The amount of food taken at a single feeding may vary and may not be a large amount, but the 3 meals and 2 to 3 snacks help ensure that your baby is exposed to a variety of foods and receives adequate nutrition. Snacks can be an opportunity to try new foods.
- Giving your baby foods of varying textures (eg, pureed, blended, mashed, finely chopped, and soft lumps) will help her successfully go through the change from gumming to chewing foods. Slowly introducing solid textures during this time may decrease the risk of feeding problems, refusing to chew, or vomiting. Gradually increase table foods. Avoid mixed textures, like broth with vegetables, because they are the most difficult for infants and toddlers to eat.
- Encourage your baby to drink from a cup with help. Juice may be served as part of a snack but should be limited to 4 oz per day. Avoid the use of sweetened drinks, such as sodas and artificially flavored "fruit" drinks. These drinks provide calories but no nutrients.

- Foods associated with lifelong sensitization (peanuts, tree nuts, fish, and shell-fish) should not be introduced until after 1 year or even later.

SAMPLE QUESTIONS:

What are your plans for continuing to breastfeed? What questions or concerns do you have?

ANTICIPATORY GUIDANCE:

- Weaning ages vary considerably from child to child. Some are ready to wean earlier than others and will show this by decreasing their interest in breast-feeding as they increase their interest in the foods they see their parents eating.
- At 9 months, breast milk with complementary food continues to be the baby's best source of nutrition. Try to continue breastfeeding through the first year of the baby's life, or for as long as both you and your baby want to continue.

SAFETY

Car safety seats, burns (hot stoves, heaters), window guards, drowning, poisoning (safety locks), guns

Parents may be tempted to prematurely change their 9-month-old baby's rear-facing car safety seat to a forward-facing seat. Death and serious injury are significantly less likely for infants and young children who are rear facing compared to forward facing. For the best protection, children should ride rear facing to the highest weight or height allowed for rear facing by the manufacturer of the seat. As infants approach 20 pounds or their head is 1 inch below the top of the infant-only seat, counsel parents to consider switching from their infant-only seat to either a rear-facing convertible seat or an infant-only seat approved for weights greater than 22 pounds.

Remind parents that their own safe driving behaviors (including using safety belts at all times and not driving under the influence of alcohol or drugs) are important to the health of their children.

Questions about proper installation should be referred to a certified Child Passenger Safety Technician in the community.
Child Safety Seat Inspection Station Locator: www.seatcheck.org
Toll-free Number: 866-SEATCHECK (866-732-8243)

SAMPLE QUESTIONS:

Is your baby fastened securely in the back seat in a rear-facing car safety seat for every ride in a vehicle? Do you know when to turn the baby's car safety seat forward facing? Do you know where to get help with using your car safety seat? Does everyone in the family use a safety belt every time they ride in a vehicle?

ANTICIPATORY GUIDANCE:

- A baby's car safety seat must never be placed in the front seat of a vehicle with a passenger air bag. Air bags deploy with great force against a car safety seat and cause serious injury or death. Babies are best protected in the event of a crash when they are in the back seat and in a rear-facing car safety seat.
- Keep your baby's car safety seat rear facing in the back seat of the vehicle until your baby is at least 1 year old and weighs at least 20 pounds. It is preferable to wait even longer, until the baby reaches the highest weight or height allowed by the manufacturer of the seat.
- Infants who reach 20 pounds or 26 to 29 inches before 1 year should use a convertible seat or infant-only seat that is approved for use rear facing to higher weights and heights (up to 30 pounds and 32 inches for infant-only seats and up to 35 pounds and at least 36 inches for convertible seats). Your baby will be safest if he rides rear facing to the highest weight or height allowed by the manufacturer.
- The back seat is the safest place for children to ride.
- Do not start the engine until everyone is buckled in.
- Your own safe driving behaviors are important to the health of your children. Use a safety belt at all times and do not drive after using alcohol or drugs.

Now that their baby is more active, discuss with parents the changes they can make to make their home safer for their child. No home is ever "childproof," but parents can initiate changes to make the environment safer.

SAMPLE QUESTION:
Now that your child can move on his own more, what changes have you made in your home to ensure his safety?

ANTICIPATORY GUIDANCE:

- Do not leave heavy objects or containers of hot liquids on tables with tablecloths. Your baby may pull on the tablecloth. Turn handles of pans or dishes so they do not hang over edge of stove or table.
- Use appropriate barriers around space heaters, wood stoves, and kerosene heaters.
- The kitchen is the most dangerous room for children. A safer place for your child while you are cooking, eating, or unable to provide your full attention is the playpen, crib, or stationary activity center, or buckled into a high chair.
- Keep electrical cords out of your child's reach. Mouth burns can result from chewing on the end of a live extension cord or on a poorly insulated wire.
- To prevent children from falling out of windows, keep furniture away from windows and install operable window guards on second- and higher-story windows. Use gates at the top and bottom of stairs.
- Watch your toddler constantly whenever he is near water. Your child can drown in even a few inches of water, including in the bathtub, play pools, buckets, or toilets. A supervising adult should be within an arm's reach, providing "touch supervision," whenever young children are in or around water.

- Do not let young brothers or sisters watch over your toddler in the bathtub, house, yard, or playground.
- Empty buckets, tubs, or small pools immediately after you use them.
- To prevent poisoning, keep household products, such as cleaners, chemicals, and medicines, locked up and out of your child's sight and reach. Keep the number of the Poison Control Center (1-800-222-1222) posted next to every telephone.

Review gun safety with parents. The AAP recommends that guns be removed from the places where children live and play. Parents who own guns may be more receptive to this discussion when guns are considered along with the other household hazards than when they are the sole focus of a discussion.

SAMPLE QUESTIONS:
Does anyone in your home have a gun? If so, is the gun unloaded and locked up? Is the ammunition stored and locked separately from the gun? Have you considered not owning a gun because of the danger to children and other family members?

ANTICIPATORY GUIDANCE:
- Homicide and suicide are more common in homes that have guns. As your child becomes more active, the potential dangers of a gun become even greater. The best way to keep your child safe from injury or death from guns is to never have a gun in the home.
- If it is necessary to keep a gun in your home or if the homes of people you visit have guns, they should be stored unloaded and locked, with the ammunition locked separately from the gun.

Poison Control Center
(1-800-222-1222)

References

1. American Academy of Pediatrics, Committee on Psychosocial Aspects of Child and Family Health. The prenatal visit. *Pediatrics*. 2001;107:1456-1458

2. National Society of Genetic Counselors. Your Family History—Your Future. Available at: http://www.nsgc.org/consumer/familytree/. Accessed May 22, 2007

3. American Academy of Pediatrics, Committee on Fetus and Newborn. Hospital stay for healthy term newborns. *Pediatrics*. 2004;113:1434-1436

4. Braveman P, Egerter S, Pearl M, Marchi K, Miller C. Problems associated with early discharge of newborn infants. Early discharge of newborns and mothers: a critical review of the literature. *Pediatrics*. 1995;96:716-726

5. American Academy of Pediatrics, American College of Obstetricians and Gynecologists. *Guidelines for Perinatal Care*. 5th ed. Elk Grove Village, IL: American Academy of Pediatrics; and Washington, DC: American College of Obstetricians and Gynecologists; 2002

6. Beal AC, Chou SC, Palmer RH, Testa MA, Newman C, Ezhuthachan S. The changing face of race: risk factors for neonatal hyperbilirubinemia. *Pediatrics*. 2006;117:1618-1625

7. Dennery PA, Seidman DS, Stevenson DK. Neonatal hyperbilirubinemia. *N Engl J Med*. 2001;344:581-590

8. Huang MJ, Kua KE, Teng HC, Tang KS, Weng HW, Huang CS. Risk factors for severe hyperbilirubinemia in neonates. *Pediatr Res*. 2004;56:682-689

9. Setia S, Villaveces A, Dhillon P, Mueller BA. Neonatal jaundice in Asian, white, and mixed-race infants. *Arch Pediatr Adolesc Med*. 2002;156:276-279

10. Kaplan M, Hammerman C. Glucose-6-phosphate dehydrogenase-deficient neonates: a potential cause for concern in North America. *Pediatrics*. 2000;106:1478-1479

11. Galbraith AA, Egerter SA, Marchi KS, Chavez G, Braveman PA. Newborn early discharge revisited: are California newborns receiving recommended postnatal services? *Pediatrics*. 2003;111:364-371

12. Maisels J, Kring E. Early discharge from the newborn nursery: effect on scheduling of follow-up visits by pediatricians. *Pediatrics*. 1997;100:72-74

13. Gardner HG, and American Academy of Pediatrics, Committee on Injury, Violence, and Poison Prevention. Office-based counseling for unintentional injury prevention. *Pediatrics*. 2007;119:202-206

14. Rickert VI, Johnson CM. Reducing noctural awakening and crying episodes in infants and young children: a comparison between scheduled awakening and systematic ignoring. *Pediatrics*. 1988;81:203-212

Early Childhood

1 to 4 Years

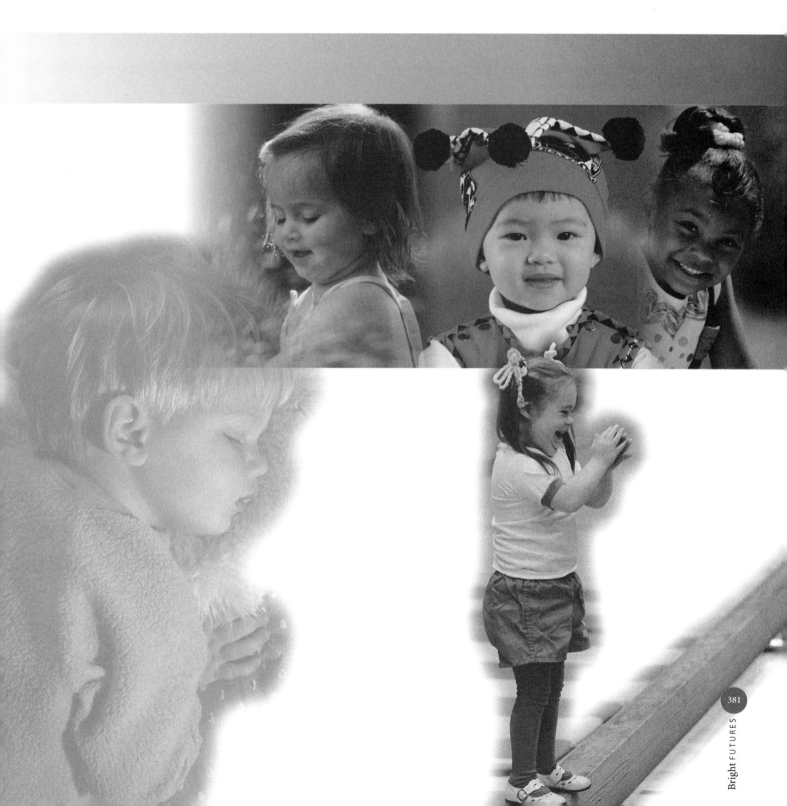

Early Childhood: 12 Month Visit

CONTEXT

The 12-month-old stands proudly, somewhat bowlegged, belly protruding. Walking, one of the most exciting developmental milestones, occurs near the toddler's first birthday, bringing with it increasing independence. During his first year of life, the infant was rarely in conflict with his environment. He might have been demanding when he cried, he required considerable care, and he changed the balance in the family. However, he spent most of his first year getting to know and trust his parents and his environment. As a toddler, he becomes increasingly competent in acting upon the world around him, all on his own. His world broadens, bringing both excitement and challenge.

Autonomy and independent mobility are developmental achievements of which the parents and toddler are justifiably proud, but the toddler constantly encounters barriers posed by his environment. He cannot go as fast as he would like without tripping, he cannot always reach desired objects, and he can fall and hurt himself. New hazards, such as access to hot liquids (eg, coffee cups left on surfaces within reach) and stairs, are now within his reach. Although they may be charmed by his exploits, a toddler's parents and other caregivers must watch him constantly to keep him safe.

As the toddler's autonomy, independence, and cognitive abilities increase, he begins to exert his own will. In response, his parents' perceptions of his demands change dramatically, influenced by their own upbringing and childhood experiences. Do the parents understand their toddler's needs and attempt to meet them? The 12-month-old's dramatic struggle for autonomy will test his parents' ability to let go, permit independence, and enjoy aspects of his behavior that are out of their direct control. The toddler's messy attempts to feed himself can be difficult for his parents as they sort out their own desire for order and neatness with his need for self-care.

Fortunately, the toddler is endowed with a social feedback loop to recognize both pleasure and displeasure from significant caregivers. Adults build on this characteristic by providing appropriate responses to a toddler's actions. Adult laughter in response to a well-played game of "peek-a-boo" holds the key to future good times in other interactive games, but laughter following a plate of food thrown on the floor sends the same positive message and invites later disruptive behavior. Turning away, ignoring, or expressing displeasure at the plate of food thrown on the floor sends a more appropriate message and helps prevent later disruptive behaviors.

Positive activities, such as cuddling, holding, praising, and firm enforcement of rules about not biting, hitting, and kicking, help the toddler develop emotional expression. Consistency is the keystone for dealing with a 12-month-old, and establishing regular routines becomes all-important.

Although the toddler's level of activity increases significantly during this period, his rate of weight gain decreases, and struggles over eating arise for many parents. A toddler frequently eats a large amount at one meal and very little at the next. However, hunger guides him and he eats a sufficient amount over time. The key is to offer nutritious foods consistently and not worry about whether all the food is finished each time.

Responding sensitively to the 12-month-old's behavior is a complex task. Some parents who did well with the more dependent, younger infant are less sure of their role now. Toddlers beginning their second year of life seem to thrive when parents accommodate their demands yet maintain a strong parenting presence, including a full measure of patience, enough self-confidence to set limits, the judgment to know which needs are most important, and the ability to realize that their 12-month-old's negative behavior is not directed against them. Reading aloud is a positive way of spending time together and can be worked into the child's daily routines (eg, at bedtime, nap time, and mealtime). By letting the child choose the book, the parent can support the child's growing independence and, by reading aloud and naming the

pictures, the parent can help the child learn language and satisfy his curiosity about the world. Parents need to be positive role models for their toddler, both physically (eg, by eating nutritiously and wearing safety belts in the car) and emotionally (eg, by being calm and consistent in setting limits and handling tantrums). Parents who enjoy their toddler's growing independence can best provide a stable home base as the toddler's curiosity and mobility carry him into an expanding world.

Children this age are uncomfortable about being restrained in their activity. The physical exam may be more successfully performed while the child is on a parent's lap or standing on the floor. Speaking directly to the child and taking a playful stance about the exam will make it easier for the child to cooperate. If the child becomes upset, it is a good idea to remind the parent that this is an expected reaction at this age. As part of the complete physical exam, perform the noninvasive procedures first, with the eyes, ears, nose, mouth, and abdomen examined last.

PRIORITIES FOR THE VISIT

The first priority is to attend to the concerns of the parents. In addition, the Bright Futures Early Childhood Expert Panel has given priority to the following topics for discussion in this visit:

- Family support (adjustment to the child's developmental changes and behavior, family-work balance, parental agreement/disagreement about child issues)
- Establishing routines (family time, bedtime, teeth brushing, nap times)
- Feeding and appetite changes (self-feeding, nutritious foods, choices, "grazing")
- Establishing a dental home (first dental checkup, dental hygiene)
- Safety (home safety, car safety seats, drowning, guns)

HEALTH SUPERVISION

History

Interval history may be obtained according to the concerns of the family and the health care professional's preference or style of practice. The following questions can encourage in-depth discussion:

- Tell me how things are going at home and how your family is adapting to your 12-month-old.
- Where are you currently living? Does anyone else care for your child other than you?
- What concerns do you still have from your last visit?
- What new concerns do you have about your child today?
- I see you are concerned about _____.
- What major changes or stresses have occurred in your family since your last visit?

Observation of Parent-Child Interaction

During the visit, the health care professional should observe:

- How does the parent interact with the toddler (eg, anxiously, calmly, reciprocally, in a controlling manner, or inattentively)?
- Does the child check back with the parent visually?
- When the health care professional gives the child a book, does the parent follow the child's gaze?
- Does he bring an object of interest to show or share with the parent?
- How does the parent react when the health care professional praises the child? How does the parent react to being praised?
- If siblings are in the room, how do they interact with the toddler?
- Does the parent seem positive when speaking about the child?

Surveillance of Development

Do you have any specific concerns about your child's development, learning, or behavior?

SOCIAL-EMOTIONAL

■ **Tell me about your child's typical play.**
  • Plays interactive games (eg, "peek-a-boo," "pat-a-cake")
  • Imitates activities
  • Hands you a book when he wants to hear a story

■ **Does your child feel free to explore or stay very close to your side?**
  • Waves "bye-bye"
  • Has a strong attachment with parent or significant caregiver
  • Shows distress on separation from parent

COMMUNICATIVE

■ **How does your child communicate?**
  • Demonstrates prodeclarative pointing (points to a desired object and watches to see whether the parent sees it)
  • Imitates vocalizations and sounds
  • Speaks 1 to 2 words
  • Jabbers with inflections of normal speech

COGNITIVE

■ **What do you think your child understands?**
  • Follows simple directions
  • Identifies persons upon request (eg, "Where is ___?")

PHYSICAL DEVELOPMENT

■ **Tell me how your child uses his hands and legs.**
  • Bangs 2 cubes held in hands
  • Stands alone

Physical Examination

A complete physical examination is included as part of every health supervision visit.

When performing a physical examination, the health care professional's attention is directed to the following components of the examination that are important for a child this age:

- **Measure and plot:**
  - Length
  - Weight
  - Head circumference
- **Plot:**
  - Weight-for-length

- **Eyes**
  - Examine pupils for red reflexes
  - Perform cover/uncover test for conjugate ocular mobility
- **Mouth**
  - Observe for caries, plaque, demineralization (white spots), and staining
- **Neurologic**
  - Observe gait
- **Genitals**
  - Determine whether testes are fully descended

Screening

UNIVERSAL SCREENING	ACTION	
Anemia	Hematocrit or hemoglobin	
Lead (High prevalence area or on Medicaid)	Lead screen	

SELECTIVE SCREENING	RISK ASSESSMENT*	ACTION IF RA +
Oral health	Does not have a dental home	Referral to dental home or, if not available, oral health risk assessment
	Primary water source is deficient in fluoride	Oral fluoride supplementation
Blood pressure	Children with specific risk conditions or change in risk	Blood pressure
Vision	Parental concern or abnormal fundoscopic examination or cover/uncover test	Ophthalmology referral
Hearing	+ on risk screening questions	Referral for diagnostic audiologic assessment
Lead (Low prevalence area and not on Medicaid)	+ on risk screening questions	Lead screen
Tuberculosis	+ on risk screening questions	Tuberculin skin test

*See the Rationale and Evidence chapter for the criteria on which risk screening questions are based.

Immunizations

Consult the CDC/ACIP or AAP Web sites for the current immunization schedule.
CDC National Immunization Program (NIP): http://www.cdc.gov/vaccines
American Academy of Pediatrics *Red Book:* http://www.aapredbook.org

ANTICIPATORY GUIDANCE

The following sample questions, which address the Early Childhood Expert Panel's Anticipatory Guidance Priorities, are intended to be used selectively to invite discussion, gather information, address the needs and concerns of the family, and build partnerships. Use of the questions may vary from visit to visit and from family to family. Questions can be modified to match the health care professional's communication style. The accompanying anticipatory guidance for the family should be geared to questions, issues, or concerns for that particular child and family.

FAMILY SUPPORT

Adjustment to the child's developmental changes and behavior, family-work balance, parental agreement/disagreement about child issues

It is best to review plans for discipline before a need arises. Discuss plans for "time-outs" when needed to calm the situation, and "time ins" when the unwanted behavior ceases. At this age, "time-outs" may take place in a playpen or crib to protect a child from injury and should be brief (1 to 2 minutes).

Forewarn parents about possible temper tantrums in the future and the child's tendency to be clingy sometimes and to merrily go her own way at other times. Recommend the use of praise to strengthen good behaviors and offer suggestions for how parents might deal with biting, hitting, or other possibly harmful activity.

A child this age starts to recognize what is permitted and may touch something forbidden. At the same time, she will look back at the parent to test a reaction. This is a normal and positive move toward internalizing rules. Temper tantrums are more frequent as the child tries to master new skills and struggles with her move toward independence and autonomy.

SAMPLE QUESTIONS:
When your child is troublesome, what do you do? What do you do when she doesn't cooperate? What do the others in your family do? Do you need help in managing your child's behavior? Sometimes raising a child can be frustrating. Does anyone ever get angry with her? What happens then? Do you ever spank her? How do you reward your child?

ANTICIPATORY GUIDANCE:
- Try not to punish your child with spanking, shouting, or long explanations. A firm "No!" is the best way to deal with minor irritations (just as "Yes!" is a great way to reward good behavior). You may want to consider a brief time-out. Put the child in her crib or playpen for 1 to 2 minutes only, until the undesirable behavior stops.
- Distracting your child with something new that gets her attention or directing the child to a new activity are excellent ways to reduce unwanted behaviors. She wants to be near you and hear your voice—reading aloud to her is a great strategy for this purpose. (It's also a way to help her love books.)
- Time with family and special caregivers is the best treat you can give your child.

Parents need time away from their toddler to pursue their own interests, have regular time alone to rest, and maintain other important relationships. During this time, they also may need extra help from community resources.

Parenting is difficult sometimes. If it is culturally appropriate, having someone to talk to about parenting issues can help mothers and fathers get through the rough spots and appreciate the joys of watching their young child grow and develop.

SAMPLE QUESTIONS:
Who cares for your child other than you? Have you shared your child's health information with them?

ANTICIPATORY GUIDANCE:
- Make sure that you discuss your child's medical needs and your feelings about healthy diet, discipline, and oral health with all of your child's caregivers.
- Make sure that any environment where the child stays has the same, or better, safety standards as your home and that the transportation to and from sites other than home is safe.
- Share any information that we discuss with other caregivers.

SAMPLE QUESTIONS:
What activities do you enjoy doing outside of the home? How often do you get together with friends? What things do you do with friends? Do you need help in finding other community resources, such as a faith-based organization, recreational centers, or volunteer opportunities? Who do you talk to about parenting matters?

ANTICIPATORY GUIDANCE:
- Maintain or expand ties to your community through social, faith-based, cultural, volunteer, and recreational organizations or programs.
- Learn about and consider participating in parent-toddler playgroups.
- Consider joining a parent education class or parent support group.

ESTABLISHING ROUTINES

Family time, bedtime, teeth brushing, nap times

Establishing family traditions is extremely important for long-term self-recognition.

Establishing routines around bedtime, meals, and playing is important, even at this age. Stranger anxiety reaches a peak in the next few months.

SAMPLE QUESTIONS:
What do you all do together? What do your child's brothers and sisters do with him? Tell me about your family's traditions. What are some of the new things that your child is doing? How does your child react to changes in his routines or to strangers? What is your child's routine for meals and snacks?

ANTICIPATORY GUIDANCE:

- Avoid watching TV during "family time." Instead, play with your child and his brothers and sisters each day through games, storytelling, reading aloud, pointing and naming, listening to music, laughing, and exercising.
- At this age, your child may feel anxious around unfamiliar people. When meeting someone new, allow time for him to warm up. Try to use a consistent child care provider.
- Schedule 3 meals and 2 to 3 snacks at regular intervals during the day. This is another good way to establish a consistent daily routine. Regular meal and snack times also provide a constant supply of nutrients to fuel his many activities. Protecting your toddler against getting too hungry also will help prevent tantrums due to hunger.

A 1-year-old should be sleeping 12 to 14 hours a day. Bedtime should be at the same time each night and should become a nightly routine. Reading and singing before bedtime are examples of sleep-promoting activities. A favorite toy or object also may help reassure and calm the child. Night-lights also may be beneficial. For both nap time and bedtime, he should be put in the crib awake so that he can make the transition from awake to asleep on his own.

Another important routine to establish during this age is daily tooth brushing as soon as teeth erupt.

SAMPLE QUESTIONS:

How are sleeping routines going? Is it difficult getting your child to go to sleep? What time is bedtime? How do you manage naps? How does your child move around? How are you and your child adjusting to his increasing mobility? How frustrated is he about getting himself where he wants to go? How often do you brush your toddler's teeth?

ANTICIPATORY GUIDANCE:

- Establish a nightly bedtime routine that begins with quiet time for your child to relax before bed, and ends with your child soothing himself in his own crib. Reading and singing to your child will help him get to sleep. A favorite toy or a night-light also can help. Make sure to space nap times so that your child is tired at bedtime.
- Toddlers should continue to have at least one nap during the day. It is important to establish a regular nap time routine.
- Another important daily routine is teeth brushing. Establish a regular time each day for this task, such as after breakfast and before bed.

FEEDING AND APPETITE CHANGES

Self-feeding, nutritious foods, choices, "grazing"

Meals should be relaxed, safe, and enjoyable family times. Encourage fine-motor skills, such as using a cup or spoon and eating finger foods.

SAMPLE QUESTION:

Tell me about mealtime in your home.

ANTICIPATORY GUIDANCE:

- Cover your floor and don't worry about messes—young children learn from experimenting.
- Avoid small, hard foods like peanuts or popcorn, on which your child can choke, and cut any firm, round food (eg, hot dogs, raw carrots, or grapes) into thin slices.
- Include your toddler in family meals by providing a high chair or booster seat at table height. Make mealtimes pleasant and companionable. Encourage conversation.

The child should be developing toddler eating skills—biting off small pieces of food, feeding herself, and holding and drinking from a cup. Toddlers learn to like foods by touching, smelling, and mouthing them repeatedly.

SAMPLE QUESTION:

How is your child doing with feeding herself during meals and snacks?

ANTICIPATORY GUIDANCE:

- Give your toddler a spoon for eating and a cup for drinking. Be sure that they are easy for her small hands to hold.

This is a good time for parents to establish positive eating patterns for their child by providing meals and snacks at regular intervals, giving appropriate amounts of foods, and emphasizing nutritious foods. Discuss the importance of providing healthy snacks rich in complex carbohydrates, and only moderate amounts of sweets and high-fat or low-nutrient snacks. Remind parents that they are responsible for providing a variety of nutritious foods and that their child is responsible for how much to eat.

SAMPLE QUESTIONS:

How has your child's appetite been? What questions do you have about choosing healthy foods for your child?

ANTICIPATORY GUIDANCE:

- The toddler's rate of weight gain will be slower than in the first year. She may eat less now than when she was an infant.
- Toddlers tend to "graze." Her appetite will vary; she will eat a lot one time, and not much the next time.
- Let your toddler decide what and how much to eat from an assortment of nutritious foods you offer. Trust your child's ability to know when she is hungry and full. If she asks for more, provide a small, additional portion. If she stops eating, accept her decision.
- Feed your toddler 3 meals and 2 or 3 planned nutritious snacks a day. Be sure that your toddler's caregiver also provides nutritious foods.
- Have healthy snacks on hand, such as:
  - Fresh fruit (eg, apples, oranges, and bananas), cut in small pieces
  - Applesauce, cheese, or small pieces of whole-grain bread or crackers
  - Homemade popsicles that you make from 100% fruit juice

  Many fresh foods are fast and easy to prepare and cost less than prepared foods.

ESTABLISHING A DENTAL HOME

First dental checkup, dental hygiene

Every child should have a dental home, which should be established soon after the first tooth erupts or by 12 months of age. The dental home must be able to meet the unique needs of each child, including accurate risk assessment for dental diseases and conditions; an individualized preventive dental health program based on risk assessment; anticipatory guidance about growth and development, including teething, digit, or pacifier habits; a plan for responding to emergency dental trauma; comprehensive dental care in accordance with accepted guidelines and periodicity schedules; and referral to other dental specialists when indicated.

SAMPLE QUESTIONS:
Tell me about how you care for your child's teeth. Have you taken your child to a dentist?

ANTICIPATORY GUIDANCE:
- Be sure to get your child to the dentist by 12 months of age or after he gets his first tooth. A dentist will help you keep your child's teeth healthy and will be available in case there is ever an emergency with his teeth, such as a broken tooth or severe pain.
- Brush his teeth with plain water twice each day, using a soft toothbrush.
- If he is still using a bottle, offer only water in the bottle.

SAFETY

Home safety, car safety seats, drowning, guns

The toddler is becoming increasingly mobile and needs protection against common and uncommon hazards. Review all aspects of safety at this visit because safety is one of the most important aspects of care at this age.

If the family lives with other family members or friends, the family may not feel that it has the power to control the environment and may need help in advocating for a safe environment for their child. This also may be true for families who are living in homeless shelters or other types of temporary or uncertain housing.

SAMPLE QUESTIONS:
What have you done to "childproof" your home? The grandparents' homes? The caregiver's home? Do you have cabinet latches? Are tables free of heavy items that your child could pull down on herself?
How safe do you think your community is? How safe and comfortable do you and your family feel inside your home? Outside your home? How can we help so that your family feels safe? Who else can help your family feel safe?

ANTICIPATORY GUIDANCE:
- Lock away medications and all cleaning, automotive, laundry, and lawn products out of sight and out of reach. Climbing toddlers can reach even high shelves.

- Keep your toddler out of rooms where there are hot objects that may be touched, including hot oven doors and heaters, or put a barrier around them.
- Now that your toddler is walking, get down on the floor yourself and check for hazards.
- Keep plastic bags, latex balloons, or small objects, such as marbles, away from your toddler.
- Be sure there are no dangling telephone, electrical, blind, or drapery cords in your home.
- Make sure televisions, furniture, and other heavy items are secure so that your child can't pull them over. If they seem unsteady, anchor bookcases, dressers, and cabinets to the wall and put floor lamps behind other furniture.
- Keep sharp objects, such as knives and scissors, out of your toddler's reach.

SAMPLE QUESTION:
How often do you let your child's brothers and sisters help you take care of her?

ANTICIPATORY GUIDANCE:
- Never leave young siblings in charge of their baby sister or brother. Allow them to help with daily tasks, like feeding, under the supervision of a responsible adult.

Never underestimate the ability of a toddler to climb. Parents must be vigilant in preventing injuries from climbing.

SAMPLE QUESTIONS:
Do you have stair guards and window guards? Where is the mattress positioned in the crib?

ANTICIPATORY GUIDANCE:
- Some children can climb out of the crib at this age. Be sure that the crib mattress is on the lowest rung and that the sides are up when she is in it.
- Use gates at the top and bottom of stairs and watch your toddler closely when she is on stairs. To prevent children from falling out of windows, keep furniture away from windows and install operable window guards on second- and higher-story windows.

Child Safety Seat Inspection Station Locator: www.seatcheck.org. **Toll-free Number: 866-SEATCHECK (866-732-8243).**

Talk with parents to ensure that their child is fastened securely in a car safety seat and that they know when to switch from a rear-facing to a forward-facing seat.

Questions about proper installation should be referred to a certified Child Passenger Safety Technician in the community.
Child Safety Seat Inspection Station Locator: www.seatcheck.org
Toll-free Number: 866-SEATCHECK (866-732-8243)

SAMPLE QUESTIONS:
Is your child fastened securely in a car safety seat in the back seat every time she rides in a vehicle? Are you having any problems using your car safety seat?

ANTICIPATORY GUIDANCE:
- Never place your child's rear-facing safety seat in the front seat of a vehicle with a passenger air bag. The back seat is the safest place for children to ride.
- The rear-facing position provides the best protection for your child's neck and head in the event of a crash. For optimal protection, your child should remain

rear facing until she reaches the highest weight or height allowed for use by the manufacturer of a convertible seat or infant-only seat that is approved for use rear facing to higher weights and heights (up to 30 pounds and 32 inches for infant only and up to 35 pounds and at least 36 inches for convertible seats). Do not switch your child to a forward-facing car safety seat before she is at least 1 year old and weighs at least 20 pounds.
- Be sure your child's car safety seat is properly installed in the back seat according to the manufacturer's instructions and the vehicle owner's manual. There should be no more than a finger's width of space between her collarbone and the harness strap.

The child's increased mobility, combined with a heightened curiosity, makes for an extremely dangerous situation around bodies of water. Explain to parents that children can drown in a small amount of water, even in buckets or a few inches of water in a tub.

SAMPLE QUESTION:
Are there swimming pools or other potential water dangers near or in your home?

ANTICIPATORY GUIDANCE:
- Watch your toddler constantly whenever she is near water. Your child can drown in even a few inches, including water in the bathtub, play pools, buckets, or toilets. A supervising adult should be within an arm's reach, providing "touch supervision," whenever young children are in or around water.
- Do not let young brothers or sisters watch over your toddler in the bathtub, house, yard, or playground.
- Empty buckets, tubs, or small pools immediately after you use them.
- Be sure that swimming pools in your community, apartment complex, or home have a 4-sided fence with a self-closing, self-latching gate.
- Children should always wear a Coast Guard-approved life jacket when on a boat or other watercraft.

Guns should be removed from places in which children live and play, or unloaded and locked, with ammunition locked and stored separately. Many young children are killed by guns each year; most are injured by a sibling, a friend, or themselves.

SAMPLE QUESTIONS:
Does anyone in your home have a gun? Does a neighbor, family friend, or any home where your child might play have a gun? If so, is the gun unloaded and locked up? Where is the ammunition stored? Have you thought about not owning a gun because of the danger to children and other family members?

ANTICIPATORY GUIDANCE:
- The best way to keep your child safe from injury or death from guns is to never have a gun in the home.
- If it is necessary to keep a gun in your home, it should be stored unloaded and locked, with the ammunition locked separately from the gun.

Early Childhood: 15 Month Visit

CONTEXT

The 15-month-old is a whirlwind of activity and curiosity, with no apparent sense of internal limits. Children this age require constant attention and guidance from parents and caregivers. The child's first tentative steps are now headlong dashes to explore new places. The energy needed to master the challenge of walking now focuses on exploring new horizons. The impact of the dramatic developmental changes at 15 months, such as independent mobility, growing self-determination, and more complex cognitive abilities, provides parents with pleasure and delight in the newfound exuberance and determination of their toddler.

With these exciting new developments, the young toddler often forms elevated desires and expectations, as manifested, for example, by a new level of resistance to being dressed, diapered, or put to bed, and a growing desire to explore and do things on his own. These expectations and desires may outstrip his physical abilities, which leads to a new and often displayed emotion—frustration. He gets upset when he is unable to accomplish a task, when he cannot make someone understand his rudimentary communication, and when he cannot do precisely as he wishes. If crying and even screaming fail to elicit the desired response, his protests may escalate to full-blown temper tantrums or episodes of holding his breath.

The toddler's new mobility, exploratory skills, and exuberance increase his risk of injury. He is likely to run into the street or climb a flight of stairs without a moment's hesitation. Lacking a sense of danger or a fear of falling, the 15- to 18-month-old will try to scale playground equipment or poke a finger into an electrical socket. Minor injuries may surprise him, but they rarely deter him for long. His explorations may bring him into contact with dangerous chemicals kept under the sink or medicines in unlocked cabinets if parents are not careful to secure these storage areas.

The child at 15 months is likely to be wary of the health care professional and the exam. Anxiety connected with the toddler's wariness toward nonfamily members can be lessened if the exam is performed with the child on his parent's lap and the health care professional positioned approximately at eye level with the child. A warming-up phase can be encouraged by initially offering the child a toy while speaking with the parent, and by starting with the least intrusive aspects of the exam. The tools used in the exam can be made less fearful by first showing them to the child or by modeling their use, such as by putting the measuring tape first around the health care professional's own head, or examining the parent's ear. The child's increasing comfort will be signaled by his giving way to the impulse to explore the new environment of the examining room.

This critical period of learning for both the parents and the toddler is most productive when parents help their child begin to make healthy choices by serving nutritious foods without pressuring him to eat; offering him the freedom to explore within safe bounds; responding to his needs while limiting his constant demands; encouraging his beginning participation in daily routines, such as brushing his teeth; and learning to cope with their own anger and frustration as they help their toddler master his. At the 15 Month Visit, the health care professional helps parents learn the parenting skills they need to achieve the delicate balancing act of providing a safe and structured environment that also allows their toddler the freedom and independence to learn and explore.

15 Month Visit

PRIORITIES FOR THE VISIT

The first priority is to attend to the concerns of the parents. In addition, the Bright Futures Early Childhood Expert Panel has given priority to the following topics for discussion in this visit:

- Communication and social development (individuation, separation, attention to how child communicates wants and interests, signs of shared attention)
- Sleep routines and issues (regular bedtime routine, night waking, no bottle in bed)
- Temper tantrums and discipline (conflict predictors, distraction, praise for accomplishments, consistency)
- Healthy teeth (brushing teeth, bottle usage)
- Safety (car safety seats, parental use of safety belts, poison, fire safety)

HEALTH SUPERVISION

History

Interval history may be obtained according to the concerns of the family and the health care professional's preference or style of practice. The following questions can encourage in-depth discussion:

- What questions or concerns do you have about your child?
- How would you describe your child's personality these days?
- What things about your child are you most proud of?
- What do you find most difficult? Challenging? Wonderful? What do other people find difficult? Challenging? Wonderful?
- What major changes or stresses have occurred in your family since your last visit?

Observation of Parent-Child Interaction

During the visit, the health care professional should observe:

- What is the emotional tone between parent and child?
- How does the parent support the toddler's need for safety and reassurance in the exam room?
- Does the toddler check back with the parent visually or bring an object to show the parent?
- How do the parent and toddler play with toys (reciprocally, directively, or inattentively)?
- Does the parent react positively when the health care professional praises the child?
- If siblings are in the room, how do they react to the toddler?

Surveillance of Development

Do you have any specific concerns about your child's development, learning, or behavior?

SOCIAL-EMOTIONAL

■ **Tell me about your child's typical play.**
- Listens to a story
- Imitates activities
- May help in the house

COMMUNICATIVE

■ **How does your child communicate?**
- Indicates what he wants by pulling, pointing, or grunting
- Brings objects over to show you
- Hands you a book when he wants to hear a story

■ **What words does he say with meaning?**
- Says 2 to 3 words (not Dada/Mama) with meaning

COGNITIVE

■ **What do you think your child understands?**
- Understands and follows simple commands
- Scribbles

PHYSICAL DEVELOPMENT

■ **How does your child get from one place to another?**
- Walks well, stoops, and recovers
- Is able to take steps backwards

■ **How does your child use his hands?**
- Puts block in cup
- Drinks from a cup

Physical Examination

A complete physical examination is included as part of every health supervision visit.

When performing a physical examination, the health care professional's attention is directed to the following components of the examination that are important for a child this age:

- **Measure and plot:**
  - Length
  - Weight
  - Head circumference
- **Plot:**
  - Weight-for-length

- **Eyes**
  - Examine pupils for red reflexes
  - Perform cover/uncover test for conjugate ocular mobility
- **Mouth**
  - Observe for caries, plaque, demineralization (white spots), and staining
- **Neurologic**
  - Observe health care professional interaction and stranger avoidance

Screening

UNIVERSAL SCREENING	ACTION	
None		
SELECTIVE SCREENING	**RISK ASSESSMENT***	**ACTION IF RA +**
Blood pressure	Children with specific risk conditions or change in risk	Blood pressure
Vision	Parental concern or abnormal fundoscopic examination or cover/uncover test	Ophthalmology referral
Hearing	+ on risk screening questions	Referral for diagnostic audiologic assessment

*See the Rationale and Evidence chapter for the criteria on which risk screening questions are based.

Immunizations

Consult the CDC/ACIP or AAP Web sites for the current immunization schedule.
CDC National Immunization Program (NIP): http://www.cdc.gov/vaccines
American Academy of Pediatrics *Red Book:* http://www.aapredbook.org

ANTICIPATORY GUIDANCE

The following sample questions, which address the Early Childhood Expert Panel's Anticipatory Guidance Priorities, are intended to be used selectively to invite discussion, gather information, address the needs and concerns of the family, and build partnerships. Use of the questions may vary from visit to visit and from family to family. Questions can be modified to match the health care professional's communication style. The accompanying anticipatory guidance for the family should be geared to questions, issues, or concerns for that particular child and family.

COMMUNICATION AND SOCIAL DEVELOPMENT

Individuation, separation, attention to how child communicates wants and interests, signs of shared attention

This is an age at which parents must encourage their toddler's autonomous behavior, curiosity, sense of emerging independence, and feeling of competence. At the same time, they must provide clear guidance about appropriate limits of safe and socially acceptable behavior.

Speak positively and honestly about the strengths of the family. Praise the child for being friendly and cooperative. Compliment parents for encouraging their child's autonomy while making sure she is safe and for helping the child through the visit. If siblings are present, compliment them on their strengths as well.

Assess the degree of parental stress in connection with the child's behavior.

SAMPLE QUESTIONS:
What are some of the new things that your child is doing? How does your child show that she has a will of her own? How do you react?

ANTICIPATORY GUIDANCE:
- Whenever possible, allow your child to choose between 2 options, both of which are acceptable to you. For example, let her decide between a banana and applesauce for a snack, or between 2 of her favorite books. Allowing her to make choices in some areas will decrease power struggles in others.

Both stranger anxiety and separation anxiety pose frustrating challenges for many parents. Taking the time to explain that they originate in new cognitive gains often helps parents to remain patient with their young toddler.

SAMPLE QUESTION:
How does your child react to strangers?

ANTICIPATORY GUIDANCE:
- "Stranger anxiety" and anxiety connected with separation from family members is still common at this age.
- Never make fun of her fear. Do not force her to confront people who scare her, such as Santa Claus or clowns. Accept her fear and speak reassuringly.
- Some children are slow to warm up. They show this by being cautious or withdrawn. Others are outgoing. They show this by being friendly and interactive, or even by being aggressive (eg, hitting or biting).

During this time of intense demands by their toddler, parents frequently experience fatigue and frustration in the moment-to-moment effort of providing both support and safe limits. Seeking out opportunities to discuss child-raising issues with other parents can help alleviate stress and give parents new ideas for positive ways to handle difficult moments with their child.

SAMPLE QUESTIONS:

What do you do when you become angry or frustrated with your child? How often do you get out of the house without your child (aside from going to work)?

ANTICIPATORY GUIDANCE:

- Take some time for yourself and spend some individual time with your partner. Seek support and understanding about being a parent from people you trust.
- If your child has special needs, it is even more important to find support from other families like yours.

15-month-olds usually speak few words, but are able to understand many. Parents need to learn strategies to promote communication and language development. By reading aloud and naming the pictures, the parent can help the child learn language and satisfy her curiosity about the world. Consideration should be given to children who are exposed to 2 languages simultaneously.

SAMPLE QUESTIONS:

How does your child communicate what she wants? Who or what does she call by name? What gestures does she use to communicate effectively? For example, does she point to something she wants and then watch to see if you see what she's doing? Does she wave "bye-bye"? What language do you speak at home? What language does your child use to communicate her needs? What words does she use?

ANTICIPATORY GUIDANCE:

- A child's understanding of how words can be used to share experiences and feelings will be increased by the conversations, songs, verbal games, and books you share with her. Books do not have to be "read." You can use simple words to just talk about the pictures and story.
- Help your child learn the language of feelings by using words that describe feelings and emotions.
- Narrate your child's gestures. For example, if she points to a cookie, say, "Jane is pointing at the cookie. Do you want the cookie?"
- Use simple, clear phrases to give your child instructions.
- Encourage your child to repeat words. Respond with pleasure to her attempts to imitate words. Listen to and answer the child's questions.

SLEEP ROUTINES AND ISSUES

Regular bedtime routine, night waking, no bottle in bed

Reinforce the importance of maintaining nap time and nighttime sleep routines. For toddlers who are still experiencing some night waking or fussing, a review of the bedtime ritual and sleep history is warranted. Prepare parents for the common reoccurrence of night waking at 18 to 20 months of age. This is normal and is in keeping with the child's new capacity for thinking and remembering both fears and desires. For more difficult and entrenched night waking, a more in-depth assessment and plan may be needed.

SAMPLE QUESTIONS:
How is your child sleeping? When does he go to sleep? What is your bedtime routine? How many hours a day and night does he sleep?

ANTICIPATORY GUIDANCE:
- Continue to put your child to bed at the same time each night. Maintaining a consistent bedtime routine, in the room where your child will be sleeping, will help prepare him for bedtime.
- Tuck him in when he is drowsy, but still awake.
- Some children at this age, even though they have been sleeping well, may go through a short period of night waking. If he wakens, do not give him enjoyable attention; a brief visit with reassurance from you is all that is needed for him to return to sleep. Provide your child with a stuffed animal, blanket, or favorite toy that he can use to help console himself at bedtime, should he wake.
- Do not give him a bottle to sleep with, or bring him into bed with you as a means to get him back to sleep.

TEMPER TANTRUMS AND DISCIPLINE

Conflict predictors, distraction, praise for accomplishments, consistency

Some of the trigger points for tantrums and conflict between parent and toddler can be avoided through creative strategies.

Review with parents whether some conflicts can be avoided by "toddler proofing" the home or by accepting the messiness that usually accompanies the eating and playing of a 15-month-old.

SAMPLE QUESTIONS:
Is your child having frequent temper tantrums? What seems to trigger them, and how do you typically respond to them? What kinds of things do you find yourself saying "No" about? Do you have any questions about what should and should not be allowed for your child?

ANTICIPATORY GUIDANCE:

- Distracting your toddler by offering her an alternative activity may prevent needless conflicts or tantrums. When reading, let her choose the book. Let her control turning the pages.
- Use discipline as a means of teaching and protecting, not punishing.
- Praise your toddler for good behavior and accomplishments.

Discuss parental challenges and goals with respect to discipline and behavior management.

Review the impact of temperamental differences on behavior.

SAMPLE QUESTIONS:

How are you and your partner managing your child's behavior? Who else is helping you raise your child? How often do you talk with each other about your child-rearing ideas? How are your approaches basically similar and how are they different? What do you do when you disagree?

ANTICIPATORY GUIDANCE:

- Develop strategies with your partner to consistently manage the power struggles that result from your toddler's need to control her environment.
- Use discipline as a means of teaching and protecting, not punishing. Set limits for your toddler by using distraction, gentle restraint, and, when necessary, a brief time-out. Separate your toddler from the cause of the problem, stay close to her, and stick to structure and routines.
- Teach your toddler not to hit, bite, or use other aggressive behaviors. Model this behavior yourself by not spanking your toddler and by handling conflict with your partner constructively and nonviolently. Spanking increases the chance of physical injury, and your child is unlikely to understand the connection between the behavior and the punishment.

HEALTHY TEETH

Brushing teeth, bottle usage

Many children exhibit their independence by demanding to brush their own teeth, but children younger than 4 years may not have the manual dexterity to do so. When a child can tie his shoes, then he has the manual dexterity to brush his own teeth.

SAMPLE QUESTIONS:

Has your toddler been to the dentist? Who brushes your child's teeth?

ANTICIPATORY GUIDANCE:

- Schedule your toddler's first dental visit if it has not already occurred.
- Children this age have not yet developed the hand coordination to clean their own teeth adequately. Brush the child's teeth twice each day (after breakfast and before bed) with a soft toothbrush and plain water.

Early childhood caries is rampant in many populations. Bacterial transmission from parent to child is a primary mechanism for introducing caries-promoting bacteria into children's mouths. Counsel parents on ways to reduce bacterial transmission to their child.

Prolonged exposure to cow's or breast milk or fruit juice causes harm to teeth because bacteria in the mouth convert the sugars in milk or juice to acids. The acids attack the enamel and lead to dental caries.

SAMPLE QUESTIONS:

Does your child take a bottle to bed? If so, what is in the bottle? How many bottles of formula or fruit juice does your child get every day? How much water does your child drink? Did you know that you can do things to prevent your child from developing tooth decay?

ANTICIPATORY GUIDANCE:

- Many toddlers develop tooth decay (also called early childhood caries) because bacteria that cause tooth decay can be passed on to your toddler through your saliva when you kiss him or share a cup or spoon. To protect your baby's teeth and prevent decay, make sure you brush and floss your own teeth, don't share utensils, and don't clean his pacifier in your mouth.
- If you are having difficulty weaning your child from the nighttime bottle, do not use formula, milk, or juice in the nighttime bottle. Put only water in the bottle.

SAFETY

Car safety seats, parental use of safety belts, poison, fire safety

Talk with parents to ensure that their child is fastened securely in a car safety seat and that they know when to switch from a rear-facing to a forward-facing seat.

Questions about proper installation should be referred to a certified Child Passenger Safety Technician in the community.
Child Safety Seat Inspection Station Locator: www.seatcheck.org
Toll-free Number: 866-SEATCHECK (866-732-8243)

Child Safety Seat Inspection Station Locator: www.seatcheck.org. Toll-free Number: 866-SEATCHECK (866-732-8243).

SAMPLE QUESTIONS:

Is your child fastened securely in a car safety seat in the back seat of the car every time she rides in a vehicle? Are you having any problems using your car safety seat?

ANTICIPATORY GUIDANCE:

- Never place your child's rear-facing safety seat in the front seat of a vehicle with a passenger air bag. The back seat is the safest place for children to ride.
- The rear-facing position provides the best protection for your child's neck and head in the event of a crash. For optimal protection, your child should remain rear facing until she reaches the highest weight or height allowed for use rear facing by the manufacturer of a convertible seat or infant-only seat that

is approved for use rear facing to higher weights and heights (up to 30 pounds and 32 inches for infant-only seats and up to 35 pounds and at least 36 inches for convertible seats).

■ When your child reaches the top weight and height allowed for use by the manufacturer of the convertible seat rear facing, remember to make the necessary changes when using the seat in a forward-facing position.

■ Be sure your child's car safety seat is properly installed in the back seat according to the manufacturer's instructions and the car's owner's manual. There should be no more than a finger's width of space between your child's collarbone and the harness strap.

■ Remember your child's safety depends upon you. Always use your safety belt, too.

Review home safety issues with parents, including poisons, fire, burns, and falling objects. Unintentional injuries are the leading cause of death among young children. Parents must use constant vigilance and regularly review the safety of the home to protect their children from harm.

**Poison Control Center
1-800-222-1222**

SAMPLE QUESTIONS:

When did you last examine your home to be sure that it is safe? Would you like a list of home safety issues to review? What emergency numbers do you have posted near your phone?

ANTICIPATORY GUIDANCE:

■ Remove poisons and toxic household products from your home or keep them high and out of reach in locked cabinets. Have safety caps on all medications and lock them away.

■ Keep the number of the Poison Control Center (1-800-222-1222) near every telephone, and call immediately if there is a poisoning emergency. Do not make your child vomit.

■ Use gates at the top and bottom of stairs. To prevent children from falling out of windows, keep furniture away from windows and install operable window guards on second- and higher-story windows.

■ Make sure that any other caregivers, such as relatives or child care providers, follow these same safety guidelines.

SAMPLE QUESTIONS:

How do you keep hot liquids out of your toddler's reach? What is the temperature of your hot water? Do you have smoke detectors on each floor in the home where your child lives? When did you last change the batteries in the smoke detectors? Do you have a plan for getting everyone out of the house and a meeting place once outside? Do you have a neighbor from whose house you can call the fire department?

ANTICIPATORY GUIDANCE:

- Do not leave heavy objects or containers of hot liquids on tables with table-cloths that your child might pull down.
- Turn pan handles toward the back of the stove. Keep your child away from hot stoves, fireplaces, irons, curling irons, and space heaters.
- Keep small appliances out of reach and keep electrical cords out of your child's reach.
- Make sure you have a working smoke detector on every level of your home, especially in the furnace and sleeping areas. Test smoke detectors every month. It is best to use smoke detectors that use long-life batteries, but, if you do not, change the batteries at least once a year.
- Develop an escape plan in the event of a fire in your home.
- Keep cigarettes, lighters, matches, and alcohol out of your child's sight and reach.
- The hottest temperature at the faucet should be no higher than 120°F. In many cases, you can adjust your water heater. Before bathing your child, continue to test the water temperature with your wrist to make sure it is not too hot.

Early Childhood: 18 Month Visit

CONTEXT

The 18-month-old requires gentle transitions, patience, consistent limits, and respect. One minute he insists on independence; the next minute he is clinging fearfully to his parent. Much of the energy and drive that were channeled into physical activity are now directed toward more complex tasks and social interaction. Having learned the concept of choice, the toddler becomes assertive about his own wishes. His understanding of language develops rapidly, bringing with it new ways of labeling and remembering his experiences, and a new avenue for understanding the expectations of his parents and for communicating his wants and needs.

Though his communicative and social skills are developing rapidly, an 18-month-old usually still has a quite limited verbal and behavioral repertoire for expressing himself. Thus, the all-purpose word "No!" signals his desire for choice and autonomy, and the seeming defiance and negativism of an 18-month-old are actually assertions of an emerging sense of his own identity. Through this period, he needs to have strong emotional ties to his parents. To venture into the world and test his newfound assertiveness, he must know that he has a safe, emotionally secure place at home. Parents appreciate knowing that the sometimes assertive, sometimes clingy, and sometimes irritable behaviors of their formerly happy and fearless explorer are a common transitional phase.

The behavior of an 18-month-old may be frustrating at times, but his delight in his own emerging competence and achievements bring a sense of joy and accomplishment to all around him. Extra patience and a sense of humor can help parents with the tough task of continually reinforcing the limits they have set. The 18-month-old lights up a room as he applauds himself and looks around for parental acclaim and reinforcement.

Children typically remain highly resistant to the physical exam at this age. Examining a doll or stuffed animal before examining the child often has a calming effect. To keep the child as comfortable as possible, perform the less-invasive procedures first. Observe, then palpate the child. Give the child the opportunity to hold the stethoscope or otoscope before it is used. Give the child as many choices as possible about where and how the exam will be conducted (eg, on the parent's lap or on the exam table? Which eye should be examined first?).

18 Month Visit

PRIORITIES FOR THE VISIT

The first priority is to attend to the concerns of the parents. In addition, the Bright Futures Early Childhood Expert Panel has given priority to the following topics for discussion in this visit:

- Family support (parental well-being, adjustment to toddler's growing independence and occasional negativity, queries about a new sibling planned or on the way)
- Child development and behavior (adaptation to nonparental care and anticipation of return to clinging, other changes connected with new cognitive gains)
- Language promotion/hearing (encouragement of language, use of simple words and phrases, engagement in reading/singing/talking)
- Toilet training readiness (recognizing signs of readiness, parental expectations)
- Safety (car safety seats; parental use of safety belts; falls, fires, and burns; poisoning; guns)

HEALTH SUPERVISION

History

Interval history may be obtained according to the concerns of the family and health care professional's preference or style of practice. The following questions can encourage in-depth discussion:

- How are you doing?
- How are things going in your family?
- Let's talk about some of the things you most enjoy about your child. On the other hand, what seems most difficult?
- What major changes have occurred in your family since your last visit? Tell me about any stressful events.
- What questions or concerns do you have about your child?

Observation of Parent-Child Interaction

During the visit, the health care professional should observe:

- How do the parent and child communicate?
- If handed a book, does the child show the parent pictures (shared attention)?
- Does the parent ask the child many questions or give many directions?
- What is the tone of the parent-child interactions and the feeling conveyed?
- How does the parent guide the child to learn safe limits?
- Does the parent seem positive when speaking about the child?

Surveillance of Development

Do you have any specific concerns about your child's development, learning, or behavior?

SOCIAL-EMOTIONAL
- **How does your child act around other children?**
  - Is interactive or withdrawn; friendly or aggressive (eg, hitting, biting)
  - Laughs in response to others
  - Explores alone but with parent in close proximity
  - Is spontaneous with affection
  - Helps in house

COMMUNICATIVE
- **How does your child communicate?**
  - Vocalizes and gestures; speaks 6 words
  - Points to indicate to someone else what he wants

COGNITIVE
- **What do you think your child understands?**
  - Points to 1 body part
  - Follows simple instructions without gestured cues ("sit down")
  - Shows interest in a doll or stuffed animal by hugging it or pretend feeding
  - Knows the names of his favorite books

PHYSICAL DEVELOPMENT
- **Do you think your child hears all right? Sees all right?**

- **How does your child get from one place to another?**
  - Walks up steps, runs

- **How does your child use his hands?**
  - Stacks 2 or 3 blocks
  - May imitate a crayon stroke and scribbles
  - Uses a spoon and cup without spilling most of the time

Physical Examination

A complete physical examination is included as part of every health supervision visit.

When performing a physical examination, the health care professional's attention is directed to the following components of the examination that are important for a child this age:

- **Measure and plot:**
  - Recumbent length
  - Weight
  - Head circumference
- **Plot:**
  - Weight-for-length

- **Neurologic**
  - Observe gait (walking and running), hand control, and arm and spine movement
- **Eyes**
  - Examine pupils for red reflexes
  - Perform cover/uncover test for conjugate ocular mobility
- **Skin**
  - Observe for Nevi, café au lait spots, birthmarks, or bruising
- **Mouth**
  - Observe for caries, plaque, demineralization (white spots), staining, and injury

Screening

UNIVERSAL SCREENING	ACTION	
Development	Structured developmental screen	
Autism	Autism Specific Screen	
SELECTIVE SCREENING	**RISK ASSESSMENT***	**ACTION IF RA +**
Oral health	Does not have a dental home	Referral to dental home or, if not available, oral health risk assessment
	Primary water source is deficient in fluoride	Oral fluoride supplementation
Blood pressure	Children with specific risk conditions or change in risk	Blood pressure
Vision	Parental concern or abnormal fundoscopic examination or cover/uncover test	Ophthalmology referral
Hearing	+ on risk screening questions	Referral for diagnostic audiologic assessment
Anemia	+ on risk screening questions	Hematocrit or hemoglobin
Lead	If no previous screen or change in risk	Lead screen
Tuberculosis	+ on risk screening questions	Tuberculin skin test

*See Rationale and Evidence chapter for the criteria on which risk screening questions are based.

Immunizations

Consult the CDC/ACIP or AAP Web sites for the current immunization schedule.
CDC National Immunization Program (NIP): http://www.cdc.gov/vaccines
American Academy of Pediatrics *Red Book:* http://www.aapredbook.org

ANTICIPATORY GUIDANCE

The following sample questions, which address the Early Childhood Expert Panel's Anticipatory Guidance Priorities, are intended to be used selectively to invite discussion, gather information, address the needs and concerns of the family, and build partnerships. Use of the questions may vary from visit to visit and from family to family. Questions can be modified to match the health care professional's communication style. The accompanying anticipatory guidance for the family should be geared to questions, issues, or concerns for that particular child and family.

FAMILY SUPPORT

Parental well-being, adjustment to toddler's growing independence and occasional negativity, queries about a new sibling planned or on the way

Talk with the parents about their own preventive and health-promoting practices (eg, using safety belts, avoiding tobacco, eating a nutritious diet, exercising, following appropriate health screening advice, and staying safe in relationships). Discuss the parents' and family's adaptation to the toddler's independent behavior. Inquire about any recent or forthcoming changes in the family.

Acknowledge that other parents and children may be living in the household and those children may not be siblings (eg, they may be cousins or children of friends). This may present challenges as the parent may not be the only adult to intervene when situations arise.

SAMPLE QUESTIONS:
Tell me about your own health and mood. How often do you take time for yourself? How often do you and your partner spend time together? What activities do you do together as a family? Tell me if you have ever been in a relationship where you have been hurt, threatened, or treated badly? What did you do when this happened?

ANTICIPATORY GUIDANCE:
- Create opportunities for your family to share time together and for family members to talk and play with your toddler. Family mealtimes and vacations are ideal opportunities.
- Keep family outings relatively short and simple. Lengthy activities tire your toddler and may lead to irritability or a temper tantrum.
- Spend individual time with each child in your family.
- Acknowledge conflicts between siblings. Whenever possible, attempt to resolve conflicts without taking sides. For example, if a conflict arises about a toy, the toy can be put away. Do not expect your toddler to share her toys.
- Allow older children to have toys and other objects that they do not have to share with the toddler. Give them a storage space that the toddler cannot reach.
- Do not allow hitting, biting, or other aggressive behavior. Brief time-outs are a good way to tell your toddler these behaviors are not appropriate.
- If you feel unsafe in your home, seek help in moving your children and yourself to a safe place.

SAMPLE QUESTION:
Are you thinking about having another child?

ANTICIPATORY GUIDANCE:

- If you're expecting a new baby, it's important to prepare your child by reading stories about a family with a new baby, big brothers, or sisters. Enroll your child in a big brother or sister class at a local hospital to help her know where you will be when the baby is born. Tell her who will care for her while you are having the new baby. Continue to give her lots of love and attention.
- Try not to make any changes or new developmental demands on your toddler close to the time of the new baby's birth. Be prepared for your child to regress in new skills, such as using the potty or giving up the bottle.

Balancing support for a child's growing physical and cognitive independence while establishing and maintaining consistent limits is difficult for parents.

It is important that family members agree on how best to support the child's emerging independence while maintaining consistent limits.

Many communities offer a variety of options to help parents manage their child's behavior during this challenging period. It is important that parents learn about options that are culturally appropriate and affordable.

SAMPLE QUESTIONS:
Tell me how you set limits for your child and discipline her. Describe how you and your partner (and other caregivers) work out ways to be consistent in setting limits for her. What have been the most challenging aspects of managing her behavior? Do you need help finding out and signing up for community resources, such as faith-based organizations, recreational centers, or volunteer opportunities? Do you need help paying for health insurance?

ANTICIPATORY GUIDANCE:

- Reinforce limits and appropriate behavior. Try to be consistent in expectations and discipline. Remember, at this age, children often cling to parents again as a way to reassure themselves of their secure emotional base.
- Learn about and consider participating in parent-toddler playgroups.
- Maintain or expand ties to your community through social, faith-based, cultural, volunteer, and recreational organizations or programs.
- If you need financial assistance to help pay for health care expenses, ask about resources or referrals to the state Medicaid programs or other state assistance and health insurance programs.

Food is an area in which toddlers frequently express their newly independent views, especially their likes and dislikes. This is NORMAL.

SAMPLE QUESTIONS:
What does your child do when you offer new foods? Tell me about any concerns you might have about having enough food for your family.

ANTICIPATORY GUIDANCE:
- Your toddler may become more aware and suspicious of new or strange foods, but do not limit the menu to foods she likes.
- You may have to offer your toddler a new food several times before she accepts it. Do not give up after one or 2 tries.
- Let your toddler experiment with a variety of foods from each food group by touching and mouthing them.
- Ask about resources or referrals for food and/or nutrition assistance (eg, Commodity Supplemental Food Program, Food Stamp Program, Early Head Start, WIC) if you need help.

CHILD DEVELOPMENT AND BEHAVIOR

Adaptation to nonparental care and anticipation of return to clinging, other changes connected with new cognitive gains

Adaptation to nonparental care may bring a return of clinging.

Assertiveness in exploring the environment and persistence in pursuit of desires are normal developmental features of this age.

Taking the time to explain that these changes originate in new cognitive gains often helps parents remain patient with their young toddler.

SAMPLE QUESTIONS:
What are some of the new things that your child is doing? Who helps you raise your child?

ANTICIPATORY GUIDANCE:
- Your child may be anxious in new situations. Clinging to you is one way for him to express his desire to be with you.
- Spend some time playing with your toddler each day. Focus on activities that he expresses interest in and enjoys.
- Praise your toddler for good behavior and accomplishments.
- Decide what limits are important to you and your toddler. Be specific when setting limits and, whenever possible, make agreements with other adult caregivers about limits for your child.
- Keep time-outs and other disciplinary measures brief. In simple language, tell your toddler what he did wrong. When possible, use positive directives as well. Be as consistent as possible when enforcing limits. Remember that the goal is teaching, not punishing.

- When your child is upset, help him change his focus to another activity, book, or toy. This strategy of distraction and substitution can often calm him.
- Consider attending parent education classes or parent support groups. Many libraries and bookstores also have books and pamphlets about parenting. Your community may even have a parenting advice telephone hotline that can help you.

LANGUAGE PROMOTION/HEARING

Encouragement of language, use of simple words and phrases, engagement in reading/singing/talking

The development of language and communication during the early childhood years is of central importance to the child's later growth in social, cognitive, and academic domains. Communication is built upon interaction and relationships. Health care professionals have the opportunity to educate parents about the importance of language stimulation, including singing songs, reading, and talking to their child. Parent-child play, in which the child takes the lead and the parent is attentive and responsive, elaborating but not controlling, is an excellent technique for enhancing both the parent-child relationship and the child's language development. Because young children are active learners, they find joy in exploring and learning new words.

Parents may ask health care professionals about the effects of being raised in a bilingual home. They may be reassured that this situation permits the child to learn both languages simultaneously.

SAMPLE QUESTIONS:
How does your child communicate what she wants? Who or what does she call by name? What gestures does she use to communicate effectively? For example, does she point to something she wants and then watch to see if you see what she's doing? Does she wave "bye-bye"?

ANTICIPATORY GUIDANCE:
- Encourage your toddler's language development by reading and singing to her, and by talking about what you both are seeing and doing together. Books do not have to be "read." Talk about the pictures or use simple words to describe what is happening in the book. Do not be surprised if she wants to hear the same book over and over. Words that describe feelings and emotions will help your child learn the language of feelings.
- Ask your child simple questions, affirm her answers, and follow up with simple explanations.
- Use simple, clear phrases to give your child instructions.

TOILET TRAINING READINESS

Recognizing signs of readiness, parental expectations

Toilet training is part of developmentally appropriate learning. Many parents need guidance about when to begin toilet training. The average age for a child to be toilet trained during the day is 30 months.

SAMPLE QUESTIONS:
Have you thought about toilet training? What are your plans for it? Is anyone urging you to toilet train your child?

ANTICIPATORY GUIDANCE:
- Wait to start toilet training until your toddler is dry for periods of about 2 hours, knows the difference between wet and dry, can pull his pants up and down, wants to learn, and can indicate when he is about to have a bowel movement.
- It is helpful to read books with your child about using the potty, to take him into the bathroom with the appropriate-sex parent or older sibling to learn the routine, and to praise attempts to sit on the potty with his clothes on. Many children enjoy a special trip to select "big kid" underwear for when they feel ready to stop using diapers during the day.

SAFETY

Car safety seats; parental use of safety belts; falls, fires, and burns; poisoning; guns

Talk with parents to ensure that they know how to securely fasten their child in a car safety seat and when to switch from a rear-facing to a forward-facing seat.

Questions about proper installation should be referred to a certified Child Passenger Safety Technician in the community.
Child Safety Seat Inspection Station Locator: www.seatcheck.org
Toll-free Number: 866-SEATCHECK (866-732-8243)

SAMPLE QUESTIONS:
How is the car safety seat working? Is your child fastened securely in a car safety seat in the back seat every time she rides in a vehicle? Does everyone use a safety belt?

ANTICIPATORY GUIDANCE:
- Never place your child's rear-facing safety seat in the front seat of a vehicle with a passenger air bag. The back seat is the safest place for children to ride.

Child Safety Seat Inspection Station Locator: www.seatcheck.org. Toll-free Number: 866-SEATCHECK (866-732-8243).

EARLY CHILDHOOD
18 MONTH VISIT

- The rear-facing position provides the best protection for your child's neck and head in the event of a crash. For optimal protection, your child should remain rear facing until she reaches the highest weight or height allowed for use rear facing by the manufacturer of a convertible seat or infant-only seat that is approved for use rear facing to higher weights and heights (up to 30 pounds and 32 inches for infant-only seats and up to 35 pounds and at least 36 inches for convertible seats).
- When your child reaches the top weight and height allowed for use by the manufacturer of the convertible seat rear facing, remember to make the necessary changes when using the seat in a forward-facing position.
- Be sure your child's car safety seat is properly installed in the back seat according to the manufacturer's instructions and the car's owner's manual. There should be no more than a finger's width of space between your child's collarbone and the harness strap.
- Do not start your vehicle until everyone is buckled up. Children watch what parents do, so it is important to model safe behaviors for your child.

The active, climbing toddler challenges parents to provide a safe environment. Highlighting new safety hazards helps parents meet this important responsibility.

SAMPLE QUESTIONS:

Does your child like to climb? What floor in your house or apartment do you live on? Do you have window guards on all windows on the second floor and higher?

ANTICIPATORY GUIDANCE:

- Remember that many toddlers are excellent climbers. Make sure to use gates at the top and bottom of stairs. To prevent children from falling out of windows, keep furniture away from windows and install operable window guards on second- and higher-story windows.
- Watch over your toddler closely when she is on stairs.
- When you or other adults are backing the car out of the garage or driving the car forward or backward in the driveway, be certain another adult is holding your child a safe distance away so that she is not run over. The driver may not be able to see her.

SAMPLE QUESTIONS:

How do you keep hot liquids out of your toddler's reach? Do you have smoke detectors on each floor in the home where your child lives? When did you last change the batteries in the smoke detectors? Do you have a plan for getting everyone out of the house and a meeting place once outside? Do you have a neighbor from whose house you can call the fire department?

ANTICIPATORY GUIDANCE:

- Do not leave heavy objects or containers of hot liquids on tables with tablecloths that your child might pull down.
- Turn pan handles toward the back of the stove. Keep your child away from hot stoves, fireplaces, irons, curling irons, and space heaters.

- Keep small appliances out of reach and keep electrical cords out of your child's reach.
- Make sure you have a working smoke detector on every level of your home, especially in the furnace and sleeping areas. Test smoke detectors every month. It is best to use smoke detectors that use long-life batteries, but, if you do not, change the batteries at least once a year.
- Develop an escape plan in the event of a fire in your home.
- Keep cigarettes, lighters, matches, and alcohol out of your child's sight and reach.

Confirm with parents that they have important telephone numbers (eg, the Poison Control Center) available in many places in their home.

SAMPLE QUESTIONS:
How recently have you examined your home to be sure that it is safe? Do you know the telephone number for the Poison Control Center?

ANTICIPATORY GUIDANCE:
- Remove poisons and toxic household products from the home or keep them in locked cabinets. Have safety caps on all medications and lock them away as well. Never refer to medicine as candy. Because children like to mimic what you do, do not take your medicine in front of your child.
- Keep the number of your local Poison Control Center (1-800-222-1222) near every telephone, and call immediately if there is a poisoning emergency. Do not make your child vomit.

Poison Control Center
1-800-222-1222

Guns should be removed from places in which children live and play, or be unloaded and locked, with ammunition stored separately. Many young children are killed by guns each year and most are injured by themselves, a sibling, or a friend.

SAMPLE QUESTIONS:
Does anyone in your home have a gun? Does a neighbor, family friend, or any home where your child might play have a gun? If so, is the gun unloaded and locked up? Where is the ammunition stored? Have you thought about not owning a gun because of the danger to children and other family members?

ANTICIPATORY GUIDANCE:
- The best way to keep your child safe from injury or death from guns is to never have a gun in the home.
- If it is necessary to keep a gun in your home, it should be stored unloaded and locked, with the ammunition locked separately from the gun.

Early Childhood: 2 Year Visit

CONTEXT

The 2-year-old is spirited, delightful, joyful, carefree, and challenging! Although families may be frustrated when their 2-year-old cannot communicate his needs successfully, helping the child master the use of language holds many rewards for both the family and the child. The 2-year-old is not yet skilled at interacting with other children. Rather than sharing, he engages in parallel play alongside his peers as he learns to be sociable. It is important that adults not expect the 2-year-old to sit in a circle with other children or listen to a long story. These abilities will develop between 2 and 3 years of age.

The 2-year-old enjoys feeding himself, reading a book, and imitating his parents doing household chores. Watching him go through his daily routine is amusing. To fully understand new activities, he tries them repeatedly. What happens when water gets splashed outside the tub? How far will the teddy bear fall down the stairs? What does mud feel like? Sometimes parents find it difficult to realize that curiosity, rather than a rejection of their standards, compels their child's repetitious explorations.

Although the 2-year-old seems determined to assert his independence, when he is presented with a choice (eg, between apple slices and orange slices), he usually ceases his activity and has a difficult time choosing. After finally making a decision, he often wants to change it. Despite his apparent yearning for independence, the 2-year-old frequently hides behind his parent's legs when approached by other adults. He may develop fears at this age. For the first time, loud sounds, animals, large moving things, and other objects and events that are unpredictable and out of the child's control appear to be threatening. Fear of the dark may develop as the child struggles with the transition between waking consciousness and sleep. Unexplained events may resonate fearfully with the child's developing imagination (eg, he may develop a new fear of going down the drain along with the bath water, or a fear of thunder and lightning). A transitional object (eg, a blanket or special stuffed animal) helps the child through anxious times, including the transition into sleep. With steady parental support and reassurance, the child gains confidence and gradually overcomes such fears.

Toilet training is often high on the list of priorities that parents have for their 2-year-old child. Many, but not all, children this age have the developmental prerequisites to accomplish this major milestone. An essential ingredient to the success of this endeavor is the child's own desire. Parents often welcome the health care professional's encouragement to recognize the signs of the child's readiness, to develop an approach to training, and to recognize their own limits in effecting this change.

At this age, many of the child's actions are still governed by his parents' reactions. He has learned what to do to get his parents to respond, either negatively or positively, and may play one against the other. He will throw tantrums to get his way if he knows that his parents will react strongly. Similarly, if his parents overreact when he has difficulty expressing himself clearly, this normal phase of speech development becomes prolonged.

At age 2, the child is ready to be taught simple rules about safety and behavior in the family, but he is only beginning to be able to internalize them. It remains essential for parents to ensure the safety of the environment and to continue to adequately supervise their active toddler. Parents who provide gentle reassurance, calmly and consistently maintain limits despite repeated tantrums, and reinforce positive behaviors help their child begin to develop healthy self-confidence and social skills.

The health care professional should not ask a child this age questions that may be answered with "No." A negative response is a 2-year-old's only way of maintaining a modicum of control. Simple statements addressed to the child are usually more successful, such as, "Now it's time for me to listen to your heart." For many children, the exam may be best accomplished on the parent's lap. Where a choice truly exists, ask the child for help (eg, "Which ear do you want me to look into first?").

PRIORITIES FOR THE VISIT

The first priority is to attend to the concerns of the parents. In addition, the Bright Futures Early Childhood Expert Panel has given priority to the following topics for discussion in this visit:

- Assessment of language development (how child communicates, expectations for language)
- Temperament and behavior (sensitivity, approachability, adaptability, intensity)
- Toilet training (what have parents tried, techniques, personal hygiene)
- Television viewing (limits on viewing, promotion of reading, promotion of physical activity and safe play)
- Safety (car safety seats, parental use of safety belts, bike helmets, outdoor safety, guns)

HEALTH SUPERVISION

History

Interval history may be obtained according to the concerns of the family and the health care professional's preference or style of practice. The following questions can encourage in-depth discussion:

- How is your child doing?
- What questions or concerns do you have about him?
- Can you tell me about something funny or maddening or wonderful that your child has done lately?
- How are things going in your family?
- What major changes or stresses in your family have occurred since your last visit?

Observation of Parent-Child Interaction

During the visit, the health care professional should observe:

- How do the parent and child communicate?
- What is the tone of the interaction and the feelings conveyed?
- Does the parent teach the child the name of a person or object during the visit?
- Does the child feel free to explore the room?
- How does the parent set appropriate limits, if needed?
- Does the parent seem positive when speaking about the child?

Surveillance of Development

Do you have any specific concerns about your child's development, learning, or behavior?

SOCIAL-EMOTIONAL

■ **Tell me about your child's typical play.**
- Imitates adults
- Increases pretend play (eg, rocking, feeding, or putting baby doll to bed)
- Plays alongside other children (parallel play)
- Refers to self more often as "I" or "me"
- May have established a special attachment to a transitional object

COMMUNICATIVE

■ **How does your child communicate?**
- Has vocabulary of at least 50 words
- Uses 2-word phrases
- Asks parent to read a book

COGNITIVE

■ **What do you think your child understands?**
- Follows 2-step commands
- Names one picture, such as a cat, horse, bird, dog, or man
- Completes sentences and rhymes in familiar books
- Corrects you if you change a word in a book he knows
- In response to, "Where is _____?", points to object or animal in a book

PHYSICAL DEVELOPMENT

■ **How does your child use his hands?**
- Stacks 5 or 6 blocks
- Makes or imitates horizontal and circular strokes with crayon
- Turns book pages one at a time
- Imitates food preparation: scrubs, tears, breaks, dips, snaps, beats an egg, "washes" dishes
- Throws ball overhand

■ **How does your child get from one place to another?**
- Goes up and down stairs one step at a time
- Kicks a ball
- Jumps up

Physical Examination

A complete physical examination is included as part of every health supervision visit.

When performing a physical examination, the health care professional's attention is directed to the following components of the examination that are important for a child this age:

- **Measure:**
  - Standing height (preferred) or recumbent length
  - Weight
  - Head circumference
- **Calculate and plot:**
  - BMI, if standing height; otherwise, plot weight-for-length

- **Eyes**
  - Examine pupils for red reflexes
  - Perform cover/uncover test for conjugate ocular mobility
- **Mouth**
  - Observe for caries, plaque, demineralization (white spots), staining, injury, and gingivitis
- **Neurologic**
  - Observe running, scribbling, socialization, and ability to follow commands
  - Assess language acquisition and clarity

Screening

UNIVERSAL SCREENING	ACTION	
Autism	Autism Specific Screen	
Lead (High prevalence area or on Medicaid)	Lead screen	
SELECTIVE SCREENING	RISK ASSESSMENT*	ACTION IF RA +
Oral health	Does not have a dental home	Referral to dental home or, if not available, oral health risk assessment
	Primary water source is deficient in fluoride	Oral fluoride supplementation
Blood pressure	Children with specific risk conditions or change in risk	Blood pressure
Vision	Parental concern or abnormal fundoscopic examination or cover/uncover test	Ophthalmology referral
Hearing	+ on risk screening questions	Referral for diagnostic audiologic assessment
Anemia	+ on risk screening questions	Hematocrit or hemoglobin
Lead (Low prevalence area and not on Medicaid)	+ on risk screening questions	Lead screen
Tuberculosis	+ on risk screening questions	Tuberculin skin test
Dyslipidemia	+ on risk screening questions	Fasting lipid profile

*See the Rationale and Evidence chapter for the criteria on which risk screening questions are based.

Immunizations

Consult the CDC/ACIP or AAP Web sites for the current immunization schedule.
CDC National Immunization Program (NIP): http://www.cdc.gov/vaccines
American Academy of Pediatrics *Red Book:* http://www.aapredbook.org

ANTICIPATORY GUIDANCE

The following sample questions, which address the Early Childhood Expert Panel's Anticipatory Guidance Priorities, are intended to be used selectively to invite discussion, gather information, address the needs and concerns of the family, and build partnerships. Use of the questions may vary from visit to visit and from family to family. Questions can be modified to match the health care professional's communication style. The accompanying anticipatory guidance for the family should be geared to questions, issues, or concerns for that particular child and family.

ASSESSMENT OF LANGUAGE DEVELOPMENT

How child communicates, expectations for language

A 2-year-old is rapidly developing language skills and experiences joy in reciprocal communication. This is a time to assess how the child communicates and to set expectations with the parents about their child's language development. Parents are keen observers of the child's behavior and often correctly identify sensory problems.

SAMPLE QUESTIONS:
How does your child communicate what she wants? What do you think your child understands? How well do you think your child hears and sees? If your child uses 2 languages, how intelligible is she in each?

Ask the Child
"What's that?" (pointing to a picture); "Which one is the ___?" (in a book); "Give me the ___." (from among several objects).

ANTICIPATORY GUIDANCE:
- Model appropriate language.
- Two-year-old children should begin using 2-word sentences or phrases, such as, "want milk," "have cookie," and "go home."
- Two-year-old children also should be able to follow simple 1- or 2-step commands, such as, "Pick up the doll and bring it to me."
- Read to your child every day. Many toddlers love the same story over and over. This is normal. Ask your child to point to pictures of objects, animals, or people on the page. If the story is familiar, pause every now and then for your child to insert a phrase or sound to help tell the story or to finish a familiar sentence or phrase.
- Encourage your child's language development by reading books and singing songs to her, and by talking about what you both are seeing and doing together.
- Many children struggle to respond quickly at this age, so talk and question slowly so that your child has the opportunity to respond without pressure. Praise all efforts to respond and repeat what is said in an affirming way.
- If you need to have your child look at you before you know she is listening to you, let us know. Hearing problems are important to identify early and are more common in children with many ear infections.
- If you notice your child squinting, holding books very close to her face, or failing to look at things you are pointing out to her, let us know. She may have a vision problem.

TEMPERAMENT AND BEHAVIOR

Sensitivity, approachability, adaptability, intensity

The parent or caregiver has the best understanding of the child and can provide much useful information about the child's development at this stage. Discuss with parents their expectations about their child's understanding and behavior. Two-year-old children still have limited abilities to internalize rules for behavior.

Through their interactions with their child, parents can nurture good behavior, self-confidence, and a desire to learn and explore.

Discuss with the parent typical variations in behavioral style, including such temperamental qualities as general activity level, sensitivity or reactivity to changes in the environment, tendency to approach or withdraw in new situations, adaptability to change in routine, intensity of response, and the predominance of a positive or negative mood, especially in social situations.

SAMPLE QUESTIONS:
What are some of the new things that your child is doing? What do you and your partner enjoy most about your child? What seems to be most difficult? Do you have special times that you set aside to be with your child?

ANTICIPATORY GUIDANCE:
- Praise your child for good behavior and accomplishments.
- Spend individual time with your child, playing with him, hugging or holding him, taking walks, painting, and doing puzzles together. Focus on activities that he expresses interest in and enjoys.
- Listen to and respect your child.
- Appreciate your child's investigative nature, and avoid excessively restricting his explorations. Guide him through fun learning experiences.
- Give your child opportunities to assert himself. Encourage self-expression.
- Help your child express such feelings as joy, anger, sadness, fear, and frustration.
- Promote a sense of competence and control by inviting your child to make choices limited to 2 equally acceptable options when possible. For example, allow him to choose between 2 kinds of fruit when picking out a snack.

SAMPLE QUESTION:
How does your child act around family members?

ANTICIPATORY GUIDANCE:
- Your child varies in how he reacts to different situations and he will quickly learn the different ways in which his parents and other family members respond to his actions and requests. Encourage family members to be consistent, patient, and respectful in how they respond to him.

EARLY CHILDHOOD
2 YEAR VISIT

425

The child enjoys playing independently but has not yet developed the skills necessary to interact with other children.

SAMPLE QUESTIONS:
Tell me about your child's typical play. How does your child act around other children? If your child is in group child care, how does he do with the other children? Are your child care arrangements working for your family and for your child?

ANTICIPATORY GUIDANCE:
- Encourage your child to play with other children, but do not expect him to share the play or toys yet.

TOILET TRAINING

What have parents tried, techniques, personal hygiene

Toilet training is part of developmentally appropriate learning. Each child progresses through toilet training differently and parents need to understand signs of readiness and how to support and encourage their child during this process.

Explore family attitudes about toilet training, including parental experiences and expectations.

SAMPLE QUESTION:
How is your child's toilet training progressing?

ANTICIPATORY GUIDANCE:
- Encourage toilet training when your child is dry for about 2 hours at a time, knows the difference between wet and dry, can pull her pants up and down, wants to learn, and can tell you when she is about to have a bowel movement.
- Here are some ways to help your child be successful: Dress her in easy-to-remove pants, establish a daily routine, place her on the potty every 1 to 2 hours, and provide a relaxed environment by reading or singing songs while she is on the potty.
- Children use the toilet more frequently than adults, often up to 10 times a day. Plan for frequent toilet breaks when traveling with your child, even if you are out for a short time.

SAMPLE QUESTIONS:
Does your child wash her hands after toileting? Before eating?

ANTICIPATORY GUIDANCE:
- Help your child wash her hands after diaper changes or toileting and before eating. Make sure to wash your own hands often.
- Clean potty chairs after each use.
- Teach your child to sneeze/cough into her shoulder. Teach your child to wipe her nose with a tissue and then wash her hands.
- Soap and water is sufficient for cleaning your child's toys.
- If your child is in child care, provide personal items, such as blankets, cups, combs, and brushes, for individual use.

TELEVISION VIEWING

Limits on viewing, promotion of reading, promotion of physical activity and safe play

The AAP recommends that children older than 2 limit television and video viewing to no more than 1 to 2 hours of quality programming per day.

If a child watches TV, parents should ensure that the programs are appropriate. Many cartoon shows are violent, soap operas often feature issues that are inappropriate for young children, and talk shows and sporting events are overwhelming for many young children. Even educational shows can be too stimulating for young minds.

SAMPLE QUESTIONS:
Does your child watch TV or videos? If so, what TV shows does your child watch?

ANTICIPATORY GUIDANCE:
- **If you let your child watch TV, watch together and talk about what you see.**
- **Be aware that the TV show may be appropriate for your child, but the commercials may not be.**
- **Limit TV watching to no more than 1 to 2 hours per day. Choose alternatives for together time, such as reading, listening to music, or playing games.**

The main ideas behind promoting physical activity at this age are to be physically active in a safe environment and to establish a habit of being active, both as an individual and a family.

SAMPLE QUESTIONS:
What kind of physical activities does your child enjoy? What types and amounts of physical activity does your child enjoy when he's with other caregivers (eg, at child care and by other family members)?

ANTICIPATORY GUIDANCE:
- Ask about the types and amounts of physical activity the child enjoys when he's with other caregivers (eg, child care, other family members).
- Enjoy being physically active as a family (eg, walk, hike, bike, play tag).
- Make sure that other caregivers also make time for physical activity with your child.

SAFETY

Car safety seats, parental use of safety belts, bike helmets, outdoor safety, guns

Talk with parents to ensure that they know how to securely fasten their child in a car safety seat. Adults should model car safety by always using a safety belt themselves.

Questions about proper installation should be referred to a certified Child Passenger Safety Technician in the community.
Child Safety Seat Inspection Station Locator: www.seatcheck.org
Toll-free Number: 866-SEATCHECK (866-732-8243)

SAMPLE QUESTIONS:
How is the car safety seat working? Is your child fastened securely in a car safety seat in the back seat every time she rides in a vehicle? Does everyone use a safety belt?

EARLY CHILDHOOD
2 YEAR VISIT

Child Safety Seat Inspection Station Locator: www.seatcheck.org. Toll-free Number: 866-SEATCHECK (866-732-8243).

ANTICIPATORY GUIDANCE:

- Be sure that the car safety seat is properly installed in the back seat according to the manufacturer's instructions and the vehicle owner's manual. There should be no more than a finger's width of space between your child's collarbone and the harness strap.
- The back seat is the safest place for children to ride.
- Do not start your vehicle until everyone is buckled up. Children watch what parents do, so it is important for you to model safe behaviors by always wearing your safety belt.

The young toddler is beginning to play outside as well as inside. This new opportunity for physical activity introduces new hazards. Outdoor safety should be tailored to the local environment where the child lives (rural vs urban hazards). Modeling is the best way to ensure that a child develops lifelong safe behaviors.

SAMPLE QUESTION:
Would you like a list of outdoor health and safety tips for your toddler?

ANTICIPATORY GUIDANCE:

- Young children should never be left unsupervised in or around vehicles.
- When your toddler is playing outside, make sure she stays within fences and gates and remember to watch her closely.
- Keep your toddler away from moving machinery, lawn mowers, overhead garage doors, driveways, and streets.
- When you or other adults are backing out of the garage or driving the car forward or backing in the driveway, be certain another adult is holding your child so that she is not run over. The driver may not be able to see her.

SAMPLE QUESTION:
Does your child wear a bike helmet when she rides her tricycle?

ANTICIPATORY GUIDANCE:

- Be sure that your child wears a helmet approved by the CPSC when riding on a tricycle or in a seat on an adult's bicycle. Wear a helmet yourself. Make sure everyone's helmets properly fit according to the manufacturer's instructions.

Guns should be removed from places in which children live and play, or unloaded and locked, with ammunition stored separately. Many young children are killed by guns each year and most are injured by themselves, a sibling, or a friend.

SAMPLE QUESTIONS:
Does anyone in your home have a gun? Does a neighbor, family friend, or any home where your child might play have a gun? If so, is the gun unloaded and locked up? Where is the ammunition stored? Have you thought about not owning a gun because of the danger to children and other family members?

ANTICIPATORY GUIDANCE:

- The best way to keep your child safe from injury or death from guns is to never have a gun in the home.
- If it is necessary to keep a gun in your home, it should be stored unloaded and locked, with the ammunition locked separately from the gun.

Early Childhood: 2½ Year Visit

CONTEXT

At age 2½, significant advances in all developmental trajectories are readily observable. Compared with the 2-year-old child, motor coordination (gross and fine) is much improved. The child now can walk on tiptoes and can jump with both feet. He modulates his movement, speeding up and slowing down as he desires, negotiating turns while running, and coming to a sudden stop. His finger movements are now better differentiated from whole-hand movements. For example, he is more able to manage puzzle pieces, string beads, and put snap-blocks together.

A strong incentive for the health care professional to see children routinely at 2½ years is the opportunity to check on the child's development of language and social communication. Where the 2-year-old is typically just starting the process of creatively joining a few words in combination, the 2½-year-old uses a wide variety of short phrases of 3 and 4 words (many, if not most, of which are understandable to family members). Vocabulary has expanded dramatically, and the child often accompanies his actions with short, verbal descriptions, such as, "Me make it go" and "I take my coat off." At 2½, children typically enjoy the playful use of words, including rhyming games and simple songs with rhythm and accompanying movement, and the child's pleasure in such interactions with others becomes an important measure of his social development. As at 2 years,

receptive language usually develops well in advance of expressive abilities and makes for new receptivity to book reading and stories. Children this age like stories that tell about everyday activities, such as getting dressed, playing with toys, eating meals with the family, and bedtime. He likes to hear the same story read to him over and over, and often insists on it being read the same way each time.

Play behaviors also have become more elaborate at 2½ years. The child this age enjoys acting out the behaviors seen in other family members, such as feeding a dolly, talking on the phone, or sweeping the floor. A new sense of order, sometimes repetitive and perfectionistic, emerges at this age, as shown in the child's interest in lining up toys or placing crayons in a specific color order. In social situations, play with peers continues to be more often parallel than collaborative. Yet, with some play activities that have an easily recognized theme and sequence of actions (eg, the tea party), 2½-year-olds delight in independent play with peers.

This age is often the time when parents begin to consider what sort of early education experience will be best for their child. The 2½ Year Visit is an ideal time to review the child's developmental readiness, behavioral style, and parental goals for such a placement, and to support parents in their efforts to determine the best programmatic match for their child.

PRIORITIES FOR THE VISIT

The first priority is to attend to the concerns of the parents. In addition, the Bright Futures Early Childhood Expert Panel has given priority to the following topics for discussion in this visit:

- Family routines (parental consistency, day and evening routines, enjoyable family activities)
- Language promotion and communication (interactive communication through song, play, and reading)
- Promoting social development (play with other children, limited reciprocal play, imitation of others, choices)
- Preschool considerations (readiness for early childhood programs, playgroups, or playdates)
- Safety (water safety, car safety seats, outdoor health and safety [pools, play areas, sun exposure], pets, fires and burns)

HEALTH SUPERVISION

History

Interval history may be obtained according to the concerns of the family and the health care professional's preference or style of practice. The following questions can encourage in-depth discussion:

- What new things is your child doing now?
- How are you and your family doing these days?
- What questions or concerns do you have about your child today?

Observation of Parent-Child Interaction

During the visit, the health care professional should observe:

- How actively do the parent and child communicate with each other?
- Does the child use questions and phrases at an appropriate age level?
- If given a book, do the child and the parent look at it together, discuss it, and interact?
- How well does the parent calm the child during the visit?
- Do the child and parent appear to have their feelings under control?

Surveillance of Development

Do you have any specific concerns about your child's development, learning, or behavior?

SOCIAL-EMOTIONAL
- **What is your child's play like?**
  - Imaginary play, such as with dolls and toys, is increasing
  - Play is starting to include other children to an increasing degree, such as play tea parties or chase games
- **Is your child expressing much fearfulness?**
  - Has fears about unexplained changes in his physical environment and unexpected events (common in children of this age)

COMMUNICATIVE
- **How does your child communicate?**
  - Uses short phrases of 3 to 4 words
  - Is understandable to others 50% of the time

COGNITIVE
- **What do you think your child understands?**
  - Knows the correct action for a selected animal or person (eg, cat meows, horse gallops, bird flies, dog barks, man talks)
  - Has friends
  - Points to 6 body parts

PHYSICAL DEVELOPMENT
- **What activities is he able to do?**
  - Jumps up and down in place
  - Throws ball overhand
  - Washes and dries hands
  - Brushes teeth with help
  - Puts on clothes with help
  - Copies a vertical line

Physical Examination

A complete physical examination is included as part of every health supervision visit.

When performing a physical examination, the health care professional's attention is directed to the following components of the examination that are important for a child this age:

- **Measure and plot:**
  - Standing height (preferred) or recumbent length
  - Weight
  - Head circumference

- **Calculate and plot:**
  - BMI, if standing height; otherwise, plot weight-for-length
- **Eyes**
  - Examine pupils for red reflexes
  - Perform cover/uncover test for conjugate ocular mobility
- **Neurologic**
  - Observe coordination, language acquisition and clarity, and socialization
  - Assess vocalizations

Screening

UNIVERSAL SCREENING	ACTION	
Development	Structured developmental screening	
SELECTIVE SCREENING	**RISK ASSESSMENT***	**ACTION IF RA +**
Oral health	Does not have a dental home	Referral to dental home or, if not available, oral health risk assessment
	Primary water source is deficient in fluoride	Oral fluoride supplementation
Blood pressure	Children with specific risk conditions or change in risk	Blood pressure
Vision	Parental concern or abnormal fundoscopic examination or cover/uncover test	Ophthalmology referral
Hearing	+ on risk screening questions	Referral for diagnostic audiologic assessment

*See Rationale and Evidence chapter for the criteria on which risk screening questions are based.

Immunizations

Consult the CDC/ACIP or AAP Web sites for the current immunization schedule.
CDC National Immunization Program (NIP): http://www.cdc.gov/vaccines
American Academy of Pediatrics *Red Book:* http://www.aapredbook.org

ANTICIPATORY GUIDANCE

The following sample questions, which address the Early Childhood Expert Panel's Anticipatory Guidance Priorities, are intended to be used selectively to invite discussion, gather information, address the needs and concerns of the family, and build partnerships. Use of the questions may vary from visit to visit and from family to family. Questions can be modified to match the health care professional's communication style. The accompanying anticipatory guidance for the family should be geared to questions, issues, or concerns for that particular child and family.

FAMILY ROUTINES

Parental consistency, day and evening routines, enjoyable family activities

As children develop more effective language skills, they and their parents experience increasing pleasure in talking together. Consistent guidance, regularly playful experiences during the day, and clear limits about bedtime all help a child develop a sense of security and self-control.

Parents need to reconnect regularly with friends and personal interests and work beyond the family at this time.

SAMPLE QUESTIONS:
What kinds of things do you do outside the family? If you work outside of the home, where do you work? How well do you and your family agree on limits and discipline for your child?

ANTICIPATORY GUIDANCE:
- Reading to your child from culturally and developmentally appropriate books and stories at least once a day is a habit that both of you will grow to look forward to.
- Try some activities outside the family. Choose activities that help reduce stress, give you pleasure, and reward your efforts.
- Reach agreement with all family members on how best to support your child's emerging independence while maintaining consistent limits.

Routine participation in activities as a family (eg, physical activities and going to museums or the park) helps build family togetherness.

SAMPLE QUESTIONS:
Tell me about how you have fun with your family? What activities do you and your family participate in together?

ANTICIPATORY GUIDANCE:
- Encourage family exercise, such as walking, jogging, swimming, or bicycling (with helmet).
- Expand your child's experiences by visiting museums, zoos, and other educational centers. Make sure they have programs designed for young children.

Mealtimes are part of a family routine that enhances a child's language, math, and motor skills as well as promotes communication and other socialization abilities. Consistent evening and bedtime routines help young children transition from the active daytime to a good night's sleep.

SAMPLE QUESTIONS:

What meals does your child eat with the family? What types of evening and bedtime routines are you using at home? How consistently do you follow these routines?

ANTICIPATORY GUIDANCE:

- Family meals are an excellent way to support language and social development in the young child. Eat together as often as possible—at least 4 to 5 times a week.
- Try not to have vigorous play or watch stimulating videos or TV programs with your child in the evening. Quiet evening activities will help your child recognize that bedtime is coming and smoothes the way to the bedtime routine and settling in early for high-quality sleep. A good night's sleep is essential to good daytime behavior and to preventing tantrums.

LANGUAGE PROMOTION AND COMMUNICATION

Interactive communication through song, play, and reading

At $2\frac{1}{2}$ years of age, children vary considerably in their spoken language skills. Most, however, are already speaking in short, complete sentences. They typically are forming 3- to 4-word sentences, most of which should be understandable to family members.

Speech tends to be unidirectional at this age, with the child most often asserting his needs and desires and describing his activities.

SAMPLE QUESTIONS:

Is your child speaking in sentences? How frustrated does he become when others cannot understand what he is saying? Does he enjoy having stories read to him? Does he enjoy participating with you in songs, rhymes, and games involving rhythm and movement, such as "Itsy, Bitsy Spider"?

ANTICIPATORY GUIDANCE:

- Read books together every day. Reading aloud will help him be ready for preschool, and then for school.
- At this age, children typically are able to follow the story line of simple books, and may ask you to read the same book again and again.
- Limit TV and video watching to no more than 1 to 2 hours each day.
- Monitor the types of shows your child watches.
- Take your child to the library and its story time regularly.
- Young children process spoken language more slowly than adults do. Be sure to give your toddler plenty of time to respond when you say something to him.
- When your child is speaking, listen attentively and clearly repeat what he says, using correct grammar. If necessary, clarify what he means, using correct grammar.

PROMOTING SOCIAL DEVELOPMENT

Play with other children, limited reciprocal play, imitation of others, choices

Children this age should feel comfortable and engaged when playing side-by-side with peers and older children. However, their capacity for cooperative, reciprocal play is quite limited.

If the child is not yet in a child care or preschool program, parents should be encouraged to help organize playdates and/or a regular playgroup to help promote the child's social development.

SAMPLE QUESTIONS:
How often does your child play with other children? How do these playtimes go?

ANTICIPATORY GUIDANCE:
- Provide opportunities for your toddler to play with other toddlers near your child's age. Be sure to supervise these times, because your child is not ready to share or play cooperatively.
- Having 2 of each toy is a good way to avoid battles over toys. If you have a close friend whose child plays with yours, consider purchasing the same toys for your children. This can help prevent battles.

At this age, children usually enjoy initiating actions and decisions, and the frequent upsets and frustrations experienced by the 2-year-old are usually decreasing by $2\frac{1}{2}$. At the same time, they definitely need and appreciate consistent parental guidance about safe, acceptable behavior and limits.

SAMPLE QUESTIONS:
Does your child enjoy making independent decisions about what to eat and wear or where to play? What are some of the new things that your child is doing?

ANTICIPATORY GUIDANCE:
- Offering toddlers limited choices between one of 2 equally acceptable, healthy options helps build your child's independence. Having more than 2 options to choose from is overwhelming and frustrating for your toddler. Once your child decides, confirm the choice and move along.
- Try to arrange one-on-one time with each of your children every day.
- Continue to follow daily routines for eating, sleeping, and playing.

EARLY CHILDHOOD
2 1/2 YEAR VISIT

PRESCHOOL CONSIDERATIONS

Readiness for early childhood programs, playgroups, or playdates

Discuss the child's developmental readiness for an early childhood program. In determining the appropriateness of the match between child and program, have parents review the features of the program (eg, duration of care, size of group, and type and closeness of supervision), temperamental qualities of the child, goals and philosophy of the program, and the family's goals for the child. For children with special needs who are receiving services under IDEA Part C, ensure that the family is working with the family service coordinator to transition the child's services to Part B. This transition needs to occur before the child's third birthday.

SAMPLE QUESTIONS:
What are your plans for child care or preschool in the year ahead? Do you need help locating or selecting a quality early education experience for your child?

ANTICIPATORY GUIDANCE:
- Child care and preschool settings offer young children the opportunity to develop social skills with other children on a daily basis. They also help children learn skills that will help them make the transition to kindergarten.
- If you choose not to enroll your child in child care or preschool, visit a teacher's store or bookstore to look at books for ideas about preparing your child for the transition to school.

Full "toilet independence" may be a requirement for attendance at preschool or child care programs. This usually is not achieved before the child is at a developmental age of $2\frac{1}{2}$ years. Children $2\frac{1}{2}$ and older who are not yet toilet trained are likely to respond best to an approach that includes encouragement, with respect for the child's own decision and determination to succeed.

SAMPLE QUESTION:
Where do things stand with toilet training?

ANTICIPATORY GUIDANCE:
- Use an approach that encourages your child to make the decision to use the potty. Do not force, punish, or shame him for accidents or reluctance to try. Instead, use praise for all efforts and interest, offer choices about trying the potty, and keep reading stories about potty training with your toddler.
- Here are some ways to help your child be successful: Dress him in easy-to-remove pants, establish a daily routine, place him on the potty every 1 to 2 hours, and provide a relaxed environment by reading or singing songs while he is on the potty.

SAFETY

Water safety, car safety seats, outdoor health and safety (pools, play areas, sun exposure), pets, fires and burns

Parents still must supervise their child closely to ensure her safety around water. All children require constant supervision by an adult whenever they are near water. Swim lessons do not prevent children from drowning, and children generally are not developmentally ready for formal swimming lessons until they are at least 4 years old.

SAMPLE QUESTIONS:
Are there swimming pools or other potential water dangers near your home? Does your child enjoy swimming?

Ask the Child:
Do you like swimming?

ANTICIPATORY GUIDANCE:
- Watch your toddler constantly whenever she is near water, including bathtubs, play pools, buckets, and the toilet. A supervising adult should be within an arm's reach, providing "touch supervision," whenever young children are in or around water.
- Do not expect young brothers or sisters to supervise your toddler in the bathtub, house, or yard.
- Empty buckets, tubs, or small pools immediately after use.
- Be sure that swimming pools in your community apartment complex or home have a 4-sided fence with a self-closing, self-latching gate.

Child Safety Seat Inspection Station Locator: www.seatcheck.org. Toll-free Number: 866-SEATCHECK (866-732-8243).

Talk with parents to ensure that they know how to securely fasten their child in a car safety seat. Adults should model car safety by always using a safety belt themselves.

Questions about proper installation should be referred to a certified Child Passenger Safety Technician in the community.
Child Safety Seat Inspection Station Locator: www.seatcheck.org
Toll-free Number: 866-SEATCHECK (866-732-8243)

SAMPLE QUESTIONS:
How is the car safety seat working for you? Is your child fastened securely in a car safety seat in the back seat every time she rides in a vehicle? Does everyone use a safety belt?

ANTICIPATORY GUIDANCE:
- Be sure your child's car safety seat is properly installed in the back seat according to the manufacturer's instructions and your vehicle's owner's manual. There should be no more than a finger's width of space between your child's collarbone and the harness strap.
- The back seat is the safest place for children to ride.
- Do not start your vehicle until everyone is buckled up. Children watch what parents do, so it is important for you to model safe behaviors by always wearing your safety belt.

Unintentional injury is the number one cause of death among young children. Because the urge to explore and learn is so strong, and young children do not have good judgment, parents must use constant vigilance and regularly review the safety of the environment to protect their young child from harm.

SAMPLE QUESTION:
Would you like a list of outdoor health and safety considerations for your toddler?

ANTICIPATORY GUIDANCE:
- When your toddler is playing outside, make sure she stays within fences and gates unless you or the adult supervisor are watching her closely.
- Carefully supervise young children using playground equipment, and make sure that the surface under play equipment is soft enough to absorb a fall.
- Keep your toddler away from moving machinery, lawn mowers, overhead garage doors, driveways, alleys, and streets.
- Be sure that your toddler wears a helmet that is approved by the CPSC when riding in a seat on an adult's bicycle or on a tricycle. Wear a helmet yourself.
- Limit time spent in the sun. Put sunscreen (SPF 15 or higher) on your toddler before she goes outside. Use a broad-brimmed hat to shade her ears, nose, and lips.
- Teach your toddler to ask permission before approaching dogs, especially if the dogs are unknown or are eating.

Young children require constant supervision around fires. They are fascinated by fire and its colors. They also may play with matches in an attempt to imitate parents who smoke. When playing, they often forget safety rules and can easily run into grills, stoves, and open fires.

SAMPLE QUESTIONS:
Where are the smoke detectors located in the home where your child lives? When did you last change the batteries in the smoke detectors? What is your plan for getting everyone out of the house and to a meeting place once outside? Do you have a neighbor from whose house you can call the fire department?

ANTICIPATORY GUIDANCE:
- Make sure you have a working smoke detector on every level of your home, especially in the furnace and sleeping areas. Test smoke detectors every month. It is best to use smoke detectors that use long-life batteries, but, if you do not, change the batteries at least once a year.
- Develop an escape plan in the event of a fire in your home.
- Install a carbon monoxide detector/alarm, certified by UL, in the hallway near every separate sleeping area of the home.
- Put matches well out of sight and reach of your child, or keep them in a locked cabinet.
- Watch your child closely when you are near a hot grill, the stove, or an open fire. Place a barrier around open fires, fire pits, or campfires.

Early Childhood: 3 Year Visit

CONTEXT

Around his third birthday, a very self-determined individualist makes his presence known. His successes or failures at controlling the world around him will influence his behavior. As he makes his own simple choices, he is able to learn from trial and error and has a new sense of right and wrong. He looks forward to something pleasant or perceives an encounter as disagreeable. Unpredictability still reigns, however, as he decides whether to fight or to talk his way out of situations in which he feels unsure of himself.

Speech and motor activity are now focused on investigating or modifying the environment. The 3-year-old has developed understandable speech—a major achievement. He can now negotiate with his parents (eg, "Story first and then nap."). He also makes choices, deciding between green and blue socks or between a tea party and playing outside. Body shape has developed from the pudgy baby mold to a more grown-up image. Awareness of gender differences has begun to emerge, in terms of both physical differences and society's expectations. Most 3-year-olds can easily state, "I am a girl" or "I am a boy." The 3-year-old's physical abilities have improved as well, giving him better control over what his hands are touching or where his feet take him. With his greater quickness and agility come new safety concerns (for instance, teaching new rules and cautions around cars and streets).

The 3-year-old's increasingly well-developed capacity to communicate his interests, desires, and preferences opens up a new world of social interaction. With children his age, language provides a new means for discovering mutual interests. At home, he proudly shows his ability to independently carry out activities of everyday living, such as feeding, bathing, and dressing. These activities still require supervision even though he wants to do it "all by myself." Food selection, for example, should remain a parental decision with minimal deviation allowed from the family's meals and food choices.

Including the child in interactions within the family, asking the child for opinions, and allowing the child to contribute to discussions within the family encourage his self-esteem and reinforces his special place in the family. Frequent family transitions often occur during this year, including pregnancy or birth of a sibling and the progression into a preschool or other educational setting. These transitions call for additional support and education by the health care professional.

PRIORITIES FOR THE VISIT

The first priority is to attend to the concerns of the parents. In addition, the Bright Futures Early Childhood Expert Panel has given priority to the following topics for discussion in this visit:

- Family support (family decisions, sibling rivalry, work balance)
- Encouraging literacy activities (singing, talking, describing, observing, reading)
- Playing with peers (interactive games, play opportunities)
- Promoting physical activity (limits on inactivity)
- Safety (car safety seats, pedestrian safety, falls from windows, guns)

HEALTH SUPERVISION

History

Interval history may be obtained according to the concerns of the family and the health care professional's preference or style of practice. The following questions can encourage in-depth discussion:

- How are you feeling as a parent?
- How are things going with your family and at preschool or child care?
- What major stresses or changes have occurred in your family since your last visit?
- What questions or concerns would you like to share with me about your child?
- What is something funny, or wonderful, or maddening that your child has done lately?

Observation of Parent-Child Interaction

During the visit, the health care professional should observe:

- How do the parent and the child communicate?
- How much of the communication is verbal? Nonverbal?
- Does the parent use baby talk?
- Does the parent give the child choices (eg, "Do you want to sit or stand?")?
- Does the parent encourage the child's cooperation during the visit?
- Does unacceptable behavior elicit appropriate responses from the parent?

Surveillance of Development

Do you have any specific concerns about your child's development, learning, or behavior?

SOCIAL-EMOTIONAL

■ **How does your child help with taking care of himself?**
- Has self-care skills (eg, self-feeding and self-dressing to the extent this is desired and permitted within individual family and cultural norms)

■ **Tell me about your child's typical play.**
- Imaginative play is becoming more elaborate, with specific themes or story lines demonstrated
- Enjoys interactive play

COMMUNICATIVE

■ **How does your child communicate what he wants?**
- Carries on a conversation with 2 to 3 sentences spoken together
- Is understandable to others 75% of the time
- Names a friend

COGNITIVE

■ **What do you think your child understands?**
- Knows the name of and the use of a cup, ball, spoon, and crayon
- Identifies self as a girl or a boy

PHYSICAL DEVELOPMENT

■ **What activities is he able to do?**
- Builds a tower of 6 to 8 cubes
- Throws a ball overhand
- Rides a tricycle
- Walks up stairs alternating feet
- Balances on 1 foot for 1 second

■ **Tell me what your child is drawing.**
- Copies a circle
- Draws a person with 2 body parts (head and one other part)

■ **How is toilet training going?**
- Is toilet trained during the daytime for both bowel and bladder

Physical Examination

A complete physical examination is included as part of every health supervision visit.

When performing a physical examination, the health care professional's attention is directed to the following components of the examination that are important for a child this age:

- **Measure:**
  - Blood pressure
- **Measure and plot:**
  - Height
  - Weight

- **Calculate and plot:**
  - BMI
- **Eyes**
  - Attempt to perform ophthalmoscopic examination of optic nerve and retinal vessels
- **Mouth**
  - Observe for caries, plaque, demineralization (white spots), staining, injury, and gingivitis
- **Neurologic**
  - Observe language acquisition and speech clarity
  - Note adult-child interaction

Screening

UNIVERSAL SCREENING	ACTION	
Visual acuity	Objective measure with age-appropriate visual acuity measurement (using HOTV; tumbling E tests; Snellen letters; Snellen numbers; or Picture tests such as Allen figures or LEA symbols)[†]	

SELECTIVE SCREENING	RISK ASSESSMENT*	ACTION IF RA +
Oral health	Does not have a dental home	Referral to dental home
	Primary water source is deficient in fluoride	Oral fluoride supplementation
Hearing	+ on risk screening questions	Referral for diagnostic audiologic assessment
Anemia	+ on risk screening questions	Hematocrit or hemoglobin
Lead	If no previous screen and + on risk screening questions or change in risk	Lead screen
Tuberculosis	+ on risk screening questions	Tuberculin skin test

†If patient is uncooperative, rescreen within 6 months.
*See Rationale and Evidence chapter for the criteria on which risk screening questions are based.

Immunizations

Consult the CDC/ACIP or AAP Web sites for the current immunization schedule.
CDC National Immunization Program (NIP): http://www.cdc.gov/vaccines
American Academy of Pediatrics *Red Book:* http://www.aapredbook.org

ANTICIPATORY GUIDANCE

The following sample questions, which address the Early Childhood Expert Panel's Anticipatory Guidance Priorities, are intended to be used selectively to invite discussion, gather information, address the needs and concerns of the family, and build partnerships. Use of the questions may vary from visit to visit and from family to family. Questions can be modified to match the health care professional's communication style. The accompanying anticipatory guidance for the family should be geared to questions, issues, or concerns for that particular child and family.

FAMILY SUPPORT

Family decisions, sibling rivalry, work balance

It is often helpful to engage parents in a discussion about their experiences as children to help them gain insight into why they parent their children as they do and to help them learn alternative strategies if they tend to use unhelpful or harmful strategies.

SAMPLE QUESTIONS:

Has anything changed at home since your last visit? Tell me how family members show affection for one another? Anger? Describe what you do together as a family. How often do you do these things?

Ask the Child

Who loves you? How do you know? What do you do when you are really mad? What do your parents do? What do you like to do best with your parents?

ANTICIPATORY GUIDANCE:

- Don't be surprised if you talk, act, and think in the same ways as your parents did when you were a child. After all, that was your primary experience. You can use this awareness to think about how you want to come across to your own children. What did you like about your parents' style and how would you like to be different?
- Show affection in your family.
- Handle anger constructively in your family by settling disputes with respectful discussion, exercise, or time alone to cool down.
- Don't allow your child to hit, bite, or use other violent behavior. Stop it immediately and explain how the behavior makes the other person feel. Help your child apologize.
- Reinforce limits and appropriate behavior. Enlist all caregivers in efforts to be consistent in expectations and discipline.
- Use time-outs or remove the source of conflict.
- Give your child opportunities to make choices, such as what clothes to wear, books to read, and places to go.

EARLY CHILDHOOD
3 YEAR VISIT

443

Siblings play a special role in the socialization and development of self-esteem in the young child. Many parents require advice on how to handle sibling rivalry.

SAMPLE QUESTIONS:
How do your children get along with one another? How are you preparing your child for the birth of a new baby?
Ask the Child
What do you like to do best with your brothers and sisters?

ANTICIPATORY GUIDANCE:
- Help your children develop good relationships with each other. Acknowledge conflicts between siblings and, whenever possible, try to resolve them without taking sides.
- Spend some individual time with each child in your family.

In many families, both parents work full-time or part-time. Encourage working parents to maintain family time and to be active together.

SAMPLE QUESTIONS:
If you or your partner work outside the home, how does work affect you and your family? Who takes care of your children? How much time does it allow for family activities?

ANTICIPATORY GUIDANCE:
- Take time for yourself and spend time alone with your partner.
- Create opportunities for your family to share time together and for family members to talk, read, and play with your child.

ENCOURAGING LITERACY ACTIVITIES

Singing, talking, describing, observing, reading

Encourage interactive reading (reading in which parent and child talk together about the text and pictures as well as the parent reading the book to the child) between parent and child every day and provide specific advice for parents with no or low literacy. Gaining an awareness of syllables and sounds (phonological awareness) is an important readiness activity for early literacy.

SAMPLE QUESTIONS:
How often are you able to read to your child? How do you include your child in reading books?
Ask the Child
What is your favorite book?

ANTICIPATORY GUIDANCE:
- Encourage your child's language development and awareness of sounds by reading books, singing songs, and playing rhyming games. Look for ways to practice reading wherever you go (eg, STOP signs or boxes at the supermarket).
- Ask your child questions about the story or pictures. Let him "tell" part of the story.

Language continues to develop rapidly at this age. Children should be using plurals, pronouns, sentences of 4 or 5 words, and short paragraphs. Speech is understandable to others 75% of the time. They also should be able to name most common objects, know gender differences, and understand 2-step instructions, such as, "Pick up your doll and put it on the chair."

SAMPLE QUESTIONS:

How does your child tell you what he wants? What do you think your child understands? What language(s) does your family speak at home? How well do family members understand your child's speech?

ANTICIPATORY GUIDANCE:

- Encourage your child to talk with you about his preschool, friends, experiences, and observations.
- Use books as a way to talk together. You don't always have to read the text to your child. You can just look at the pictures and talk about the story.

PLAYING WITH PEERS

Interactive games, play opportunities

Playtime with peers provides valuable opportunities for learning social skills that are important to a successful transition to school. Encourage parents whose children are not in preschool to arrange playdates for their child.

SAMPLE QUESTIONS:

What are some of the new things that your child is doing? What do you and your partner enjoy most about her these days? What seems most difficult? Tell me about your child's typical play. How does your child interact with children her age? At child care or otherwise? Does she engage in imaginative play with other children?

Ask the Child

What is your favorite toy?

ANTICIPATORY GUIDANCE:

- Encourage your child to play with her favorite toys. Toys should be appropriate for her age.
- Expect her to engage in increasingly elaborate fantasy play, using dolls, toy animals, and other toys, on her own and with others.
- Spend time alone with your child, doing something you both enjoy.
- Provide opportunities for your child to safely explore the world around her.
- If your child is not in child care or preschool, make sure she has opportunities to play with other children.
- Encourage interactive games with peers and help her understand the importance of taking turns.

PROMOTING PHYSICAL ACTIVITY

Limits on inactivity

By this age, many children have mastered running and marching, and have begun to master galloping. Children need to play every day; it is their "job." It is helpful if adults guide children in learning how to master physical activity skills. Adults show children ways to move their bodies, how to move around and through objects, and how to improve their large- and small-muscle movements. Although preschool-aged children naturally do this when they play, adult guidance improves their fitness levels (stability, agility, endurance, and coordination).

Children should not be inactive for more than 60 minutes at a time, except when sleeping. Counsel parents to limit screen time to no more than 1 to 2 hours per day. Children should not have televisions or DVD players in their bedrooms.

Talk with parents of children with special health care needs (whether physically or cognitively delayed) to ensure that they have opportunities to be physically active.

SAMPLE QUESTIONS:
Tell me about what you and your child enjoy doing together each day. How much time does your child spend watching TV or videos each day? Does he have a TV in his bedroom? If your child is in child care or preschool, what types of physical activity are offered daily?
Ask the Child
Let me see how fast you can run. What are your favorite games? Do you like to play inside or outside?

ANTICIPATORY GUIDANCE:
- Create opportunities for your family to share time and exercise together.
- Promote physical activity in a safe environment at home and in preschool.
- Limit all forms of screen time to no more than 1 to 2 hours total per day. Do not put a TV or DVD player in your child's bedroom.
- Monitor the TV programs your child watches. Be aware that commercials strongly influence even young children to want things that are not healthy for them.

SAFETY

Car safety seats, pedestrian safety, falls from windows, guns

Talk with parents to ensure that they and their child's caregivers know how to securely fasten their child in a car safety seat. Adults should model car safety by always using a safety belt themselves.

Questions about proper installation should be referred to a certified Child Passenger Safety Technician in the community.
Child Safety Seat Inspection Station Locator: www.seatcheck.org
Toll-free Number: 866-SEATCHECK (866-732-8243)

Child Safety Seat Inspection Station Locator: www.seatcheck.org. **Toll-free Number: 866-SEATCHECK (866-732-8243).**

446

Bright FUTURES

SAMPLE QUESTIONS:

Is your child fastened securely in a car safety seat in the back seat every time she rides in a vehicle? Are you having any problems using your car safety seat?

Ask the Child

Where do you sit when you ride in the car? Do you have a special seat?

ANTICIPATORY GUIDANCE:

- Continue to use a size-appropriate forward-facing safety seat that is properly installed in the back seat according to the manufacturer's instructions and the vehicle owner's manual.
- When your child reaches the highest weight or height allowed by the manufacturer, her shoulders are above the top harness slots, or her ears come to the top of the car safety seat, consider whether she is mature enough for the greater flexibility of movement allowed by a belt-positioning booster seat. If not, use a forward-facing seat with a harness with a higher weight limit or a travel vest.
- The back seat is the safest place for children to ride.

Death from unintentional injuries is the number one cause of death among young children. Because the urge to explore and learn is so strong, and young children do not have good judgment, parents must use constant vigilance and regularly review the safety of the environment to protect them from harm.

Remind parents about the importance of installing operable window guards on all windows on the second floor and higher.

SAMPLE QUESTIONS:

Who watches your child when you cannot? Does your child play in a driveway or close to the street? What floor in your house or apartment do you live on? Do you have window guards on all windows on the second floor and higher?

Ask the Child

When you play outside, who watches you? Who watches you when your parents are gone?

ANTICIPATORY GUIDANCE:

- Never leave your child alone in the car, house, or yard.
- Do not expect young brothers or sister to watch over your child.
- Supervise all play near streets or driveways. Your child is not ready to cross the street alone.
- Remember that many young children are excellent climbers. To prevent children from falling out of windows, keep furniture away from windows and install operable window guards on second- and higher-story windows.

Young children are curious about everything, including guns, and have no concept of the consequences of firing a weapon. Encourage parents to remove guns from their home. If it is necessary to keep a gun in the home, encourage parents to store it unloaded and locked, with the ammunition locked separately from the gun.

SAMPLE QUESTION:

Is there a gun in your home or in the homes where your child might play or go for child care?

ANTICIPATORY GUIDANCE:

- Remember that young children simply do not understand how dangerous guns can be, despite your warnings. The best way to keep your child safe from injury or death from guns is to never have a gun in your home.
- Children this age are naturally curious and will get into everything! Just as you need to keep medications, cleaning solutions, and insecticides out of children's reach, loaded guns should never be anywhere where your child can get to them. If it is necessary to keep a gun in your home, it should be stored unloaded and locked, with the ammunition locked separately from the gun.
- Ask if there are guns in homes where your child plays. If so, make sure they are stored unloaded and locked, with the ammunition locked separately, before allowing your child to play in the home.

Early Childhood: 4 Year Visit

CONTEXT

Rapidly developing language skills, combined with an insatiable curiosity, enlarge the world of the 4-year-old and give him a sense of independence. Able to dress and undress himself and maintain bowel and bladder control (although he may not be dry at night), the 4-year-old feels grown up beyond his years. Though his thinking remains self-focused, he is sensitive to the feelings of others. He identifies such emotions as joy, happiness, sadness, anger, anxiety, and fear, in others as well as himself. Now he plays collaboratively and he has budding friendships with his peers.

Talkative and animated, the 4-year-old is a delightful conversationalist, able to tell an involved story or relate a recent experience. He frequently demands to know why, what, when, and how. His seemingly boundless energy and increased motor skills find release in group games and physical activities, such as running, climbing, swinging, sliding, and jumping. Yet, he also needs opportunities to rest and play quietly by himself. Imaginative play, including make-believe and dress up, reflect the fantasy and "magical thinking" of this age. Television, computer games, and even educational videos may hold a strong appeal for this new fascination with fantasy and may hold excessive power over his time and attention unless limited by parents and child care providers.

Because 4-year-olds are curious about their own bodies and those of the opposite sex, sexual exploration is typical at this age.

Modesty and a desire for privacy begin to emerge. Every culture looks at sexual behaviors and explorations in different ways. It is the responsibility of the health care professional to understand the cultural norms of the child's family when addressing the topic of sexuality. In fact, in some cultures, it is inappropriate to discuss this subject, and that belief must be respected. Whenever possible, health care practices should employ staff from the communities served and ask everyone to become knowledgeable about the cultural beliefs of the community.

The child enjoys and looks forward to the social and learning opportunities at preschool. "Scrappy" behavior with peers can present a problem at preschool or during play, but the 4-year-old can learn to be assertive without being aggressive. Making allowances for the appropriateness of the match between the child and the program, the 4-year-old's experiences in the early education and child care settings provide an important measure of his social development and his developing readiness for elementary school.

The 4-year-old's family finds his behavior frustrating and challenging at times. He is still trying to understand how and why things work as they do and he is interested in seeing the consequences of his actions on family members. How many times will his parents say "No" before they get angry? How far off the sidewalk can he stray before they chase after him? How many toys can he take before his sister protests? In his efforts to learn about appropriate social interaction and expected behavior in the family, he frequently tests the limits of his parents and siblings. On the other hand, the 4-year-old responds well to praise and clearly stated rules.

Reassure the child at the beginning of the physical exam through talking and through touch. The child should be able to discuss the function of the eyes and ears, memories of the last visit, or how to take a bath. It may be possible to perform the exam moving from head to toe. Talking about the physical findings is instructive to the child and parent and demystifies the office visit. The child at 4 often participates in the exam to a much greater degree than at past visits. Speaking to the child about what is being examined and how, and including the child in conversation about his ears, eyes, muscles, and other body parts, successfully engages the 4-year-old's curiosity and gains his cooperation.

PRIORITIES FOR THE VISIT

The first priority is to attend to the concerns of the parents. In addition, the Bright Futures Early Childhood Expert Panel has given priority to the following topics for discussion in this visit:

- School readiness (structured learning experiences, opportunities to socialize with other children, fears, friends, fluency)
- Developing healthy personal habits (daily routines that promote health)
- Television/media (limits on viewing, promotion of physical activity and safe play)
- Child and family involvement and safety in the community (activities outside the home, community projects, educational programs, relating to peers and adults, domestic violence)
- Safety (belt positioning booster seats, supervision, outdoor safety, guns)

HEALTH SUPERVISION

History

Interval history may be obtained according to the concerns of the family and the health care professional's preference or style of practice. The following questions can encourage in-depth discussion:

- How is your child doing at preschool or child care?
- What questions or concerns do you have about him? His health? His ability to get along with other people?
- How are things going for your family?
- How are things going for your child?
- What changes or stresses have occurred in your family lately?

Observation of Parent-Child Interaction

During the visit, the health care professional should observe:

- How do the parent and the child communicate?
- Does the parent allow the child to answer the health care professional's questions directly, or does the parent intervene?
- Does the child separate from the parent for the weighing and measuring and the physical exam?
- Does the child dress and undress himself?
- Does the parent pay attention to the child's behavior, matching unacceptable behavior with consequences?
- How do the parent, the 4-year-old, and any siblings interact? Who sits where? Does the parent pay attention to all of the children?
- If offered 2 or more books to choose from, does the parent advise and encourage, and then let the child choose?

Surveillance of Development

Do you have any specific concerns about your child's development, learning, or behavior?

SOCIAL-EMOTIONAL

■ **How does your child describe himself?**
  • Describes features of himself, including gender, age, interests, and strengths

■ **How does your child act around other children?**
  • Is responsive or withdrawn
  • Is friendly or hostile/aggressive
  • Is cooperative or defiant
  • Acts appropriately for the community's or family's cultural values

■ **Tell me about your child's typical play.**
  • Plays with favorite toys *(describe play)*
  • Listens to stories
  • Engages in fantasy play

COMMUNICATIVE

■ **How does your child communicate?**
  • Gives first and last name
  • Sings a song or says a poem from memory
  • Knows what to do if cold, tired, or hungry
  • Is clearly understandable with most speech efforts

COGNITIVE

■ **What do you think your child understands?**
  • Names 4 colors
  • Is aware of gender (of self and others)
  • Plays board/card games
  • Draws a person with 3 parts
  • Tells you what he thinks is going to happen next in a book

PHYSICAL DEVELOPMENT

■ **What physical activities is your child able to do?**
  • Hops on one foot
  • Balances on one foot for 2 seconds
  • Builds a tower of 8 blocks
  • Copies a cross

■ **How does your child help with eating and dressing?**
  • Pours, cuts, and mashes own food
  • Brushes own teeth
  • Dresses self, including buttons

Physical Examination

A complete physical examination is included as part of every health supervision visit.

When performing a physical examination, the health care professional's attention is directed to the following components of the examination that are important for a child this age:

- **Measure**
  - Blood pressure

- **Measure and plot:**
  - Height
  - Weight
- **Calculate and plot:**
  - BMI
- **Neurologic**
  - Observe fine and gross motor skills
  - Assess language acquisition, speech fluency and clarity, thought content, and abstraction

Screening

UNIVERSAL SCREENING	ACTION	
Visual acuity	Objective measure with age-appropriate visual acuity measurement (using HOTV; tumbling E tests; Snellen letters; Snellen numbers; or Picture tests such as Allen figures or LEA symbols)	
Hearing	Audiometry	
SELECTIVE SCREENING	RISK ASSESSMENT*	ACTION IF RA +
Anemia	+ on risk screening questions	Hematocrit or hemoglobin
Lead	If no previous screen and + on risk screening questions or change in risk	Lead screen
Tuberculosis	+ on risk screening questions	Tuberculin skin test
Dyslipidemia	+ on risk screening questions and not previously screened with normal results	Fasting lipid profile

*See Rationale and Evidence chapter for the criteria on which risk screening questions are based.

Immunizations

Consult the CDC/ACIP or AAP Web sites for the current immunization schedule.

CDC National Immunization Program (NIP): http://www.cdc.gov/vaccines
American Academy of Pediatrics *Red Book:* http://www.aapredbook.org

EARLY CHILDHOOD
4 YEAR VISIT

453

ANTICIPATORY GUIDANCE

The following sample questions, which address the Early Childhood Expert Panel's Anticipatory Guidance Priorities, are intended to be used selectively to invite discussion, gather information, address the needs and concerns of the family, and build partnerships. Use of the questions may vary from visit to visit and from family to family. Questions can be modified to match the health care professional's communication style. The accompanying anticipatory guidance for the family should be geared to questions, issues, or concerns for that particular child and family.

SCHOOL READINESS

Structured learning experiences, opportunities to socialize with other children, fears, friends, fluency

A 4-year-old best understands explanations that are short and to the point, and that refer to the direct experiences of the child.

SAMPLE QUESTIONS:
What do you think your child understands? For example, can she understand:
- *Concepts of "same" and "different"?*
- *2- or 3-step instructions?*

ANTICIPATORY GUIDANCE:
- Because children this age ask many questions, it is easy to offer too much information. It is best to keep answers short, simple, and factual.

At 4 years of age, children are very sensitive. They wear their feelings on their sleeves and are easily encouraged or hurt by what people say or do to them.

SAMPLE QUESTIONS:
How does your child act around others? Is she:
- *Responsive or withdrawn?*
- *Friendly or hostile/aggressive?*
- *Cooperative or defiant?*
- *Dependent or self-reliant?*
Are her current behaviors consistent with her past temperamental style?

ANTICIPATORY GUIDANCE:
- Watching your child interact with other children provides a valuable window into her social understanding and skills.
- Listen to and always treat your child with the respect you offer a fellow adult. Insist that all family members treat one another with respect and model respectful behavior for your children.
- Model apologizing if you are wrong or have hurt someone's feelings. Help your child apologize for hurting others' feelings, too. Praise her when she demonstrates sensitivity to the feelings of others.

SAMPLE QUESTIONS:

How interested is your child in other children? How confident is she socially and emotionally? Who are her special playmates?

Ask the Child

Who do you like to play with? Do you have a favorite friend?

ANTICIPATORY GUIDANCE:

- Praise your child for her cooperation and accomplishments.
- Help your child express such feelings as joy, anger, sadness, fear, and frustration.
- Spend time alone with your child doing something you both enjoy.
- Provide opportunities for your child to play with other children in playgroups, preschool, or other community activities.

Readiness for school is a lengthy process that begins at birth. Advise parents about ways to prepare their child for a successful transition to school. Early literacy skills are emerging as children show interest in letters and play with sounds making rhymes of real and nonsense words.

SAMPLE QUESTIONS:

How is your child learning and getting ready for school? What thoughts have you had about starting her in school in the year ahead?

ANTICIPATORY GUIDANCE:

- Read interactively with your child. Reading with your child is important to help her like reading and be ready for school.
- As your child shows interest in words, engage her by pointing out letters, particularly the ones that begins her name ("It's a T like in Taylor!"), and playing with sounds by making rhymes of real and nonsense words ("oodles and boodles of noodles and foodles").
- Enlarge your child's experiences through trips and visits to parks and other places of interest. Take her often to the library. Ask whether she can get a library card and let her choose books that interest her.
- Consider some type of structured learning environment for your child, whether in Head Start, preschool, Sunday school, or a community program or child care center.
- Let's talk about how to determine when your child is ready for school.

SAMPLE QUESTIONS:

How happy are you with your child care arrangements? What does your child care provider or teacher say about your child? On most days, does she seem happy to go? How many other children are in her class and how is she coping socially?

Ask the Child

What do you like to do best at child care/preschool?

ANTICIPATORY GUIDANCE:

- If your child is in child care, continue to provide personal items, such as blankets, clothing, combs, and brushes, for her own use.
- Visit your child's preschool or other child care program. You can learn a lot about what really goes on at the program if you arrive unannounced.
- Show interest in your child's preschool and/or child care activities.

Children may show some lack of fluency (stuttering) when speaking.

As children develop speech and language skills, they often experience normal disfluencies such as repetitions of whole words, and false starts and revisions in sentences. Most children outgrow stuttering. Indications for speech evaluation include stuttering for more than 6 months and no improvement during this time. Referral may be appropriate if the parent describes the child as struggling to get words out and showing signs of distress about difficulties with speaking.

SAMPLE QUESTIONS
How does your child communicate what she wants and knows? Can she:
- *Speak clearly enough so that strangers understand her almost 100% of the time?*
- *Use the past as well as the present tense?*
- *Use sentences of 4 or 5 words and short paragraphs?*
- *Describe a recent experience?*

Ask the Child
Do you have a favorite story book that you like to hear?

ANTICIPATORY GUIDANCE:
- Help your child develop her language skills by encouraging her to talk with you about her preschool, friends, experiences, or observations.
- Read together daily and ask your child questions about the stories.
- Provide plenty of time for your child to tell stories or respond to questions. Hurrying a child's response increases stuttering.
- Allow children to finish sentences and thoughts, do not interrupt, speak in a relaxed tone, and pause before responding.

DEVELOPING HEALTHY PERSONAL HABITS

Daily routines that promote health

The 4-year-old typically enjoys being recognized as being "big enough" to assume greater independence in daily routines. Nightmares and night terrors are common at this age. Discuss the parents' approach to sleep disturbances. Family stresses and TV viewing habits should be evaluated in children with sleep disturbances.

SAMPLE QUESTIONS:
How is he sleeping at night? Does he still require a nap on most days? Are you encouraging him to take a more active role in daily routines connected with mealtimes, cleanliness, and help around the house?

Ask the Child
Are you eating good food to keep you strong? Are you getting good at brushing your teeth and washing your hands? Can you fasten your own safety belt?

ANTICIPATORY GUIDANCE:
- Create a calm bedtime ritual that includes reading or telling stories to promote language development and pre-reading skills and to help your child sleep peacefully.

- A poor appetite or limited food preference is not a major concern if your child's growth rate has been normal. Create a pleasant atmosphere at mealtimes by turning off the TV and having table conversation that includes your child.
- Be sure that your child brushes his teeth twice a day with a pea-sized amount of fluoridated toothpaste. He should spit out the toothpaste after brushing, but not rinse his mouth with water. Supervise tooth brushing each time.

TELEVISION/MEDIA

Limits on viewing, promotion of physical activity and safe play

Television and video viewing, especially when a child has a unit in her own room, has been associated with overweight in children.

Television and other media viewing also have been shown to increase violence in children, create conflicts over purchase of advertised products, and decrease time for physically active play. Judicious use of educational media can improve school readiness in children.

Children should spend less than 2 hours total a day watching any type of media. They should not have a TV in their bedroom.

SAMPLE QUESTIONS:
How many video players and televisions are in your house? Does your child have one in her bedroom?
Ask the Child
What is your favorite TV show or video? Why do you like it?

ANTICIPATORY GUIDANCE:
- Limit television and video viewing to no more than 2 hours per day. Be sure the programs are appropriate. If you allow your child to watch TV, watch with her and talk together about the programs.

Unless a child has a developmental delay, she should be able to run, march, and gallop, and try to jump by this age.

SAMPLE QUESTIONS:
Does your child play with other children? Does she play outdoors as well as indoors? Is your community safe for her to play outdoors?
Ask the Child
Let me see you hop. What else do you like to do when you play?

ANTICIPATORY GUIDANCE:
- Encourage your child to be active in many ways, including running, marching, and jumping. Praise her for her ability to do these activities.
- As often as possible, be physically active as a family. Go on walks, play in the park or on a safe street, or ride bikes. Use this time to help your child get to know her community.
- Make sure your child has plenty of opportunity for active play at child care or preschool.

CHILD AND FAMILY INVOLVEMENT AND SAFETY IN THE COMMUNITY

Activities outside the home, community projects, educational programs, relating to peers and adults, domestic violence

Talk with the parents about possible programs for their child, including preschool, Head Start, special education programs, or other community programs.

SAMPLE QUESTIONS:

Do you need help in finding and signing up for educational opportunities for your child? What activities do you participate in outside of the home? What help do you need in finding other community resources, such as a faith-based group, recreational centers, or volunteer opportunities? What help do you need in finding safe places in your community where your child can play and participate in other activities?

ANTICIPATORY GUIDANCE:

- Maintain or expand ties to your community through social, faith-based, cultural, volunteer, and recreational organizations or programs.
- Participate in community projects that provide opportunities for physical activity for the whole family (eg, walk-a-thons, community cleanup day, or a community garden project).
- Find out what you can do to make your community safe.
- Advocate for and participate in a neighborhood watch program.
- Advocate for adequate housing and for safe play spaces and playgrounds.

Parents should know the adults with whom their children will come in contact. Parents should keep their children away from any adult or older child they think may be dangerous.

SAMPLE QUESTIONS:

How safe do you feel in your community? Do you or other trusted adults watch over your child when he is in the neighborhood? How cautious is your child around strangers?

ANTICIPATORY GUIDANCE:

- Anticipate your child's normal curiosity about his body and the differences between boys and girls.
- Use correct terms for all body parts, including genitals.
- Explain to your child that certain parts of the body (those areas normally covered by a bathing suit) are private and should not be touched by others without his permission.
- We used to be worried about strangers. Now we know that abusers are often a person the child should be able to trust. Teach your child rules for how to be safe with other adults, using these 3 principles: (1) no adult should tell a child to keep secrets from parents, (2) no adult should express interest in private parts, and (3) no adult should ask a child for help with his or her own private parts.

Some health care professionals prefer to use a written screen or a screen administered by a nurse to assess for potential domestic violence when verbal children are present. This will help increase disclosure and minimize increasing risk of violence in the family.

Provide information on the impact of domestic violence on children and on community resources that provide assistance. Recommend resources and support groups. Many states have laws that require all cases of domestic violence be reported when there is a child in the home.

SAMPLE QUESTIONS:

Because violence is so common in many people's lives, I've begun to ask about it. I don't know if this is a problem for you, but many children I see have parents who have been hurt by someone else. Some are too afraid or uncomfortable to bring it up, so I've started asking about it routinely.

Do you always feel safe in your home? Are you scared that your partner or someone else may try to hurt you or your child? What will you do if you feel this way? Do you have a plan? How do you handle the feeling? Would you like information about who to contact or where to go if you need help?

ANTICIPATORY GUIDANCE:

- One way that I and other health care professionals can help you if your partner is hitting or threatening you is to support you and provide information about local resources that can help you.

SAFETY

Belt positioning booster seats, supervision, outdoor safety, guns

Child Safety Seat Inspection Station Locator: www.seatcheck.org. Toll-free Number: 866-SEATCHECK (866-732-8243).

Around this age, most children will transition to a belt-positioning booster seat. Adults should model car safety by always using a safety belt themselves.

Questions about proper installation should be referred to a certified Child Passenger Safety Technician in the community.
Child Safety Seat Inspection Station Locator: www.seatcheck.org
Toll-free Number: 866-SEATCHECK (866-732-8243)

SAMPLE QUESTIONS:

Is your child fastened securely in a car safety seat or belt-positioning booster seat in the back seat every time she rides in a vehicle?

Ask the Child

Where do you sit when you ride in the car? Do you have a special seat?

ANTICIPATORY GUIDANCE:
- Continue to use a size-appropriate forward-facing car safety seat that is properly installed in the back seat according to the manufacturer's instructions and the vehicle owner's manual until your child reaches the highest weight or height allowed by the manufacturer, her shoulders are above the top harness slots, or her ears come to the top of the car safety seat. When she reaches one of these limits, consider whether she is mature enough for the greater flexibility of movement allowed by a belt-positioning booster seat. If not, use a forward-facing seat with a harness with a higher weight limit or a travel vest.
- The back seat is the safest place for children to ride.

Young children lack the neurologic maturity, skills, and knowledge needed to safely cross the street. They have not developed neurologically enough to have the skills to see cars in their peripheral vision, localize sounds, and judge vehicle distance and speed. In general, children are not ready to cross the street alone until they are 10 years old or older. Parents must use constant vigilance and regularly review the safety of the environment to protect their young child from harm.

SAMPLE QUESTIONS:
Where does your child play when she goes outdoors? Who watches your child when you cannot?
Ask the Child
When you play outside, who watches you? Who watches you when your parents are gone?

ANTICIPATORY GUIDANCE:
- Never leave your child alone when she is outside.
- Supervise all play near streets or driveways. Your child is not ready to cross the street alone.

Young children are curious about everything, including guns, and have no concept of the consequences of firing a weapon. Encourage parents to remove guns from their home. If it is necessary to keep a gun in their home, encourage them to store it unloaded and locked, with the ammunition locked separately from the gun.

SAMPLE QUESTION:
Is there a gun in your home or in the homes where your child might play or go for child care?

ANTICIPATORY GUIDANCE:
- The best way to keep your child safe from injury or death from guns is to never have a gun in the home.
- Remember that young children simply do not understand how dangerous guns can be, despite your warnings.

- Children this age are naturally curious, and will get into everything! Just as you need to keep medications, cleaning solutions, and insecticides out of children's reach, loaded guns should never be anywhere where the child can get to them. If it is necessary to keep a gun in your home, it should be stored unloaded and locked, with the ammunition locked separately from the gun.
- Ask if there are guns in homes where your child plays. If so, make sure they are stored unloaded and locked, with the ammunition locked separately, before allowing your child to play in the home.

Middle Childhood

5 to 10 Years

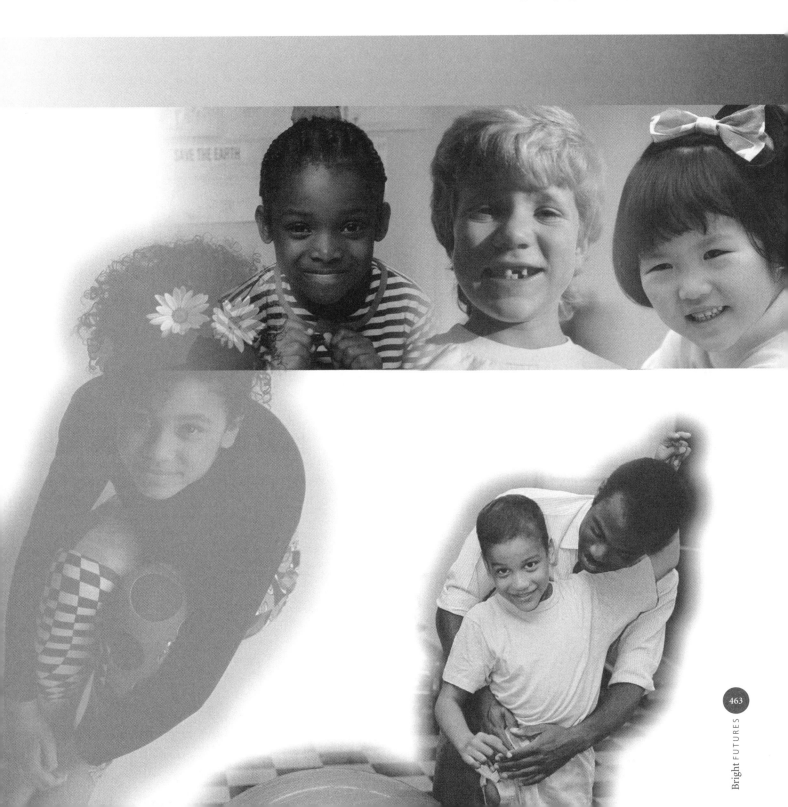

Middle Childhood: 5 and 6 Year Visits

CONTEXT

As the middle childhood stage begins, children are growing steadily and their physical competence continues to increase. Their improved language and communication skills match social competence to physical ability. They are prepared to move out of home care and child care or preschool. They are ready for school.

Starting school is a major milestone for the 5- or 6-year-old child and for his family. As he prepares to enter kindergarten or elementary school, key developmental issues emerge, such as his readiness for school and his ability to separate from his parents. The 5-year-old who has attended preschool or has been in child care out of the home may be able to separate from his parents more easily than children who have stayed at home. Most 6-year-olds will have attended kindergarten and acquired the social skills necessary for learning in a full-day, first-grade setting. By observing how the child responds to new situations, the parents, teacher, and health care professional can anticipate how temperament and experience may affect school readiness and competence. The 5 and 6 Year Visits permit observation of his ability to follow directions, as well as his language skills, maturity level, and motor ability.

Starting school brings new opportunities, challenges, and rules for children. School activities require increased impulse control. Children are expected to obey rules, get along with others, and avoid disruptive behavior. Paying attention to teachers and other adults can be difficult for some children. Acquiring skills in listening, reading, and math excites some children and challenges others. Children entering kindergarten will have many opportunities to make friends and meet other families. They may go on school field trips or participate in after-school activities. Some children can have difficulty adjusting to eating at school with self-service lunches or structured times for lunch and snacks. Most will manage these new challenges gracefully, while others struggle to learn appropriate behaviors during these transitions. Parents should listen to their child's feelings, reassure him, and praise his efforts and accomplishments.

A child's progress in school is an important factor in his development at this age. School-based assessments, report cards, and IEPs are used to track a child's progress. Children with special health care needs or children with developmental disability or delay likely will have been receiving services through your community's early childhood special education services program. Inquiry regarding transition from this program to kindergarten is appropriate.

Not every child is immediately successful in the school experience. Adjustment difficulties or psychosocial stressors must be addressed. Disorders of attention and learning are typically undetected until school entry. Federal education law requires school systems to evaluate children who are experiencing learning or developmental difficulties. Families may need help finding advocates for the exact services they need.

465

Each family will have its own perspective on how a child is performing in school. A child will perform best if he feels there is consistency between the expectations of the school and his family regarding educational performance and behavior at school. Parents sometimes need help in understanding the significance of particular academic struggles. In addition, the concept of a learning disability may not make sense within certain cultural beliefs about health or abilities.

Families who are newly immigrated may not understand the educational system in this country and may need guidance about what to expect and how they can be involved in supporting their child in school. If English is not spoken at home, health care professionals should assess the child's exposure to English and what resources are needed to support the important learning tasks ahead of her.

An increasing amount of time is spent with friends and others outside the home. Parents should meet these new friends and their families. Parents need to encourage their child's friendships and respect the growing influence of peers. Rules and behavioral expectations will vary among families, especially across cultures. As they acquire new experiences, 5- and 6-year-olds normally begin to test whether the rules can change now that they are older. Some rules can be loosened, but others must be maintained in the interest of sustaining appropriate behavior, providing emotional security and personal safety, and promoting moral upbringing.

Certain hazards, such as matches, cigarette lighters, gas stoves, and fireplaces, often fascinate 5- and 6-year-olds. Thus, parents should remember to keep matches and lighters out of reach, and remind children that these items are not toys. Parents should be cautioned specifically about the dangers of keeping guns in the home. It is critical that children continue to use appropriate car safety seats and booster seats.

The child's community affects safety concerns because the setting and seasonal climate determine common activities and risks. Traffic crashes and playing around cars are health risks for the young child, with a higher proportion of minority children experiencing death or injury than children of other races and ethnicities. Children living in poverty may have limited access to appropriate play areas or activities, and may be out in the neighborhood playing in unsafe venues. Families with limited economic resources may be able to find places in the community where they can receive help in obtaining low-cost bike helmets, car safety seats, and other safety equipment.

By his sixth birthday, a child is eager to act independently, but he is not yet able to consistently make good decisions. He likes to climb trees or fire escapes and play in the yard or on the sidewalk with other children, but he is still learning about safety. Children must learn to be safe at home, at school, on the playground, and in the neighborhood. Families will need to continue to set appropriate boundaries and other limits while encouraging and promoting their child's growing independence. Before he is ready to start exploring the community on his own, he must be able to remember and understand safety rules well enough to interpret them and adapt them for different situations. Children need rules for interacting with and avoiding strangers, as well as instructions on telephone numbers to call for help in case of emergencies. At this age, most children are riding bicycles or using in-line skates and may be learning to use skateboards and to swim. Parents need to teach, and frequently review with their child, the safety rules for playing on the playground, riding a bicycle in the neighborhood, and engaging in other recreational activities. Children this age are not yet ready to cross the street alone, and adult supervision also is needed for swimming and

5 and 6 Year Visits

other water sports. A child's bicycle should be suited to his ability level and adjusted to his size. He should always wear an approved helmet and protective equipment when riding, skateboarding, in-line skating, or playing in organized sports.

Newly found skills generate interest in testing physical prowess. How fast can he run? How far can he throw? As he learns how his body works, the 5- and 6-year-old gains the confidence and skills needed to enjoy physical activities or to participate in individual or team sports. A team sport focused on skill building and learning "sportsmanlike" behavior, rather than winning or keeping score, is a good way to encourage further engagement in physical activities. Parents should be sure that coaches' demands are reasonable. For children who are from cultures where gender roles and modesty issues preclude girls from participating in typical sports activities, opportunities for cooperation and physical development can be found in activities such as ethnic dance groups, scouting, or same-sex physical activities that are arranged by the cultural community.

As the child's cognitive skills continue to develop, his ability to understand and communicate becomes more sophisticated. At this age, health care professionals can talk directly with the child about his family, friends, and excitement or fears about going to school and becoming more independent. This provides an opportunity for the health care professional to develop a partnership directly with the child and to encourage him to assume responsibility for his clothes, toys, or other belongings, selected chores, and good health habits. These responsibilities will help promote autonomy, independence, and a sense of competence.

PRIORITIES FOR THE VISIT

The first priority is to attend to the concerns of the parents. In addition, the Bright Futures Middle Childhood Expert Panel has given priority to the following topics for discussion in this visit:

■ School readiness (established routines, after-school care and activities, parent-teacher communication, friends, bullying, maturity, management of disappointments, fears)
■ Mental health (family time, routines, temper problems, social interactions)
■ Nutrition and physical activity (healthy weight; appropriate well-balanced diet; increased fruit, vegetable, whole-grain consumption; adequate calcium intake; 60 minutes of exercise a day)
■ Oral health (regular visits with dentist, daily brushing and flossing, adequate fluoride)
■ Safety (pedestrian safety, booster seat, safety helmets, swimming safety, child sexual abuse prevention, fire escape/drill plan and smoke detectors, carbon monoxide detectors/alarms, guns)

HEALTH SUPERVISION

History

Interval history may be obtained according to the concerns of the family and the health care professional's preference or style of practice. The following questions can encourage in-depth discussion:

■ Do you have any concerns about your child's physical well-being or special health care needs?
■ Do you have any concerns about your child starting school or your child's school performance?
■ Do you have any concerns about your child's development (eg, walking, talking, drawing, or writing her name or ABCs)?
■ Do you have any concerns about your child's mood or behavior (eg, attention, hitting, temper, worries, not participating in play with others, irritability, mood, or activity level)?

Observation of Parent-Child Interaction

During the visit, the health care professional should observe:

■ Do both the parent and the child ask questions and speak directly with the health care professional, or does the parent dominate?
■ Do the parent and child make eye contact with each other and with the health care professional?
■ Does the parent attend to the child and listen to what the child has to say?
■ Does the parent praise, support, and seem proud of the child's abilities and accomplishments, or is the parent impatient and critical?

- Does the parent have realistic expectations, given the child's age and developmental abilities?
- Does the child communicate with respect and in a friendly way with his parents?

The health care professional also should observe for the child's ability to interact with adults other than parents:

- Is the child friendly, cooperative, and comfortable in speaking with others?
- Is the child unwilling to speak or excessively shy?
- What is the child's level of concentration, attention, or activity?
- Is the child's language understandable? Are the child's syntax, vocabulary, grammar, and speech content appropriate for his age?

Surveillance of Development

Children Transitioning to Kindergarten

Starting school is a major milestone for child and family. Parents may have concerns about their child's readiness for this big step. Although many parents tend to focus on the child's knowledge of the alphabet, numbers, or drawing skills as evidence of school readiness, teachers are most concerned about the child's language skills and social readiness to separate from parents easily and get along with other children. If parents are considering holding their child back, it is important to explore their rationale. The desire to give their child an advantage over younger children by placing their child in a pre-kindergarten class may actually cause more harm than benefit. For children who have low school-readiness test results, it is often more helpful to place them in kindergarten with well-chosen supports than to hold them back. Older children who are held back from school may become bored and be mismatched with their peers in terms of behavior and interests.

The child with special health care needs transitions from early childhood special education services to the classroom setting. The child's IEP should be revised before this move, and the health care professional should discuss appropriate changes with the family.

Children Currently Attending School

Adjustment to new school experiences are both the measure and the end-point of developmental accomplishment. Health care professionals may measure school success by parent and child report or by review of the child's most recent report card. The health care professional must be alert for diagnoses such as ADHD and learning disorders. For children with special health care needs, it is important for the health care professional to review a copy of the IEP or any special accommodations.

Do you have any specific concerns about your child's development, learning, or behavior?

- **A 5- or 6-year-old child**
  - Balances on one foot, hops, and skips
  - Is able to tie a knot, has mature pencil grasp, can draw a person with at least 6 body parts, prints some letters and numbers, and is able to copy squares and triangles
  - Has good articulation, tells a simple story using full sentences, uses appropriate tenses and pronouns, can count to 10, and names at least 4 colors
  - Follows simple directions, is able to listen and attend, and undresses and dresses with minimal assistance

Physical Examination

A complete physical examination is included as part of every health supervision visit.

When performing a physical examination, the health care professional's attention is directed to the following components of the examination that are important for a child this age:

- **Measure:**
  - Blood pressure
- **Measure and plot:**
  - Height
  - Weight
- **Calculate and plot:**
  - BMI

- **Eyes**
  - Attempt to perform ophthalmoscopic examination of optic nerve and retinal vessels
- **Mouth**
  - Observe for caries, gingival inflammation, and malocclusion
- **Neurologic**
  - Observe fine and gross motor skills, including gait
  - Assess language acquisition, speech fluency and clarity, thought content, and ability to understand abstract thinking

Screening — 5 Year

UNIVERSAL SCREENING	ACTION	
Vision	Objective measure with age-appropriate visual acuity measurement (using HOTV; tumbling E tests; Snellen letters; Snellen numbers; or Picture tests, such as Allen figures or LEA symbols)	
Hearing	Audiometry	
SELECTIVE SCREENING	RISK ASSESSMENT*	ACTION IF RA +
Anemia	+ on risk screening questions	Hemoglobin or hematocrit
Lead	If no previous screen and + on risk screening questions or change in risk	Lead screen
Tuberculosis	+ on risk screening questions	Tuberculin skin test
*See Rationale and Evidence chapter for the criteria on which risk screening questions are based.		

Screening — 6 Year

UNIVERSAL SCREENING	ACTION	
Vision	Objective measure with age-appropriate visual acuity measurement (using HOTV; tumbling E tests; Snellen letters; Snellen numbers; or Picture tests, such as Allen figures or LEA symbols)	
Hearing	Audiometry	
SELECTIVE SCREENING	RISK ASSESSMENT*	ACTION IF RA +
Oral Health	Does not have a dental home	Referral to dental home
	Primary water source is deficient in fluoride	Oral fluoride supplementation
Anemia	+ on risk screening questions	Hemoglobin or hematocrit
Lead	If no previous screen and + on risk screening questions or change in risk	Lead screen
Tuberculosis	+ on risk screening questions	Tuberculin skin test
Dyslipidemia	+ on risk screening questions and not previously screened with normal results	Fasting lipid profile
*See Rationale and Evidence chapter for the criteria on which risk screening questions are based.		

Immunizations

Consult the CDC/ACIP or AAP Web sites for the current immunization schedule.

CDC National Immunization Program (NIP): http://www.cdc.gov/vaccines

American Academy of Pediatrics *Red Book:* http://www.aapredbook.org

ANTICIPATORY GUIDANCE

The following sample questions, which address the Middle Childhood Expert Panel's Anticipatory Guidance Priorities, are intended to be used selectively to invite discussion, gather information, address the needs and concerns of the family, and build partnerships. Use of the questions may vary from visit to visit and from family to family. Questions can be modified to match the health care professional's communication style. The accompanying anticipatory guidance for the family should be geared to questions, issues, or concerns for that particular child and family.

SCHOOL READINESS

Established routines, after-school care and activities, parent-teacher communication, friends, bullying, maturity, management of disappointments, fears

Determine whether newly immigrated families understand the local educational system, which may be very different from that in their country of origin. Check whether any language barriers exist to parent/caregiver interactions with the school.

For the child with special health care needs, discuss the child's specific needs related to the school setting. Encourage parents to maintain an active role in the IEP process. Remind parents to bring a copy of the IEP to each health supervision visit.

Bullying and teasing can interfere with normal development and school performance. Assist parents in being observant for signs of bullying.[1]

For the Child Entering Kindergarten and Elementary School:
SAMPLE QUESTIONS:
Did your child go to preschool? Tell me about her preschool experience. Is there anything the school or teacher should know related to any special needs your child may have?
For the child
Tell me about your new school. (Probe for feelings and concerns about starting school.)

ANTICIPATORY GUIDANCE:
- Prepare your child for school. Talk about new opportunities, friends, and activities at school. Tour your child's school with her and meet her teacher.
For the child
- Ask your teacher to explain things if you do not know what you are supposed to do. It helps all the kids in class know what they are supposed to do.

For the Child Currently Enrolled in School:
SAMPLE QUESTIONS:
What concerns do you have about your child's ability to do well in academic work? Follow the rules at school? What are your plans for your child's after-school activities? (Probe for type of adult supervision, appropriate mix of active and sedentary activities, and food provided.)

For the child

Tell me about your new school. (Probe for feelings and concerns about elementary school.) *Tell me about your best friend. What kinds of things do you and your best friend do together? Do kids ever call you mean names or tease you?*

ANTICIPATORY GUIDANCE:

- Attend back-to-school nights, parent-teacher meetings, and other school functions. These will give you a chance to get to know your child's teacher and become familiar with the school so you can talk more knowledgeably with her about her experiences at school.
- If you enroll your child in an after-school program or hire a caregiver for the after-school period, be sure your child is in a safe environment. Talk with caregivers about their attitudes and behavior about discipline. Do not let them discipline your child by hitting or spanking her.

For the child

- Talk with your parents every day about things that you like and any things that may worry you at school.
- If anyone is being mean to you, tell your teacher and your parents. They can help you deal with it.

MENTAL HEALTH

Family time, routines, temper problems, social interactions

Family routines create a sense of safety and security for the child. Assigning regular household chores is good because it engenders a sense of responsibility in the child and helps him feel as though he is an essential part of the family.

Parents should encourage self-discipline and impulse control.

SAMPLE QUESTIONS:

What are some of the family routines you have at home? What chores is your child responsible for at home? How does your child handle angry feelings? How do you and your partner (or other caregiver) handle discipline?

For the child

What regular jobs do you have at home? What family traditions do you enjoy? What things make you sad? Angry? Scared? How do you handle these feelings? Do you talk to your parents about your concerns? What happens in your house if your dad or mom doesn't approve of something you're doing? When do your mom or dad get angry with you?

ANTICIPATORY GUIDANCE:

- Talk with your partner about important routines you and your partner loved as children. Decide together which of these routines, or new ones, you want for your family. Observe them consistently. Your child will look forward to these special traditions.
- Show affection in your family.
- Listen to and respect your child as well as your partner. Serve as a positive ethical and behavioral role model.
- Teach your child the difference between right and wrong. The goal of discipline is teaching appropriate behavior, not punishment.
- Promote a sense of responsibility in your child by assigning chores and expecting them to be done, including for children with special health care needs. For all children, chores should be determined by what is needed and what is appropriate for the child's ability.
- Model anger management by talking about your anger and letting off steam in positive ways.
- Help your child manage anger and resolve conflicts without violence. Do not allow hitting, biting, or other violent behavior.
- Encourage self-discipline and impulse control in your child by modeling these behaviors and by praising his efforts at self-control.

For the child

- Chores are an important part of being in a family. You help make things go well at home and learn new skills you can be proud of. If you need a break from a chore, talk about it with your parents.
- Everyone gets angry at times, but it's never OK to hit, bite, kick, or punch another person. Better ways to deal with feeling angry are to talk about what has upset you with the person who made you angry, to get outside and run or play hard, or just walk away from the person who is making you angry.

NUTRITION AND PHYSICAL ACTIVITY

Healthy weight; appropriate well-balanced diet; increased fruit, vegetable, and whole-grain consumption; adequate calcium intake; 60 minutes of exercise a day

Discuss healthy weight by using the BMI chart to show children and their families where they are in relationship to weight/stature/age. If the child's BMI is greater than the 85th percentile, it is appropriate to begin more in-depth counseling on nutritious food choices and physical activity.

As 5- and 6-year-old children begin to broaden their experiences beyond home, they are increasingly expected to make their own choices about what to eat. This is a good time to counsel families about appropriate food choices that promote nutritional adequacy and to reinforce positive nutrition habits established earlier. Provide guidance or a referral if the family needs nutrition help because of cultural, religious, or financial reasons.

SAMPLE QUESTIONS:

What concerns do you have about your child's eating (eg, getting her to drink enough milk and eat fruits and vegetables)? What does your child usually eat for snacks? How often does she drink soda and juice? Are there ever times when your family does not have enough to eat?

For the child

What fruits and vegetables did you eat yesterday? How many sodas do you drink each day? How many glasses of juice do you drink each day? How much milk did you drink yesterday? What other dairy foods, such as yogurt or cheese, did you eat? What do you eat for breakfast?

ANTICIPATORY GUIDANCE:

- Breakfast is an important meal. Research shows that eating breakfast helps children learn and behave better at school.
- Help your child learn to choose appropriate foods, including plenty of fruits and vegetables every day. Aim for at least 5 servings of fruits or vegetables every day by including them in most of your meals and snacks.
- Limit high-fat and low-nutrient foods and drinks, such as candy, salty snacks, fast foods, and soda.
- Make sure your child is getting enough calcium daily. Children ages 4 to 8 need about 2 cups of low-fat milk each day. Low-fat yogurt and cheese are good alternatives to milk. Limit juice to 4 to 6 oz per day of 100% fruit juice. Do not serve fruit drinks.

For the child

- Eating breakfast helps you learn better and feel better at school, so always eat something healthy for breakfast.
- Fruits and vegetables are an important part of healthy eating. Ask your parents to let you help choose fruits and vegetables at the store and to help prepare them for meals and snacks.
- Be sure to drink at least 2 cups of low-fat milk a day or eat cheese or yogurt because they are important for strong bones and teeth.

Encourage parents to support their children in being physically active and to be physically active together as a family.

Encourage parents of children with special health care needs to allow their children to participate in regular physical activity or cardiovascular fitness within the limits of their medical conditions.

Emphasize the importance of safety equipment when the child participates in physical activity. In unsafe neighborhoods, help families identify appropriate community activities for their child (eg, Boys and Girls Clubs, 4-H, community centers, and faith-based programs).

SAMPLE QUESTIONS:

How much physical activity does your child get every day? How many hours per day does she play outside? Do you and your child participate in physical activities together? About how much time does your child spend each weekday watching TV or videos, or playing computer games? How about on weekends?

MIDDLE CHILDHOOD
5 AND 6 YEAR VISITS

For the child
Do you play together with your family? How much time each day do you spend watching TV or videos or playing computer games?

ANTICIPATORY GUIDANCE:
- Encourage your child to be physically active for at least 60 minutes total every day. It doesn't have to happen all at once, but can be split up into several periods of activity over the course of the day.
- Find physical activities your family can enjoy and incorporate into their daily lives.
- Limit the amount of time your child watches TV and plays video games or is on the computer (other than for homework) to no more than 2 hours altogether each day. Remove any TVs from your child's bedroom.
- To minimize your child's exposure to violence and other age-inappropriate material, be aware of the content included in music, video games, and TV programs that your child watches.

For the child
- It's a good idea to get outside and play several times every day.
- Turn off the TV, get up, and play. For every half hour you watch TV or play a video game, match it with a half hour of active play.
- When you see something on TV or in a game that makes you uncomfortable or frightened, turn off the TV or video game and tell your parents about it.

ORAL HEALTH

Regular visits with dentist, daily brushing and flossing, adequate fluoride

By 5 years, the child already should have an established dental home. He should be having regularly scheduled visits with his dentist at least twice each year. He should also receive a fluoride supplement if the fluoride level in community (at home and at school) water supplies is low.

SAMPLE QUESTIONS:
How many times a day does your child brush and floss his teeth?

For parents of children with special health care needs:
Does your child need help with brushing his teeth? Do you use any special oral health equipment, such as a mouth prop to keep his mouth open, to complete this task?

For the child
Do you brush and floss your teeth every day? How many times? When do you brush your teeth?

ANTICIPATORY GUIDANCE:
- Be sure that your child brushes his teeth twice a day with a pea-sized amount of fluoridated toothpaste and flosses once a day with your help. Be sure to supervise brushing and flossing. Help him if necessary.

- If your child does not have a regular dentist (also called a dental home), it's important to get one.

For the child

- It is important to brush your teeth at least twice a day and to floss at least once a day, especially when your new teeth come in, because they are the teeth you'll have forever.

SAFETY

Pedestrian safety, booster seat, safety helmets, swimming safety, child sexual abuse prevention, fire escape/drill plan and smoke detectors, carbon monoxide detectors/alarms, guns

Car safety is a critical area to address because many deaths at this age are due to crashes involving vehicles when child passengers are inadequately restrained. Riding bikes safely and pedestrian safety are other issues of importance for counseling parents.

Young children lack the neurologic maturity, skills, and knowledge needed to safely cross the street. They have not developed neurologically to have the skills to see cars in their peripheral vision, localize sounds, and judge vehicle distance and speed, and, in general, are not ready to cross the street alone until age 10 or older. To protect their young child from harm, parents must use constant vigilance and regularly review the safety of the environment. Parents often overestimate the cognitive and sensory integration of young children and need advice on how to teach and provide adequate supervision for injury prevention.

SAMPLE QUESTION:

What have you done to prepare your child for crossing the street on the way to school or for taking a school bus?

ANTICIPATORY GUIDANCE:

- Begin to teach your child safe street habits. Teach your child to stop at the curb, and then look to the left, to the right, and back to the left again. Teach your child never to cross the street without a grown-up.
- Children need to learn where to wait for the school bus and should have adult supervision for getting on and off the bus.

The back seat is the safest place for all children to ride until age 13, and they should use a belt-positioning booster seat until the safety belt fits well, usually between the ages of 8 and 12 and when the child is about 4'9" tall. Assist families who cannot afford appropriate car safety seats by connecting them with community resources. Children with behavior problems or special health care needs may benefit from the use of seats with full harnesses to higher weights or restraints designed for special needs (www.preventinjury.org).

Questions about proper installation should be referred to a certified Child Passenger Safety Technician in the community.
Child Safety Seat Inspection Station Locator: www.seatcheck.org
Toll-free Number: 866-SEATCHECK (866-732-8243)

MIDDLE CHILDHOOD
5 AND 6 YEAR VISITS

SAMPLE QUESTIONS:

Does your child always use a car safety seat or belt-positioning booster seat securely fastened in the back seat of a vehicle?

For the child

What type of seat do you sit in when you ride in a car? Do you sit in the back seat?

ANTICIPATORY GUIDANCE:

- Be sure the vehicle lap and shoulder belt are positioned across the child in the belt-positioning booster seat in the back seat of the vehicle. Your child should use a car safety seat or a booster seat until the lap belt can be worn low and flat on her upper thighs and the shoulder belt can be worn across her shoulder rather than the face or neck, and she can bend at the knees while sitting against the vehicle seat back (usually between 8 and 12 years old and at about 4'9" tall). The back seat is the safest place for all children younger than 13 to ride.

For the child

- Always sit in your booster seat and ride in the back seat of the car because that is where you are safest.

SAMPLE QUESTIONS:

Does your child use safety equipment when biking, skating, skiing, in-line skating, snowboarding, or horseback riding? (Tailor the list of activities appropriate to the area and the family.)

For the child

Do you always wear a helmet when biking, skating, skiing, in-line skating, snow boarding, or horseback riding? (Tailor these questions as appropriate.)

ANTICIPATORY GUIDANCE:

- Be sure your child always wears appropriate safety equipment when biking, skating, skiing, in-line skating, snowboarding, or horseback riding. *(Tailor the list of activities appropriate to the area.)*
- Make sure your child wears a properly fitted, approved helmet every time she rides a bike. Never let your child ride in the street. Your child is too young to ride in the street safely.

For the child

- Being active is good for you, but being safe while being active is just as important. One of the best ways to protect yourself is to wear the right safety equipment, especially a helmet, every time you go biking, skating, skiing, in-line skating, snowboarding, or horseback riding. *(Tailor the activities as appropriate.)*

Child Safety
Seat Inspection
Station Locator:
www.seatcheck.org.
Toll-free Number:
866-SEATCHECK
(866-732-8243).

An adult should supervise whenever children are in or near water.

SAMPLE QUESTIONS:

Does your child know how to swim? Does she know about water safety?

For the child

Do you know how to swim?

What rules do your parents have about swimming?

478

ANTICIPATORY GUIDANCE:

- Now is the time to teach your child to swim.
- Do not let your child play around any water (lake, stream, pool, or ocean) unless an adult is watching. Even if your child knows how to swim, never let her swim alone. NEVER let your child swim in any fast-moving water.
- Teach your child to never dive into water unless an adult has checked the depth of the water. When on any boat, be sure your child is wearing an appropriately fitting, US Coast Guard-approved life jacket.
- Be sure that swimming pools in your community, apartment complex, or home have a 4-sided fence with a self-closing, self-latching gate.
- Continue to put sunscreen (SPF 15 or higher) on your child before she goes outside to play or swim.

For the child

- Swimming lessons are an important way to become safe in the water. Ask your parents about learning to swim.
- Never swim without an adult around.
- Always wear a life jacket in a boat.

As children now spend increasing amounts of time with other adults, parents should discuss personal safety in a manner that is informative and empowering without provoking unnecessary anxiety.

Because the majority of sexual abuse and misuse is intrafamily, safety messages must focus on privacy, autonomy, and avoiding victimization and not just on the risks from strangers.

SAMPLE QUESTIONS:

Have you talked to your child about ways to avoid sexual abuse?

For the child

What are your "privates"? Why do we call them that? What would you do if a grown-up made you scared? Who could you tell? Who would help you?

ANTICIPATORY GUIDANCE:

- Teach your child that it is never all right for an adult to tell a child to keep secrets from parents, to express interest in private parts, or to ask a child for help with his or her private parts.

For the child

- We call the parts of your body that are usually under a bathing suit "privates" because we keep them covered and because you are the only one in charge of them.
- It is never OK for an older child or an adult to show you his or her private parts, to ask you to show your privates, to touch you there, to scare you, or to ask you not to tell your parents about what he or she did with you. Always get away from the person as quickly as possible and tell your parent or another adult right away.

Home fire safety is best achieved with prevention (teaching children not to play with matches or lighters), protection (smoke detectors), and planning (reaction and escape).

SAMPLE QUESTIONS:

Where are the smoke detectors in your home? (Probe for multiple locations.) *Do you have carbon monoxide detectors/alarms in your home? Do you have an emergency escape plan in case of fire and does your child know what to do in case the alarm rings?*

For the child

What should you do if a fire starts in your home? What should you do if your clothes catch on fire?

ANTICIPATORY GUIDANCE:

- Install smoke detectors on every level in your house, especially in furnace and sleeping areas, and test the detectors every month. It is best to use smoke detectors that use long-life batteries, but, if you do not, change the batteries once a year.
- Install a carbon monoxide detector/alarm, certified by UL, in the hallway near every separate sleeping area of the home.
- Make an escape plan in case of fire in your home. Your fire department can tell you how. Teach your child what to do when the smoke detector rings. Practice what you and your child would do if you had a fire.
- Keep all matches and lighters out of reach of children.

For the child

- Never play with matches or lighters or let others do so.
- If your clothes catch on fire, don't run. Stop, drop, and roll.

Discuss gun safety in the home and danger to family members and children. Homicide and completed suicide are more common in homes in which guns are kept. To keep children safe, the AAP recommends that guns be removed from where children live and play. If it is necessary to keep a gun, it should be stored unloaded and locked, with the ammunition locked separately from the gun.

At this age, children lack the maturity or cognitive capacity to reliably follow advice concerning guns. The health care professional's guidance should be addressed to the parents.

SAMPLE QUESTIONS:

If there is a gun in your home, is it unloaded and locked up? Where is the ammunition stored? Have you considered not owning a gun because it poses the danger to children and other family members?

ANTICIPATORY GUIDANCE:

- The best way to keep your child safe from injury or death from guns is to never have a gun in the home.

- If it is necessary to keep a gun in your home, keep it unloaded and in a locked place, with ammunition locked separately. Keep the key where children cannot have access.
- Ask if there are guns in homes where your child plays. If so, make sure they are stored unloaded and locked, with the ammunition locked separately, before allowing your child to play in the home.
- Remember that young children simply do not understand how dangerous guns can be, despite your warnings.

Middle Childhood: 7 and 8 Year Visits

CONTEXT

Now prepubertal, bigger, more interactive, and involved with friends, the emotionally developed 7- and 8-year-old child now uses his increasing cognitive strengths and communication skills to plot a developmental trajectory toward mature independence and autonomy. His newly formed superego, or conscience, allows the understanding of rules, relationships, and social mores. Moral development progresses. Early experiences with separation foster individuation. Coping skills develop, supporting the child's social activities, friendships outside the family, and school and community competencies. This process continues into young adulthood.

A 7- or 8-year-old child begins to look outside the family for new ideas and activities. He may encounter beliefs and practices that differ from those of his family. He will try to make sense of these differences and may begin to experience some conflict between the beliefs and values at home and those of his peers. A child's peer group becomes increasingly important; he identifies with children of the same gender who have similar interests and abilities. He may have a best friend, a milestone in interpersonal development. The growing influence of peers may present a challenge to the family.

Children at these ages increasingly spend time away from family with school and social activities. Opportunities for formal after-school activities, such as scouts, team sports, and arts activities, are beginning to be readily available. A 7- or 8-year-old child also can begin to take on new family responsibilities, such as making his own bed, picking up his clothes, setting the table, and helping with meals. These responsibilities can help him develop a sense of personal competence. His sense of accomplishment and pride helps him become confident in attempting activities that require increased responsibility.

By 8 years, a child is able to use logic and to focus on multiple aspects of a problem. Busy with school projects, book reports, and creating collections that reflect his interests in sports, animals, or other topics, he wants to learn how things work and he has many questions about the world around him. He also is beginning to recognize that others' viewpoints may differ from his own.

School performance remains a functional marker of a child's development and accomplishments across all developmental domains (social-emotional, communicative, cognitive, and physical). By now, a child should have completed the transition to the classroom setting. Behaviors necessary for learning, such as cooperation and attention, are demonstrated.

If the child has a special health care need or a disability, the health care professional should be concerned with how well the child is coping with his special predicament, given the new developmental, social, and environmental demands of becoming older. A child with special health care needs may be on a different or similar developmental trajectory when compared with age and classroom peers. Cultural and family values and beliefs about the cause of special health care needs and expectations for individuals with illnesses and disabilities will influence both current adjustments and planning for transition to adulthood.

For children with special health care needs and for children receiving supplemental or special education services, a review of services with parents is appropriate. Parents can provide a copy and discuss their child's IEP or Section 504 Plan for in-classroom accommodations. These documents should be checked for accurate attention to medical co-morbidities, appropriate accommodations, and for comprehensive approaches to learning. The role of psychotropic medications may need to be reviewed. Children with special health care needs should have a Care Plan that is developed in conjunction with the parents and shared with the school nurse and after-school caregivers. The Care Plan should address any chronic medications, emergency medications, alterations of diet or activity, and signs of a worsening health condition.

Children from cultures other than the predominant one of their community will continue to struggle with individuality and assimilation. By 7 and 8 years of age, a child living in linguistically isolated households (defined by the Census Bureau as those in which no one older than 14 speaks English at least "very well") may be taking on responsibilities beyond those typical for his age in dealing with family needs. He is required to be a bridge between the family and the unfamiliar school, neighborhood, or social services. For example, he may be serving as an interpreter for adults in communicating with the school, with agencies, or on issues such as keeping the electricity on in the house. These are weighty tasks for a 7- or 8-year-old.

Health supervision visits with 7- and 8-year-olds provide an opportunity for the health care professional to talk directly with the child and build a trusting relationship with him. As he continues to grow and develop, he will need to feel comfortable asking questions and discussing concerns with the health care professional if he is to begin to assume personal responsibility for his health.

The child is now cementing health habits, including those related to nutrition, physical activity, and safety. This visit provides an excellent opportunity to foster self-responsibility for positive health behaviors. The child needs to eat a variety of nutritious foods, brush his teeth twice a day, participate in physical activities, limit screen time, and make safety a priority by, for example, using a booster seat and safety belt when riding in a vehicle and by wearing a helmet when biking. Parents continue to be role models for their children in health behaviors. Many health care professionals will now note the importance of not smoking or drinking alcohol. A discussion of the initiation of puberty and value of ongoing sexuality education within the family is appropriate at this age and developmental stage.

PRIORITIES FOR THE VISIT

The first priority is to attend to the concerns of the parents. In addition, the Bright Futures Middle Childhood Expert Panel has given priority to the following topics for discussion in this visit:

- School (adaptation to school, school problems [behavior or learning issues], school performance/progress, involvement in school activities and after-school programs, bullying, parental involvement, IEP or special education services)
- Development and mental health (independence, self-esteem, establishing rules and consequences, temper problems, managing and resolving conflicts, puberty/pubertal development)
- Nutrition and physical activity (healthy weight, appropriate food intake, adequate calcium, water instead of soda, adequate physical activity in organized sports/after-school programs/fun activities, limits on screen time)
- Oral health (regular visits with dentist, daily brushing and flossing, adequate fluoride)
- Safety (knowing child's friends and their families, supervision with friends, safety belts/booster seats, helmets, playground safety, sports safety, swimming safety, sunscreen, smoke-free home/vehicles, guns, careful monitoring of computer use [games, Internet, e-mail])

HEALTH SUPERVISION

History

Interval history may be obtained according to the concerns of the family and the health care professional's preference or style of practice. The following questions can encourage in-depth discussion:

Questions to the Parent:
- What are your concerns about your child's physical well-being or special health care needs?
- Do you have any concerns about your child's development or learning?
- Please share any concerns you may have about your child's mood or behavior (eg, attention, hitting, temper, worries, not participating in play with others, irritability, mood, or activity level)?
- Are there any changes at home since last year?

Questions to the Child:
- How are you?
- How is school going?
- What would you like to discuss about your health today?

Observation of Parent-Child Interaction

During the visit, the health care professional should observe:

- Do both the parent and the child ask questions?
- Does the parent allow the child to communicate with the health care professional directly, or does the parent interfere in the interaction?
- Does the parent have realistic expectations, given the child's age and developmental abilities?
- Does the child communicate with respect and in a friendly way with his parents?
- Do the parent and child make eye contact with each other and with the health care professional?

The health care professional also should observe for the child's ability to interact with adults other than parents:

- Is the child friendly and cooperative?
- Is the child unwilling to speak or excessively shy?
- Is the child's language understandable (eg, is the child's syntax, vocabulary, grammar, and content appropriate for his age)?
- Does the child appear angry or depressed?
- Does the child follow directions?
- What is the child's level of concentration, attention, or activity?
- Does the child seem proud to describe his friendships, activities, and emerging skills?

Surveillance of Development

As children move into the second and third grades, issues of inattention, hyperactivity, and impulsiveness can interfere with the learning of complex concepts as well as with fitting into most school environments. Aggressive and oppositional behaviors may become maladaptive behaviors rather than behaviors of adjustment to the expectations and demands of school. Demanding learning tasks may reveal learning disabilities.

Sorting among the issues created by parent and cultural expectations, the fit of the child with teacher and school expectations, and school performance deficits in light of the child's previous developmental and social history is challenging but of critical importance to the child's well-being. School failure has significant negative impact on a child's self-esteem and confidence. Therefore, the nature of problems revealed in poor school performance needs to be identified as soon as possible through referrals for the assessment and diagnosis of learning disabilities and mental health disorders so that appropriate treatments can begin.

For children with special health care needs and for children receiving supplemental or special education services, a review of services with parents is appropriate. It is helpful for parents to provide a copy of their child's IEP or Section 504 Plan for discussion. Review these documents carefully for accurate attention to medical co-morbidities, appropriate accommodations for the child's special needs, and for comprehensive approaches to learning. Also, review medications that may need to be administered during the school day, including psychotropic medications, and ensure completion of appropriate school forms. Consider switching the child to extended-release medications if the child is embarrassed by taking medications at school. Some parents may wish to avoid contacting the school about ADHD medications because of concerns about stigma. Yet, parents should be informed that teacher-parent communication about behavior and medications will help the parent and the health care professional make the right decisions about dosing.

Do you have any specific concerns about your child's development, learning, or behavior?

A 7- or 8-year-old child
- Demonstrates physical, cognitive, emotional, social, and moral competencies
- Engages in behaviors that promote wellness and contribute to a healthy lifestyle
- Has a caring, supportive relationship with family, other adults, and peers[2]

Physical Examination

A complete physical examination is included as part of every health supervision visit. Respect the child's privacy by using appropriate draping during the examination. Ask siblings to wait in the waiting room, if possible.

When performing a physical examination, the health care professional's attention is directed to the following components of the examination that are important for a child this age:

- **Measure**
  - Blood pressure

- **Measure and plot:**
  - Height
  - Weight
- **Calculate and plot:**
  - BMI
- **Musculoskeletal**
  - Observe hip, knee, and ankle function
- **Mouth**
  - Observe for caries, gingival inflammation, and malocclusion
- **Breasts and Genitalia**
  - Assess for sexual maturity rating

Screening — 7 Year

UNIVERSAL SCREENING	ACTION	
None		
SELECTIVE SCREENING	RISK ASSESSMENT*	ACTION IF RA +
Vision	+ on risk screening questions	Snellen test
Hearing	+ on risk screening questions	Audiometry
Anemia	+ on risk screening questions	Hemoglobin or hematocrit
Tuberculosis	+ on risk screening questions	Tuberculin skin test

*See Rationale and Evidence chapter for the criteria on which risk screening questions are based.

Screening — 8 Year

UNIVERSAL SCREENING	ACTION	
Vision	Snellen test	
Hearing	Audiometry	
SELECTIVE SCREENING	RISK ASSESSMENT*	ACTION IF RA +
Anemia	+ on risk screening questions	Hemoglobin or hematocrit
Tuberculosis	+ on risk screening questions	Tuberculin skin test
Dyslipidemia	+ on risk screening questions and not previously screened with normal results	Fasting lipid profile

*See Rationale and Evidence chapter for the criteria on which risk screening questions are based.

Immunizations

Consult the CDC/ACIP or AAP Web sites for the current immunization schedule.
CDC National Immunization Program (NIP): http://www.cdc.gov/vaccines
American Academy of Pediatrics *Red Book:* http://www.aapredbook.org

ANTICIPATORY GUIDANCE

The following sample questions, which address the Middle Childhood Expert Panel's Anticipatory Guidance Priorities, are intended to be used selectively to invite discussion, gather information, address the needs and concerns of the family, and build partnerships. Use of the questions may vary from visit to visit and from family to family. Questions can be modified to match the health care professional's communication style. The accompanying anticipatory guidance for the family should be geared to questions, issues, or concerns for that particular child and family.

SCHOOL

Adaptation to school, school problems (behavior or learning issues), school performance/progress, involvement in school activities and after-school programs, bullying, parental involvement, IEP or special education services

School is the most readily observable marker of a child's social, linguistic, and cognitive development. Encourage parents to be supportive, observant, and involved in this essential component of their child's life.

SAMPLE QUESTIONS:
How is your child enjoying school? Do you have any concerns about bullying of your child? How do you help your child solve conflicts on the playground or elsewhere?

For the child
How do you like school? What kind of grades are you getting this year? How about last year? Are you happy with them? What kinds of school and after-school activities do you do? Are you picked on by other kids at school or has anyone there ever tried to hurt you? What would you do if someone said they were going to hurt you?

ANTICIPATORY GUIDANCE:
- If your child is not doing well in school, ask the teacher about evaluation for special help or tutoring that may be available.
- If your child is anxious about going to school, talk with her about the possibility that she is being bullied by another child. Try to obtain a complete picture of what is happening, and when and where. Contact your child's teacher and the principal to seek their assistance in dealing with the bully.

For the child
- Doing well in school is important to how you feel about yourself. However, doing well means something different for each person. What matters is that you try your best and ask for help when you need it.
- If someone picks on you or tries to hurt you, tell them in a firm voice to stop bothering you and walk away. Tell an adult you trust, your teacher, or your parents about what is happening. Have them help you avoid these situations and stop the bad behavior of others.

DEVELOPMENT AND MENTAL HEALTH

Independence, self-esteem, social interactions, establishing rules and consequences, temper problems, managing and resolving conflicts, puberty/pubertal development

Self-esteem is a key feature of a fulfilling life and has an enormous influence on mental health. Children develop a positive sense of self if they think they are making a contribution. Words of encouragement are important and provide energizing motivation. Help parents think about how they can encourage their child to be responsible by modeling responsibility themselves, by keeping promises, showing up on time, and completing tasks on time.

Parents can help make their child feel secure by giving hugs, participating in activities together, and talking. Children with warm, nurturing parents are more likely to have high self-esteem. Hypercritical parents who have unrealistically high expectations, and uninvolved parents who do not encourage their children to achieve and to try new experiences, can damage their child's self-esteem.

SAMPLE QUESTIONS:
What are your child's favorite activities? What concerns and worries has your child shared with you? What types of discipline do you use most often? What responsibilities does your child have at home (eg, helping care for younger siblings, helping prepare meals together, raking an elderly neighbor's leaves)? Are temper tantrums a frequent problem for your child? How does he deal with frustration?

For the child
What new things have you tried in the past year? Who do you usually talk to about your worries and things that made you mad?

ANTICIPATORY GUIDANCE:
- Encourage competence, independence, and self-responsibility in all areas by not doing things for your child, but by helping him do things well himself, and by supporting him in helping others through volunteering.
- Show affection and pride in your child's special strengths and use praise liberally.
- Be a positive role model for your child in terms of activities, values, attitudes, and morality.
- Do not hit, shake, or spank your child or permit others to do so. Instead, talk with your child about establishing reasonable consequences for breaking the rules, and follow through with the agreed-upon consequences each time a rule is broken.

For the child
- Everyone has worries and things that make them mad. These feelings don't feel good. The best way to deal with them is to talk with someone who listens well and who will help you learn how to deal with them in good ways. Often, just talking about unpleasant feelings helps them go away.

Parents of various cultural and religious backgrounds may differ in their opinions about puberty. Explore their beliefs and respect them, while also explaining that their child's curiosity about this issue is normal.

SAMPLE QUESTIONS:

What have you told your child about how to care for his changing body?

For the child

Do you know what puberty is? Has anyone discussed with you how your body will change in the time called puberty?

ANTICIPATORY GUIDANCE:

- Answer questions simply and honestly at a level appropriate to your child's understanding. If your child receives family life education at school or in the community, discuss the information with him.

For the child

- Lots of changes happen to you and your body during puberty, and some of those changes can be surprising or hard to figure out. It's always OK to ask your parent or another adult you trust if you have any concerns or worries.
- Even embarrassing questions can be important ones. It's OK to talk about your body's development.

NUTRITION AND PHYSICAL ACTIVITY

Healthy weight, appropriate food intake, adequate calcium, water instead of soda, adequate physical activity in organized sports/after-school programs/fun activities, limits on screen time

Counsel families about appropriate food choices that promote nutritional adequacy and reinforce positive nutrition habits. Guidance or a referral is appropriate if the family needs nutrition help because of cultural, religious, or financial reasons. Encourage parents to support their children in being physically active and to be physically active together as a family.

Discuss healthy weight by using the BMI chart to show children and their families where they are in relationship to weight/stature/age. If the child's BMI is greater than the 85th percentile, it is appropriate to begin more in-depth counseling on nutritious food choices and physical activity.

SAMPLE QUESTIONS:

What do you think of your child's weight and growth over the past year? What concerns do you have about your child's eating (eg, getting her to drink enough milk and eat fruits and vegetables)? How often does she drink soda or juice drinks? How often does she drink or eat a food rich in calcium, such as milk, calcium-fortified juice, cheese, or yogurt? How often do you eat together as a family? Are there ever times when your family does not have enough to eat?

For the child

How many sodas a day do you drink? Do you drink milk? Is it low fat?

ANTICIPATORY GUIDANCE:

- Help your child learn to choose appropriate foods, including plenty of fruits and vegetables every day. Aim for at least 5 servings of fruits or vegetables every day by including them in most of your meals and snacks.
- Serve your child a balanced breakfast or make sure that the school provides one.
- Limit high-fat and low-nutrient foods and drinks, such as candy, salty snacks, fast foods, and soda.
- Make sure your child is getting enough calcium daily. Children aged 4 to 8 need about 2 cups of low-fat milk a day. Low-fat yogurt and cheese are good alternatives to milk.
- Limit juice to 4 to 6 oz per day of 100% fruit juice. Do not serve fruit drinks.
- Share family meals together as often as possible. Make mealtimes pleasant and companionable; encourage conversation and turn off the TV during mealtimes.

For the child

- Eating healthy foods is important to helping you do well in school and sports.
- Dairy foods are important for strong bones and teeth. Be sure to drink at least 2 glasses of milk each day. You can also eat cheese and yogurt instead of drinking milk.

All children should be able to participate in some type of physical activity daily. Current recommendations state that children should be physically active for at least 60 minutes on most, if not all, days. For a child with special health care needs, encourage parents to allow her to participate in regular physical activity or cardiovascular fitness within the limits of her medical or physical conditions.

This is the age when children become involved in organized sports.

Emphasize the importance of safety equipment when the child participates in physical activity.

SAMPLE QUESTIONS:

How much physical activity does your child get every day? About how much time does your child spend each weekday watching television or videos, or playing computer games? How about on weekends?

For the child

How often do you go outside to play? How much time each day do you spend watching TV or videos or playing computer games?

ANTICIPATORY GUIDANCE:

- Encourage your child to be physically active at least 60 minutes total every day. It doesn't have to be all at once. Find physical activities that your family enjoys. Include them in your daily lives.
- Limit the amount of time your child watches TV and plays video games or is on the computer (other than homework) to no more than 2 hours total each day. Do not let your child have a TV or computer in her room.

For the child

- It's a good idea to get outside and play hard several times every day.
- Turn off the TV and get up and play. For every half hour you watch TV or play a video game, match it with a half hour of active play.

ORAL HEALTH

Regular visits with dentist, daily brushing and flossing, adequate fluoride

Children should have an established dental home. They should have regularly scheduled visits with their dentist at least twice each year. Fluoride supplementation should be provided if the fluoride level in community (at home and at school) water supplies is low.

Your child's dentist may schedule a first visit to the orthodontist to evaluate the need for braces.

SAMPLE QUESTIONS:

How many times a day does your child brush and floss his teeth? How often does your child see the dentist? Does your child need help brushing his teeth?

For the child

Do you brush and floss your teeth every day? How many times? Do you always wear a mouth guard when you play contact sports?

ANTICIPATORY GUIDANCE:

- Your child already should have an established dental home (a dentist he sees regularly). He should be having regularly scheduled visits to the dentist. If your child does not have a dental home, we can help you find one.
- Be sure that your child brushes his teeth twice a day with a pea-sized amount of fluoridated toothpaste and flosses once a day with your help. Be sure to supervise the brushing and flossing, and help your child if necessary.
- Give your child a fluoride supplement if recommended by your dentist.

For the child

- It is important to brush your teeth at least twice a day and to floss at least once a day, to protect your teeth.
- If you are playing sports, always wear your mouth guard to protect your teeth.

SAFETY

Knowing child's friends and their families, supervision with friends, safety belts/ booster seats, helmets, playground safety, sports safety, swimming safety, sunscreen, smoke-free home/vehicles, guns, careful monitoring of computer use (games, Internet, e-mail)

As children now spend more time with other children and families, parents must help their children develop safe play habits. Play should be supervised by a responsible adult aware of children's activities and available in case of problems.

Parents should discuss personal safety in a manner that is informative and empowering without provoking unnecessary anxiety. Child sexual abuse prevention requires that children have knowledge and age-appropriate skills to keep themselves safe.

SAMPLE QUESTIONS:

Do you know your child's friends? Their families? Does your child know how to get help in an emergency if you are not present? Does your child have a back-up plan if you are not home when she gets there after school? Have you discussed with your child ways to prevent sexual abuse?

For the child

Do you know what to do if you get home and Mom or Dad is not there? What would you do if you felt unsafe at a friend's house? What would you do if a grown-up made you scared? Who could you tell? Who would help you? Has anyone ever touched you in a way that made you feel uncomfortable? Has anyone ever tried to harm you physically?

ANTICIPATORY GUIDANCE:

- Teach your child that the safety rules at home apply at other homes as well.
- Be sure that your child is supervised in a safe environment before and after school and at times when school is out.
- Anticipate providing less direct supervision as your child demonstrates more maturity.
- Be sure your child understands safety rules for the home, including emergency phone numbers, and that she knows what to do in case of a fire or other emergency. Teach your child how to dial 911.
- Help your child to understand it is always OK to ask to come home or call you if she is not comfortable at someone else's house.
- Teach your child that it is never all right for an adult to tell a child to keep secrets from parents, to express interest in private parts, or to ask a child for help with his or her private parts.

For the child

- Don't open the door to anyone you don't know. It's best not to have friends over unless your parents give you permission for them to be there.
- Be sure you play safe wherever you play. Every family should have the same safety rules.
- It's always OK to ask a grown-up for help if you are scared or worried. And it's OK to ask to go home and be with your Mom or Dad.
- We call the parts of your body that are usually under a bathing suit "privates" because we keep them covered and because you are the only one in charge of them.
- It is never OK for an older child or an adult to show you his or her private parts, to ask you to show your privates, to touch you there, to scare you, or to ask you not to tell your parents about what he or she did with you. Always get away from the person as quickly as possible and tell your parent or another adult right away.

Remind parents of the ongoing importance of automobile and bicycle safety. Children should use belt-positioning booster seats until the safety belt fits well. Stress the need for parental modeling of safe behaviors by wearing their own safety belts and bike helmets.

Questions about proper installation should be referred to a Certified Child Passenger Safety technician in the community.
Child Safety Seat Inspection Station Locator: www.seatcheck.org
Toll-free Number: 866-SEATCHECK (866-732-8243)

Child Safety Seat Inspection Station Locator: www.seatcheck.org. Toll-free Number: 866-SEATCHECK (866-732-8243).

SAMPLE QUESTIONS:
Does everyone in the family always wear a safety belt?
For the child
What type of seat do you sit in when you are in the car? Do you sit in the back seat every time you ride in the car?

ANTICIPATORY GUIDANCE:
- Continue to use a belt-positioning booster seat with the lap and shoulder safety belt until the lap/shoulder belt fits, which means the lap belt can be worn low and flat on the upper thighs, the shoulder belt can be worn across the shoulder rather than the face or neck, and your child can bend at the knees while sitting against the vehicle seat back. This usually happens when your child is between the ages of 8 and 12 and at about 4'9" tall.
- The back seat is the safest place for children younger than 13 to ride.

For the child
- Always sit in your booster seat and ride in the back seat of the car because that is where you are safest.

Reinforce the importance of safety in sports and other physical activities, emphasizing the need for wearing protective gear (eg, helmet, mouth guard, eye protection, and knee and elbow pads).

Children younger than 16 should not ride an all-terrain vehicle.

SAMPLE QUESTIONS:

Do you enforce the use of helmets? Do you always wear helmets yourself?

For the child

Do you always wear a helmet when biking, skating, skiing, in-line skating, snow boarding, or horseback riding? (List activities appropriate to the area and child.)

ANTICIPATORY GUIDANCE:

- Make sure your child always wears a helmet while riding a bike. Now is the time to teach your child "Rules of the Road." Be sure she knows the rules and can use them.
- Watch your child ride. See if she is in control of the bike. See if your child uses good judgment. Your 8-year-old child is not old enough to ride at dusk or after dark. Make sure your child brings the bike in when the sun starts to set.
- Make sure your child also always wears protective equipment when skating, skiing, in-line skating, snowboarding, horseback riding, skateboarding, or riding a scooter. *(List activities appropriate to the area and family.)*

For the child

- Being active is good for you, but being safe while being active is just as important. One of the best ways to protect yourself is to wear the right safety equipment, especially a helmet, when you are biking, skating, skiing, in-line skating, snowboarding, or horseback riding. *(List activities as appropriate.)*

An adult should supervise whenever children are in or near water. Reinforce the continuing importance of using sunscreen on the child when the child is outside.

SAMPLE QUESTIONS:

Does your child know how to swim?

For the child

Do you know how to swim? What rules do your parents have about swimming?

ANTICIPATORY GUIDANCE:

- Teach your child to swim. Knowing how to swim does not make children "drown proof," so even if your child knows how to swim, never let her swim alone.
- Do not let your child play around any water (lake, stream, pool, or ocean) unless an adult is watching. NEVER let your child swim in any fast-moving water.
- Teach your child to never dive into water unless an adult has checked the depth of the water.
- When on any boat, be sure your child is wearing an appropriately fitting, US Coast Guard-approved life jacket.

- Be sure that swimming pools in your community, apartment complex, or home have a 4-sided fence with a self-closing, self-latching gate.

For the child

- Swimming lessons are an important way to become comfortable in the water. Ask your parents about learning to swim.
- Never swim without an adult around.

SAMPLE QUESTIONS:

What type of sunscreen do you use on your child when she goes outside?

ANTICIPATORY GUIDANCE:

- Use sunscreen (SPF 15 or higher) on your child before she goes outside to play or swim. Read the directions carefully and apply the correct amount of sunscreen. Apply it at least 15 minutes before she goes out in the sun and reapply it every 2 hours.

Encourage parents to keep their home and vehicles smoke-free. Refer parents who smoke and request assistance in quitting to community resources for smoking cessation.

SAMPLE QUESTIONS:

Does anyone smoke in your home or vehicle? If so, who?

ANTICIPATORY GUIDANCE:

- Exposure to secondhand smoke greatly increases the risk of heart and lung diseases in your child. For your health and your child's health, please stop smoking if you are a smoker, and insist that others not smoke around your child.

For the child

- Don't try cigarettes. They are bad for your lungs and heart, and your skin and teeth. Walk away from kids who offer you cigarettes or other things to smoke.

Discuss gun safety in the home and the danger of guns to family members and children. Homicide and completed suicide are more common in homes in which guns are kept. The AAP recommends that guns be removed from where children live and play, and that, if it is necessary to keep a gun, it should be stored unloaded and locked, with the ammunition locked separately from the gun.

Children this age are curious. Because guns can lead to serious injury or death, parents cannot rely on their own children, no matter how well-behaved they are, to avoid handling a weapon that they find. At this age, children still lack the maturity or cognitive capacity to reliably follow advice concerning guns.

SAMPLE QUESTIONS:

If there is a gun in your home, is it unloaded and locked up? Where is the ammunition stored? Have you considered not owning a gun because it poses a danger to children and other family members?

For the child
What would you do if you saw a gun?

ANTICIPATORY GUIDANCE:

- If it is necessary to keep a gun in your home, it should be stored unloaded and locked, with the ammunition locked separately from the gun. Keep the key where children cannot have access.
- Remember that children simply do not understand how dangerous guns can be, despite your warnings.

For the child

- Adults are supposed to keep their guns away from children. If you see a gun that is unlocked, don't touch it, but do tell your parent right away.

Internet safety is similar to neighborhood safety. Younger children never play outside unsupervised or leave the yard. More mature children will be allowed to go to known safe places like a playground, but not allowed to wander into inappropriate or unsafe areas. Internet use should parallel safe play outdoors. Younger children should only be online supervised, and, with increasing maturity, limited browsing can be permitted.

Information about safe Internet use and the AAP-Microsoft Family Safety Settings can be found at www.aap.org.

SAMPLE QUESTIONS:
How much do you know about your child's Internet use (eg, what sites she's visiting, what games she's playing, who she's talking to, and how much time she's spending on the computer)? Do you have rules for the Internet? Have you installed an Internet filter?

For the child
What would you do if you came to an Internet site that you thought wasn't a good idea or that scared you?

ANTICIPATORY GUIDANCE:

- Your family computer should be in a place where you can easily observe your child's use.
- Check the Internet history regularly to be sure you approve of your child's Internet choices.
- Just as you monitor your child's activity in the neighborhood and community, it is important to be aware of her Internet use. A safety filter allows some parental supervision.[3]

For the child

- It is important to only go online when your parents say it's OK. And never go to Internet sites unless you know they are good choices.
- Never chat online unless you tell your parents. No one should ever make you feel scared online.
- Do not give your personal information (like your full name or address or phone number) on a Web site unless your parents say it is OK.

Middle Childhood: 9 and 10 Year Visits

CONTEXT

Puberty is beginning in some children. Pubertal onset is marked by breast development at about age 10 for girls, and by testicular enlargement at about age 11 for boys. These changes are accompanied by a growth spurt. Individual, as well as racial, differences are noted with pubertal onset. This is an opportunity for the health care professional to learn about family and cultural beliefs about puberty and about how the family's cultural and religious values will guide the discussion of sexuality and physical changes of puberty.

By the time a child is 9 or 10, he has become a member of a peer group and is playing sports, involved in social and community activities, competing at video games, and listening to his favorite music. Most of his friends are the same gender, and these friends have assumed great importance in his life. The child's growing independence from the family is now more apparent.

Parents can acknowledge the child's desire for independence by offering him opportunities to earn privileges by demonstrating his responsibility (eg, parents may identify appropriate chores, while allowing the child to decide when to complete them and the consequences if the chores are or are not completed). The value placed on independence and how it is defined are determined by culture, the economic realities of the family, and the safety of the general environment. In some families, conflict arises if the parents misinterpret this normal realignment of allegiance toward peers as a rejection of family values, past support, and guidance.

Supporting and enhancing the child's self-esteem and self-confidence are critical during this period. Children who feel good about themselves are better equipped to withstand negative peer pressure than children who have a lot of self-doubt. Families need to spend time with the child, talking with him, showing affection, and praising his efforts and accomplishments. In some cultures, it is deemed inappropriate to praise children, and they will have alternative approaches to enhance their child's sense of competence and self-esteem. It is important to have this discussion with parents in the context of the family's culture. Caregivers who are depressed may have difficulty providing such emotional support. The health care professional can help by identifying the child's strengths and promoting communication between him and his family.

School performance continues to mark the child's accomplishments across all developmental domains (social-emotional, communicative, cognitive, and physical). Inquire about school success. It may be of value to review the child's most recent report card. Increasing requirements for autonomy and self-motivation may lead to academic deterioration for children who functioned well with supervised and structured academic tasks. Is the child having any academic or social problems? How does he get along with teachers and peers? Is the child participating in extracurricular activities or is he involved with clubs? At this age, many children become

9 and 10 Year Visits

9 and 10 Year Visits

involved in a variety of outside activities, including sports, music, scouting, and community or faith-based activities. A child can easily become overscheduled, and parents need to balance enriching activities with sufficient "down time" and family time.

Injury prevention should be emphasized during this stage of development. The 9- or 10-year-old child may engage in dangerous risk-taking behaviors (eg, dares, drinking, smoking, inhaling, or gang involvement) as a result of peer pressure. If the peer group includes older children, the child may encounter pressure to perform acts and take risks for which he is not developmentally prepared. Recognizing and discussing this possibility may help parents teach their children about dealing with peer pressure.

Parents need to know their children's friends and the friends' parents. For parents and caregivers with limited English proficiency, supervising their child in the broader community can be a challenge. Health care professionals can help provide connections to supports in the community that will enhance the parents' role. Children this age should still be in environments where appropriate adult supervision exists so as to limit opportunities for experimentation with cigarettes, alcohol and other drugs, and other developmentally inappropriate activities. The amount of unsupervised time and the incidence of drug use are directly related.

The health care professional may want to meet alone with the child or the child may want to meet alone with the health care professional. It may be most appropriate to give the child the choice. At this age, some children may feel a need to have a parent close by during the visit to help describe any individual or family concerns; while others may feel they are "pre-teenagers" and should be seen without parental supervision. However the health care professional may need for parents to verify and expand some of the child's answers. Cultural norms should be taken into account in making this decision.

PRIORITIES FOR THE VISIT

The first priority is to attend to the concerns of the parents. In addition, the Bright Futures Middle Childhood Expert Panel has given priority to the following topics for discussion in this visit:

- School (school performance, homework, bullying)
- Development and mental health (emotional security and self-esteem, family communication and family time, temper problems and setting reasonable limits, friends, school performance, readiness for middle school, sexuality [pubertal onset, personal hygiene, initiation of growth spurt, menstruation and ejaculation, loss of "baby fat" and accretion of muscle, sexual safety])
- Nutrition and physical activity (weight concerns, body image, importance of breakfast, limits on high-fat foods, water rather than soda or juice, eating as a family, physical activity)
- Oral health (regular visits with dentist, daily brushing and flossing, adequate fluoride)
- Safety (safety belts, helmets, bicycle safety, swimming, sunscreen, tobacco/alcohol/drugs, knowing child's friends and their families, supervision of child with friends, guns)

HEALTH SUPERVISION

History

Interval history may be obtained according to the concerns of the family and the health care professional's preference or style of practice. The following questions can encourage in-depth discussion:

Questions to the Parent:
- What concerns do you have about your child's physical well-being or special health care needs?
- Do you have any concerns about your child's development or learning?
- Tell me about any concerns you may have about your child's mood or behavior (eg, attention, hitting others, temper, worries, not having good friends, irritability, mood, or activity level)?

Questions to the Child:
- How have you been?
- How is everything going for you?
- What issues or concerns would you like to discuss today?

Observation of Parent-Child Interaction

During the visit, the health care professional should observe:

- Do both the parent and the child ask questions?
- Does the parent allow the child to communicate with you directly, or does the parent interfere in your interaction with the child?

Surveillance of Development

School performance is a functional marker of a child's development and accomplishments across all developmental domains (social-emotional, communicative, cognitive, and physical). Increasing requirements for autonomy and self-motivation sometimes lead to academic deterioration for children who functioned well with supervised and structured academic tasks.

The child's intellectual abilities as well as learning problems become more apparent during this period of the child's development. Many learning problems become evident in the later elementary school years, as expectations for class performance increase. School failure or new struggles require investigation, as they frequently indicate an unrecognized learning disability, ADHD, or the impact of stressors, such as family dysfunction and divorce, bullying at school, or depression in the child or parent. Some children and parents also become apprehensive about the transition to middle school.

For children and youth with special health care needs and for children receiving supplemental or special education services, a review of services with parents is appropriate. It is helpful for parents to provide a copy of their child's IEP or Section 504 Plan for discussion. Review these documents carefully for accurate attention to medical co-morbidities, appropriate accommodations for the child's special needs, and for comprehensive approaches to learning. Also, review medications that may need to be administered during the school day, including psychotropic medications, and ensure completion of appropriate school forms. Consider switching the child to extended-release medications if the child is embarrassed by taking medications at school. Some parents may choose to avoid contacting the school about ADHD medications because of concerns about stigma. Yet, parents should be informed that teacher-parent communication about behavior and medications will help the parents and the health care professional make the right decisions about dosing.

Do you have any specific concerns about your child's development, learning, or behavior?

A 9- or 10-year-old child
- Demonstrates physical, cognitive, emotional, social, and moral competencies
- Engages in behaviors that promote wellness and contribute to a healthy lifestyle
- Demonstrates increasingly responsible and independent decision making
- Has a caring, supportive relationship with family, other adults, and peers
- Experiences a sense of self-confidence, hopefulness, and well-being[2]

Physical Examination

A complete physical examination is included as part of every health supervision visit. Respect the child's privacy by using appropriate draping during the examination. Ask siblings to wait in the waiting room, if possible.

When performing a physical examination, the health care professional's attention is directed to the following components of the examination that are important for a child this age:

- **Measure:**
  - Blood pressure

- **Measure and plot:**
  - Height
  - Weight
- **Calculate and plot:**
  - BMI
- **Skin**
  - Observe tattoos, piercings, and any signs of abuse or self-inflicted injuries
  - Inspect nevi or birthmarks; note any changes
- **Spine**
  - Examine back
- **Breasts and Genitalia**
  - Assess for sexual maturity rating

Screening — 9 Year

UNIVERSAL SCREENING	ACTION	
None		
SELECTIVE SCREENING	**RISK ASSESSMENT***	**ACTION IF RA +**
Vision	+ on risk screening questions	Snellen test
Hearing	+ on risk screening questions	Audiometry
Anemia	+ on risk screening questions	Hemoglobin or hematocrit
Tuberculosis	+ on risk screening questions	Tuberculin skin test

*See Rationale and Evidence chapter for the criteria on which risk screening questions are based.

Screening — 10 Year

UNIVERSAL SCREENING	ACTION	
Vision	Snellen test	
Hearing	Audiometry	
SELECTIVE SCREENING	**RISK ASSESSMENT***	**ACTION IF RA +**
Anemia	+ on risk screening questions	Hemoglobin or hematocrit
Tuberculosis	+ on risk screening questions	Tuberculin skin test
Dyslipidemia	+ on risk screening questions and not previously screened with normal results	Fasting lipid profile

*See Rationale and Evidence chapter for the criteria on which risk screening questions are based.

Immunizations

Consult the CDC/ACIP or AAP Web site for the current immunization schedule.
CDC National Immunization Program (NIP): http://www.cdc.gov/vaccines
American Academy of Pediatrics *Red Book:* http://www.aapredbook.org

ANTICIPATORY GUIDANCE

The following sample questions, which address the Middle Childhood Expert Panel's Anticipatory Guidance Priorities, are intended to be used selectively to invite discussion, gather information, address the needs and concerns of the family, and build partnerships. Use of the questions may vary from visit to visit and from family to family. Questions can be modified to match the health care professional's communication style. The accompanying anticipatory guidance for the family should be geared to questions, issues, or concerns for that particular child and family.

SCHOOL

School performance, homework, bullying

At this age, the child may be expected to display self-confidence with a sense of mastery and pride in school and extracurricular activities, participate in group activities, understand and comply with most rules at school, and assume reasonable responsibility for her schoolwork. Reinforce the strengths of the child and parents with comments such as, "I'm so pleased that you are making good progress with math."

SAMPLE QUESTIONS:
What issues about school would you like to discuss? What extracurricular activities do you encourage your child to participate in?

For the child
How is school going? What are some of the things you are good at doing? What are you proud of? What kinds of school and after-school activities are you involved in? What concerns do you have about being bullied or teased or being hurt physically or sexually?

ANTICIPATORY GUIDANCE:
- If your child is not doing well in school, ask the teacher about special help or tutoring that may be available.
- Praise your child's efforts and accomplishments in school. Show interest in her school performance and after-school activities.
- Provide a well-lit, quiet space for homework. Remove distractions such as television. Set routine times for homework.
- If your child tells you that she is being bullied, discuss it with her teacher or guidance counselor.

For the child
- Doing well in school is important to how you feel about yourself. However, doing well means something different for each person. What matters is that you try your best and ask for help when you need it.
- Joining clubs and teams, church groups, and friends for activities is a fun way to stay healthy and enjoy being with other kids outside of school.
- If someone picks on you or tries to hurt you, tell them in a firm voice to stop bothering you, and walk away. Tell your teacher, your parents, or another adult you trust about what is happening. Have them help you avoid these situations and stop their harmful behavior.

DEVELOPMENT AND MENTAL HEALTH

Emotional security and self-esteem, family communication and family time, temper problems and setting reasonable limits, friends, school performance, readiness for middle school, sexuality (pubertal onset, personal hygiene, initiation of growth spurt, menstruation and ejaculation, loss of "baby fat" and accretion of muscle, sexual safety)

At this age, the child may be expected to display self-confidence, understand and comply with most rules at home, and assume reasonable responsibility for his chores.

SAMPLE QUESTIONS:

How happy a person is your child? Has your child been having any recent stresses in the family or school? How do you discipline your child? How often do you share a clear "no use" message about alcohol, tobacco, and other drugs with your child? What are your household rules and the consequences for not observing them? How respectful of others do you think your child is? Do you talk to your child about your values and attitudes about sex?

For the child

Tell me about some of the things you are good at doing. What are some of the things that make you sad? Angry? Worried? How do you handle that?

How do your parents or other adults help you when you get upset or angry? How do your parents discipline you? What do you and your friends like to do together? What do you do when your friends pressure you to do things you don't want to do? If you said, "No," what do you think your friends would do? Do you have friends or know other children at school who use or try to get other kids to use cigarettes, alcoholic drinks, drugs, or having sex?

ANTICIPATORY GUIDANCE:

- Promote self-responsibility.
- Assign age-appropriate chores, including responsibility for personal belongings and for some household or yard tasks.
- Provide personal space at home, even if limited, for your child.
- Promote independence by encouraging developmentally appropriate decision making.
- Anticipate the normal range of early adolescent behaviors, including the pervasive influence of peers, a change in the communication between you and your child, sudden challenges to parental rules and authority, conflicts over issues of independence, refusal to participate in some family activities, moodiness, and a new desire to take risks.
- Serve as a positive ethical and behavioral role model.
- Handle anger constructively in the family. Do not allow either physical or verbal violence; encourage compromise. Do not permit yourself or others to use corporal punishment.
- Encourage and role model the admission of mistakes and asking of forgiveness.

- Supervise your child's activities with peers. Encourage your child to bring friends into your home and help them feel welcome there.
- Help your child learn appropriate and respectful behavior. Reinforce the importance of respectful behavior toward others.
- Counsel your child to not use alcohol, tobacco, drugs, and inhalants.

For the child

- Talking with a safe and trusted adult is an important way to handle anger, disappointment, and worry.
- Good friends are important. They never ask you to do harmful or scary things; they want what is best for you. If you find that a good friend has become a bad friend, try talking with him. If that person is unwilling to change, stop spending time with him.
- Everyone gets angry. It's normal. Here are some ways you can deal with anger. You can avoid getting defensive, calm yourself, acknowledge the importance of the other person's point of view, listen without interrupting, repeat your understanding of what the issues are, and demonstrate your desire to understand the angered person.
- It's normal to have up moods and down moods, but, if you feel sad most of the time, enjoy very few things, or find yourself wishing you were dead, we should talk about it. Almost everyone worries at times about how they look and whether they are developing normally.
- Every person has to decide whether or not to try alcohol, drugs, cigarettes, and sex. Chances are, you know at least some of the dangers of trying each of these, but there are many more dangers you likely don't know or don't want to think about. It's not enough to just say, "No." If you really mean "No!" to any one of these choices, you need to clearly say why you feel that way.

Children are now initiating sexual development. They are aware of sexual themes and content in media. Access to accurate and culturally appropriate information on sexual development and sexuality is essential from multiple sources (home, school, and health care professionals).

Parents are encouraged to engage their children in an ongoing conversation regarding sexual development. Questions can be answered simply, and additional discussion should be welcomed.

SAMPLE QUESTIONS:
How well do you and your partner agree on how to talk with your child about issues related to sexual development and sexuality? Does your child know any gay men or lesbian women? How about children brought up by same-sex couples? How would you respond if your child asked you about this topic?

For the child
What questions do you have about the way your body is developing? Have you ever been pressured to touch someone in a way that made you feel uncomfortable? Has anyone ever tried to touch you in a way that made you feel uncomfortable?

ANTICIPATORY GUIDANCE:

- Be prepared to answer questions about sexuality and to provide concrete examples of the types of behavior that are not acceptable to you.
- Encourage your child to ask questions. Answer them at a level appropriate to his understanding. Discuss these issues even if sexual activity seems unlikely.
- Teach your child the importance of delaying sexual behavior.
- If your child receives family life education at school or in the community, discuss the information and review materials with him.
- Teach your child that it is never all right for an adult to tell a child to keep secrets from parents, to express interest in private parts, or to ask a child for help with his or her private parts.

For the child
- For boys and girls:
  - Around age 8 or 9, you will notice your body starting to change. Some of the first things that happen are that you develop body odor, and the skin on your face becomes oilier and may break out in pimples or acne. You will need to bathe every day, use deodorant, and wash your face well in the morning and at night.
- For girls:
  - The next changes you will notice are that your breasts will start to get bigger. It's normal for one side to be bigger than the other at first. As your breasts grow, you will need to wear a bra.
  - Hair will grow on your underarms and pubic area, becoming thicker, darker, and curlier over time. You also will start to grow taller at a very fast rate. This is called the growth spurt. Now is a good time to have pads (sanitary napkins) available to use in your underwear when your periods start.
  - Girls can have their first period, or menses, as early as 10, but usually by 13. Every girl is different. Periods often come at unpredictable times at first, but they eventually will come about once every 4 weeks. A small amount of blood, sometimes more brown in color than red, will come from your vagina and appear on your underwear. Use the pads to catch the blood. Change your pad every few hours and wrap the used pad in toilet paper or place it in a small paper bag to be discarded. Most pads cannot be flushed down toilets. Always wash your hands after changing your pad.
- For boys:
  - The next change you will notice is that your testicles will begin to grow larger. Hair will grow on your underarms and pubic area, becoming thicker, darker, and curlier over time. Soon, your penis will become longer and wider and your testicles will continue to grow. You also will start to grow taller at a very fast rate. This is called the growth spurt. Your voice will also start to crack and deepen as your larynx or voice box grows longer. You may find a wet, sticky discharge, called an ejaculation, on your pajama bottoms in the morning. This is called a wet dream. Ejaculations are not the same as passing urine. Ejaculations contain sperm and a special fluid. This happens because of strong surges of hormones that occur while you sleep.

- For boys and girls:
  - It is never OK for an older child or an adult to show you his or her private parts, to ask you to show your privates, to touch you there, to scare you, or to ask you not to tell your parents about what he or she did with you. Always get away from the person as quickly as possible and tell your parent or another adult right away.

NUTRITION AND PHYSICAL ACTIVITY

Weight concerns, body image, importance of breakfast, limits on high-fat foods, water rather than soda or juice, eating as a family, physical activity

Children this age are at risk of overweight or obesity. Carefully assess BMI and discuss results with parents. Meal skipping increases in this age group. Often, a child will eat snacks and not be hungry at mealtimes. This habit may lead to unhealthy eating practices.

In addition, at this age, girls begin to think of dieting and weight loss. Evaluate the child's risk of severe dieting or tendencies toward an eating disorder.

SAMPLE QUESTIONS:
Do you have any concerns about your child's weight? Do you have any concerns about her eating behaviors or food intake (eg, getting her to drink enough milk and eat fruits and vegetables)? How often does she drink soda and/or juice? How often do you have a family meal together? Are there ever times when your family does not have enough to eat?

For the child
What concerns do you have about your weight? How do you feel about how you look? How often have you cut back on how much you eat or tried a diet to lose weight? What fruits and/or vegetables did you eat yesterday? Did you eat breakfast this morning? How often do you drink soda, sports drinks, or juices?

ANTICIPATORY GUIDANCE:
- Help your child learn to choose appropriate foods, including plenty of fruits and vegetables every day. Aim for at least 5 servings of fruits or vegetables every day by including them in most of your meals and snacks.
- Limit high-fat or low-nutrient foods and beverages, such as candy, salty snacks, fast foods, or soft drinks.
- Make sure your child is getting enough calcium daily. Children aged 9 to 18 need about 3 cups of low-fat milk a day. Low-fat yogurt and cheese are good alternatives to milk.
- Share family meals together regularly. Make mealtimes pleasant and companionable; encourage conversation. Avoid having the TV on during mealtimes.

For the child

- I am happy to answer your questions and explain your weight and height measurements. The key to good health is a balance between calorie intake from foods and calorie output in activity.
- Healthy eating prevents weight problems and helps learning. Eating a healthy breakfast every day is especially important.
- Every day, try to eat fruits, vegetables, whole-grain breads and cereals, low-fat or fat-free dairy products, and lean meats. Drink low-fat or fat-free milk or water instead of soda and sugared drinks. Choose small portions instead of large ones, or share a large portion (especially foods that are high in fat or sugar) with someone else.
- Weight loss is almost never a good idea while your body is rapidly growing in puberty. If you are considering going on a diet to lose weight, let's talk about it first.
- If you are considering taking dietary supplements, please discuss these plans with me to make sure they are safe and really will help you reach your goals.

All children should be able to participate in some type of physical activity. Talk to parents of children with special health care needs about the benefits and risks associated with physical activity. Emphasize the importance of safety equipment when the child participates in physical activity.

At this age, children become involved in organized sports. Educate parents about appropriate sports for age and ability. Discuss with the family the attributes of a quality program and coach.

SAMPLE QUESTIONS:
Do you have concerns about your child's activity level (either too much or too little)?
For the child
Tell me about the physical activities you do inside and outside of school. How often do you do them?

ANTICIPATORY GUIDANCE:
- Support your child's sport and physical activity interests, and play with your child.
- Limit all screen time (TV, videos, video games, and computer time other than for homework) to no more than 2 hours total per day.

For the child
- Try to get at least 1 hour of moderate- to high-intensity exercise every day. Find ways to become more active, such as walking or biking instead of riding in a car, and taking the stairs, not elevators. Be active with your friends to increase the fun. Being physically active every day helps you feel good and focus on your schoolwork.
- It helps to plan times each day that are dedicated to a physical activity you enjoy, making activity part of your routine, rather than an exception.

ORAL HEALTH

Regular visits with dentist, daily brushing and flossing, adequate fluoride

Children should have an established dental home. They should have regularly scheduled visits with their dentist at least twice each year. Fluoride supplementation should be provided if the fluoride level in community (at home and at school) water supplies is low.

SAMPLE QUESTIONS:
Who is your child's regular dentist? Is the water you drink fluoridated? Is your child involved in physical activities, such as contact sports, that could potentially result in dental injuries? (Probe for use of protective gear.) *How would you handle a dental emergency?*

For the child
Do you brush and floss your teeth every day?

ANTICIPATORY GUIDANCE:
- Be sure that your child brushes his teeth twice a day with a pea-sized amount of fluoridated toothpaste and flosses once a day with your help. Be sure to supervise brushing and flossing every day and help if necessary.
- By the time your child is 10, he already should have an established dental home (a dentist he sees regularly). He should see the dentist at least twice a year. If your child does not have a dental home, try to get one.
- Give your child fluoride supplements if recommended by your dentist.

For the child
- To protect your teeth, it is important to brush your teeth at least twice each day and to floss at least once a day.
- If you are playing sports, always wear your mouth guard to protect your teeth.

SAFETY

Safety belts, helmets, bicycle safety, swimming, sunscreen, tobacco/alcohol/drugs, knowing child's friends and their families, supervision of child with friends, guns

A child should use a booster seat until the safety belt fits properly, which means the lap belt can be worn low and flat on the upper thighs, the shoulder belt can be worn across the shoulder rather than the face or neck, and the child can bend at the knees while sitting against the vehicle seat back (usually between the ages of 8 and 12 and about 4'9" tall).

Questions about proper installation should be referred to a Certified Child Passenger Safety technician in the community.
Child Safety Seat Inspection Station Locator: www.seatcheck.org
Toll-free Number: 866-SEATCHECK (866-732-8243)

The back seat is the safest place for children younger than 13 to ride.

Child Safety Seat Inspection Station Locator: www.seatcheck.org. Toll-free Number: 866-SEATCHECK (866-732-8243).

MIDDLE CHILDHOOD 9 AND 10 YEAR VISITS

SAMPLE QUESTIONS:

Does everyone in the family use a safety belt?

For the child

Do you use a booster seat or safety belt every time you ride in the car?

Do you sit in the back seat every time you ride in the car?

ANTICIPATORY GUIDANCE:

- Do not start your vehicle until everyone's safety belt is buckled.

For the child

- The back seat of the car is still the safest place for you to sit until you are at least 13.
- Using a booster seat or wearing a safety belt every time you get in the car is the best way to protect yourself from injury and death in a crash.

Reinforce the importance of safety in sports and other physical activities, emphasizing the need for wearing protective gear (helmet, mouth guard, eye protection, and knee and elbow pads).

SAMPLE QUESTIONS:

Do you enforce the use of helmets? Do you model this behavior?

For the child

How often do you wear a helmet and protective gear when biking, skating, skiing, in-line skating, snowboarding, or horseback riding? (Tailor the list of activities appropriate to the area and the child.)

ANTICIPATORY GUIDANCE:

- Make sure your child always wears protective equipment when biking, skating, skiing, snowboarding, horseback riding, skateboarding, riding a scooter, or in-line skating. *(Tailor the list to activities appropriate to the area and family.)*

For the child

- Being active is good for you, but being safe while being active is just as important. One of the best ways to protect yourself is to wear the right safety equipment, especially a helmet when you are biking, skating, skiing, in-line skating, snowboarding, or horseback riding. *(Tailor the list to activities as appropriate.)*

511

An adult should supervise children when they are near water. Reinforce the continuing importance of using sunscreen on your child when she is outside.

SAMPLE QUESTIONS:
Does your child know how to swim?
For the child
Do you know how to swim? What rules do your parents have about swimming?

ANTICIPATORY GUIDANCE:
- Teach your child to swim.
- Do not let your child play around any water (lake, stream, pool, or ocean) unless an adult is watching. Even if your child knows how to swim, never let her swim alone. NEVER let your child swim in any fast-moving water.
- Teach your child to never dive into water unless an adult has checked the depth of the water.
- When on any boat, be sure your child is wearing an appropriately fitting, US Coast Guard-approved life jacket.
- Be sure that swimming pools in your community, apartment complex, or home have a 4-sided fence with a self-closing, self-latching gate.

For the child
- Swimming lessons are an important way to become comfortable in the water. Ask your parents about learning to swim.
- Never swim without an adult around.

SAMPLE QUESTION:
What type of sunscreen do you use on your child when she goes outside?

ANTICIPATORY GUIDANCE:
- Use sunscreen (SPF 15 or higher) on your child before she goes outside to play or swim. Read the directions carefully and apply the correct amount of sunscreen. Apply it at least 15 minutes before she goes out in the sun, and reapply it every 2 hours.

Tobacco, alcohol, and drugs are new risks for children as they approach middle school. Children need clear messages about the dangers of substance use.

SAMPLE QUESTIONS:
Is smoking, alcohol, or drug use a concern in your family? Is your child exposed to substance use?

ANTICIPATORY GUIDANCE:
- Children are constantly exposed to smoking, drinking, and drug-use behaviors through TV and other media. They need clear messages that substance use is substance abuse.
- If alcohol is used in the home, its use should be appropriate and discussed with children.
- If you or anyone in the house smoke, try to quit. If quitting is not possible, discuss the difficulty of addiction with your child.

For the child

■ Do any of your friends smoke, drink alcohol or beer, or use drugs? Will you ever smoke, drink alcohol, or use drugs?

As their children are now spending increasing amounts of time with other children and families, parents must help their children develop safe play habits. Play should be supervised by a responsible adult who is aware of children's activities and available in case of problems.

SAMPLE QUESTIONS:

Do you know your child's friends? Their families? Does your child know how to get help in an emergency if you are not present?

For the child

What would you do if you felt unsafe at a friend's house?

ANTICIPATORY GUIDANCE:

■ Teach your child that the safety rules at home apply at other homes as well.
■ Help your child understand it is always OK to ask to come home or call her parent if she is not comfortable at someone else's house.

For the child

■ Be sure you play safe wherever you play. Every family should have the same safety rules.
■ It's always OK to ask a grown-up for help if you are scared or worried. And it's OK to ask to go home and be with your Mom or Dad.

The safest home is one without a gun. A gun kept in the home is far more likely to kill or injure someone known to the family than to kill or injure an intruder. A gun kept in the home triples the risk of homicide. The risk of completed suicide is far more likely if a gun is kept in the home.

There is evidence that programs designed to teach children to avoid contact with guns are not effective in overcoming the child's innate curiosity and social pressure to handle guns. At this age, children still lack the maturity or cognitive capacity to reliably follow advice concerning guns.

SAMPLE QUESTIONS:

Who, among family members and friends, owns a weapon or gun? Have you considered not owning a gun because it poses a danger to children and other family members?

For the child

What have your parents taught you about guns and what not to do with them?

ANTICIPATORY GUIDANCE:

■ Homicide and completed suicide are more common in homes that have guns. The best way to keep your child safe from injury or death from guns is to never have a gun in the home.
■ If it is necessary to keep a gun in your home, it should be stored unloaded and locked, with the ammunition locked separately from the gun. Keep the key where children cannot have access.

■ Ask if there are guns in homes where your child plays. If so, make sure they are stored unloaded and locked, with the ammunition locked separately, before allowing your child to play in the home.

■ Talk to your child about guns in school or on your streets. Find out if your child's friends carry guns.

For the child

■ Adults are supposed to keep their guns away from children. If you see a gun that is unlocked, don't touch it, but tell your parent right away.

■ If you are starting to hunt with adults in your family, learn how to use guns and hunting knives safely, and use them only under adult supervision.

References

1. Olweus Bullying Prevention Program. Available at: http://www.clemson.edu/olweus/index.html. Accessed November 18, 2006

2. Association of Maternal and Child Health Programs. *A Conceptual Framework for Adolescent Health*. Washington, DC: Association of Maternal and Child Health Programs, National Network of State Adolescent Health Coordinators; 2005:5-6

3. Microsoft strives to help make Internet use safer, more family-friendly. Available at: http://www.aap.org/advocacy/releases/mar06microsoft.htm. Accessed November 21, 2006

Adolescence

11 to 21 Years

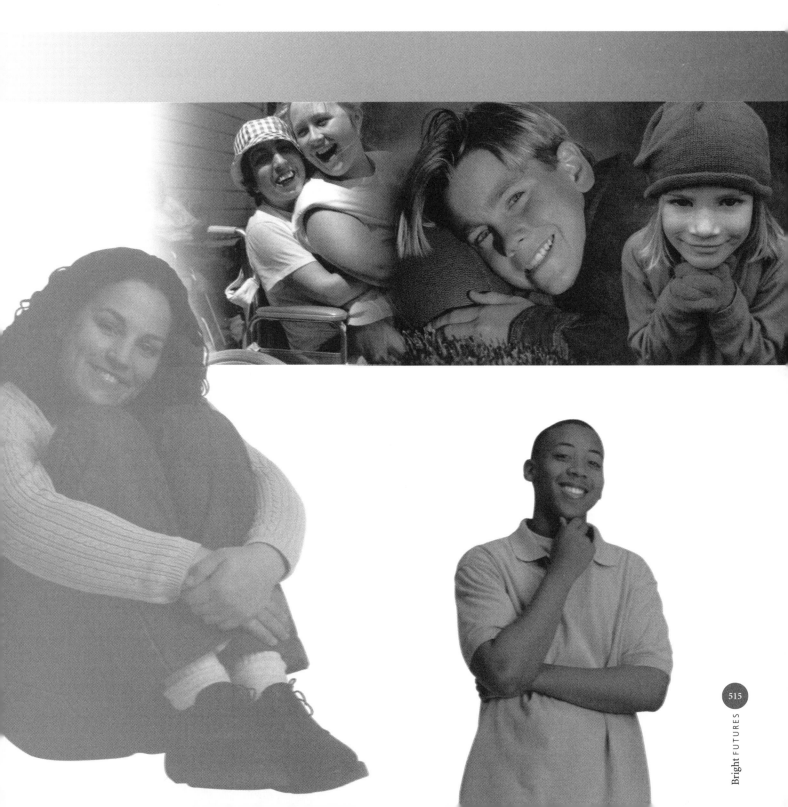

Health Supervision: Early Adolescence (11 to 14 Year Visits)

CONTEXT

The early adolescent is embarking on a journey of remarkable transitions and transformations—physically, cognitively, emotionally, and socially—and the pace at which these physical and emotional changes occur varies widely. The onset of puberty is one indicator that the adolescent phase of life is beginning. Because puberty typically involves breast development at about age 9 or 10 for girls, and testicular enlargement for boys at about age 11, many youth have some degree of pubertal developmental as they enter early adolescence. These changes are accompanied by a growth spurt. For girls, the maximal growth rate is reached about 6 to 12 months before menarche. Boys have a later growth spurt and, during their growth spurt, have a greater peak height velocity[1] than girls. Other physical changes also become apparent. The skin of both boys and girls becomes oily as apocrine glands begin to secrete. Secondary sex characteristics (ie, female breasts, male genitalia, and pubic hair) develop, notable changes in body fat and musculature occur, and a boy's voice begins to change. Many of these physical changes are more closely associated with the stage of sexual maturity than with chronological age. Menarche often occurs between SMR stages 3 and 4. The AAP and ACOG recommend that health care professionals view the menstrual cycle as a "vital sign"[2] and include education about the normal timing and characteristics of menstruation and other pubertal markers as an important component of health supervision for young girls and their parents.

Puberty, perhaps the key developmental milestone of early adolescence, is an important focus for all cultures. Health care professionals should seek to understand the meaning of it in the cultures of the families they serve. Early adolescents with special health care needs can experience puberty at the usual time or they can have an earlier or delayed onset of pubertal change based on their health condition. All children should receive appropriate education about the changes of puberty and what to expect for themselves and classmates.

Along with these physical changes, early adolescents' cognitive abilities are developing. As they mature, these youth develop increased capacity for logical, abstract, and idealistic thinking. Schooling shifts from the emotionally secure environment of elementary school, where students have only a single teacher and the same classmates, to the more challenging social environment of middle school and high school, with intense course work, multiple teachers, multiple groups of classmates, and rising expectations for academic and social advancement. These academic demands provide many opportunities for early adolescents to explore their burgeoning interests and for their sense of achievement and self-esteem to blossom. They also can unmask a previously undiagnosed learning disorder or attention-deficit problems, or can affect the adolescent's ability to cope, which, in turn, can lead to depression and other mental health issues.

517

As academic work increases in complexity, parents may feel challenged and unsure about how to help. These issues can be even more difficult among youth with special health care needs, who may be challenged physically, cognitively, or socially to engage in school activities and fit in with their peers.

Socially, early adolescents experience dramatic changes over relatively few years as they mature. They need to belong to a peer group and they desire the independence or freedom to do what they want and with whom they want. However, these changes do not occur at the same time or at the same pace among all youth. In an attempt to keep pace with individual physical changes that can outpace or lag behind that of their friends, young adolescents often will use clothing (eg, designer T-shirts), accessories (eg, body piercing), and hairstyles (eg, color rinses) as a way to fit in with peers. Youth with special health care needs experience the same social changes, although their reactions may be influenced by the nature of their conditions and acceptance or rejection of their condition by friends, family, and community (eg, stigma of being HIV positive or having a very obvious physical difference).

For many, early adolescence can be a difficult time socially. Parents and educators must remain alert and take extra steps to ensure inclusion as social networks form and re-form, and activities sometimes take place in geographically dispersed parts of the community. Young adolescents cannot obtain a driver's license until age 16, so they walk, ride their bikes, use public transportation, or depend upon others, including other friends, to drive them to such popular hangouts as shopping malls, movie theatres, music concerts, and parks. Parental monitoring remains critical to ensure that young teens remain safe while gradually becoming more independent.

As early adolescents mature, they spend time without adult supervision both at home and away. This freedom presents opportunities to mature in new responsibilities and develop strong decision-making skills. Indeed, many early adolescents begin babysitting other children, including their younger siblings. This new freedom presents challenges because of the attractions of risky behaviors. The temptation to experience something that one believes is pleasurable, "cool," or that builds status is hard to resist if the youth lacks insight to the consequences, has poor negotiation skills, and has ample opportunity to experiment. New brain research is demonstrating that the "neurological structures that underlie the functions of controlling impulses and making decisions are still maturing during adolescence."[3] Discretion and decision making is further inhibited under the influence of alcohol or drugs. As social creatures, adolescents enjoy being with their friends, having fun, and going places. Shored up by the power and energy of their peer group, early adolescents may shun caution to satisfy their curiosity. If they are eager to impress a new friend or "crush," a naive, uninitiated youth may feel overly confident about engaging in risky behavior.

Adolescents' relationships with their parents and other adults may begin to change during the early stages of this period. In some families, an orderly progression to independent decision making can be noted. For many young people, however, mood swings and attempts at independence can trigger volatile arguments and challenges to rules. Occasional arguments with parents are common. Authoritative parents who have a balanced approach with unconditional love, combined with clear boundaries (family rules, limits, and expectations) and consistent enforcement of discipline are building a strong protective bond between themselves and their adolescent. Research data consistently show that parents who are authoritative (defined as "accepting, firm, and democratic") have adolescents who are less depressed, enter into risk-taking behaviors at later ages, and succeed better academically than parents who use authoritarian approaches.[4] Having a positive relationship with parents, engagement in school and community activities, and having a sense of spirituality are major assets associated with positive youth development.[5]

Adolescents from racial and ethnic backgrounds that differ from the majority population may have to juggle the demands and values of their family and community culture with the demands and values of the mainstream culture. In families who have immigrated, this tension may be exacerbated because the children may speak English better than their parents, and may be more engaged in the predominant social environment. This role reversal is particularly difficult during the adolescent years when youth need support and guidance and when parents need to be able to assert their ability to protect and guide the youth. As adolescents work to establish their identity, dealing with being bicultural can be confusing and stressful.

Early adolescents also may experience a variety of unexpected dramatic personal changes, such as divorce, parental death, or family relocation. These events, coming on top of the other emotional, social, and academic pressures that are typically experienced during early adolescence, will require these youth to develop mature coping mechanisms. Family members and other adults play an essential role in helping early adolescents develop coping mechanisms, and these personal challenges provide opportunities for emotional growth, leading to increased resiliency (a trait that will prove valuable throughout adolescence and into adulthood).

Health behaviors and lifestyle habits that are formed in adolescence often continue into adulthood. Therefore, early adolescence is a key period for engaging the adolescent's active participation in promoting optimal nutrition, physical activity, academic initiative, family connectedness, mental health and emotional well-being, injury prevention, risk reduction, avoidance of substance use and sexual activity, and involvement in community service.[6-10] Parents who also practice these behaviors reinforce their child's willingness and ability to promote their own healthy lifestyles. Health care professionals should be sensitive to patient's concerns about body image and the emergence of disordered patterns of eating, from anorexia to obesity. Evaluating the level of body satisfaction and practices that the adolescent uses to maintain body weight (eg, dieting or binge eating and exercise patterns) will help the health care professional recognize early symptoms of eating disorders or patterns that promote unhealthy body weight.

Health care routines also change according to adolescents' development and their unique cultural circumstances. Beginning with the Early Adolescence Visits, many health care professionals conduct the first part of the medical interview with the parent in the examination room, and then spend time with the adolescent alone. This approach helps early adolescents build a unique relationship with their health care professional, promotes confidence and full disclosure of health information, and enhances self-management. When explained within the context of healthy adolescent development, parents usually support this approach.

PRIORITIES FOR THE VISIT

The first priority is to address the concerns of the adolescent and his parents. In addition, the Bright Futures Adolescence Expert Panel has given priority to the following additional topics for discussion in the 4 Early Adolescence Visits. The goal of these discussions is to determine the health needs of the youth and family that should be addressed by the health care professional. The following priorities are consistent throughout adolescence. However, the questions used to effectively obtain information and the anticipatory guidance provided to the adolescent and family can vary.

Including all the priority issues in every visit may not be feasible, but the goal should be to address issues important to this age group over the course of the 4 visits. These issues include:

- Physical growth and development (physical and oral health, body image, healthy eating, physical activity)
- Social and academic competence (connectedness with family, peers, and community; interpersonal relationships; school performance)
- Emotional well-being (coping, mood regulation and mental health, sexuality)
- Risk reduction (tobacco, alcohol, or other drugs; pregnancy; STIs)
- Violence and injury prevention (safety belt and helmet use, substance abuse and riding in a vehicle, guns, interpersonal violence [fights], bullying)

HEALTH SUPERVISION

History

Interval history can be obtained according to the health care professional's preference or style of practice. The following questions can encourage in-depth discussion to determine changes in health status that would warrant further physical or emotional assessment.

To the Youth:
- Since your last visit here, how have you been? What health problems, concerns, or questions have you had?

To the Parent:
- What questions do you have about your child's physical well-being, growth, or pubertal development?
- What questions or concerns do you have about your child's emotional well-being, feelings, behavior, or learning?
- What have you and your child discussed about feelings and behaviors that are contributing to his emotional well-being and a healthy lifestyle?
- What have you and your child discussed about avoiding risky behaviors? Does your child have any behaviors that you are concerned about?

Observation of Parent-Youth Interaction

The parent of the early adolescent often accompanies the youth to the visit, but some time during each Early Adolescence Visit will be with the youth alone. The health care professional can observe parent-child interactions, including:

- How comfortably do the youth and parent interact, both verbally and nonverbally?
- Who asks and answers most of the questions?
- Does the youth express an interest in managing his own health issues (including youth who have special health care needs)?

Cultural norms and values shape parent-youth interactions. To accurately interpret observations, the health care professional should learn about the norms and expectations of the populations served. Different cultures have different norms about how youth and adults interact and whether youth speak directly to adults or offer their own opinions in front of adults.

In addition to observation, the health care professional can help guide the parent and the youth's interaction to encourage the youth's participation in his health decisions. For example, if the parent is answering all the questions, then the health care professional can redirect questions straight to the youth with wording such as, "What are your thoughts on what your mom/dad said?"

Surveillance of Development

The developmental tasks of early adolescence can be addressed through information obtained in the medical examination, by observation, by asking specific questions, and through general discussion. The following areas can be assessed to understand the developmental health of the adolescent. A goal of this assessment is to determine whether the adolescent is developing in an appropriate fashion and, if not, to provide information, assistance, or intervention. In the assessment, determine whether the youth is making progress on these developmental tasks:

- Demonstrates physical, cognitive, emotional, social, and moral competencies
- Engages in behaviors that promote wellness and contribute to a healthy lifestyle
- Forms a caring, supportive relationship with family, other adults, and peers
- Engages in a positive way in the life of the community
- Displays a sense of self-confidence, hopefulness, and well-being
- Demonstrates resiliency when confronted with life stressors
- Demonstrates increasingly responsible and independent decision making[11]

Physical Examination

A complete physical examination is included as part of every health supervision visit.

When performing a physical examination, the health care professional's attention is directed to the following components of the exam that are important for 11- to 14-year-olds:

- **Measure:**
  - Blood pressure
- **Measure and plot:**
  - Height
  - Weight
- **Calculate and plot:**
  - BMI
- **Skin**
  - Inspect for acne, acanthosis nigricans, atypical nevi, tattoos, piercings, and signs of abuse or self-inflicted injury
- **Spine**
  - Examine back

- **Breast**
  Female
  - Assess sexual maturity rating
  Male
  - Observe for gynecomastia
- **Genitalia**
  Female
  - Perform visual inspection for sexual maturity rating and observation for signs of STIs (eg, warts, vesicles, vaginal discharge)
  - Perform pelvic exam, if clinically warranted, based on sexual activity (eg, for Pap smear within 3 years of onset of sexual activity) and/or specific problems (eg, pubertal aberrancy, abnormal bleeding, abdominal or pelvic pain)
  Male
  - Perform visual inspection for sexual maturity rating and observations for signs of STIs (ie, warts, vesicles)
  - Examine testicles for hydrocele, hernias, varicocele, or masses

Screening

UNIVERSAL SCREENING	ACTION	
Vision (once in early adolescence)	Snellen test	

SELECTIVE SCREENING	RISK ASSESSMENT*	ACTION IF RA +
Vision at other ages	+ on risk screening questions	Snellen test
Hearing	+ on risk screening questions	Audiometry
Anemia	+ on risk screening questions	Hemoglobin or hematocrit
Tuberculosis	+ on risk screening questions	Tuberculin skin test
Dyslipidemia	+ on risk screening questions and not previously screened with normal results	Lipid screen
STIs	Sexually active	Screen for chlamydia and gonorrhea; use tests appropriate to the patient population and clinical setting
	Sexually active and + on risk questions	Syphilis blood test HIV[†12]
Pregnancy	Sexually active without contraception, late menses, or amenorrhea	Urine hCG
Cervical dysplasia	Sexually active, within 3 years of onset of sexual activity	Pap smear, conventional slide or liquid-based
Alcohol or drug use	+ on risk screening questions	Administer alcohol and drug screening tool

*See Rationale and Evidence chapter for the criteria on which risk screening questions are based.

†The CDC has recently recommended universal voluntary HIV screening for all sexually active people, beginning at age 13. At the time of publication, the AAP and other groups had not yet commented on the CDC recommendation, nor recommended screening criteria or techniques. The health care professional's attention is drawn to the voluntary nature of screening and that the CDC allows an opt out in communities where the HIV rate is <0.1%. The management of positives and false positives must be considered before testing.

Immunizations

Consult the CDC/ACIP or AAP Web sites for the current immunization schedule.
CDC National Immunization Program (NIP): http://www.cdc.gov/vaccines
American Academy of Pediatrics *Red Book:* http://www.aapredbook.org

ANTICIPATORY GUIDANCE

The following sample questions, which address the Adolescent Expert Panel's Anticipatory Guidance Priorities for this visit, are intended to be used selectively to invite discussion, gather information, address the needs and concerns of the family, and build partnerships. Questions can be modified to match the health care professional's communication style. Any anticipatory guidance for the family should be geared to questions, issues, or concerns for that particular adolescent and family.

PHYSICAL GROWTH AND DEVELOPMENT

Physical and oral health, body image, healthy eating, physical activity

The benefits of brushing the teeth with a fluoridated toothpaste extend to all ages. Fluoride is beneficial because it remineralizes tooth enamel and inhibits bacterial growth, thereby preventing caries. Flossing daily is important to prevent gum disease. Youth should have regularly scheduled visits with their dentist at least twice each year. They also should receive a fluoride supplement if the fluoride level in community (at home and at school) water supplies is low.

SAMPLE QUESTIONS:

Ask the parent

When was the last time your child had a dental visit? Do you have trouble getting dental care?

Ask the youth

How often do you brush your teeth? When was your last dental visit?

ANTICIPATORY GUIDANCE:

For the parent

- Help your child establish a daily oral health routine of brushing and flossing.
- Continue dental appointments twice a year or according the individual schedule for your child that is set within her dental home.
- Give your child a fluoride supplement if recommended by your dentist.

For the youth

- Brush your teeth at least twice daily with fluoridated toothpaste and floss every day.

Many young adolescents going through puberty develop a vastly enhanced sensitivity to their physical appearance, how it is changing, and how it compares with their peers and with the idealized body image portrayed in the media. Health care professionals can evaluate patient concerns about body image and the emergence of disordered patterns of eating, from anorexia to obesity. Evaluating the level of body satisfaction and practices that the adolescent uses to maintain body weight will help the health care professional recognize early symptoms of eating disorders or patterns that promote unhealthy weight.

SAMPLE QUESTIONS:

Ask the parent

Do you have any questions or concerns about your child's nutrition, weight, or physical activity?

Ask the youth

How do you feel about the way you look? Do you feel that you are underweight? Overweight? Just right? How much would you like to weigh? Are you doing anything to change your weight? How?

ANTICIPATORY GUIDANCE:

For the parent

- Support a healthy weight in your child by emphasizing a balance between eating a healthy diet and getting regular physical activity.
- Support your child's evolving self-image by commenting on the positive things she does or has learned rather than only her physical appearance.

For the youth

- Manage weight through healthy eating habits and regular physical activity.

As the early adolescent begins to take responsibility for what she eats, her parents can support this decision making by providing healthy foods at home and opportunities for her to participate in food shopping and meal preparation. This can help the young person learn how to avoid high-fat, high-sugar foods in other situations, such as in school and restaurants. Family meals facilitate communication and optimal nutrition. Advocating for healthy food in school cafeterias and vending machines also can be an important strategy.

Refer the family to supports, such as Food Stamps, food banks, or the USDA Food Distribution Programs, if the family is having trouble getting sufficient food.

Adequate calcium intake is an important concern for early adolescents, who are experiencing their growth spurts and need calcium to support optimal bone growth. Educate parents and youth on ways to ensure sufficient calcium intake through daily choices of dairy foods, such as low-fat or fat-free milk, yogurt, and cheese. For youth who do not or cannot use dairy products, suggest other sources of calcium, such as some non-dairy foods (eg, dark green, leafy vegetables; cooked dried beans; and canned salmon) and calcium-fortified foods (eg, orange juice, bread, breakfast cereals, and soy beverages).

SAMPLE QUESTIONS:

Ask the parent

Do you think your child eats healthy foods? Can you give me some examples? Do you have any difficulty getting healthy foods for your family? Do you have any concerns about your child's eating behaviors (eg, not drinking milk or skipping meals)? How frequently are you able to eat meals together as a family? How are you helping your child get enough calcium every day?

Ask the youth

Which meals do you usually eat each day?

Do you ever skip a meal? If so, how many times a week? How many servings of milk or other dairy foods (eg, yogurt or cheese) did you have yesterday? How many servings of other calcium-containing foods (eg, dark green, leafy vegetables, or calcium-fortified orange juice or cereal) did you have yesterday? How many fruits did you eat yesterday? How many vegetables? Does your family ever not have enough food? How often do you drink juice or soft drinks? Are there any foods you won't eat? If so, which ones? What changes would you like to make in the way you eat?

ANTICIPATORY GUIDANCE:

For the parent

■ Support positive nutrition habits by keeping a variety of healthy foods at home and encouraging your child to make healthful food choices.
  - Provide lots of fruits and vegetables, especially the really colorful ones.
  - Serve whole-grain breads, cereals, and other grain products.
  - Provide 3 or more daily servings of low-fat (1%) or non-fat milk and other low-fat dairy products.
  - Serve lean meats, chicken, fish, and other sources of protein and iron.
  - Limit high-fat or low-nutrient foods and beverages, such as candy, chips, and soft drinks.
  - Eat together as a family as often as possible.
  - Use community nutrition programs and food resources, if necessary.

For the youth

■ Eat 3 nutritious meals a day. Breakfast is an especially important meal. Select a nutritious lunch from the cafeteria or pack a balanced lunch.

■ Eat meals with your family as often as you can.

■ Focus on food choices that help you stay healthy.

■ Drink plenty of water; choose water instead of soda.

■ Getting enough calcium and vitamin D is important for keeping your bones strong. Make sure to have 3 servings of low-fat or non-fat milk, yogurt, or cheese every day. If you don't eat dairy foods, try other sources of calcium.

■ Limit high-fat or low-nutrient foods and beverages, such as candy, chips, and soft drinks.

Current recommendations state that children and adolescents should engage in 60 minutes of physical activity on most, if not all, days of the week. Early adolescents can explore new opportunities for physical activity because they have leisure-time play, physical education, and sports at school, and community sports. Attention to balancing physical activity and inactivity is needed. Early adolescence is a time that interest in computers, movies, and DVDs increases, which presents opportunities for physical inactivity. Computers are often an essential social and recreational outlet for youth with special health care needs, so guidance about limiting screen time may need to be modified for these patients.

SAMPLE QUESTIONS:

Ask the parent

Does your child participate in regular physical activity on most, if not all, days of the week? Are there opportunities for safe recreation in your neighborhood? How can you help your child become more physically active? How much time each day does your child watch TV, videotapes, or DVDs? How much time does she spend at the computer? Do you and your child participate in physical activities together? If so, which ones? How often?

Ask the youth

Do you participate in any physical activities, such as walking, biking, hiking, skating, swimming, or running? Which physical activities do you participate in? How often? For how long each time? How much time each day do you spend watching TV, videotapes, or DVDs? How many hours a day do you use a computer? Do you participate in any physical activities with your parents, such as biking, hiking, skating, swimming, or running?

ANTICIPATORY GUIDANCE:

For the parent

- Support your child's healthy weight and physical fitness by:
  - Encouraging and facilitating recommended levels of physical activity
  - Helping her limit screen time (TV, video, DVD, computer, other than for homework) by setting rules and providing alternatives

For the youth

- Be physically active as part of play, games, physical education, planned physical activities, recreation, and organized sports. Try to be physically active for 1 hour on most, if not all, days of the week. You don't have to do it all at once. You can break it up into shorter times of activity throughout the day. Doing a mix of physical activities you enjoy is a great way to reach the 60 minute-a-day goal.
- Drink plenty of water to maintain hydration lost during physical activity to prevent heat-related illnesses, such as heat cramps, exhaustion, and heat stroke.
- Cut back on physical inactivity by limiting the time you spend watching TV, videotapes, or DVDs, or using a computer other than for homework, to no more than 2 hours a day.

SOCIAL AND ACADEMIC COMPETENCE

Connectedness with family, peers, and community; interpersonal relationships; school performance

Young people are more likely to make healthy choices if they stay connected with family members, and if clear rules and limits are set.

Remind parents that, although their child's friends are becoming increasingly important to him, they should not underestimate their own ability to positively influence his opinions and decisions. This shift in the balance can be difficult for parents to deal with, but it is an important time to continue to cement family relationships. This effort will pay off later because close family ties are an important protective, risk-reducing factor in middle and late adolescence. Connection to parents and other responsible adults is associated with a reduced number of risk behaviors. Asking parents whether they understand their child's world and daily life is particularly important for immigrant parents.

SAMPLE QUESTIONS:

Ask the parent

How are you getting along as a family? What do you do together? Do you understand your child's world and daily life?

Ask the youth

How do you get along with your family? What do you like to do together? How closely connected do you feel to your family's cultural and faith life?

ANTICIPATORY GUIDANCE:

For the parent

- Discuss youth responsibilities in the family and how they change with age.
- Clearly communicate rules and expectations.
- Get to know your child's friends and encourage him to make good decisions about choosing friends.
- Discuss your expectations for dress, friends, media, and activities, and supervise your child.
- Spend time with your child. Express a willingness for questions and discussion. Develop a pattern of communication and support him as an independent person. Make time every day to talk (mealtime, bedtime, drive time, or check-in time) about lots of things, not just about difficult or unpleasant topics.

For the youth

- This is an important time to stay connected with your parents. You might not always agree on everything, but work with your family to solve problems, especially around difficult situations or topics.
- How to make friends and keep them is an important life skill.
- Spend time with family members. Help out at home.
- Follow your family rules, such as for curfews and riding in a car (eg, who you accept rides from and whether the driver has been drinking or doing drugs).

Youth who take part in a range of activities that interest them are more confident, manage their time better, and do better in school than those who do not. These activities can nurture strengths and assets that will help an early adolescent successfully navigate this developmental stage.

SAMPLE QUESTIONS:

Ask the parent

What does your child do after school?

Ask the youth

What are your interests outside of school? Who are the important adults in your life? What are your responsibilities at home?

ANTICIPATORY GUIDANCE:

For the parent

- Provide opportunities for your child to find activities, other than academics, that truly interest him, especially if your child is struggling academically.
- Help your child see things from another person's point of view, becoming more aware of other peoples' situations in your community.

For the youth

- This is a good time to start figuring out what interests you have. Art, drama, mentoring, volunteering, construction, gardening, and individual and organized sports are only a few possibilities. Consider learning new skills that can be helpful to your friends, family, or community, such as lifesaving, CPR, or peer mentoring.

The transition from elementary school to middle school and then to high school is an exciting time because it brings new experiences and responsibilities and increased freedom. It also has its difficult moments, as youth grapple with new social and academic situations and challenges. Success in school is associated with a reduced number of risky behaviors and it increases positive social relationships.

Poor academic achievement may be a sign of depression, anxiety, attention, or learning problems.

SAMPLE QUESTIONS:

Ask the parent

Is your child getting to school on time? How is your child doing in school? Is he completing his homework? How are his grades?

Ask the youth

What do you enjoy at school? What is your favorite subject? How are you doing in school? Are you having particular difficulty with any subjects?

ANTICIPATORY GUIDANCE:

For the parent

- Emphasize the importance of school.
- Praise positive efforts.
- Recognize success and achievements.
- Monitor and guide your child as he assumes more responsibility for his schoolwork.
- Many youth need help with organization and setting priorities as they transition through middle school and into high school.
- Encourage reading by helping your youth find books and magazines about subjects that interest him.
- Have him bring a book when you know he'll be waiting somewhere or in a situation requiring patience.

For the youth
- Take responsibility for getting your homework done and getting to school on time.
- If you are having difficulty at school or problems on the way to and from school, talk with your parent or another trusted adult about it.

EMOTIONAL WELL-BEING

Coping, mood regulation and mental health, sexuality

The ability to solve problems, make good decisions, and cope with stress is an important skill for youth. Health care professionals can support parents in helping their children set priorities, manage stress, and make progress toward goals.

SAMPLE QUESTIONS:
Ask the parent
Do you think your child worries too much or appears overly anxious? How do you help your child cope with stress? How do you teach her to make decisions and solve problems?

Ask the youth
Do you worry a lot or feel overly stressed out? How do you cope with stress?

ANTICIPATORY GUIDANCE:
For the parent
- Involve your child in family decision making, as appropriate, to give her experience with solving problems and making decisions.
- Encourage your child to think through solutions rather than giving her all the answers.

For the youth
- Everyone has stress in their lives, such as school deadlines or occasional difficulties with friends. It's important for you to figure out how to deal with stress in the ways that work best for you. If you would like some help with this, I would be happy to give you some ideas.

Many adolescents may not present with classic adult symptoms of depression. Irritability or pervasive boredom may be symptoms of depression in this age group. Because adolescents are more likely to report suicidal thoughts or attempts than their parents, it is important to question them directly about suicidal thoughts or attempts if there is any concern about depression or other mental health problems.

Anxiety falls along a spectrum of intensity, and symptoms may cause significant distress and affect the early adolescent's functioning at school, at home, or with friends.

Posttraumatic stress disorder is frequently overlooked and can present with symptoms of depression and anxiety. Past traumatic events can include being in a motor vehicle crash, experiencing physical or sexual abuse or other major life events, or witnessing violence.

Fighting and bullying behaviors can indicate the presence of a conduct disorder and may co-occur with problems with substance abuse, depression, or anxiety.

Worsening or poor academic achievement may be a sign of depression, anxiety, attention or learning problems, or drug use/abuse.

Not adhering to parental rules and requests can indicate problems with the parent-youth relationship or with other authority figures. Disagreements over cultural values can lead to distress and high levels of conflict in the family and can affect the child's functioning and developing identity and may increase the risk of abuse.

Any youth with substance abuse problems also may be struggling with a mental health problem. These youth need to be evaluated for both substance abuse and mental health problems because they occur more often together in adolescents than they do in adults.

SAMPLE QUESTIONS:
Ask the parent
Is your child frequently irritable? Have you noticed any changes in your child's weight or sleep habits? Does your child have recurring thoughts or memories about an unpleasant event in the past, such as a motor vehicle crash or being hurt by someone? Do you and your child have frequent conflict about what your culture expects of her behavior and how her friends behave? Do you have any concerns about your child's emotional health? Has anyone in the family had mental health problems or committed suicide?

Ask the youth
Have you been feeling bored all the time? Do you feel sad? Have you had difficulty sleeping or do you often feel irritable? Do you ever feel so upset that you wished you were not alive or that you wanted to die? Do you find yourself continuing to remember or think about an unpleasant experience that happened in the past? Do you find that you and your parents are often in conflict about what your culture expects of you and what your friends are doing?

ANTICIPATORY GUIDANCE:
For the parent
- As your child's health care professional, I am just as interested in her emotional well-being and mental health as I am in her physical health. If you are concerned about your child's behavior, moods, mental health, or substance use, please talk with me.

For the youth
- Everyone has difficult times and disappointments, but these usually are temporary and you can keep on track with school, family, friends, and a generally positive attitude toward life.
- Sometimes, though, people your age may feel like they're too sad, depressed, hopeless, nervous, or angry to be able to do these things. If you feel that way now, I'd like to talk about it with you. If you ever feel that way, it is important for you to seek help. Turn to your parents, me, or another adult you trust when you feel sad, down, or alone.

Concerns about puberty often preoccupy early adolescents, and these concerns can be a frequent topic of discussion during the visit. Health care professionals are uniquely positioned to discuss the young persons' individual pubertal developmental trajectory. This can be especially helpful for early-maturing and late-maturing teens. For example, reassurance about the normality of most breast development in boys, and asymmetrical breast development in females, is helpful. Because of its importance at this developmental stage, health care professionals should educate young girls and their parents about menarche and subsequent cycle length as well as issues related to hygiene, dysmenorrhea, and irregular bleeding. During early adolescence, youth also may have questions about gender identity, sexual attraction, and relationships.

In general, it is helpful to advise parents to be open to listening and discussing sexuality with their children. Being sensitive to cultural issues related to sexuality and paying close attention to understanding parents' views can help parents perceive the health care professional as a credible resource. Consider partnering with members of the family's community to identify strategies to support adolescents who are not following the traditions of their family. Some families will perceive it to be inappropriate for a health care professional to talk to teens about this topic, so it is useful to provide them with information and sources of support in their community.

SAMPLE QUESTIONS:

Ask the parent

Have you and your child discussed the physical changes that occur during puberty? Would you like more information about puberty and the emotional changes that occur? What are your house rules about curfews, dating, and friends?

Ask the youth

Do you know what to expect as your body changes during puberty?
For girls: *Have you had your first period? If you have menstruated, tell me more about your periods (eg, how often, how heavy?)*
Have you talked with your parents about dating and sex?

ANTICIPATORY GUIDANCE:

For the parent

- Youth go through the physical changes of puberty at different times; so, if you or your child has any questions about her particular developmental path, please ask me.
- Talk to your child about your knowledge, expectations, and values about dating, activities, relationships, marriage, parenting, and family.
- Talk to your child often, and clearly share your expectations and beliefs about sex and relationships.

For the youth

- It's important for you to have accurate information about sexuality, your physical development, and your sexual feelings. Please ask me if you have any questions.
- *For girls:* I want to make sure you understand about your periods (your menstrual cycles). Please ask me if you have any questions.

RISK REDUCTION

Tobacco, alcohol, or other drugs; pregnancy; STIs

Provide information and/or role-play on how to resist peer pressure to smoke, drink alcohol, or use drugs.

SAMPLE QUESTIONS:

Ask the parent

Does anyone in your home smoke? What has your child been taught at home or in school about alcohol and drugs? Do you regularly supervise your child's social and recreational activities? Does your child understand what you consider appropriate behavior? How do you check for the use of alcohol, tobacco, or other drugs? What have you and your child discussed about the risks of using alcohol, tobacco, and other drugs? What are the expected consequences or disciplinary action that you would take (or have taken) if you discovered that your child was using tobacco, alcohol, or other drugs?

Ask the youth

Have you (or your friends) ever experimented with smoking? Chewing tobacco? Drinking alcohol? Taking drugs? Using anabolic steroids? Do you ever sniff, "huff," or breathe anything to get high?

If the adolescent reports substance use, ask about duration, amount, and frequency.

ANTICIPATORY GUIDANCE:

For the parent

- Know where and with whom your child is spending leisure time.
- Clearly discuss rules and expectations for acceptable behavior.
- Praise your child for not using tobacco, alcohol, or other drugs. Reinforce this decision through positive and open conversations about these issues.
- Consider locking your liquor cabinet and putting your prescription medicines in a place where your child cannot get them.

For the youth

- Do not smoke, use tobacco, drink alcohol, or use drugs, inhalants, anabolic steroids, or diet pills. Smoking marijuana and other drugs can hurt your lungs; alcohol and other drugs are bad for brain development.
- Avoid situations in which drugs or alcohol are readily available.
- Support friends who choose not to use tobacco, alcohol, drugs, steroids, or diet pills.
- If you smoke, use drugs, or drink alcohol, let's talk about it. I can suggest ways to help you quit.
- If you do drink alcohol, do not drink when swimming, boating, riding a bike or motorcycle, or operating farm equipment.
- If you are worried about any family members' drug or alcohol use problems, you can talk with me.

Abstinence for those who have not had sex, and as an option to those who are sexually experienced, is the best protection from pregnancy, STIs, and the emotional distress of disrupted relationships. Knowing how to protect oneself and one's partner from pregnancy and STIs is critical for those who are sexually active.

SAMPLE QUESTIONS:

Ask the parent

How do you plan to help your child deal with pressures to have sex? How does your culture help you do this?

Ask the youth

Have you had sex? Was it wanted or unwanted? Have you ever been forced or pressured to do something sexual that you haven't wanted to do? How many partners have you had in the past year? Were your partners male or female, or have you had both male and female partners? Were your partners younger, older, or your age? Did you use a condom and/or other contraception?

ANTICIPATORY GUIDANCE:

For the parent

- Encourage abstinence from sexual activity or a return to abstinence.
- Help your child make a plan to resist pressures to use substances or have sex. Be there for him when he needs support or help.
- Support safe activities at school, with community and faith organizations, and with volunteer groups to encourage personal and social development.
- If you are uncomfortable talking about teen development, sexual pressures, teen pregnancy, and STIs, learn more through reliable resources.
- Talk about relationships and sex when issues arise on television, at school, or with friends. Be open and nonjudgmental, but honest, about your personal views.

For the youth

- Abstaining from sexual intercourse, including oral sex, is the safest way to prevent pregnancy and STIs.
- Figure out ways to make sure you can carry through on your decisions regarding your sexual behaviors. Plan how to avoid risky places and relationships. For example, don't use drugs or alcohol, because these can raise the risk of unwanted sex or other risky behaviors.
- If you are sexually active, protect yourself and your partners from STIs and pregnancy.

VIOLENCE AND INJURY PREVENTION

Safety belt and helmet use, substance abuse and riding in a vehicle, guns, interpersonal violence (fights), bullying

Everyone should wear safety belts when riding in a car, and helmets or other protective gear when participating in activities such as biking, skating, or water sports.

If parents and peers wear safety belts and bicycle helmets, the early adolescent is more likely to do so.

Children younger than 16 should not ride an ATV.

SAMPLE QUESTIONS:

Ask the parent

Do you always wear a safety belt and bicycle helmet? Do you insist that your child use appropriate safety equipment when participating in physical activities, such biking, team sports, or water sports?

Ask the youth

Do you always wear a safety belt? Do you always wear a helmet or other protective gear when you bike, play team sports, or do water sports?

ANTICIPATORY GUIDANCE:

For the parent

- It's important that you and everyone else always wear a safety belt and helmet.
- Children younger than 16 should not ride an ATV because they do not yet have the physical coordination or judgment to handle these vehicles.

For the youth

- Always wear a safety belt in a vehicle.
- Always wear a helmet and other protective gear when you are biking, skateboarding, or skating.
- Always wear protective gear when engaged in team sports.
- Always wear water-flotation clothing or an appropriately fitting US Coast Guard-approved life jacket when engaged in water sports.

The use of alcohol and other drugs has been associated with car crash deaths in teens. Sometimes, young adolescents don't have control over the substance use of people with whom they ride (eg, rides home from an adult after babysitting or rides with older friends and siblings). Counsel parents to develop strategies with their adolescent on how to avoid these situations.

SAMPLE QUESTIONS:

Ask the parent

Have you discussed with your child how she should get home safely if she is with someone who has been using drugs or alcohol?

Ask the youth

Have you ever ridden in a vehicle with someone who has been drinking or using drugs? Do you have someone you can call for a ride if you feel unsafe riding with someone?

ANTICIPATORY GUIDANCE:

For the parent

- Help your child make a plan for what to do in case she ever feels unsafe riding in a vehicle because the driver has been drinking or using drugs, or if any situation is out of hand.

For the youth

- Do not ride in a vehicle with someone who has been using drugs or alcohol. Call your parents or another trusted adult and get help.

The AAP recommends that homes be free of guns and that if it is necessary to keep a gun, it should be stored unloaded and locked, with the ammunition locked separately from the gun.

Guns should be removed from the homes of adolescents who have a history of aggressive or violent behaviors, suicide attempts, or depression.

SAMPLE QUESTIONS:

Ask the parent

Is there a gun in your house? Is it locked, and is the ammunition locked and stored separately? Is there a gun in the homes where you and your child visit, such as the homes of grandparents, other relatives, or friends?

Ask the youth

Do you ever carry a gun or knife (even for self-protection)?

ANTICIPATORY GUIDANCE:

For the parent

- The best way to keep your adolescent safe from injury or death from guns is to never have a gun in the home. If it is necessary to keep a gun in your home, it should be stored unloaded and locked, with the ammunition locked separately from the gun. Keep the key where adolescents cannot have access.

For the youth

- Fighting and carrying weapons can be dangerous. Would you like to discuss how to avoid these situations?

Fighting and bullying behaviors can indicate the presence of conduct disorders or may co-occur with problems of substance abuse, depression, or anxiety. Interpersonal violence includes physical attacks and sexual coercion. Young adolescents can benefit from a discussion of safety in all these aspects.

SAMPLE QUESTIONS:

Ask the parent

Are there frequent reports of violence in your community or school? Is your child involved in that violence? Do you think your child is safe in the neighborhood? Has your child ever been injured in a fight? Has your child been bullied or hit by others? Has your child demonstrated bullying or aggression toward others? Have you talked to your child about dating violence and how to be safe?

Ask the youth

Have you ever been involved with a group who did things that could have gotten them into trouble? What do you do when someone tries to pick a fight with you? What do you do when you are angry? Have you been in a physical fight in the past 6 months? Do you know anyone in a gang? Have you ever been touched in a way that made you feel uncomfortable or that was unwelcome? Have you ever been touched on your private parts against your wish or without your consent? Has anyone ever forced you to have sex? Are you in a relationship with a person who threatens you physically or hurts you?

ANTICIPATORY GUIDANCE:

For the parent

- Teach your child nonviolent conflict-resolution techniques.
- Talk to your child about your family's expectations for time with friends and rules about dating.

For the youth

- Confide in parents/guardians, health care professionals, or other trusted adults (such as teachers) if anyone bullies, stalks, or abuses you or threatens your safety.
- Learn to manage conflict nonviolently. Walk away if necessary.
- Avoid risky situations. Avoid violent people. Call for help if things get dangerous.
- When dating, or in any situations related to sexual behavior, remember that "No" means NO. Saying "No" is OK.
- Healthy dating relationships are built on respect, concern, and doing things both of you like to do.

Health Supervision: Middle Adolescence (15 to 17 Year Visits)

CONTEXT

Middle adolescents continue to rapidly develop in many directions simultaneously—physically, cognitively, emotionally, and socially. For the most part, these adolescents are in high school. School and its associated activities, such as academics, sports, clubs, and the arts, become the central focus of life for many middle adolescents. Many youth also begin working after school or on weekends. Youth with special health care needs are often "mainstreamed" and, therefore, able to take advantage of the educational opportunities of large schools. In addition, some children with cognitive challenges may be eligible for extended educational opportunities in high school until they reach age 21.[13] These experiences provide a wonderful opportunity for middle adolescents to solidify life skills and positive habits that will serve them well as they encounter new experiences and new opportunities for experimenting with risk behaviors.

As much as high school is a positive formative experience for many adolescents, other middle adolescents have a different experience. In 2003, 11% of 18- to 24-year-olds had not completed high school and were not enrolled.[14] Health care professionals should learn the drop-out rates in their area and which youth may be at highest risk.

Appearance is an especially important issue during middle adolescence. Health care professionals should be sensitive to patient's concerns about body image and the emergence of disordered patterns of eating, from anorexia to obesity.[15] Evaluating the level of body satisfaction and practices that the adolescent uses to maintain body weight (eg, dieting or binge eating and exercise patterns) will help the health care professional recognize early symptoms of eating disorders or patterns that promote unhealthy body weight.

By middle adolescence, adolescent peers are an important source of health information to teens and are a key reference group. Peers frame behaviors that adolescents feel are appropriate and may offer insight into practices that pose a health risk. For example, adolescents who engage in competitive sports, such as gymnastics or wrestling, may be vulnerable to misinformation about unhealthy or even unsafe nutrition choices and behaviors (eg, replacing food with chewing gum or drinking excessive amounts of water to maintain a low body weight).

Beginning at age 14, adolescents are entering the developmental period of highest risk for mental health problems.[16] The most common mental health concerns for adolescents are mood disorders (depression and anxiety), learning disorders and attention deficit disorders, and conduct disturbances. Emotional well-being is related to the patient's biophysical development. As the teen moves into high school, skills used successfully in junior high may be insufficient or ineffective for the increased rigor of the high-school curriculum. Support is critical for the teen and family with school concerns or behavioral issues that emerge with this new academic environment and developmental stage. Health care professionals must be cognizant of this and refer their adolescent patients for neuropsychological assessment and/or behavioral counseling as needed.

Many adolescents also experiment with risk behaviors, such as drug use or unsafe sexual behaviors. Chronically ill adolescents may question whether medications they have used during middle childhood are still needed. Many adolescents receive driver's permits/licenses now, which allow them increased freedom and unsupervised time. By the end of this developmental period, the health care professional should have discussed topics such as tobacco use, alcohol and illicit drug experimentation, healthy sexual development, abstinence, and the importance of responsible and safe driving.[17] Discussions also may include ways in which the youth's culture, religion, and family can be viewed as supports in making healthy behavior choices.

During this developmental stage, the adolescent's interpersonal relationships evolve, and interest in dating, sexual intimacy, and related behaviors increases. These issues can be particularly complex for the lesbian, gay, bisexual, transgendered, or questioning youth. The health care professional should create a clinical environment where clear messages that are sensitive to personal issues, including sexual orientation, can be given whenever the adolescent feels ready to discuss them. Experimentation with sexual behaviors, including oral sex and vaginal intercourse, can occur at this age. Frank and candid conversations about these issues and behavior within the context of the youth's cultural perspective are important.

The legal age of majority varies from state to state as do the circumstances in which minors can consent to their own health care. Some minor adolescents may be deemed *emancipated* (eg, those who are married or divorced, a member of the armed forces, or living separate from parents and managing their own financial affairs). Others may be considered a *mature minor* and thus able to consent to their own care under certain conditions (eg, pregnancy-related services, reportable diseases and STIs, mental health, and substance abuse). Patient-provider confidentiality related to such care is a delicate issue, especially when supporting parental involvement. If an adolescent patient is entitled to confidential care (either because he is legally at the age of majority or he has been deemed an emancipated or a mature minor), a health care professional generally needs the adolescent's permission to discuss his case with his parents. Health care professionals should be aware of their local laws and public health regulations. Health care professionals should inform adolescent patients and their parents of the practice's terms of confidentiality, as well as any exceptions, such as patient safety. Ultimately, clinical judgment, ethical principles, and moral certitude guide decisions about individual cases.

PRIORITIES FOR THE VISIT

The first priority is to address the concerns of the adolescent and his parents. In addition, the Bright Futures Adolescence Expert Panel has given priority to the following additional topics for discussion in the 3 Middle Adolescence Visits. The goal of these discussions is to determine the health needs of the youth and family that should be addressed by the health care professional. The following priorities are consistent throughout adolescence. However, the questions used to effectively obtain information and the anticipatory guidance provided to the adolescent and family can vary.

Including all the priority issues in every visit may not be feasible, but the goal should be to address issues important to this age group over the course of the 3 visits. These issues include:

- Physical growth and development (physical and oral health, body image, healthy eating, physical activity)
- Social and academic competence (connectedness with family, peers, and community; interpersonal relationships; school performance)
- Emotional well-being (coping, mood regulation and mental health, sexuality)
- Risk reduction (tobacco, alcohol, or other drugs; pregnancy; STIs)
- Violence and injury prevention (safety belt and helmet use, driving [graduated license] and substance abuse, guns, interpersonal violence [dating violence], bullying)

HEALTH SUPERVISION

History

Interval history can be obtained according to the health care professional's preference or style of practice. The following questions may encourage in-depth discussion to determine changes in health status that would warrant further physical or emotional assessment.

To the Adolescent:
- Since your last visit here, how have you been? What health problems, concerns, or questions have you had?
- How are things going with your family, friends, school, and work?
- Do you have a question or worry about anything we should cover today?

To the Parent:
- What questions do you have about your adolescent's physical well-being or growth?
- What questions or concerns do you have about your adolescent's emotional well-being, feelings, behavior, or learning?
- What have you and your adolescent discussed about feelings and behaviors that are contributing to his emotional well-being and a healthy lifestyle?
- What have you and your adolescent discussed about avoiding risk behaviors? Does your adolescent have any behaviors that you are concerned about?

Observation of Parent-Adolescent Interaction

Much of each Middle Adolescense Visit will be the adolescent alone, but there still will be opportunities for the health care professional to observe parent-adolescent interactions, including:

- Do parents encourage self-management and independent decision making about health?
- How comfortably do the adolescent and parent interact, both verbally and nonverbally?
- Who asks and answers most of the questions?
- Does the adolescent express an interest in self-management of health issues, including youth who have special health care needs?

Cultural norms and values shape parent-adolescent interactions. To accurately interpret observations, the health care professional should learn about the norms and expectations of the populations served. Different cultures have different norms about how adolescents and adults interact and whether adolescents speak directly to adults or offer their own opinions in front of adults.

Surveillance of Development

The developmental tasks of middle adolescence can be addressed through information obtained in the medical examination, by observation, by asking specific questions, and through general discussion. The following areas can be assessed to better understand the developmental health of the adolescent. A goal of this assessment is to determine whether the adolescent is developing in an appropriate fashion and, if not, to provide information for assistance or intervention. In the assessment, determine whether the adolescent is making progress on these developmental tasks:

- Demonstrates physical, cognitive, emotional, social, and moral competencies
- Engages in behaviors that promote wellness and contribute to a healthy lifestyle
- Forms a caring, supportive relationship with family, other adults, and peers
- Engages in a positive way in the life of the community
- Displays a sense of self-confidence, hopefulness, and well-being
- Demonstrates resiliency when confronted with life stressors
- Demonstrates increasingly responsible and independent decision making[11]

Physical Examination

A complete physical examination is included as part of every health supervision visit.

When performing a physical examination, the practitioner's attention is directed to the following components of the exam that are important for 15- to 17-year-olds:

- **Measure:**
  - Blood pressure
- **Measure and plot:**
  - Height
  - Weight
- **Calculate and plot:**
  - BMI
- **Skin**
  - Inspect for acne, acanthosis nigricans, atypical nevi, tattoos, piercings, and signs of abuse or self-inflicted injury
- **Spine**
  - Examine back

- ■ **Breast**
Female
  - Assess for sexual maturity rating
Male
  - Observe for gynecomastia
- ■ **Genitalia**
Female
  - Perform visual inspection for sexual maturity rating and observation for signs of STIs (eg, warts, vesicles, vaginal discharge)
  - Perform pelvic exam, if clinically warranted, based on sexual activity (eg, for Pap smear within 3 years of onset of sexual activity) and/or specific problems (eg, pubertal aberrancy, abnormal bleeding, abdominal or pelvic pain)
Male
  - Perform visual inspection for sexual maturity rating and observations for signs of STIs (ie, warts, vesicles)
  - Examine testicles for hydrocele hernias, varicocele, or masses

Screening

UNIVERSAL SCREENING	ACTION	
Vision (once in middle adolescence)	Snellen test	

SELECTIVE SCREENING	RISK ASSESSMENT*	ACTION IF RA +
Vision at other ages	+ on risk screening questions	Snellen test
Hearing	+ on risk screening questions	Audiometry
Anemia	+ on risk screening questions	Hemoglobin or hematocrit
Tuberculosis	+ on risk screening questions	Tuberculin skin test
Dyslipidemia	+ on risk screening questions and if not previously screened with normal results	Lipid screen
STIs	Sexually active	Screen for chlamydia and gonorrhea; use tests appropriate to the patient population and clinical setting
	Sexually active and + on risk questions	Syphilis blood test HIV[†12]
Pregnancy	Sexually active without contraception, late menses, or amenorrhea	Urine hCG
Cervical dysplasia	Sexually active, within 3 years of onset of sexual activity	Pap smear, conventional slide or liquid-based
Alcohol or drug use	+ on risk screening questions	Administer alcohol- and drug-screening tool

*See Rationale and Evidence chapter for the criteria on which risk screening questions are based.

†The CDC has recently recommended universal voluntary HIV screening for all sexually active people, beginning at age 13. At the time of publication, the AAP and other groups had not yet commented on the CDC recommendation, nor recommended screening criteria or techniques. The health care professional's attention is drawn to the voluntary nature of screening and that the CDC allows an opt out in communities where the HIV rate is <0.1%. The management of positives and false positives must be considered before testing.

Immunizations

Consult the CDC/ACIP or AAP Web sites for the current immunization schedule.
CDC National Immunization Program (NIP): http://www.cdc.gov/vaccines
American Academy of Pediatrics *Red Book:* http://www.aapredbook.org

ANTICIPATORY GUIDANCE

The following sample questions, which address the Adolescent Expert Panel's Anticipatory Guidance Priorities for this visit, are intended to be used selectively to invite discussion, gather information, address the needs and concerns of the family, and build partnerships. Use of the questions may vary from visit to visit and from family to family. Not all questions need to be asked at every visit. Questions can be modified to match the health care professional's communication style. Any anticipatory guidance for the family should be geared to questions, issues, or concerns for that particular adolescent and family.

PHYSICAL GROWTH AND DEVELOPMENT

Physical and oral health, body image, healthy eating, physical activity

The benefits of brushing the teeth with a fluoridated toothpaste extend to all ages. Fluoride is beneficial because it remineralizes tooth enamel and inhibits bacterial growth, thereby preventing caries. Daily flossing also is important to prevent gum disease. To maximize topical benefit through the adolescent caries-risk period, a fluoride supplement should be prescribed up to the age of 16 if the fluoride level in community water supplies (at home and at school) is low. Youth should have regularly scheduled visits with their dentist at least twice each year.

Hearing loss may begin to be an issue with adolescents who are consistently exposed to loud noise, such as at music concerts or at sporting events in enclosed spaces. Counsel the adolescent about the advisability of wearing hearing protection in these situations.

SAMPLE QUESTIONS:
Ask the youth
Do you brush your teeth every day? Do you floss your teeth every day? When did you last see a dentist?
Ask the parent
Does your child see a dentist regularly? Do you have trouble accessing dental care?

ANTICIPATORY GUIDANCE:
For the youth
- Brush your teeth at least twice a day with fluoridated toothpaste and floss every day also. See a dentist twice a year and discuss ways to keep your teeth healthy. Use a mouth guard for all contact sports.
- Wear hearing protection when you are exposed to loud noise, such as music at concerts.

For the parent
- Continue dental appointments according the individual schedule that is set for your adolescent within his dental home.

An adolescent's body image is influenced by many emotional and physical factors that are associated with the changes of puberty. In middle adolescence, these issues can gain prominence when the normal weight gain and body shape changes associated with puberty combine with influences of media, advertising, and peers.

SAMPLE QUESTIONS:

Ask the youth

How do you feel about the way you look? Do you feel that you are underweight? Overweight? Just right? How much would you like to weigh? Are you doing anything to change your weight? How?

Ask the parent

Do you have any questions or concerns about your child's nutrition, weight, or physical activity?

ANTICIPATORY GUIDANCE:

For the youth

- With all the changes of puberty, this is a good time to start figuring out what combination of healthy eating and physical activity works to keep your body strong and healthy.

For the parent

- Support your adolescent's healthy weight by keeping a variety of healthy foods at home.
- Support your adolescent's evolving self-image by commenting on the positive things she does or has learned rather than only on her physical appearance.

As the middle adolescent takes increasing responsibility for what she eats, parents can support this decision making by providing healthy foods at home and opportunities for the adolescent to participate in food shopping and meal preparation. This can help the young person learn how to avoid high-fat and high-sugar foods in other situations, including school and restaurants. Ensuring adequate calcium intake is of continued importance. Family meals facilitate communication and optimal nutrition. Advocating for healthy food in school cafeterias and vending machines also can be an important strategy.

Refer the family to supports, such as Food Stamps, food banks, or the USDA Food Distribution Programs, if the family is having trouble getting sufficient food.

SAMPLE QUESTIONS:

Ask the youth

Which meals do you usually eat each day? Do you ever skip a meal? If so, how many times a week? How many servings of milk did you have yesterday? How many servings of other dairy foods (eg, yogurt or cheese)? How many fruits did you eat yesterday? How many vegetables? Does your family ever not have enough food? How often do you drink soft drinks? Juice? Are there any foods you won't eat? If so, which ones? What changes would you like to make in the way you eat?

Ask the parent

Do you think your adolescent eats healthy foods? Can you give me an example? Do you have any difficulty getting healthy foods for your family? Do you have any concerns about your adolescent's eating behaviors (eg, not drinking milk or skipping meals)? How frequently are you able to eat meals together as a family?

ANTICIPATORY GUIDANCE:

For the youth

- Eat 3 nutritious meals a day. Breakfast is an especially important meal. Select a nutritious lunch from the cafeteria or pack a balanced lunch.
- Eat meals with your family as often as you can.
- Focus on food choices that help you stay healthy.
- Drink plenty of water; choose water instead of soda or sports drinks.

For the parent

- Support positive nutrition habits by keeping a variety of healthy foods at home and encouraging healthful food choices.
  - Provide lots of fruits and vegetables, especially the really colorful ones.
  - Serve whole-grain breads, cereals, and other grain products.
  - Provide 3 or more daily servings of low-fat (1%) and non-fat milk and other low-fat dairy products.
  - Serve lean meats, chicken, fish, and other sources of protein and iron.
  - Limit high-fat or low-nutrient foods and beverages, such as candy, chips, and soft drinks.
  - Eat together as a family as often as possible.
  - Use community nutrition programs and food resources if necessary.

Current recommendations state that adolescents should engage in 60 minutes of physical activity on most, if not all, days of the week. The middle adolescent may need help in maintaining adequate physical activity daily. School physical education programs rarely exist by the second year of high school, sports teams begin limiting their membership to highly successful players, and participation in other clubs and school activities, as well as an increasing academic load, can limit the time available for physical activity. Depending on the safety and resources of the community, this can pose a challenge to adolescents and families. Problem solving and helping adolescents identify activities that they can pursue may be an important part of these visits.

Attention to balancing physical activity and inactivity is needed because computers, movies, and DVDs present numerous opportunities for physical inactivity. Computers are often an essential social and recreational outlet for youth with special health care needs, so guidance about limiting screen time may need to be modified for these patients.

SAMPLE QUESTIONS:

Ask the youth

Do you participate in any physical activities, such as walking, biking, hiking, skating, swimming, or running? Which physical activities do you do? How often? For how long each time? How much time each day do you spend watching television, videotapes, or DVDs? How many hours a day do you use a computer? Do you do any physical activities with your parents, such as biking, hiking, skating, dancing, swimming, or running?

Ask the parent

Does your adolescent participate in regular physical activity on most, if not all, days of the week? Does your neighborhood have opportunities for safe recreation? How can you help your adolescent become more physically active? How much time each day does your adolescent watch television, videotapes, or DVDs? How much time does she spend at the computer? Do you and your adolescent participate in physical activities together? If so, which ones? How often?

ANTICIPATORY GUIDANCE:

For the youth

- Be physically active as part of play, games, physical education, planned physical activities, recreation, and organized sports. Try to be active for 1 hour on most, if not all, days of the week. You don't have to do it all at once. You can break it up into shorter times of activity throughout the day. Doing a mix of physical activities you enjoy is a great way to reach the 60-minutes-a-day goal.
- Drink plenty of water to maintain hydration lost during physical activity to prevent heat-related illnesses, such as heat cramps, exhaustion, and heat stroke.
- Cut back on physical inactivity by limiting the time you spend watching TV, videotapes, or DVDs, or using a computer, outside of homework, to no more than 2 hours a day.

For the parent

- Help your adolescent get adequate physical activity by encouraging and facilitating recommended levels of physical activity.
- Help her limit screen time (TV, video, DVD, or computer, exclusive of homework) by setting rules and providing alternatives.

SOCIAL AND ACADEMIC COMPETENCE

Connectedness with family, peers, and community; interpersonal relationships; school performance

Young people are more likely to make healthy choices if they stay connected with family members and if clear rules and limits are set. Many family rules relate to safety and common courtesy. Following these rules will continue to be important in their relationships with friends and family when they become adults.

Friends continue to be very important in this period and adolescents tend to have a small group of friends who share similar interests and activities, including dress, hairstyle, music, and behaviors. Peer pressure can work in a positive as well as a negative direction at this time. At the older end of this age group, adolescents also take pride in their uniqueness so they can be encouraged to develop their own sense of identity and take on challenges that increase their skills and self-confidence.

SAMPLE QUESTIONS:

Ask the youth

How do you get along with your family? What do you like to do together? Do you follow your family rules and limits? How closely do you feel connected to your family's cultural and religious life? How do you get along with your friends? Do you have any concerns about this that you'd like to discuss?

Ask the parent

How are you getting along as a family? What do you do together? Do you understand your child's world and daily life? (This is important for all parents, but particularly for immigrant parents.) *What rules and expectations do you set for your child?*

ANTICIPATORY GUIDANCE:

For the youth

- In most situations, it's important to stay connected with your family as you get older. Work with your family to solve problems, especially around difficult situations or topics.
- Consider getting involved in your community about an issue that interests or concerns you.
- How to make friends and keep them is an important life skill. Evaluating whether a friendship is no longer good for you is also important.
- Spend time with family members. Help out at home.
- Take responsibility for getting your schoolwork done and being at school on time.
- Follow your family rules, such as for curfews and driving.
- Ask for help when you need it.

For the parent

- Have a positive relationship with your adolescent. Show affection. Praise his efforts and achievements.
- Model the positive behaviors you want your adolescent to have.
- Monitor and be aware. Know where your adolescent is and who his friends are. Set limits.
- Reach agreement about limits, consequences, and independent decision making.
- Provide opportunities for your adolescent to develop independent decision-making skills.

Adolescents who take part in a range of activities they enjoy are more confident, manage their time better, and do better in school than adolescents who do not. These activities can nurture the strengths and assets that will help a middle adolescent navigate these formative years.

SAMPLE QUESTIONS:

Ask the youth

What are your interests outside of school?

Ask the parent

What does your adolescent do after school?

ANTICIPATORY GUIDANCE:

For the youth

- This is a good time to start figuring out what interests you have. How about art, drama, mentoring, volunteering, construction, and individual and organized sports? Consider learning new skills that can be helpful to your friends, family, or community, such as lifesaving, CPR, or peer mentoring.

For the parent

- Provide opportunities for your adolescent to find activities, other than academics, that truly interest him, especially if your child is struggling academically.
- Help your adolescent see things from another person's point of view, becoming more aware of other peoples' situations in your community.

Success in school is associated with reduction in risky behaviors and an increase in positive social relationships.

Worsening or poor academic achievement can be a sign of depression, anxiety, or attention or learning problems.

Adolescents should be planning for college or beginning to think about potential career options. Having no plan may indicate a lack of connectedness to school and community.

SAMPLE QUESTIONS:

Ask the youth

Are you attending school? How are you doing in school? Do you have any trouble in school with reading, writing, or doing math? How are your grades? What do you plan to do after high school?

Ask the parent

Is your adolescent getting to school on time? How is your adolescent doing in school? How do you support him in getting his homework done (eg, expressing interest in his schoolwork, making sure he has dedicated time and space at home for homework)? How are his grades? What do you see your adolescent doing after he completes high school?

ANTICIPATORY GUIDANCE:

For the youth

- Take responsibility for getting your homework done and getting to school on time.
- This is a good time to discuss college or work plans and goals with your family and other appropriate adults.

For the parent

- Emphasize the importance of school.
- Praise positive efforts.
- Recognize success and achievements.
- Encourage your child to take responsibility for school-related issues, but continue to be ready to help out with organizational issues or new activities, such as applying for jobs and college.
- Encourage reading for pleasure and relaxation.
- Encourage him to look at the newspaper every day.

EMOTIONAL WELL-BEING

Coping, mood regulation and mental health, sexuality

Strategies for coping effectively with stress are an important aspect of emotional well-being. Time management skills, problem-solving skills, and refusal skills all have been identified as helpful. Some adolescents use their social support network, exercise, journaling, or meditation to help them manage.

SAMPLE QUESTIONS:

Ask the youth

How do you cope with stress? Are you feeling really stressed out all the time?

Ask the parent

How are you helping your young adult become a good decision maker? Cope with stress?

ANTICIPATORY GUIDANCE:

For the youth

- Most people your age experience ups and downs as they transition from adolescence to adulthood. They have great days and not-so-great days, and successes and failures. Everyone has stress in their lives. It's important for you to figure out how to deal with stress in the ways that work best for you. If you would like some help with this, I would be happy to give you some ideas.

For the parent

- Involve the child in family decision making, as appropriate, to give her experience with solving problems and making decisions.
- Encourage your child to think through solutions rather than giving her all the answers.

Many adolescents may not present with classic adult symptoms of depression. Pervasive boredom or irritability may be symptoms of depression in this age group. Because adolescents are more likely to report suicidal thoughts or attempts than their parents, it is important to question them directly about suicidal thoughts or attempts if there is any concern about depression or other mental health problems.

Anxiety falls along a spectrum of intensity, and symptoms may cause significant distress and affect the adolescent's functioning at school, at home, or with friends.

Posttraumatic stress disorder is frequently overlooked and can present with symptoms of depression and anxiety. Past traumatic events can include being in a motor vehicle crash, experiencing physical or sexual abuse or other major life events, or witnessing violence.

Fighting and bullying behaviors can indicate the presence of a conduct disorder and may co-occur with problems with substance abuse, depression, or anxiety.

Worsening or poor academic achievement or job performance may be a sign of depression, anxiety, attention, or learning problems, or a substance abuse problem.

Not adhering to parental rules and requests can indicate problems with the parent-youth relationship or significant problems with other authority figures.

Any adolescent with substance abuse problems also may be struggling with a mental health problem. These adolescents need to be evaluated for both substance abuse and mental health problems because they occur more often together in adolescents than they do in adults.

SAMPLE QUESTIONS:
Ask the youth
Have you been feeling sad, had difficulty sleeping, or frequently feel irritable? Do you ever feel so upset that you wish you were not alive or that you want to die? Do you worry a lot or feel overly stressed out? Do you find yourself continuing to remember or think about an unpleasant experience that happened in the past? Who do you go to for advice and help with personal decisions in your life?
Ask the parent
Have you noticed any changes in your adolescent's weight, sleep habits, or behaviors, such as becoming more isolated from her peers? Is your adolescent frequently irritable? Do you have any concerns about your adolescent's emotional health? Do you think your adolescent worries too much or appears overly anxious? Does your adolescent have reoccurring thoughts or worries about a past unpleasant event, such as a motor vehicle crash or being hurt by someone? Has anyone in the family had mental health problems or committed suicide?

ANTICIPATORY GUIDANCE:
For the youth
- Even with the ups and downs of everyday life, most people can figure out how to find and do the things they enjoy in life, such as doing their job or schoolwork; having good relationships with friends, family, and other adults; making decisions (often after talking with trusted friends and family members); having goals for the future; and adhering to their values.
- Sometimes, though, people your age may feel like they're too sad, depressed, bored, hopeless, nervous, or angry to do these things. If you feel that way now, I'd like to talk about it with you. If you ever feel that way, it is important for you to ask for help.
For the parent
- As your adolescent's health care professional, I am just as interested in her emotional well-being and mental health as I am in her physical health. If you are concerned about your adolescent's behavior, moods, mental health, or substance use, please talk with me.

Sexuality and relationships are an important issue in middle adolescence. Parents and adolescents need accurate information and support to help them communicate with each other.

SAMPLE QUESTIONS:
Ask the youth
For females: *Have you had your first period? If you have menstruated, tell me more about your periods (how often, how many, accompanied by pain?).*

Have you talked with your parents about crushes you've had, about dating and relationships, and about sex? In terms of your sexual attraction, are you attracted to males, females, or both, or are you undecided? Do you have any questions or concerns about your gender identity (your identity as a male or female)? Have you had sex?

Ask the parent
Do you monitor and supervise your adolescent's activities and friends? Do you enjoy talking with your adolescent and her friends? Have you established house rules about curfews, parties, dating, and friends? How do you plan to help your adolescent deal with pressures to have sex? Does she have any special relationships or someone she dates steadily?

ANTICIPATORY GUIDANCE:
For the youth
- It's important for you to have accurate information about sexuality, your physical development, and your sexual feelings. Please ask me if you have any questions.

For the parent
- Communicate frequently and share expectations clearly.
- Help your adolescent make a plan to resist pressures to have sex. Be there for her when she needs support or assistance.

RISK REDUCTION

Tobacco, alcohol, or other drugs; pregnancy; STIs

Provide information on how to resist peer pressure to smoke, drink alcohol, use drugs, or have sex. If the adolescent refers to substance abuse, ask about duration, amount, and frequency.

SAMPLE QUESTIONS:
Ask the youth
Do you (or your friends) smoke? Chew tobacco? Drink alcohol? Take drugs? Use anabolic steroids? Do you ever sniff, "huff," or breathe anything to get high?

Ask the parent
Does anyone in your home smoke? What has your adolescent been taught at home or in school about alcohol and drugs? Do you regularly supervise your adolescent's social and recreational activities? Does your adolescent understand what you consider appropriate behavior? How do you check for the use of tobacco, alcohol, or other drugs? What have you and your adolescent discussed about the risks of

using alcohol, tobacco, and other drugs? What consequences or disciplinary action would you take (or have you taken) if you discovered that your adolescent used tobacco, alcohol, or other drugs? Are you worried about any family members and how much they smoke, drink, or use drugs?

ANTICIPATORY GUIDANCE:
For the youth
- Do not smoke, use tobacco, drink alcohol, or use drugs, inhalants, anabolic steroids, or diet pills. Smoking marijuana and other drugs can hurt your lungs; alcohol and other drugs are bad for brain development.
- Avoid situations in which drugs or alcohol are readily available.
- Support friends who choose not to use tobacco, alcohol, drugs, steroids, or diet pills.
- If you are worried about any family member's drug or alcohol use problems, you can talk to me.
- If you smoke, use drugs, or drink alcohol, let's talk about it. Ask for help with quitting or cutting down on your use.
- If you do drink alcohol, do not drink when driving, swimming, boating, riding a bike or motorcycle, or operating farm equipment.

For the parent
- Know where and with whom your adolescent is spending leisure time. Be involved in his life.
- Clearly discuss rules and expectations for acceptable behavior.
- Praise your adolescent for not using tobacco, alcohol, or other drugs. Encourage him to stick to this decision.
- Set a good example for your adolescent through your own responsible use of alcohol and other substances.
- Consider locking your liquor cabinet and putting your prescription medicines in a place where your adolescent cannot get them.

SAMPLE QUESTIONS:
Ask the youth
Have you had sex? Was it wanted or unwanted? Have you ever felt pressured or forced to do something sexual you didn't want to do? How many partners have you had in the last year? Were your partners male or female, or have you had both male and female partners? Were your partners younger, older, or your age? Did you use other birth control instead of, or along with, a condom? Are you aware of emergency contraception? If you are having sex, are you making good choices to avoid emotional hurt for you and your partner? How are you protecting yourself against STIs and pregnancy?

Ask the parent
Have you shared your hopes, expectations, and values about relationships and sex with your adolescent? Are you worried about sexual pressures on him? How do you plan to help him deal with these issues? How does your culture help you do this?

ANTICIPATORY GUIDANCE:

For the youth

- Abstaining from sexual intercourse is the safest way to prevent pregnancy and STIs. Many people don't know that STIs can be transmitted by oral and anal sex.
- Plan how to avoid risky places and relationships. If you are sexually active, protect yourself and your partners from STIs and pregnancy by using contraceptives and condoms correctly and consistently. Consider having emergency contraception available. Make sure you understand what protection contraceptives do and don't offer.

For the parent

- Have discussions with your adolescent as he accepts responsibility for his decisions and relationships.

VIOLENCE AND INJURY PREVENTION

Safety belt and helmet use, driving (graduated license) and substance abuse, guns, interpersonal violence (dating violence), bullying

Everyone should wear safety belts when riding in a vehicle, and helmets when riding a bicycle, a motorcycle, or an ATV, and other protective gear when participating in activities such as biking, skating, or water sports. Graduated driver requirements have been shown to be effective, and it is important for parents to enforce them and for adolescents to understand their importance.

Learning to drive is a rite of passage for many adolescents and a reflection of their growing independence and maturity. Health care professionals should encourage parents to be initially involved with their adolescent's driver's education by doing practice driving sessions together and by establishing rules that foster safe, responsible driving behaviors. Parents should familiarize themselves with the provisions of the Graduated Driver License law in their state and continue to monitor their adolescent's driving skills and habits to ensure that safe behaviors persist.

SAMPLE QUESTIONS:

Ask the youth

Do you always wear a safety belt? Do you always wear a helmet or protective gear when biking, playing team sports, or doing water sports? Have you started to learn how to drive? Do you follow the driving regulations for young drivers? Do you have someone you can call for a ride if you feel unsafe driving yourself or unsafe in riding with someone else?

Ask the parent

Do you always wear a safety belt and bicycle or motorcycle helmet? Do you insist that your adolescent wear them? What kinds of restrictions have you set regarding your adolescent's driving?

ANTICIPATORY GUIDANCE:

For the youth

- Always wear a safety belt in a vehicle, and a helmet when riding a bike, a motorcycle, or an ATV, or when skateboarding.
- Always wear water-floatation clothing or an appropriately fitting US Coast Guard-approved life jacket when engaged in water sports.
- Always wear protective gear when engaged in team sports.
- Do not ride in a vehicle with someone who has been using drugs or alcohol.
- Do not drive after using alcohol or drugs.
- Limit night driving and driving with other teen passengers.
- If you feel unsafe driving yourself or riding with someone else, call someone to drive you.

For the parent

- If you wear safety belts and helmets, your adolescent is more likely to do so also. Insist that everyone in the vehicle wear a safety belt.
- Be involved with your adolescent's life. Know where she is and who her friends are.
- Set limits and expectations about driving, such as number of passengers, the amount of night driving allowed, how to minimize distracted driving, and how to avoid high-risk situations.
- Be involved in your adolescent's driving, because parents who are involved are successful at imposing limits.

The AAP recommends that homes be free of guns and that if it is necessary to keep a gun, it should be stored unloaded and locked, with the ammunition locked separately from the gun. Guns should be removed from the homes of adolescents who have a history of aggressive or violent behaviors, suicide attempts, or depression.

SAMPLE QUESTIONS:

Ask the youth

Do you ever carry a gun? Can you get a gun if you want to? Is there a gun at home?

Ask the parent

Is there a gun in your house? Is it locked and is the ammunition locked and stored separately? Is there a gun in the homes where you and your adolescent visit, such as the homes of grandparents, other relatives, or friends?

ANTICIPATORY GUIDANCE:

For the youth

- Fighting and carrying weapons can be dangerous. Would you like to discuss how to avoid these situations?

For the parent

- The best way to keep your adolescent safe from injury or death from guns is to never have a gun in the home. If it is necessary to keep a gun in your home, it should be stored unloaded and locked, with the ammunition locked separately from the gun. Keep the key where adolescents cannot have access.

Fighting and bullying behaviors can indicate the presence of conduct disorders or may co-occur with problems of substance abuse, depression, or anxiety.

Discuss youth involvement with negotiating anger or conflict with peers and adults to avoid physical fights in school or in neighborhood.

Interpersonal violence and gang involvement are key issues in this age group, and bullying or being bullied is often less of a concern.

Discuss ways to avoid dating violence.

SAMPLE QUESTIONS:

Ask the youth

What do you do when someone tries to pick a fight with you? What do you do when you are angry? Have you been in a fight in the past 12 months? Do you carry a weapon? Have you carried a weapon to school? If so, why? Do you know anyone in a gang? Do you belong to a gang? Has your girlfriend or boyfriend ever hit, slapped, or physically hurt you? Have you ever been touched in a sexual way against your wish or without your consent? Have you ever been forced to have sexual intercourse? Are you in a relationship with a person who threatens you physically or hurts you?

Ask the parent

Are there frequent reports of violence in your community or school? Is your adolescent involved in it? Has your teen ever been threatened with a gun or knife or some other physical harm, or been injured in a fight? Has your teen bullied others? Has your teen been suspended from school because of fighting or bullying or carrying a weapon? Do you know your adolescent's friends and the activities they participate in or attend? Does your adolescent have a boyfriend or girlfriend and, if so, is their relationship respectful toward each other? Would your adolescent feel comfortable enough to inform you whether anyone has ever attempted to force sex with her?

ANTICIPATORY GUIDANCE:

For the youth

- Learn to manage conflict nonviolently. Walk away if necessary.
- Avoid risky situations. Avoid violent people. Call for help if things get dangerous.
- Healthy dating relationships are built on respect, concern, and doing things both of you like to do.
- Leave a relationship when you see signs of violence.
- In dating situations, remember that "No" means NO. Saying "No" is OK.

For the parent

- Teach nonviolent conflict resolution.
- Talk to your adolescent about safe dating practices.

Health Supervision: Late Adolescence (18 to 21 Year Visits)

CONTEXT

The late adolescent stands at an exhilarating moment in life. He has progressed through a huge developmental trajectory that began 18 years ago. The accumulated physical, cognitive, emotional, and social experiences of infancy, early childhood, middle childhood, and the earlier phases of adolescence have prepared him for the final transition to adulthood. This transition is the work of late adolescence.

Physical development is generally complete by late adolescence. By this point, young adults also typically have developed a sense of self-identity and a rational and realistic conscience, and they have refined their moral, religious, and sexual values. They are able to compromise, set limits, and think through issues to make decisions. Cognitively, young adults are still developing, and new research evidence suggests that this process may continue into the third decade of life.[3] Society, however, regards late adolescents as adults, as they are legally able to drive, vote, smoke, drink alcohol (at 21), give consent, and enter into contracts. Legal infractions create a permanent criminal record for a young adult.

The experiences of late adolescence vary greatly and depend on the adolescent's resources, previous academic performance, life choices, opportunities, motivations, and cultural expectations about independence. The adolescent may be entering college (close to 17 million students are enrolled in the nation's colleges and universities,[14] and the number is expected to increase to about 18 million by the year 2009[18]), starting a first job, becoming a parent, finding employment, or serving in the military. A number of programs exist to help young adults make a successful transition into the working world. For example, Job Corps, a comprehensive residential, education, and job-training program, serves nearly 70,000 students a year. Job Corps centers throughout the country have provided more than 2 million disadvantaged young adults with the integrated academic, vocational, and social skills training they need to gain independence and get quality, long-term jobs or further their education.[19]

The experience of youth completing high school and entering the work force, the military, or universities varies widely by race/ethnicity. High-school drop-out rates for non-Hispanic white and black youth declined substantially (from 12% to 7% and 21% to 11%, respectively), from 1972 to 2001, although no statistically significant decline occurred among Hispanics/Latinos. Twenty-seven percent of Hispanic/Latino young adults dropped out before completing high school in 2001.[20]

Living situations vary widely among young adults. Older adolescents may be living at home, on their own, with a roommate or partner, or in a group setting. They may be getting married or starting their own families. A young adult with special health care needs may be in high school or at work and still living at home. In some cultures, young adults are expected to live at home until they are married.

559

It is argued that "emerging adulthood is neither adolesence nor young adulthood, but is theoretically and empirically distinct from them both."[21] Many young adults experience an apparent lengthening of the transition period from childhood to economic independence. Attending college typically results in a higher paying job, but it also delays moving into the work force full-time and entails paying historically high tuition rates. With all its benefits, this expensive lengthening of the education process makes it difficult for young people to become financially independent.

All these transitional experiences expose the adolescent to new relationships, lifestyles, driving habits, dietary patterns, and exercise habits. They may be starting new sexual relationships and defining their sexual identity. Parental and other adult supervision decreases and autonomy increases. Responsibilities and life stresses also increase, as does access to alcohol and drugs. Personal health behaviors may change. The nutrition and physical activity habits of this age group may change, too, as their food choices are no longer supervised. For some young adults, the transition to independent living creates opportunities to improve their nutrition and physical activity patterns. For others, nutritious foods may be perceived as unaffordable or inconvenient. In addition, access to formal exercise programs or team participation may be limited.

The health needs of older adolescents vary greatly based on their situations and, thus, the health care professional should inquire about these issues. The young adult's response can often lead to topics that merit further exploration and assistance. Older adolescents should have medical preventive visits annually to assess any new positive and negative influences that may be affecting their health. Unfortunately, young adults' participation in health supervision visits tends to decrease. Many people in this age group are no longer legally considered "dependents" of their parents and are unlikely to be covered under their parent's insurance policies. However, other sources of health supervision exist for young adults, depending on their life choices. For example, college and university health care centers can play an important role in addressing the health conditions and risky behaviors (eg, episodic heavy drinking/binge drinking, drinking and driving, cigarette smoking, and overweight[22,23]) of young adults. The military provides health care to active duty personnel, and many workplaces sponsor wellness and health-promotion activities.

The age of consent varies from state to state. If a patient is older than the age of consent, a health care professional cannot discuss the young adult's care with the parents or caregiver without the young adult's permission. All the anticipatory guidance information should be directed toward the young adult patient.

PRIORITIES FOR THE VISIT

The first priority is to address any specific concerns that the patient may have. The Bright Futures Adolescence Expert Panel has given priority to the following additional topics for discussion in the 4 Late Adolescence Visits. The goal of these discussions is to determine the health needs of the young adult and family that should be addressed by the health care professional. The following priorities are consistent throughout adolescence. However, the questions used to effectively obtain information and the anticipatory guidance provided to the young adult and family can vary.

Including all the priority issues in every visit may not be feasible, but the goal should be to address issues important to this age group over the span of the 4 visits. These issues include:

- Physical growth and development (physical and oral health, body image, healthy eating, physical activity)
- Social and academic competence (connectedness with family, peers, and community; interpersonal relationships; school/job performance)
- Emotional well-being (coping, mood regulation and mental health, sexuality)
- Risk reduction (tobacco, alcohol, or other drugs; pregnancy; STIs)
- Violence and injury prevention (safety belts and helmets, driving and substance abuse, access to guns, interpersonal violence [dating violence, stalking])

HEALTH SUPERVISION

History

Interval history can be obtained according to the health care professional's preference or style of practice. The following questions may encourage in-depth discussion to determine changes in health status that would warrant further physical or emotional assessment:

To the Young Adult:
- Have you been in good health since your last visit here? Do you have any medical questions, problems, or complaints?
- How are things going with your family, your friends, your job, in school?
- What are your future plans for employment, further education, or relationships?

To the Parent (if accompanying the young adult at the visit):
- Do you have any questions about your young adult's physical or emotional well-being?

Observation of Parent-Young Adult Interaction

Most of the Late Adolescence Visits will be with the young adult alone, without a parent, unless the young adult requests differently. However, if parents are present, the health care professional can observe the interactions between the parent and young adult, including:

- How comfortably do the young adult and parent interact, both verbally and nonverbally?

For all young adults who have a parent, guardian, partner, or spouse accompanying them to the visit, and especially for those with special health care needs, these visits provide an excellent opportunity to see whether the young adults are being appropriately encouraged toward managing and making independent decisions about their own health.

Surveillance of Development

The developmental tasks of late adolescence can be addressed through information obtained in the medical examination by observation, by asking specific questions, and through general discussion. The following areas can be assessed to better understand the developmental health of the young adult. A goal of this assessment is to determine whether the young adult is developing in an appropriate fashion and, if not, to provide information for assistance or intervention. In the assessment, determine whether the young adult is making progress on these developmental tasks:

- Demonstrates physical, cognitive, emotional, social, and moral competencies
- Engages in behaviors that promote wellness and contribute to a healthy lifestyle
- Forms a caring, supportive relationship with family, other adults, and peers
- Engages in a positive way in the life of the community
- Displays a sense of self-confidence, hopefulness, and well-being
- Demonstrates resiliency when confronted with life stressors
- Demonstrates increasingly responsible and independent decision making[11]

Physical Examination

A complete physical examination is included as part of every health supervision visit.

When performing a physical examination, the health care professional's attention is directed to the following components of the exam that are important for 18- to 21-year-olds:

- ■ **Measure:**
  - Blood pressure
- ■ **Measure and plot:**
  - Height
  - Weight
- ■ **Calculate and plot:**
  - BMI
- ■ **Skin**
  - Inspect for acne, acanthosis nigricans, atypical nevi, tattoos, piercings, and signs of abuse or self-inflicted injuries

- ■ **Breast**
  Female
  - Clinical Breast Examination is considered routine after age 20
- ■ **Genitalia**
  Female
  - Inspect for signs of STIs (eg, warts, vesicles, vaginal discharge)
  - Perform pelvic exam by age 21 or if clinically warranted, based on sexual activity (eg, for Pap smear within 3 years of onset of sexual activity) and/or specific problems (eg, pubertal aberrancy, abnormal bleeding or abdominal or pelvic pain)

  Male
  - Perform visual inspection for sexual maturity rating and observations for signs of STIs (ie, warts, vesicles)
  - Examine testicles for hydrocele, hernias, varicocele, or masses

Screening

UNIVERSAL SCREENING	ACTION	
Vision (once in late adolescence)	Snellen test	
Dyslipidemia (once in late adolescence)	A fasting lipoprotein profile (total cholesterol, LDL cholesterol, high density lipoprotein [HDL], cholesterol, and triglyceride). If the testing opportunity is non-fasting, only total cholesterol and HDL cholesterol will be usable.	

SELECTIVE SCREENING	RISK ASSESSMENT*	ACTION IF RA +
Vision at other ages	+ on risk screening questions	Snellen test
Hearing	+ on risk screening questions	Audiometry
Anemia	+ on risk screening questions	Hemoglobin or hematocrit
Tuberculosis	+ on risk screening questions	Tuberculin skin test
Dyslipidemia	If not age 20, + on risk screening questions and not previously screened with normal results	Lipid screen
STIs	Sexually active	Screen for chlamydia and gonorrhea; use tests appropriate for the patient population and clinical setting
	Sexually active and + on risk questions	Syphilis blood test HIV[†12]
Pregnancy	Sexually active without contraception, late or absent menses, or heavy or irregular bleeding	Urine hCG
Cervical dysplasia	Sexually active, within 3 years of onset of sexual activity or no later than age 21[24]	Pap smear, conventional slide or liquid-based
Alcohol or drug use	+ on risk screening questions	Administer alcohol and drug screening tool

*See Rationale and Evidence chapter for the criteria on which risk screening questions are based.

[†]The CDC has recently recommended universal voluntary HIV screening for all sexually active people, beginning at age 13. At the time of publication, the AAP and other groups had not yet commented on the CDC recommendation, nor recommended screening criteria or techniques. The health care professional's attention is drawn to the voluntary nature of screening and that the CDC allows an opt out in communities where the HIV rate is <0.1%. The management of positives and false positives must be considered before testing.

Immunizations

Consult the CDC/ACIP or AAP Web sites for the current immunization schedule.
CDC National Immunization Program (NIP): http://www.cdc.gov/vaccines
American Academy of Pediatrics *Red Book:* http://www.aapredbook.org

ANTICIPATORY GUIDANCE

The following sample questions, which address the Adolescent Expert Panel's Anticipatory Guidance Priorities for this visit, are intended to be used selectively to invite discussion, gather information, address the needs and concerns of the young adults, and build partnerships. Use of the questions may vary from visit to visit. It will not be feasible to ask all the questions at every visit. Questions can be modified to match the health care professional's communication style. Any anticipatory guidance for the young adult should be geared to questions, issues, or concerns for that particular young adult.

In most cases, the young adult will be alone at the visit. In some situations, especially if the young adult has a special health care need, he or she may be accompanied by a parent, guardian, partner, or spouse. The questions for parents are added to help guide the conversation if the young adult wants that person to participate in the visit.

PHYSICAL GROWTH AND DEVELOPMENT

Physical and oral health, body image, healthy eating, physical activity

The benefits of brushing the teeth with a fluoridated toothpaste extend to all ages. Fluoride is beneficial because it remineralizes tooth enamel and inhibits bacterial growth, thereby preventing caries. Flossing daily is important to prevent gum disease. Young adults should have regularly scheduled visits with their dentist at least twice each year.

Hearing loss may begin to be an issue with young adults who are consistently exposed to loud noise, such as at music concerts or in loud working environments. Counsel the young adult about the advisability of wearing hearing protection in these situations.

SAMPLE QUESTIONS:

Ask the young adult

Do you brush twice a day? Do you floss regularly? When was the last time you saw a dentist? Do you have trouble accessing dental care?

Ask the parent (if present)

Does your young adult see a dentist regularly?

ANTICIPATORY GUIDANCE:

For the young adult

- Brush your teeth at least twice daily with fluoridated toothpaste. See a dentist twice a year and discuss ways to keep your teeth healthy.
- Wear hearing protection when you are exposed to loud noise, such as music, at concerts, or in loud working conditions.

As young adults move away from home to college, the military, or their own apartments, they must take responsibility for establishing a healthy balance of physical activity and nutrition. Eating disorders are still a significant risk for young people in this age group, especially females.

SAMPLE QUESTIONS:

Ask the young adult

How do you feel about the way you look? How much would you like to weigh? Are you doing anything to change your weight? How?

Ask the parent (if present)

Do you have any questions or concerns about your young adult's nutrition, weight, or physical activity?

ANTICIPATORY GUIDANCE:

For the young adult

- It's important for you to begin to figure out the right balance for you between your eating and physical activity so you can maintain a weight that is healthy for you.

Appropriately, many 18- to 21-year-olds are making the majority of food decisions on their own. They may be living on their own, eating college cafeteria food, and eating out more often. Even if they are still living at home, their schedules often do not foster participation in family meals. Vegetarian or vegan diets require careful attention to ensure adequate intakes of protein and nutrients.

SAMPLE QUESTIONS:

Ask the young adult

Which meals do you usually eat each day? Do you ever skip a meal? If so, how many times a week? How many servings of milk did you have yesterday? How many servings of other dairy foods, such as yogurt or cheese? How many fruits did you eat yesterday? How many vegetables? Do you ever not have enough food? How often do you drink soft drinks? Are there any foods you won't eat? If so, which ones? What changes would you like to make in the way you eat?

Ask the parent (if present)

Do you think your young adult eats healthy foods? What do you consider healthy foods? Do you have any difficulty getting healthy foods for your family? Do you have any concerns about your young adult's eating behaviors, such as not drinking milk or skipping meals?

ANTICIPATORY GUIDANCE:

For the young adult

- Eat 3 nutritious meals a day. Breakfast is an especially important meal. Select a nutritious lunch from the cafeteria or pack a balanced lunch.
- Focus on food choices that help you stay healthy.
  - Eat lots of fruits and vegetables, especially the really colorful ones.
  - Focus on whole-grain breads, cereals, and other grain products.
  - Have 3 or more servings of low-fat (1%) or fat-free milk and other low-fat dairy products.
  - Eat lean meats, chicken, fish, and other sources of protein and iron.
  - Limit high-fat or low-nutrient foods and beverages, such as candy, chips, and soft drinks.
  - Drink plenty of water.

Current recommendations state that adolescents and young adults should engage in 60 minutes of physical activity on most, if not all, days of the week. Physical activity is one cornerstone of a healthy adult life and is essential to maintaining a healthy weight. Young adults who have transitioned from their usual high-school activities to many different living and working situations may benefit the most from encouragement, advice, and problem solving tailored to their individual situation.

Attention to balancing physical activity and inactivity is needed because computers, movies, and DVDs present numerous opportunities for physical inactivity. Computers are often an essential social and recreational outlet for young adults with special health care needs, so guidance about limiting screen time may need to be modified for these patients.

SAMPLE QUESTIONS:
Ask the young adult
Do you participate in any physical activities, such as walking, biking, hiking, skating, swimming, or running? How often? For how long each time? How much time each day do you spend watching TV, videotapes, or DVDs? How many hours a day do you use a computer? Do you participate in any physical activities with your family or friends, such as biking, hiking, skating, swimming, or running?

Ask the parent (if present)
Does your young adult participate in regular physical activity on most, if not all, days of the week? Are there opportunities for safe recreation in your neighborhood? How can you help your young adult become more physically active? How much time each day does your young adult watch TV, videotapes, or DVDs? How much time does she spend at the computer? Do you and your young adult participate in physical activities together? If so, which ones? How often?

ANTICIPATORY GUIDANCE:
For the young adult
- Be physically active as part of play, games, physical education, planned physical activities, recreation, and organized sports. Try to be active for 1 hour on most, if not all, days of the week. You don't have to do it all at once. You can break it up into shorter times of activity throughout the day. Doing a mix of physical activities you enjoy is a great way to reach the 60-minutes-a-day goal.
- To prevent injuries, use appropriate safety equipment (such as a helmet, a mouth guard, eye protection, wrist guards, and elbow and knee pads) when participating in physical activity.
- Drink plenty of water to maintain hydration lost during physical activity to prevent heat-related illnesses, such as heat cramps, exhaustion, and heat stroke.
- Cut back on physical inactivity by limiting the time you spend watching TV, videotapes, or DVDs, or using a computer, other than for work or school, to no more than 2 hours a day.
- If the safety of the environment or neighborhood is a concern, find other settings to participate in physical activity.

For young adults with special health care needs:

■ Engage in physical activity for cardiovascular fitness within the limits of your medical or physical condition. Adaptive physical education can be helpful, and a physical therapist can help you identify appropriate activities.

SOCIAL AND ACADEMIC COMPETENCE

Connectedness with family, peers, and community; interpersonal relationships; school/job performance

Peer relationships can positively or negatively affect a young adult's outlook and choice of behaviors. Even though young adults spend increasing amounts of time with peers, it is still important for them to have the support of their families when they need help.

SAMPLE QUESTIONS:
Ask the young adult
Do you have close friends? If not, what stands in the way? What interests do you have outside of school and work?

ANTICIPATORY GUIDANCE:
For the young adult
■ It's still important to stay connected with your family as you grow to adulthood. Talk with your family to solve problems, especially around difficult situations or topics.
■ Making friends and keeping them is an important life skill. Evaluating whether a friendship is no longer good for you also is important. As you leave high school and begin a new life with new interests, you may find that you drift away from some of your old friends. That's a normal part of growing up and becoming an adult.

Students who complete high school and are more successful in supporting themselves and living independently than adolescents who do not. Poor academic achievement can be a sign of depression, anxiety, or attention or learning problems.

SAMPLE QUESTIONS:
Ask the young adult
Have you graduated from high school? What are your plans for work or school? What help do you need from me or your parents to help you reach your goal?
Ask the parent (if present)
What educational or work plans does your young adult have? What do you see your young adult doing 1 year from now? 5 years from now? How can you help your young adult achieve his educational or work goals?

ANTICIPATORY GUIDANCE:
For the young adult
■ Take responsibility for being organized enough to get yourself to school or work on time.

■ As you head to college, the military, or your first full-time job, consider getting involved in your community about an issue that interests or concerns you.

EMOTIONAL WELL-BEING

Coping, mood regulation and mental health, sexuality

Strategies for coping effectively with stress are an important aspect of emotional well-being. Time-management skills, problem-solving skills, and refusal skills all have been identified as helpful. Some adolescents and young adults have found that their social support network, exercise, journaling, or meditation helps them manage.

SAMPLE QUESTIONS:
Ask the young adult
How do you cope with stress? Are you feeling really stressed out all the time?
Ask the parent (if present)
How are you helping your young adult become a good decision maker? Cope with stress?

ANTICIPATORY GUIDANCE:
For the young adult
■ Most people your age experience ups and downs as they make the transition from adolescence to adulthood. They have great days and not so great days, and successes and failures. Everyone has stress in their lives. It's important for you to figure out how to deal with stress in ways that work well for you. If you would like some help with this, I would be happy to give you some ideas.

Many young adults may not present with classic adult symptoms of depression. Pervasive boredom or irritability still may be symptoms of depression in this age group. It is important to question them directly about suicidal thoughts or attempts if there is any concern about depression or other mental health problems.

Anxiety falls along a spectrum of intensity, and symptoms can cause significant distress and affect the young adult's functioning at school, at home, or with friends.

Posttraumatic stress disorder is frequently overlooked and can present with symptoms of depression and anxiety. Past traumatic events can include being in a motor vehicle crash, experiencing physical or sexual abuse or other major life events, or witnessing violence.

Fighting behaviors can indicate the presence of conduct disorder and may co-occur with problems with substance abuse, depression, or anxiety.

Worsening or poor academic achievement or job performance may be signs of depression, anxiety, attention or learning problems, or a substance abuse problem.

Consistently not adhering to rules and requests from parents, teachers, or employers can indicate problems with the relationship or significant problems with other authority figures.

ADOLESCENCE
18 TO 21 YEAR VISITS

Any young adult with substance abuse problems also may be struggling with a mental health problem. These youth need to be evaluated for both substance abuse and mental health because they occur more often together in adolescents than in adults.

SAMPLE QUESTIONS:

Ask the young adult

Have you been feeling sad, have difficulty sleeping, or frequently feel irritable? Did you ever feel so upset that you wished you were not alive or that you wanted to die? Do you find yourself continuing to remember or think about an unpleasant experience that happened in the past?

Ask the parent (if present)

Have you noticed any changes in your young adult's weight or sleep habits? Is your young adult frequently irritable? Do you have any concerns about your young adult's emotional health? Do you think he worries too much or appears overly anxious? Does your young adult have reoccurring thoughts or worries about an unpleasant event from the past, such as a motor vehicle crash or being hurt by someone? Has anyone in the family had mental health problems or committed suicide?

ANTICIPATORY GUIDANCE:

For the young adult

- Even with these ups and downs, most people can figure out how to find and do the things they enjoy in life, such as doing their job or schoolwork; having good relationships with friends, family, and other adults; making decisions (often after talking with trusted friends and family members); having goals for the future; and sticking to their values.
- Sometimes, though, people your age may feel like they're too sad, depressed, hopeless, nervous, or angry to do these things. If you feel that way now, I'd like to talk about it with you. If you ever feel that way, it is important for you to ask for help.

For the young adult, the issue of sexuality is central. Some young adults still may have questions or concerns about their sexual orientation, gender identity, or sexual maturity. For some, the decision to have an intimate relationship and become sexually active may be relevant. For others, decisions about continued sexual activity versus a period of abstinence from sex, thoughts about the emotional intensity of a romantic relationships, or protection from STIs and pregnancy may be uppermost in their minds.

SAMPLE QUESTIONS:

Ask the young adult

What are your values about dating and relationships? Are you attracted to males, females, or both? Do you have any questions or concerns about your gender identity (your identity as a male or female)? Have you had sex? What are your plans and values about relationships, sex, and future family or marriage? Have you talked with your parents/family about stable relationships or marriage?

For females: *Have you menstruated? Tell me more about your periods (how often, how heavy, painful?).*

Ask the parent (if present)

Your teen is now a young adult. Are you comfortable with her development?

ANTICIPATORY GUIDANCE:

For the young adult

- Sexuality is an important part of your normal development as a young adult.
- If you have any questions or concerns about sexuality or your development, I hope you will consider me one of the people you can discuss these issues with.

RISK REDUCTION

Tobacco, alcohol, or other drugs; pregnancy; STIs

The use of tobacco, alcohol, and other drugs has adverse health effects on young adults and their still-developing brain. This focus on the health effects is often the most helpful approach and may help some young adults with quitting or cutting back on substance use. Others may be concerned about problems with substance use by their friends or family members.

It is important for all young adults to understand how to avoid pregnancy and STIs. By understanding both the physical and emotional health aspects of a young adult's sexual decision making, the health care professional can ensure that the young adult has all the accurate information necessary to foster healthy decisions. This health focus also conveys that the health care professional is not making judgments about the young adults' worth as a person, but providing guidance and support for healthy behaviors.

SAMPLE QUESTIONS:

Ask the young adult

Do you or your friends smoke? Chew tobacco? Drink alcohol? Tell me about any experiences you've had with alcohol, marijuana, or other drugs. If the young adult reports substance use, ask about duration, amount, and frequency. (Do a brief intervention for cessation or harm reduction.)

Have you had sex? Was it wanted or unwanted? How many partners have you had in the last year? Were your partners male, female, or did you have both male and female partners? Were your partners younger, older, or your age? Did you use a condom? Did you use birth control? Do you know about emergency contraception? Are you or your partner interested in having a child at this time?

Ask the parent (if present)

Does anyone in your home smoke? Do you know what social and recreational activities your young adult participates in? Does your young adult understand what you consider appropriate behavior? Are you worried about your young adult's drug or alcohol use? What have you and your young adult discussed about the risks of using alcohol, tobacco, and other drugs?

ANTICIPATORY GUIDANCE:
For the young adult

- Do not smoke, use tobacco, drink alcohol, or use drugs, anabolic steroids, or diet pills. Avoid situations in which drugs or alcohol are readily available. Smoking marijuana and other drugs can hurt your lungs. Alcohol and other drugs are bad for brain development.
- Support friends who choose not to use tobacco, alcohol, drugs, steroids, or diet pills.
- If you use drugs or alcohol, talk to me about it. I can help you with quitting or cutting down on your use. To be safe, do not drink alcohol or use drugs when driving, swimming, boating, riding a bike or motorcycle, or operating farm equipment.
- If you or your friends drink or use drugs, plan to ride with a designated driver or call for a ride.
- If you are sexually active, it's important to protect you and your partner or partners from an unwanted pregnancy and STIs by using contraceptives and condoms correctly and consistently. Consider having emergency contraception available.
- One important issue is that any sexual activity should be something you want. No one should ever force you or try to convince to do something you do not want to do.
- It can be helpful to think through ahead of time how to make sure you can carry out your decisions about sex. Two things that have helped other youth are to be careful with alcohol and drug use and to avoid risky places and relationships.

VIOLENCE AND INJURY PREVENTION

Safety belts and helmets, driving and substance abuse, access to guns, interpersonal violence (dating violence, stalking)

Everyone should wear safety belts when riding in a vehicle and wear helmets when riding a bicycle, motorcycle, or ATV. Crashes are a major cause of morbidity and mortality for young adults. Substance use by the driver can be a factor in many of these crashes. An arrest for driving while under the influence of a substance can have significant negative impact on a young adult's educational plans and insurance and employment prospects.

SAMPLE QUESTIONS:
Ask the young adult
Do you always wear a safety belt? Do you always wear a helmet when you are riding a bike, a motorcycle, or an ATV?
Ask the parent (if present)
Do you always wear a safety belt and bicycle helmet? Do you remind your young adult to wear them?

ANTICIPATORY GUIDANCE:
For the young adult
- Always wear a safety belt in a vehicle and wear a helmet when biking or riding a motorcycle or ATV.
- Do not drive after using alcohol or drugs.
- Do not ride in a vehicle with someone who has been using drugs or alcohol.
- If you feel unsafe driving yourself or riding with someone else, call someone to drive you.

The AAP recommends that homes be free of guns and that if it is necessary to keep a gun, it should be stored unloaded and locked, with the ammunition locked separately from the gun.

It is particularly important that guns be removed from the homes of young adults who have a history of aggressive or violent behaviors, suicide attempts, or depression.

SAMPLE QUESTIONS:
Ask the young adult
Do you know anyone with a weapon? Do you carry a weapon? Is there a gun at home? Have you carried a weapon to school or work? If so, why?
Ask the parent (if present)
Is there a gun in your house? Is it locked, with the ammunition locked separately?

ANTICIPATORY GUIDANCE:
For the young adult
- Fighting and carrying weapons can be dangerous. Would you like to discuss how to avoid these situations?
- The best way to keep your family safe from injury or death from guns is to never have a gun in the home. If it is necessary to keep a gun in your home, it should be stored unloaded and locked, with the ammunition locked separately from the gun. If children live with you, you must be sure that they cannot get to the key.

Fighting behaviors can indicate the presence of conduct disorders or may co-occur with problems of substance abuse, depression, or anxiety. Many young adults are unaware of the prevalence of dating violence and would benefit from understanding the warning signs and actions to take.

SAMPLE QUESTIONS:
Ask the young adult
What do you do when you get angry? Do you often get into fights? Physical or verbal? Have you been in a fight in the past 12 months? Do you know anyone in a gang? Do you belong to a gang? Have you ever been hit, slapped, or physically hurt while on a date? Have you ever been touched sexually against your wish or without your consent? Have you ever been forced to have sexual intercourse? Are you in a relationship with a person who threatens you physically or hurts you?

Ask the parent (if present)

Has your young adult been suspended from school or work because of fighting or carrying a weapon? Has your young adult ever been threatened with a gun or knife or some other physical harm? Are there frequent reports of violence in your community or school? Is your young adult involved in your community? Do you know your young adult's friends and the activities she participates in or attends? Is your young adult dating, and is the relationship mutually respectful? Would your young adult feel comfortable enough to inform you whether anyone had ever attempted to force sex with her?

ANTICIPATORY GUIDANCE:

For the young adult

- Learn to manage conflict nonviolently. Walk away if necessary.
- Avoid risky situations. Avoid violent people. Call for help if things get dangerous.
- Leave a relationship if there are any signs of violence.
- When dating, remember that "No" means NO. Saying "No" is OK.
- Healthy dating relationships are built on respect, concern, and doing things both of you like to do.

References

1. McAnarney ER, Kreipe R, Comerci G. Normal somatic adolescent growth and development. In: Bralow L, ed. *Textbook of Adolescent Medicine*. Philadelphia, PA: WB Saunders Co; 1992:46-67

2. American Academy of Pediatrics, Committee on Adolescence, American College of Obstetricians and Gynecologists, Committee on Adolescent Health Care. Menstruation in girls and adolescents: using the menstrual cycle as a vital sign. *Pediatrics*. 2006;118:2245-2250

3. Weinberger DR, Elvevag B, Giedd JN. *The Adolescent Brain: A Work in Progress*. Washington, DC: The National Campaign to Prevent Teen Pregnancy; 2005

4. Steinberg L, Mounts NS, Lamborn SD, Dornbusch SM. Authoritative parenting and adolescent adjustment across varied ecological niches. *J Res Adolesc*. 1991;1:19-36

5. Moore K, Halle T. *Preventing Problems Versus Promoting the Positive: What Do We Want for Our Children?* Washington, DC: Child Trends; 2000

6. Bradley RH, Whiteside L, Mundfrom DJ, Casey PH, Kelleher KJ, Pope SK. Early indications of resilience and their relation to experiences in the home environments of low birthweight, premature children living in poverty. *Child Dev*. 1994;65(2 Spec No):346-360

7. Murphey DA, Lamonda KH, Carney JK, Duncan P. Relationships of a brief measure of youth assets to health-promoting and risk behaviors. *J Adolesc Health*. 2004;34:184-191

8. Resnick MD. Protective factors, resiliency and healthy youth development. *Adolesc Med*. 2000;11:157-165

9. Resnick MD. Resilience and protective factors in the lives of adolescents. *J Adolesc Health*. 2000;27:1-2

10. Steinberg L. Gallagher lecture. The family at adolescence: transition and transformation. *J Adolesc Health*. 2000;27:170-178

11. Association of Maternal & Child Health Programs. *A Conceptual Framework for Adolescent Health*. Washington, DC: Association of Maternal & Child Health Programs, National Network of State Adolescent Health Coordinators; 2005:5-6

12. Centers for Disease Control and Prevention. Revised Recommendations for HIV Testing of Adults, Adolescents, and Pregnant Women in Health-Care Settings. *MMWR 2006*. September 22, 2006;55(No. RR-14)

13. Individuals with Disabilities Education Improvement Act (IDEA) of 2004, Provisions for Children and Youth with Disabilities Who Experience Homelessness. Available at: http://www.serve.org/nche. Accessed September 15, 2006

14. US Census Bureau. Statistical Abstract of the United States. Available at: http://www.census.gov/prod/www/statistical-abstract.html. Accessed September 15, 2006

15. American College of Obstetricians and Gynecologists. Eating disorders. In: *Health Care for Adolescents*. Washington, DC: American College of Obstetricians and Gynecologists; 2003:83-92

16. National Institute of Mental Health. Mental Illness Exacts Heavy Toll, Beginning in Youth. Available at: http://www.nimh.nih.gov/press/mentalhealthstats.cfm. Accessed September 15, 2006

17. American College of Obstetricians and Gynecologists. Primary and preventive health care. In: *Health Care for Adolescents*. Washington, DC: American College of Obstetricians and Gynecologist; 2003:3-23

18. National Center for Education Statistics. Projections of Education Statistics to 2014. Available at: http://www.nces.ed.gov. Accessed September 15, 2006

19. US Department of Labor. Job Corps. Available at: http://jobcorps.doleta.gov/. Accessed January 1, 2007

20. US Department of Education, National Center for Education Statistics. *Dropout Rates in the United States: 2001*. Kaufman P, Alt MN, Chapman C, eds. Washington, DC: US Government Printing Office; 2004. Publication No. NCES 2005-046

21. Arnett JJ. Emerging adulthood. A theory of development from the late teens through the twenties. *Am Psychol*. 2000;55:469-480

22. Centers for Disease Control and Prevention. Youth Risk Behavior Surveillance: National College Health Risk Behavior Survey—United States, 1995. Washington, DC: *MMWR CDC Surveill Summ*. 1997;46(SS-6):1-56

23. Neinstein LS, Johnson BA. Overview of college health issues. In: Neinstein LS, ed. *Adolescent Health Care. A Practical Guide*. Philadelphia, PA: Lippincott Williams & Wilkins; 2002:1551-1579

24. American College of Obstetricians and Gynecologists, Committee on Gynecologic Practice. Primary and preventive care: periodic assessments. ACOG Committee Opinion No. 292. *Obstet Gynecol*. 2003;102:1117-1124

Appendices

Birth to 36 months: Boys
Length-for-age and Weight-for-age percentiles

NAME _____

RECORD # _____

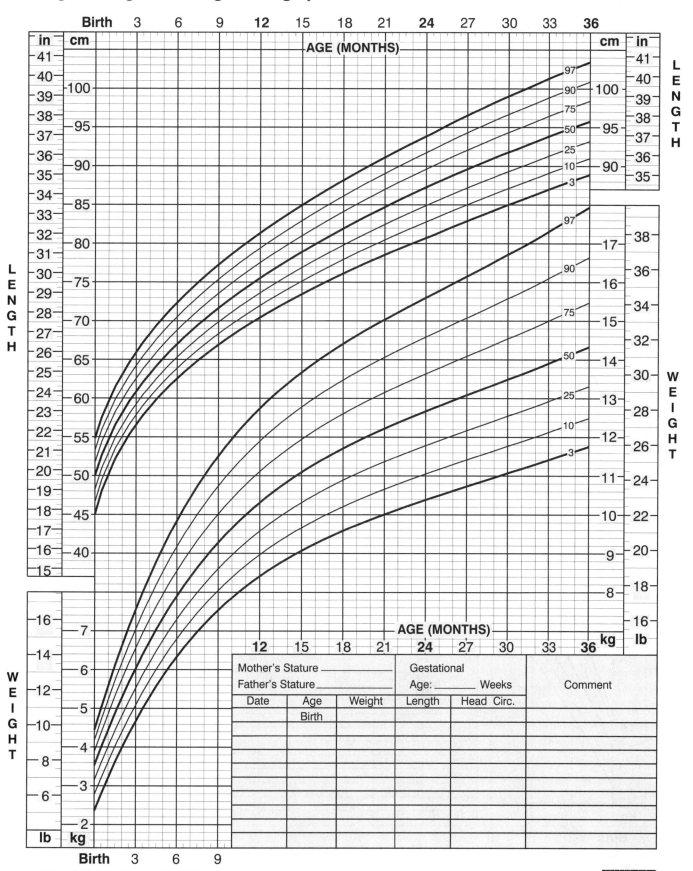

Published May 30, 2000 (modified 4/20/01).
SOURCE: Developed by the National Center for Health Statistics in collaboration with
the National Center for Chronic Disease Prevention and Health Promotion (2000).
http://www.cdc.gov/growthcharts

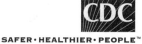

CDC

SAFER · HEALTHIER · PEOPLE™

Birth to 36 months: Girls
Length-for-age and Weight-for-age percentiles

NAME _____

RECORD # _____

AGE (MONTHS)

Birth 3 6 9 12 15 18 21 24 27 30 33 36

in	cm						cm	in

LENGTH percentiles: 97, 90, 75, 50, 25, 10, 3

WEIGHT percentiles: 97, 90, 75, 50, 25, 10, 3

AGE (MONTHS)

12 15 18 21 24 27 30 33 36 kg lb

	Gestational	
Mother's Stature _____	Age: _____ Weeks	Comment
Father's Stature _____		

Date	Age	Weight	Length	Head Circ.	
	Birth				

lb kg

Birth 3 6 9

Published May 30, 2000 (modified 4/20/01).
SOURCE: Developed by the National Center for Health Statistics in collaboration with
the National Center for Chronic Disease Prevention and Health Promotion (2000).
http://www.cdc.gov/growthcharts

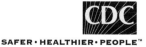

SAFER · HEALTHIER · PEOPLE™

Birth to 36 months: Boys
Head circumference-for-age and
Weight-for-length percentiles

NAME _____

RECORD # _____

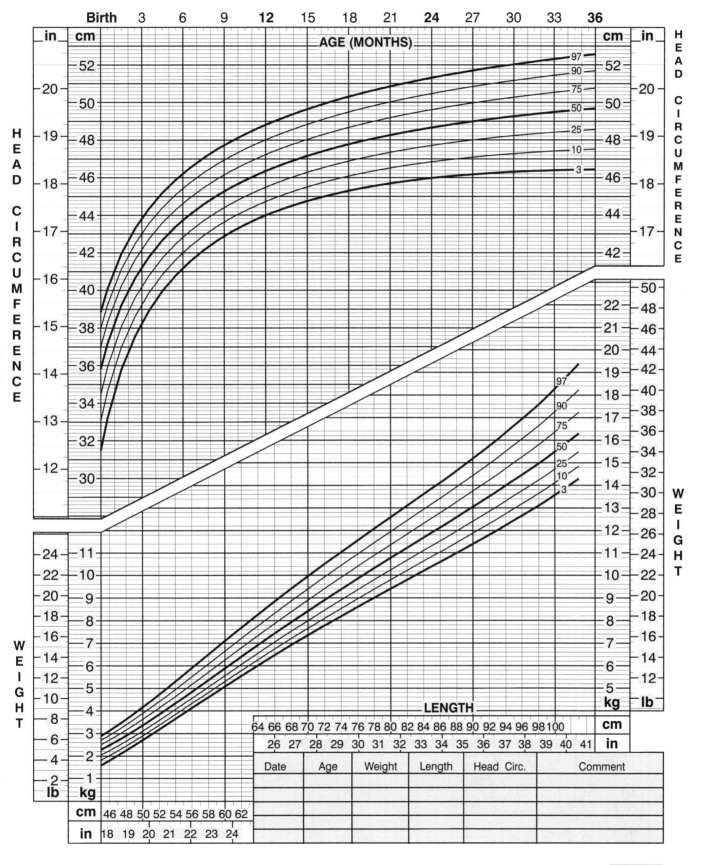

Date	Age	Weight	Length	Head Circ.	Comment

Published May 30, 2000 (modified 10/16/00).
SOURCE: Developed by the National Center for Health Statistics in collaboration with
the National Center for Chronic Disease Prevention and Health Promotion (2000).
http://www.cdc.gov/growthcharts

SAFER · HEALTHIER · PEOPLE™

581

Bright FUTURES

Birth to 36 months: Girls
Head circumference-for-age and
Weight-for-length percentiles

NAME _____

RECORD # _____

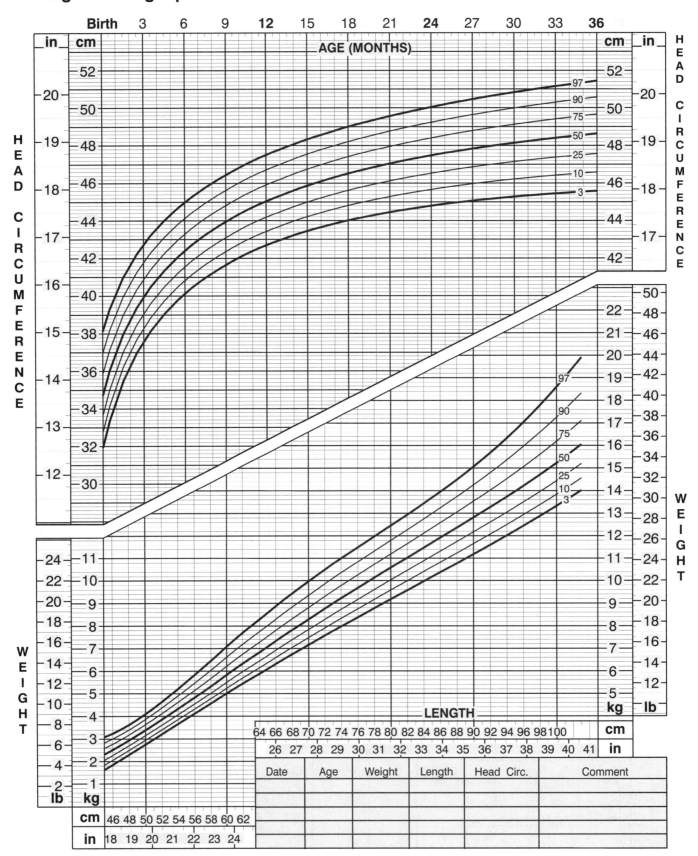

Published May 30, 2000 (modified 10/16/00).
SOURCE: Developed by the National Center for Health Statistics in collaboration with
the National Center for Chronic Disease Prevention and Health Promotion (2000).
http://www.cdc.gov/growthcharts

582

Bright FUTURES

CDC
SAFER · HEALTHIER · PEOPLE™

2 to 20 years: Boys
Stature-for-age and Weight-for-age percentiles

NAME _____

RECORD # _____

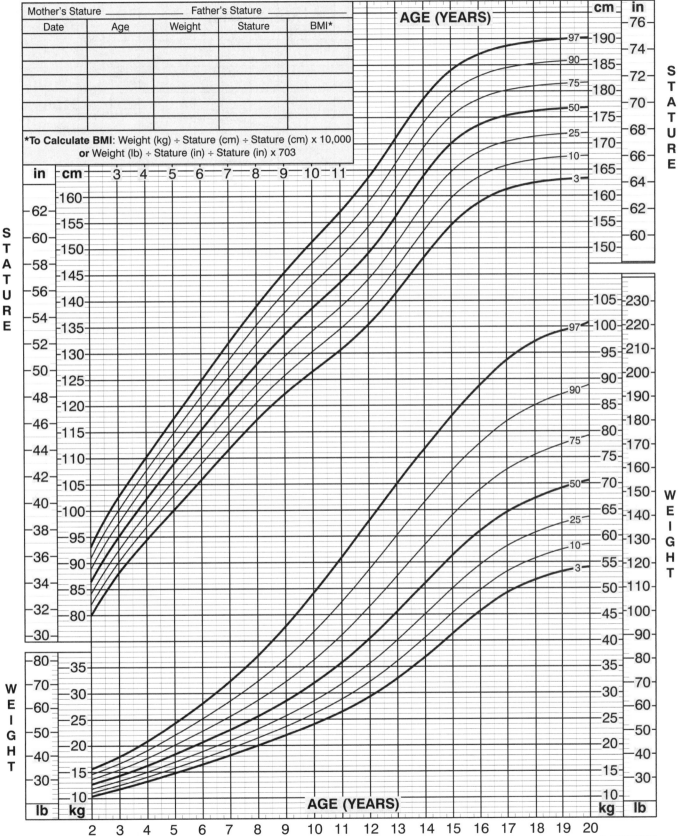

Mother's Stature _____		Father's Stature _____		
Date	Age	Weight	Stature	BMI*

*To Calculate BMI: Weight (kg) ÷ Stature (cm) ÷ Stature (cm) x 10,000
or Weight (lb) ÷ Stature (in) ÷ Stature (in) x 703

AGE (YEARS)

STATURE

WEIGHT

Published May 30, 2000 (modified 11/21/00).
SOURCE: Developed by the National Center for Health Statistics in collaboration with
the National Center for Chronic Disease Prevention and Health Promotion (2000).
http://www.cdc.gov/growthcharts

SAFER · HEALTHIER · PEOPLE™

583

Bright FUTURES

2 to 20 years: Girls
Stature-for-age and Weight-for-age percentiles

NAME _____

RECORD # _____

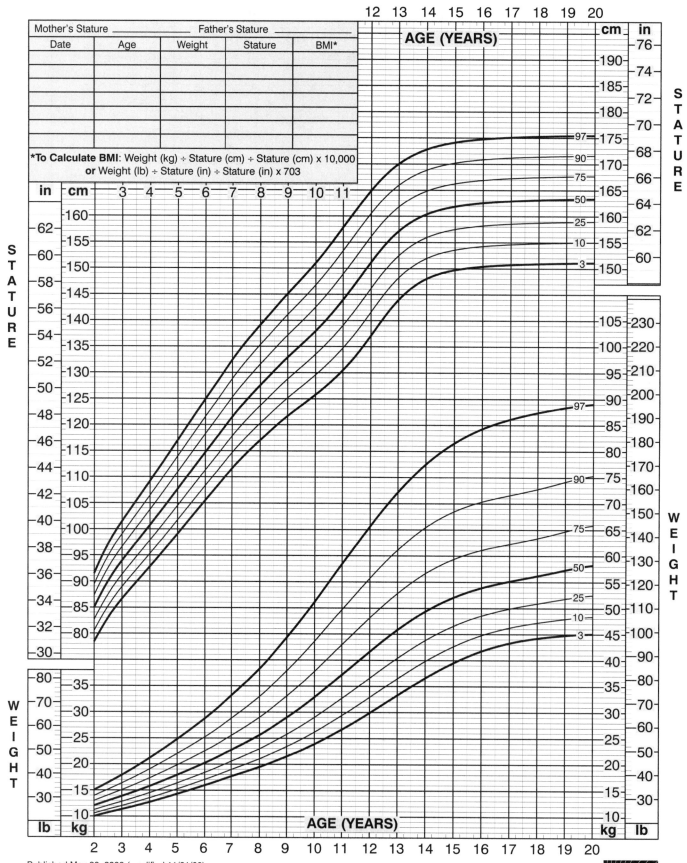

Published May 30, 2000 (modified 11/21/00).

SOURCE: Developed by the National Center for Health Statistics in collaboration with
the National Center for Chronic Disease Prevention and Health Promotion (2000).
http://www.cdc.gov/growthcharts

SAFER · HEALTHIER · PEOPLE™

CENTERS FOR DISEASE CONTROL AND PREVENTION GROWTH CHARTS

2 to 20 years: Boys
Body mass index-for-age percentiles

NAME _____

RECORD # _____

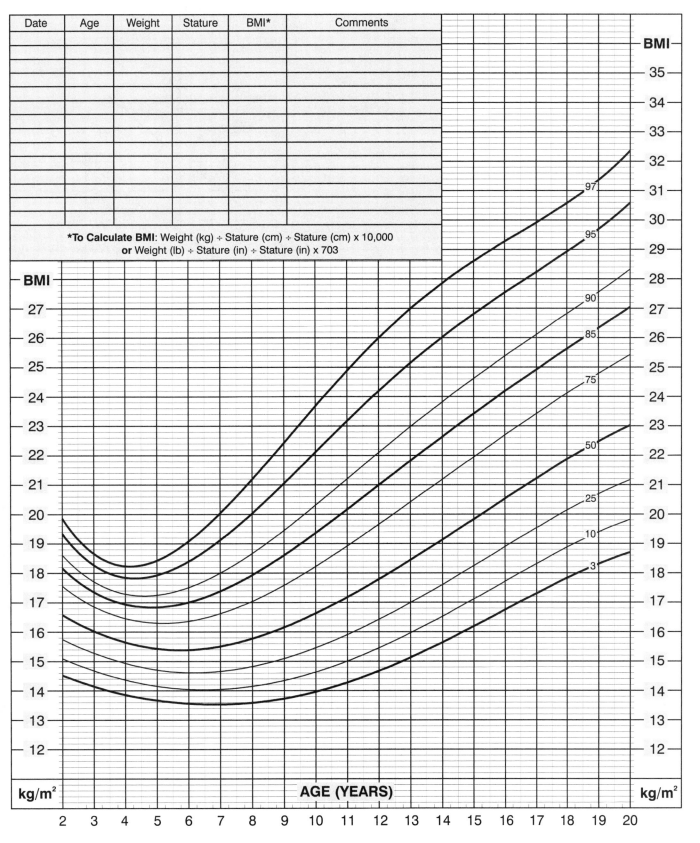

Date	Age	Weight	Stature	BMI*	Comments

*To Calculate BMI: Weight (kg) ÷ Stature (cm) ÷ Stature (cm) x 10,000
or Weight (lb) ÷ Stature (in) ÷ Stature (in) x 703

BMI

35
34
33
32
31
30
29
28
27
26
25
24
23
22
21
20
19
18
17
16
15
14
13
12

97
95
90
85
75
50
25
10
3

kg/m²

AGE (YEARS)

2 3 4 5 6 7 8 9 10 11 12 13 14 15 16 17 18 19 20

Published May 30, 2000 (modified 10/16/00).
SOURCE: Developed by the National Center for Health Statistics in collaboration with
the National Center for Chronic Disease Prevention and Health Promotion (2000).
http://www.cdc.gov/growthcharts

CENTERS FOR DISEASE CONTROL
AND PREVENTION GROWTH CHARTS

585

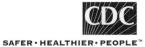

SAFER · HEALTHIER · PEOPLE™

Bright FUTURES

2 to 20 years: Girls
Body mass index-for-age percentiles

NAME _____

RECORD # _____

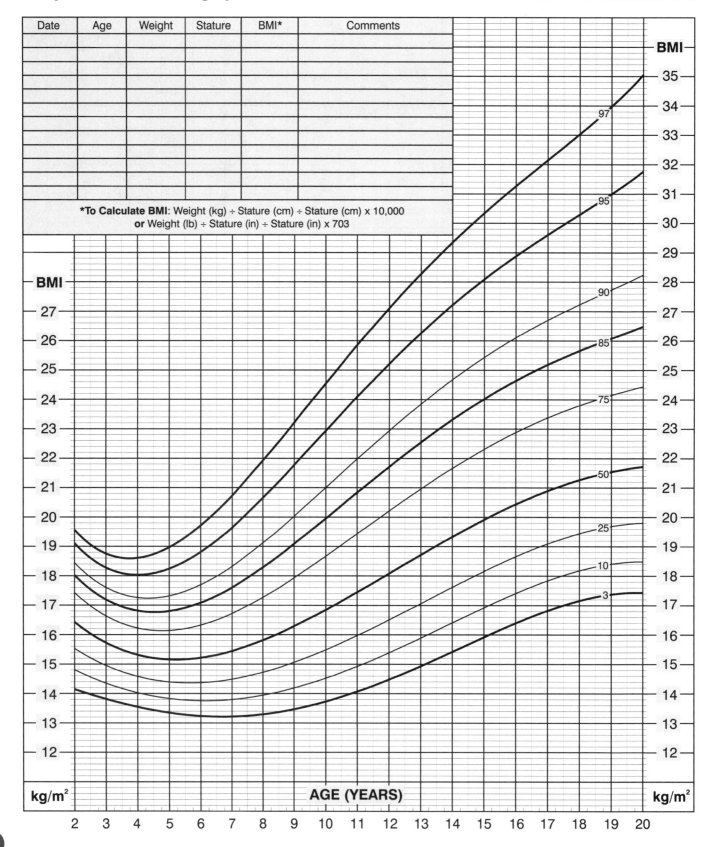

Date	Age	Weight	Stature	BMI*	Comments

*To Calculate BMI: Weight (kg) ÷ Stature (cm) ÷ Stature (cm) x 10,000
or Weight (lb) ÷ Stature (in) ÷ Stature (in) x 703

BMI

AGE (YEARS)

kg/m²   kg/m²

2 3 4 5 6 7 8 9 10 11 12 13 14 15 16 17 18 19 20

Published May 30, 2000 (modified 10/16/00).
SOURCE: Developed by the National Center for Health Statistics in collaboration with
the National Center for Chronic Disease Prevention and Health Promotion (2000).
http://www.cdc.gov/growthcharts

SAFER · HEALTHIER · PEOPLE™

CENTERS FOR DISEASE CONTROL AND PREVENTION GROWTH CHARTS

Bright FUTURES

Weight-for-stature percentiles: Boys

NAME _____

RECORD # _____

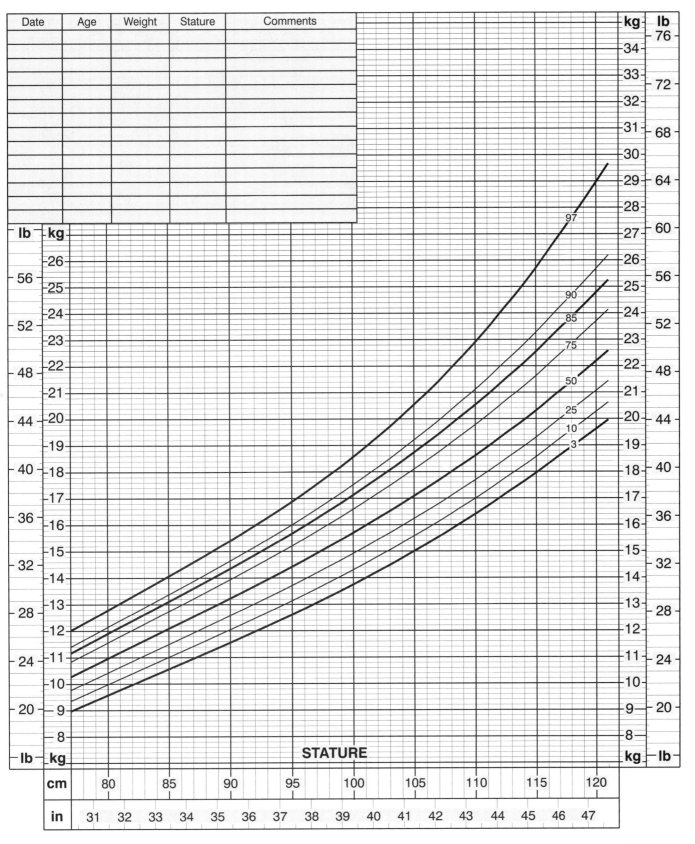

Date	Age	Weight	Stature	Comments

STATURE

cm: 80 85 90 95 100 105 110 115 120

in: 31 32 33 34 35 36 37 38 39 40 41 42 43 44 45 46 47

Published May 30, 2000 (modified 10/16/00).
SOURCE: Developed by the National Center for Health Statistics in collaboration with
the National Center for Chronic Disease Prevention and Health Promotion (2000).
http://www.cdc.gov/growthcharts

SAFER · HEALTHIER · PEOPLE™

587

Bright FUTURES

Weight-for-stature percentiles: Girls

NAME _____

RECORD # _____

Date	Age	Weight	Stature	Comments

CENTERS FOR DISEASE CONTROL AND PREVENTION GROWTH CHARTS

STATURE

97
90
85
75
50
25
10
3

cm 80 85 90 95 100 105 110 115 120

in 31 32 33 34 35 36 37 38 39 40 41 42 43 44 45 46 47

588

Published May 30, 2000 (modified 10/16/00).
SOURCE: Developed by the National Center for Health Statistics in collaboration with
the National Center for Chronic Disease Prevention and Health Promotion (2000).
http://www.cdc.gov/growthcharts

Bright FUTURES

SAFER · HEALTHIER · PEOPLE™

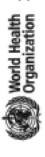

Length/height-for-age BOYS

Birth to 5 years (percentiles)

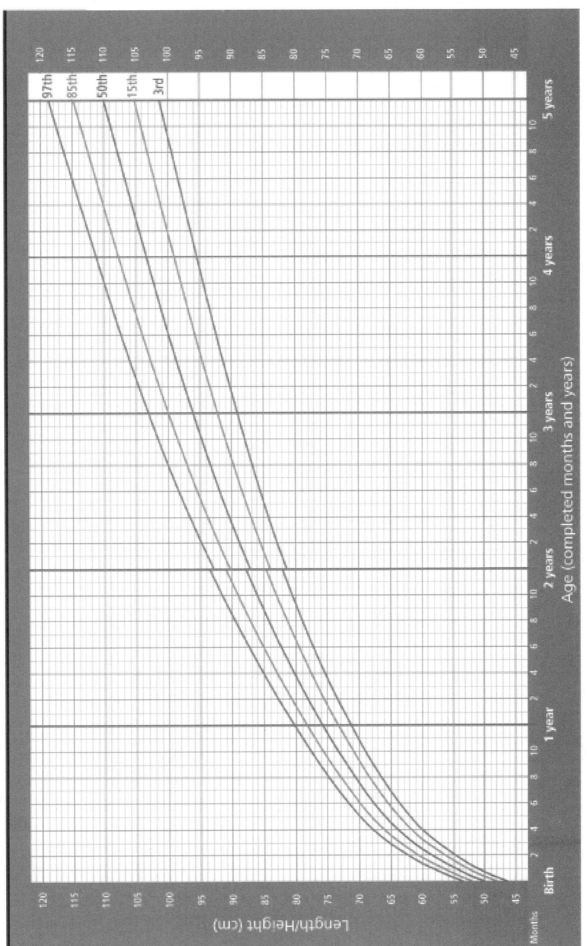

WHO Child Growth Standards

Length/height-for-age GIRLS

Birth to 5 years (percentiles)

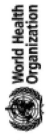
World Health Organization

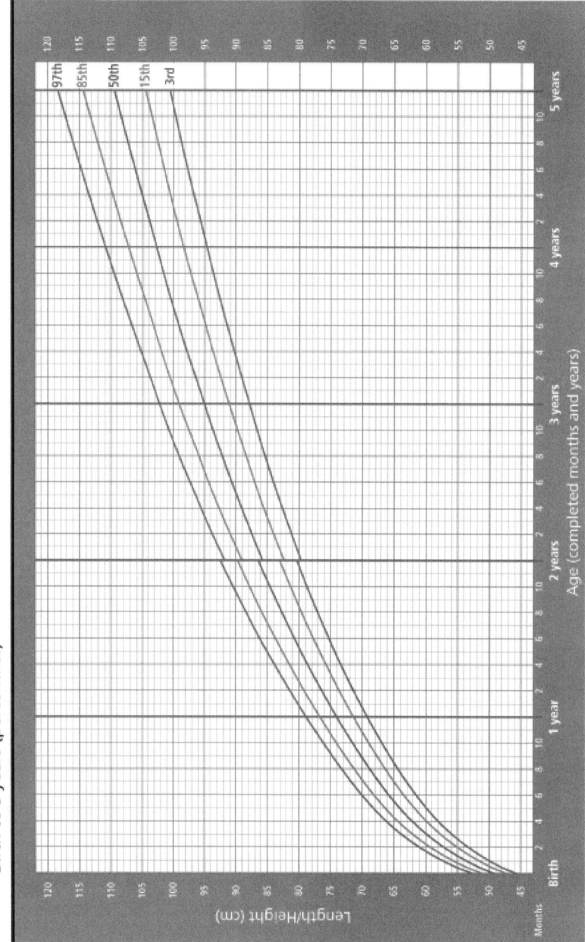

WHO Child Growth Standards

American Academy of Pediatrics
DEDICATED TO THE HEALTH OF ALL CHILDREN™

Recommendations for Preventive Pediatric Health Care

Bright Futures/American Academy of Pediatrics

Bright Futures
Prevention and health promotion for infants, children, adolescents, and their families™

Each child and family is unique; therefore, these **Recommendations for Preventive Pediatric Health Care** are designed for the care of children who are receiving competent parenting, have no manifestations of any important health problems, and are growing and developing in satisfactory fashion. **Additional visits may become necessary** if circumstances suggest variations from normal.

Developmental, psychosocial, and chronic disease issues for children and adolescents may require frequent counseling and treatment visits separate from preventive care visits.

These guidelines represent a consensus by the American Academy of Pediatrics (AAP) and Bright Futures. The AAP continues to emphasize the great importance of **continuity of care** in comprehensive health supervision and the need to avoid **fragmentation of care.**

The recommendations in this statement do not indicate an exclusive course of treatment or standard of medical care. Variations, taking into account individual circumstances, may be appropriate.

Copyright © 2008 by the American Academy of Pediatrics.

No part of this statement may be reproduced in any form or by any means without prior written permission from the American Academy of Pediatrics except for one copy for one's personal use.

		INFANCY								EARLY CHILDHOOD							MIDDLE CHILDHOOD						ADOLESCENCE											
AGE¹	PRENATAL²	NEWBORN³	3–5 d⁴	By 1 mo	2 mo	4 mo	6 mo	9 mo	12 m	15 mo	18 mo	24 mo	30 mo	3 y	4 y	5 y	6 y	7 y	8 y	9 y	10 y	11 y	12 y	13 y	14 y	15 y	16 y	17 y	18 y	19 y	20 y	21 y
HISTORY Initial/Interval	●	●	●	●	●	●	●	●	●	●	●	●	●	●	●	●	●	●	●	●	●	●	●	●	●	●	●	●	●	●	●	●
MEASUREMENTS																																
Length/Height and Weight		●	●	●	●	●	●	●	●	●	●	●	●	●	●	●	●	●	●	●	●	●	●	●	●	●	●	●	●	●	●	●
Head Circumference		●	●	●	●	●	●	●	●	●	●	●																				
Weight for Length		●	●	●	●	●	●	●	●	●	●	●																				
Body Mass Index														●	●	●	●	●	●	●	●	●	●	●	●	●	●	●	●	●	●	●
Blood Pressure³		★	★	★	★	★	★	★	★	★	★	★	★	●	●	●	●	●	●	●	●	●	●	●	●	●	●	●	●	●	●	●
SENSORY SCREENING																																
Vision		★⁷	★	★	★	★	★	★	★	★	★	★	★	●	●	●	●	★	●	★	●	●	★	★	●	★	●	★	●	★	●	★
Hearing		★	★	★	★	★	★	★	★	★	★	★	★	★	★	★	★	★	★	★	★	●	★	★	●	★	●	★	●	★	●	★
DEVELOPMENTAL/BEHAVIORAL ASSESSMENT																																
Developmental Screening⁸								●			●		●																			
Autism Screening⁹											●																					
Developmental Surveillance⁸		●	●	●	●	●	●		●	●		●		●	●	●	●	●	●	●	●	●	●	●	●	●	●	●	●	●	●	●
Psychosocial/Behavioral Assessment		●	●	●	●	●	●	●	●	●	●	●	●	●	●	●	●	●	●	●	●	●	●	●	●	●	●	●	●	●	●	●
Alcohol and Drug Use Assessment																						★	★	★	★	★	★	★	★	★	★	★
PHYSICAL EXAMINATION¹⁰		●	●	●	●	●	●	●	●	●	●	●	●	●	●	●	●	●	●	●	●	●	●	●	●	●	●	●	●	●	●	●
PROCEDURES¹¹																																
Newborn Metabolic/Hemoglobin Screening¹²		●	●																													
Immunization¹³		●	●	●	●	●	●	●	●	●	●	●	●	●	●	●	●	●	●	●	●	●	●	●	●	●	●	●	●	●	●	●
Hematocrit or Hemoglobin¹⁴					★	★	★	●	●or★¹⁶		●or★¹⁶		★	★	★	★	★	★	★	★	★	★	★	★	★	★	★	★	★	★	★	★
Lead Screening¹⁵							★	★	●or★¹⁷		●or★¹⁷		★	●or★²¹	●or★²¹	★	●²²															
Tuberculin Test¹⁷				★			★	★	★		★		★	★	★	★	★	★	★	★	★	★	★	★	★	★	★	★	★	★	★	★
Dyslipidemia Screening¹⁸												★		★	★	★	★	★	★	★	★ ←—————→								★	★	★	★
STI Screening¹⁹																						★	★	★	★	★	★	★	★	★	★	★
Cervical Dysplasia Screening²⁰																						★	★	★	★	★	★	★	★	★	★	★
ORAL HEALTH²¹							★	★	●or★²¹		●or★²¹																					
ANTICIPATORY GUIDANCE²³	●	●	●	●	●	●	●	●	●	●	●	●	●	●	●	●	●	●	●	●	●	●	●	●	●	●	●	●	●	●	●	●

1. If a child comes under care for the first time at any point on the schedule, or if any items are not accomplished at the suggested age, the schedule should be brought up to date at the earliest possible time.
2. A prenatal visit is recommended for parents who are at high risk, for first-time parents, and for those who request a conference. The prenatal visit should include anticipatory guidance, pertinent medical history, and a discussion of benefits of breastfeeding and planned method of feeding per AAP statement "The Prenatal Visit" (2001) [URL: http://aappolicy.aappublications.org/cgi/content/full/pediatrics;107/6/1456].
3. Every infant should have a newborn evaluation after birth, breastfeeding encouraged, and instruction and support offered.
4. Every infant should have an evaluation within 3 to 5 days of birth and within 48 to 72 hours after discharge from the hospital, to include evaluation for feeding and jaundice. Breastfeeding infants should receive formal breastfeeding evaluation, encouragement, and instruction as recommended in AAP statement "Breastfeeding and the Use of Human Milk" (2005) [URL: http://aappolicy.aappublications.org/cgi/content/full/pediatrics;115/2/496]. For newborns discharged in less than 48 hours after delivery, the infant must be examined within 48 hours of discharge per AAP statement "Hospital Stay for Healthy Term Newborns" (2004) [URL: http://aappolicy.aappublications.org/cgi/content/full/pediatrics;113/5/1434].
5. Blood pressure measurement in infants and children with specific risk conditions should be performed at visits before age 3 years.
6. If the patient is uncooperative, rescreen within 6 months per AAP statement "Eye Examination and Vision Screening in Infants, Children, and Young Adults" (1996) [URL: http://aappolicy.aappublications.org/cgi/reprint/pediatrics;98/1/153.pdf].
7. All newborns should be screened per AAP statement "Year 2000 Position Statement: Principles and Guidelines for Early Hearing Detection and Intervention Programs" (2000) [URL: http://aappolicy.aappublications.org/cgi/content/full/

pediatrics;106/4/798]. Joint Committee on Infant Hearing. Year 2007 position statement: principles and guidelines for early hearing detection and intervention programs. Pediatrics. 2007;120:898–921.
8. AAP Council on Children With Disabilities, AAP Section on Developmental Behavioral Pediatrics, AAP Bright Futures Steering Committee, AAP Medical Home Initiatives for Children With Special Needs Project Advisory Committee. Identifying infants and young children with developmental disorders in the medical home: an algorithm for developmental surveillance and screening. Pediatrics. 2006;118:405–420 [URL: http://aappolicy.aappublications.org/cgi/content/full/pediatrics;118/1/405].
9. Gupta VB, Hyman SL, Johnson CP, et al. Identifying children with autism early? Pediatrics. 2007;119:152–153 [URL: http://pediatrics.aappublications.org/cgi/content/full/119/1/152].
10. At each visit, age-appropriate physical examination is essential, with infant totally unclothed, older child undressed and suitably draped.
11. These may be modified, depending on entry point into schedule and individual need.
12. Newborn metabolic and hemoglobinopathy screening should be done according to state law. Results should be reviewed at visits and appropriate retesting or referral done as needed.
13. Schedules per the Committee on Infectious Diseases, published annually in the January issue of Pediatrics. Every visit should be an opportunity to update and complete a child's immunizations.
14. See AAP Pediatric Nutrition Handbook, 5th Edition (2003) for a discussion of universal and selective screening options. See also Recommendations to prevent and control iron deficiency in the United States. MMWR. 1998;47(RR-3):1–36.
15. For children at risk of lead exposure, consult the AAP statement "Lead Exposure in Children: Prevention, Detection, and Management" (2005) [URL: http://aappolicy.aappublications.org/cgi/content/full/pediatrics;116/4/1036]. Additionally, screening should be done in accordance with state law where applicable.
16. Perform risk assessments or screens as appropriate, based on universal screening requirements for patients with Medicaid or high prevalence areas.
17. Tuberculosis testing per recommendations of the Committee on Infectious Diseases, published in the current edition of Red Book: Report of the Committee on Infectious Diseases. Testing should be done on recognition of high-risk factors.
18. "Third Report of the National Cholesterol Education Program (NCEP) Expert Panel on Detection, Evaluation, and Treatment of High Blood Cholesterol in Adults (Adult Treatment Panel III) Final Report" (2002) [URL: http://circ.ahajournals.org/cgi/content/full/106/25/3143] and "The Expert Committee Recommendations on the Assessment, Prevention, and Treatment of Child and Adolescent Overweight and Obesity." Supplement to Pediatrics. In press.
19. All sexually active patients should be screened for sexually transmitted infections (STIs).
20. All sexually active girls should have screening for cervical dysplasia as part of a pelvic examination beginning within 3 years of onset of sexual activity or age 21 (whichever comes first).
21. Referral to dental home, if available. Otherwise, administer oral health risk assessment. If the primary water source is deficient in fluoride, consider oral fluoride supplementation.
22. At the visits for 3 years and 6 years of age, it should be determined whether the patient has a dental home. If the patient does not have a dental home, a referral should be made to one. If the primary water source is deficient in fluoride, consider oral fluoride supplementation.
23. Refer to the specific guidance by age as listed in Bright Futures Guidelines (Hagan JF, Shaw JS, Duncan PM, eds. Bright Futures: Guidelines for Health Supervision of Infants, Children, and Adolescents. 3rd ed. Elk Grove Village, IL: American Academy of Pediatrics; 2008).

KEY

● = to be performed   ★ = risk assessment to be performed, with appropriate action to follow, if positive   ——→ = range during which a service may be provided, with the symbol indicating the preferred age

Index

Literacy
    anticipatory guidance for, for 3 year period, 443–444
    in child development, in early childhood, 58–59
    promotion of, 44

M

Marijuana, adolescent use of, 99–103
Mastery, in building strengths of youth, 26
Masturbation, in sexual development, in early childhood, 170
Maternal and Child Health Bureau (MCHB), Bright Futures from, ix, xix
MCHB. See Maternal and Child Health Bureau
Media viewing
    anticipatory guidance for
        for 18 to 21 year period, 567–568
        for 15 to 17 year period, 547–548
        for 4 year period, 457
        for 2 year period, 427
    in building family strengths, 28–29
    in overweight and obesity, 115–117
    physical inactivity and, 148
Medical home
    child and youth care and, 4–5
    description of, 4
Mental health
    adolescent concerns of, 98–103
        attention, cognition, and learning deficits, 99
        conduct disturbances, 99
        depression and anxiety, 98–99
        substance use and abuse, 99–103
        suicide, 99
    anticipatory guidance for
        for 5 and 6 year period, 473–474
        for 9 and 10 year period, 505–508
        for 7 and 8 year period, 490–491
    challenges to, 81–84, 86–97
        anxiety disorders, 93
        ASDs identification, 89–90
        behavioral patterns, 86–87
        bullying, 93–95
        child maltreatment and neglect, 82
        conduct disturbances, 95
        domains of influence, 87–89
        early substance abuse, 95
        facing infant illness or death, 83–84
        infant well-being, 81–82
        LDs and ADHD, 92–93
        mood disorders, 93
        protective factors, 92
        shaken baby syndrome, 83
    in childhood and adolescents, 3
        prevalence and trends in, 78
        risk factors for, 77–78
        screening and referral, 78–80
        with special health care needs, 80
    promotion of, 77–103
        in adolescence, 95–103
        in early childhood, 84–90
        evidence for, 242–243
        in infancy, 80–84
        introduction to, 77
        in middle childhood, 90–95
        overview of, 77–80
Metabolic syndrome
    criteria for, 112
    overview of, 112
    prevalence of, 112–113
Methamphetamine, oral health and, 165
Mineral supplements
    for adolescent nutrition, 139–141
    for infant nutrition, 126–127
Mission, of Bright Futures, ix
Models of care, in adolescent development, 72
Mood disorders, in middle childhood, 93
Moral development, in child development, in middle childhood, 66–68
Motor skills. See Fine motor skills; Gross motor skills
Mouth injury, in adolescents, 166

N

Newborn, health supervision visit for, 271–288
    anticipatory guidance, 269–270, 276–288, 295–296, 301–302
    context, 271
    health screening, 272–275
    priorities for, 272
9 and 10 year visits, health supervision for, 499–514
    anticipatory guidance, 504–514
    context, 499–500
    health screening, 501–503
    priorities, 501
9 month visit, health supervision for, 367–379
    anticipatory guidance, 372–379
    context, 367–368
    health screening, 369–371
    priorities, 369
Nutrition
    anticipatory guidance for
        for 18 to 21 year period, 565–566
        for 11 to 14 year period, 525–526
        for 15 to 17 year period, 546–547
        for first week period, 296–299
        for 5 and 6 year period, 474–476
        for 4 month period, 344–347
        for 9 and 10 year period, 508–509
        safety, 332–333
        for 7 and 8 year period, 491–493
        for 6 month period, 360–363
        for 2 month period, 330–332
    in building family strengths, 28

Appendix C
Recommendations for
Preventive Pediatric Health Care